MALE INFERTILITY

MALE INFERTILITY

Management of Infertile Men in Reproductive Medicine

Ashok Agarwal, PhD, HCLD (Andrology)
Global Andrology Forum
Moreland Hills, OH, United States;
Emeritus Staff, Cleveland Clinic
Cleveland, OH, United States

Florence Boitrelle, MD, PhD
Department of Reproductive Biology
Preservation of Fertility, Andrology
BREED
UVSQ, Jouy-en-Josas
Île-de-France, France

Panagiotis Drakopoulos, MD, PhD
Reproductive Medicine
UZ Brussel
Brussels, Belgium

Hassan Nooman Sallam, MD, FRCOG, PhD
Department of Obstetrics and Gynaecology
Faculty of Medicine
Alexandria University;
Alexandria Fertility and ART Center
Alexandria, Egypt

Ramadan Saleh, MD
Departments of Dermatology, Venereology, and
Andrology
Sohag University;
Ajyal IVF Center
Ajyal Hospital,
Sohag, Egypt

ELSEVIER

Elsevier
1600 John F. Kennedy Blvd.
Ste 1800
Philadelphia, PA 19103-2899

MALE INFERTILITY: MANAGEMENT OF INFERTILE MEN IN
REPRODUCTIVE MEDICINE

ISBN: **978-0-323-93047-5**

Notice

Senior Content Development Manager: Somodatta Roy Choudhury
Executive Content Strategist: Nancy Anastasi Duffy
Senior Content Development Specialist: Priyadarshini Pandey
Publishing Services Manager: Shereen Jameel
Project Manager: Vishnu T. Jiji
Designer: Bridget Hoette/Miles Hitchen

Printed in India.

Last digit is the print number: 9 8 7 6 5 4 3 2 1

To my father, the late Professor RC Aggarwal for instilling the virtues of honesty, dedication, and hard work. To my wonderful wife, Meenu, and my sons, Rishi and Neil-Yogi, for their unconditional love and support. To Professor Kevin Loughlin (Harvard Medical School), the late Professor Anthony Thomas (Cleveland Clinic), and Dr. Rupin Shah (India) for their friendship, guidance, and support and for making an indelible positive impression on my life. To over a thousand researchers and students who have worked with me over the past four decades, and most importantly, the patients who have placed their trust in my work.

Ashok Agarwal, PhD, HCLD (Andrology)

To my parents, for having brought me this far and for having passed on to me the values of work and sincerity. To my husband, Pierre, and my children Julia (8) and Pierre (4), who remind me every day how important life is to live. Thank you for your love and support every day.

To my siblings, Audrey, Fabrice, Alban, and Gauthier, thank you for your unconditional support.

To Professor Agarwal and the Global Andrology Forum (GAF), I never imagined that the world of andrology could come together in this way. I am proud of what has been achieved and wish this book and the GAF long life.

Florence Boitrelle, MD, PhD

To my family, for your constant love and support. You have always been there for me, even on the tough days. To Professor Ashok Agarwal (director, Global Andrology Forum), for your guidance and support. You were the first person to encourage me to be part of this achievement. Thank you for believing in my dream.

To my wife, Eva, and my kids, Rafailia and Thanos-Paul, for their love and support, and above all to my intellectual father, Rafail, who helped me make the impossible possible.

Panagiotis Drakopoulos, MD, PhD

To the memory of my father and mother and to my wife, Magda, and my three children, and all those who have helped me along the way.

Hassan Nooman Sallam, MD, FRCOG, PhD

To my family for your constant love and support. You have always been there for me, even on the tough days. To professor Ashok Agarwal (Director, Global Andrology Forum) for your guidance and support. You were the first person to encourage me to be part of this achievement. Thank you for believing in my dream.

Ramadan Saleh, MD

CONTRIBUTORS

Ibrahim Abdel-Hamid, MD
Department of Andrology
Mansoura University
Mansoura, Egypt

Ashok Agarwal, PhD, HCLD (Andrology)
Global Andrology Forum
Moreland Hills, OH, United States;
Emeritus Staff, Cleveland Clinic
Cleveland, OH, United States

Hassan Mohammed Aljifri, MD, MBBS, MSc
Department of Urology
King Abdulaziz University Hospital
Jeddah, Saudi Arabia

Rafael Favero Ambar, MD
Department of Urology
Centro Universitário em Saúde do ABC - FMABC;
Andrology Group
Ideia Fertil Institute of Human Reproduction;
Department of Urology
Hospital do Servidor Público Estadual - IAMSPE;
Department of Andrology
Hope Clinic–Human Reproduction
São Paulo, Brazil

Christina Anagnostopoulou, BSc, MSc
Reproductive Medicine Unit - EmbryoART
Leto Maternity Hospital
Athens, Greece

Mohamed Arafa, MD
Department of Urology
Hamad Medical Corporation
Doha, Qatar;
Department of Andrology
Cairo University
Cairo, Egypt;
Department of Urology
Weill Cornell Medicine-Qatar
Doha, Qatar

Giancarlo Balercia, MD
Endocrinology Clinic
Polytechnic University of Marche
Ancona, Italy

Erlisa Bardhi, MD
Centre for Reproductive Medicine, Universitair
    Ziekenhuis Brussel,
Vrije Universiteit Brussel
Brussels, Belgium

Lluís Bassas, MD, PhD
Department of Andrology
Fundacio Puigvert
Barcelona, Spain

Marion Bendayan, MD
BREED
INRAe
Jouy-en-Josas, France

Kadir Bocu, MD, FEBU
Department of Urology
Silopi State Hospital
Sirnak, Turkey

Florence Boitrelle, MD, PhD
Department of Reproductive Biology
Preservation of Fertility, Andrology
BREED
UVSQ, Jouy-en-Josas
Île-de-France, France

Edson Borges Jr., PhD
Scientific Research
Sapientiae Institute;
Fertility Medical Group
São Paulo, Brazil

Daniela Paes de Almeida Ferreira Braga, DVM, MSc
Department of Scientific Research
Fertility - Centro de Fertilização Assistida
São Paulo, Brazil

Mohit Butaney, MD
Vattikuti Urology Institute
Henry Ford Health System
Detroit, MI, United States

Aldo E. Calogero, MD
Department of Clinical and Experimental Medicine
University of Catania
Catania, Italy

Rossella Cannarella, MD, PhD
Department of Clinical and Experimental Medicine
University of Catania
Catania, Italy;
American Center for Reproductive Medicine
Cleveland Clinic
Cleveland, OH, United States

Eric Chung, FRACS
Department of Andrology and Urology
AndroUrology Centre;
University of Queensland
Department of Urology
Princess Alexandra Hospital
Brisbane, QLD, Australia

Rosita A. Condorelli, MD, PhD
Department of Clinical and Experimental Medicine
University of Catania
Catania, Italy

Mausumi Das, MD, MRCOG, MPH
Department of Obstetrics and Gynecology, Division of
    Reproductive Medicine
Imperial College Healthcare NHS Trust & Chelsea and
    Westmisnter Hospital NHS Foundation Trust
London, United Kingdom

Thais Serzedello de Paula, MSc
Department of Urology
Federal University of São Paulo
São Paulo, Brazil

Panagiotis Drakopoulos, MD, PhD
Reproductive Medicine
UZ Brussel
Brussels, Belgium

Damayanthi Durairajanayagam, PhD
Department of Physiology, Faculty of Medicine
Universiti Teknologi MARA (UiTM)
Selangor, Malaysia

Evangelini Evgeni, MPhil, PhD
Department of Seminology
Cryogonia Cryopreservation Bank
Athens, Greece

Francesca Firmani, MD
Primary Care Complex Unit
Outpatient Endocrinology Clinic, Martinsicuro
Teramo, Italy

Nicolas Garrido Puchalt, PhD, MSc
Research Administration
IVI Foundation
Valencia, Spain

Murat Gül, MD, FEBU
Department of Urology
Selcuk University School of Medicine
Konya, Turkey

**Taha Abo-Almagd Abdel-Meguid Hamoda, MD, MSc,
MBBS**
Department of Urology
Faculty of Medicine
King Abdulaziz University
Jeddah, Saudi Arabia;
Faculty of Medicine
Minia University
El-Minia, Egypt

Ralf Reinhold Henkel, PhD
Department of Metabolism, Digestion & Reproduction
Imperial College London
London, United Kingdom;
Department of Fertility
LogixX Pharma
Theale, United Kingdom;
Department of Medical Bioscience
University of the Western Cape
Bellville, South Africa

Hussein Kandil, MBBCh, FACS, MBA
Department of Urology - Andrology
Fakih IVF Fertility Center
Abu Dhabi, United Arab Emirates

Parviz K. Kavoussi, MD, FACS
Department of Urology
Austin Fertility & Reproductive Medicine/Westlake IVF
Austin, TX, United States;
Department of Psychology: Neuroendocrinology and
    Motivation
University of Texas at Austin
Austin, TX, United States;
Department of Urology
University of Texas Health Sciences Center at San
    Antonio
San Antonio, TX, United States

Kareim Khalafalla, MD, FECSM
Department of Urology
University of Texas Health Science, McGovern Medical
    School
Houston, TX, United States;
Department of Urology
MD Anderson Cancer Center
Houston, TX, United States;
Department of Urology
Hamad Medical Corporation
Doha, Qatar

Edmund Yuey Kun Ko, MD
Department of Urology
Loma Linda University
Loma Linda, CA, United States

**Raghavender Kosgi, Mch (Urology), DNB (Urology),
FECSM**
Apollo Hospitals Jubilee Hills
Hyderabad, Telangana, India

Sandro La Vignera, MD, PhD
Department of Clinical and Experimental Medicine
University of Catania
Catania, Italy

Tan V. Le, MD
Department of Andrology
Binh Dan Hospital;
Department of Andrology and Nephro-Urology
Pham Ngoc Thach University of Medicine
Ho Chi Minh City, Vietnam

Kristian Leisegang, PhD
School of Natural Medicine
University of the Western Cape
Western Cape, South Africa

Vineet Malhotra, MD
Department of Urology and Andrology
VNA Hospital
New Delhi, India

Israel Maldonado-Rosas, BS, MS
IVF Laboratory
CITMER Reproductive Medicine
Mexico City, Mexico

Marlon Pedrozo Martinez, MD, FPUA, FPCS
University of Santo Tomas Hospital
Manila, Philippines

Melissa A. Mathes, MD
Department of Obstetrics and Gynecology
University of Nebraska Medical Center
Omaha, NE, United States

Megan McMurray, DO
Division of Urology
Southern Illinois University School of Medicine
Springfield, IL, United States

Suks Minhas, MD, FRCS(Urol)
Department of Urology
Imperial College
London, United Kingdom

Faith Tebatso Moichela, MSc, Hons, BSc
Department of Medical Biosciences
University of the Western Cape
Cape Town, South Africa

Taymour Mostafa, MD, MB BCh, MSc, DS
Department of Andrology, Sexology & STIs
Cairo University
Cairo, Egypt

Hoang P.C. Nguyen, MD, PhD
Associate Professor of Urology
Binh Dan Hospital;
Department of Andrology and Nephro-Urology
Pham Ngoc Thach University of Medicine
Ho Chi Minh City, Vietnam

Ana Navarro-Gomezlechon, BSc, MSc
Department of Andrology and Male Infertility
IVIRMA Global Research Alliance, IVI Foundation,
    Instituto de Investigación Sanitaria La Fe (IIS La Fe)
Valencia, Spain

Filipe Tenorio Lira Neto, MD, MSc, MBA
Department of Andrology
Andros Recife
Recife, Brazil

Willem Ombelet, MD, PhD
Department of Obstetrics & Gynaecology, ZOL
Genk Institute for Fertility Technology
Genk, Belgium

Chara Oraiopoulou I, BSc, MRes
Department of Embryology
Embryolab Fertility Clinic
Thessaloniki, Greece

Achilleas Papatheodorou, PhD, MMedSc
IVF Lab
Embryolab Fertility Clinic
Thessaloniki, Greece

Phu V. Pham, MD
Gastrointestinal Surgery Department
Binh Dan Hospital
Ho Chi Minh city, Vietnam

Hanae Pons-Rejraji, PhD
AMP-CECOS
CHU Estaing
CHU de Clermont Ferrand;
IMoST
UCA-Faculté de Médecine
Clermont Ferrand, France

Mahmoud Fareed Qutub, MD
Department of Urology
King Abdulaziz University Hospital
Jeddah, Saudi Arabia

Osvaldo Rajmil, MD, PhD
Senior Consultant
Department of Andrology
Puigvert Foundation;
University of Vic - Central University of Catalonia
Barcelona, Spain

Ranjith Ramasamy, MD
Department of Urology
University of Miami
Miami, FL, United States

Amarnath Rambhatla, MD
Department of Urology
Vattikuti Urology Institute, Henry Ford Health
Detroit, MI, United States

Liliana Ramirez-Dominguez, BSc
IVF Laboratory
CITMER Reproductive Medicine
Mexico City, Mexico

Ramadan Saleh, MD
Departments of Dermatology, Venereology, and
Andrology
Sohag University;
Ajyal IVF Center
Ajyal Hospital,
Sohag, Egypt

Hassan Nooman Sallam, MD, FRCOG, PhD
Department of Obstetrics and Gynaecology
Faculty of Medicine
Alexandria University;
Alexandria Fertility and ART Center
Alexandria, Egypt

Gianmaria Salvio, MD, PhD
Endocrinology Clinic
Polytechnic University of Marche
Ancona, Italy

Samantha B. Schon, MD, MTR
Division of Reproductive Endocrinology & Infertility,
    Department of Obstetrics & Gynecology
University of Michigan
Ann Arbor, MI, United States

Pallav Sengupta, MSc, PhD
Department of Physiology
Gulf Medical University
Ajman, United Arab Emirates

Amanda Souza Setti, MSc
Department of Scientific Research
Fertility Medical Group;
Department of Scientific Research
Instituto Sapientiae
São Paulo, Brazil

Rupin Shah, MS, MCh
Department of Urology
Lilavati Hospital & Research Centre
Sir HN Reliance Hospital
Mumbai, India

Kanha Charudutt Shete, DO, MM
Department of Urology
Loma Linda University
Loma Linda, CA, United States

Nicholas N. Tadros, MD, MCR, MBA
Department of Urology
Southern Illinois University
Springfield, IL, United States

Paraskevi Vogiatzi, BSc, MSc, DEA, PhD
Fertility & Reproductive Health Diagnostic Center
Andromed Health & Reproduction, Maroussi
Athens, Greece

Armand Zini, MD
Department of Surgery
McGill University
Montreal, QE, Canada

Wael Zohdy, MD, PhD, PMP, PBA, ITIL
Department of Andrology, Sexology and STIs
Cairo University
Cairo, Egypt

Sulagna Dutta, PhD
School of Life Sciences
Manipal Academy of Higher Education (MAHE)
Dubai, United Arab Emirates

Infertility is a growing concern, as highlighted in the latest World Health Organization (WHO) report this year. While infertility was long perceived as a female issue, the importance of the male contribution to a successful reproductive outcome is now well accepted, as around 50% of infertile couples are diagnosed with an abnormal work-up in the male partner. Multiple studies have also shown the trend of decreasing sperm counts over the past century, making our understanding of the etiology of male infertility a crucial issue to address.

Andrologists, urologists, gynecologists, and reproductive endocrinologists are daily confronted with questions around the causes and treatments of male infertility.

The field is quite recent, considering that the first paper on male infertility found on Scopus was published in 1941, followed by increasing annual numbers of publications. Continuously emerging research and clinical evidence support proper genome, epigenome, transcriptome, and proteome signatures to be essential for complete functionality of the sperm cell.

The book traces efforts towards improving diagnostic capability and provides essential information for healthcare professionals to utilize in routine practice for the management of male infertility. It therefore represents a guide for personalized and efficient treatment of the infertile male.

The first three sections cover definitions and epidemiology of male infertility, its causes classified as pretesticular, testicular, posttesticular, environmental, and idiopathic. The diagnostic tools used to explore fertility are also covered, including the recording of relevant medical history, physical examination, basic semen analysis with manual or automated methods, detection of sperm DNA fragmentation and sources of oxidative stress, reproductive hormone determinations towards genetic and genomic investigations and imaging techniques, and the most recent developments.

In the two next sections, medical treatments based on hormones, antioxidants, antibiotics, or alternative care such as herbs, behavioral therapy, and lifestyle changes, as well as surgical interventions useful to improve male fertility or to retrieve sperm in azoospermic patients, are discussed.

Section 6 is dedicated to medically assisted reproduction and the latest knowledge on sperm processing and selection for each of the various techniques, including intrauterine insemination, conventional in vitro fertilization, intracytoplasmic sperm injection, and sperm cryopreservation. Evolutions with a special focus on preimplantation genetic testing and cryopreservation methods are also presented. Notably, and in a fair way, it is pointed to the possibility to further improve male infertility care beyond intracytoplasmatic sperm injection (ICSI) and strive to obtain sperm with the best quality towards achieving higher success rates and safe perinatal outcomes.

Where appropriate, clinical case scenarios illustrate clinical management, and tables showing differential diagnoses summarize knowledge in a didactic and practical way.

While current American and European guidelines are provided throughout the book and also separately in Section 7, in the absence of consensus among the scientific community, expert opinions are given to further help the clinician.

Finally, the last section allows insight into the future of male infertility and research perspectives with regard to innovative therapies in the post-ICSI era. Hence the reader will discover the potential value of artificial intelligence and home semen testing for the future of male infertility assessment, and the upcoming contribution of microfluidics technology for improved sperm sorting.

Most textbooks in the field are edited by specialists of a single domain, being either urologists or andrologists. What is unique with this book is that the four editors, coming from different horizons and training, are a perfect combination to cover in a broad way all knowledge brought by multidisciplinary teams as required to achieve the best care for our patients. It is also in this quality of multidisciplinarity that I was invited to write this foreword, being trained as a gynecologist, obstetrician, and andrologist specialized in reproductive medicine.

I was very pleased to see that the editors brought together excellent and well-chosen contributors for each of the chapters where special attention was given to encompass not only the male side but also the broader couples context, pointing to essential female characteristics that may change the strategy of care.

The authors also reached a good balance between the basic knowledge of male reproductive physiology with keystones of male infertility assessment and treatment, and the more advanced information on investigational and therapeutical approaches.

Overall, this book is a valuable resource for clinicians to resolve the etiology of male infertility, provide all aspects of its management, and guide expert care in male infertility.

One of the key messages widely illustrated along its 29 chapters is "Do not just focus on the sperm and do not forget the male behind," knowing that male infertility is more and more considered a marker of current and future males's health.

Professor Christine Wyns,
MD, PhD
Department of Gynecology and Andrology
Cliniques Universitaires
Saint-Luc
Catholic University of Louvain
Brussels, Belgium

SHORT BIOGRAPHY

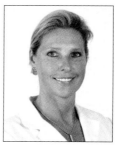

Christine Wyns obtained her doctor of medicine degree from the Catholic University of Louvain, Brussels, in 1993. She graduated in Gynecology from the Catholic University of Louvain, applied Andrology from the University of Limoges, and Health and Biomedical Sciences from the Catholic University of Louvain. Thesis presented on "Male fertility preservation after gonadotoxic treatment."

She is the director of the Reproductive Tissue and Cell Bank at University Clinics Saint Luc, Brussels, Belgium, and a professor at the Catholic University of Louvain. She is the head of the Andrology Research Laboratory, with special focus on fertility preservation for prepubertal boys.

PREFACE

Infertility affects approximately 15% of couples worldwide and negatively impacts the quality of life of the affected couples. Male factors, alone or in combination with female factors, account for at least 50% of all cases of infertility. Starting in the late 20th century, scientists have expressed concerns about the declining semen quality in males. In 1992, a study of males who had never suffered from infertility showed that the amount of sperm in semen had declined by 1% per year since 1938. Male infertility has been attributed to a variety of problems such as varicocele, genetic disorders, genital tract inflammation/infections, advanced paternal age, and environmental/lifestyle factors.

In 30% to 45% of infertility cases, the cause of abnormal semen parameters is not identified; hence a diagnosis of idiopathic male infertility is applied. Despite the fact that about half of infertility problems stem from male factors, gynecologists are often the first healthcare providers to perform the initial assessment of an infertile heterosexual couple. Therefore it is crucial that they remain updated on the main conditions that cause male infertility, as well as current diagnostic tools and treatment options in the contexts of natural and assisted conception.

The idea of this book was an offshoot of a series of webinars organized by Professor Ashok Agarwal during the COVID pandemic in 2020–21. These webinars covered various facets of infertility, male and female, in which infertility specialists from over 100 countries participated. Based on the feedback received from these webinars, we realized that it was time to produce an easy-to-read text that would summarize what has been achieved so far in the context of male infertility and what is still in the pipeline. Also, it was time to present the state-of-the-art knowledge and recent guidelines in the clinical andrology field in a concise, modern, and palatable text, compatible with the 21st century, that is suitable for both the beginner and the expert. Additionally, we need to remove barriers between both groups of subspecialties dealing with infertile couples and include gynecologists working in the field of reproductive medicine, next to the andrologists. Furthermore, the comprehensive information provided in this book makes it very interesting to all reproductive professionals, including embryologists, endocrinologists, biologists, and researchers.

The book starts with an introductory section on the definition and epidemiology of male infertility and its implications on the quality of life of the affected couple. This is followed by a section with a series of chapters detailing the causes of male infertility and laying the groundwork for the subsequent chapters. A third section on the diagnostic aspects of male infertility, including clinical, laboratory, and imaging methods necessary for proper diagnosis of male infertility, is presented. The fourth section of the book deals with different therapeutic options for treating infertile males, while the fifth section discusses the details of the classical and advanced surgical procedures available. The next section is dedicated to state-of-the-art information on various assisted reproductive techniques. The seventh section summarizes the most recent guidelines of male infertility management that are set by professional societies working in the reproductive field. Finally, the book ends with a visionary section that provides insights on the future of the ever-evolving field of male infertility.

The book is written by 68 world-renowned infertility experts from 21 countries representing 6 continents, offering their knowledge and experience in an easy-to-read manner. Each chapter starts with the key points discussed by the authors and ends with clinical scenarios offering real-life problems and their solutions, with a structured text in between. A nonexhaustive list of references follows and includes the most relevant papers published on a particular topic.

We hope the book will be a welcome addition to the library of infertility in general and male infertility in particular. The way this book is designed ensures that it will be of great help for junior as well as senior experts in their expanding subspecialties.

We wish you an enjoyable read,

Ashok Agarwal, PhD, HCLD (Andrology)
Florence Boitrelle, MD, PhD
Panagiotis Drakopoulos, MD, PhD
Hassan Nooman Sallam, MD, FRCOG, PhD
Ramadan Saleh, MD

ABOUT THE AUTHOR

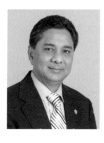

Ashok Agarwal is a highly regarded andrologist and researcher who has made significant contributions to the field of male infertility. He is a founding member and current President of the Global Andrology Forum (GAF, based in Moreland Hills, Ohio), an international organization dedicated to advancing the field of andrology and promoting male reproductive health. Ashok has served as the Director of the Andrology Laboratory and the Director of Research in Urology at Cleveland Clinic and as Professor of Surgery at Case Western Reserve University, Cleveland for about 30 years (from 1993 to 2022). He has published over 900 scientific articles, edited over 50 medical text books and has received numerous awards for his contributions to the field of andrology and male infertility. In addition to his research and clinical work, Dr. Agarwal is also a dedicated teacher and mentor, and has trained over 1000 clinicians and scientists from more than 65 countries in the field of andrology. He is widely recognized as a leader in the field of male infertility and has been invited to speak at numerous national and international conferences and events in over 75 countries.

Ashok Agarwal, PhD, HCLD (Andrology)
Global Andrology Forum
Moreland Hills, OH, United States;
Emeritus Staff, Cleveland Clinic
Cleveland, OH, United States

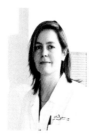

Florence Boitrelle is a medical doctor, Professor of Reproductive Biology and Andrology at the University of Paris Saclay (UVSQ, France). She is in charge of the Poissy Saint Germain en Laye (Yvelines) assisted reproductive technology centre and head of the Reproductive Biology-Andrology-CECOS department. Florence Boitrelle is a former president of the French-speaking Society of Andrology (SALF) and a member of several societies active in reproductive medicine and biology (FFER, CECOS, ESHRE, ISA, GAF). She is a member of the management committee of the GAF which brings together more than 600 andrologists worldwide. She is the author of nearly 100 articles in peer-reviewed journals.

Florence Boitrelle, MD, PhD
Department of Reproductive Biology
Preservation of Fertility, Andrology
BREED
UVSQ, Jouy-en-Josas
Île-de-France, France

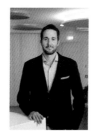

Professor Panagiotis Drakopoulos is recognized as a subspecialist in reproductive medicine and surgery by the European Society of Human Reproduction and Embryology (ESHRE) and the European Board and College of Obstetrics and Gynecology (EBCOG). He holds a PhD in reproductive medicine from the University of Brussels (Vrije Universiteit Brussel) and he is a visiting Professor at the University since 2019. He also works in private, from his office in Athens, Greece. He has authored more than 90 peer-reviewed papers. His research is focused on poor responders and ovarian stimulation strategies.

Panagiotis Drakopoulos, MD, PhD
Reproductive Medicine
UZ Brussel
Brussels, Belgium

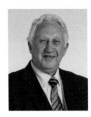

Hassan Nooman Sallam is Professor of Obstetrics and Gynaecology in Alexandria University in Egypt, clinical director of the Alexandria Fertility Center and founding chairperson of the Alexandria Regional Center for Women's Health and Development. He was a founding member of the IVF unit at King's College Hospital, London in 1981 and in St. Luke's-Roosevelt Hospital, Columbia University, New York in 1984. He is the founding chairperson of the Mediterranean Society for Reproductive Medicine, sometime examiner to the Royal College of Obstetricians and Gynaecologists (RCOG) of England and recipient of the RCOG Historical lecture in 2012. He is/was a member of editorial boards of many journals including *Human Reproduction and Reproductive Medicine and Biology online*. He has more than 100 publications in refereed journals and co-edited four books.

Hassan Nooman Sallam, MD, FRCOG, PhD
Department of Obstetrics and Gynaecology
Faculty of Medicine
Alexandria University;
Alexandria Fertility and ART Center
Alexandria, Egypt

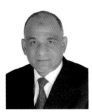

Ramadan Saleh is a Professor of Dermatology, Venereology and Andrology, in Sohag University, Egypt. He is the founder of the Ajyal IVF Center, Ajyal Hospital, Sohag, Egypt. He is a co-founder of GAF created in May 2020, and formally established in December 2021. He is an editorial board member of *The Journal of Sexual Medicine*, and an Associate Editor of the Male Urology section of Frontiers in Urology. He is a member of several professional societies and a reviewer in many international peer-reviewed journals in the field of reproductive medicine. He has published more than 120 research articles in peer-reviewed scientific journals, and co-edited three books.

Ramadan Saleh, MD
Departments of Dermatology,
Venereology, and Andrology
Sohag University;
Ajyal IVF Center
Ajyal Hospital,
Sohag, Egypt

CONTENTS

SECTION 7 Clinical Practice Guidelines for Male Infertility

Definition, Epidemiology, and Implications of Male Infertility

Definition, Epidemiology, and Implications of Male Infertility

Eric Chung

KEY POINTS

- Infertility is a disease of the male or female reproductive system defined by the failure to achieve a pregnancy after 12 months or more of regular unprotected sexual intercourse.
- Male infertility is a global population health concern, with the global rates of male infertility ranging from 2.5%–12%.
- While the distribution of male causes of infertility has not been well defined, and it is not possible to make accurate estimates because of the low quality of scientific evidence, the large geographical differences in sperm counts could be attributable to various factors such as fertility awareness, changes in lifestyles, control of sexually transmitted diseases,

environmental pollutants, and the growing availability of effective assisted reproductive technology.
- Although male infertility is not deemed a reportable disease, the manifestations of male infertility can signify a future health concern.
- Current literature suggests an association between male infertility and risk of chronic disease, comorbidity, cardiovascular disease, and cancer development. However, the volume of literature remains relatively small, with heterogeneous study populations and a lack of well-designed prospective trials to control for confounders that may preclude drawing a definitive conclusion about male infertility as a precursor of these outcomes.

INTRODUCTION

Infertility has traditionally been defined as the inability to conceive after 1 year of regular sexual intercourse without contraception or the inability of a female to sustain a full-term pregnancy.

The World Health Organization (WHO) states that infertility is a disease of the male or female reproductive system defined by the failure to achieve a pregnancy after 12 months or more of regular unprotected sexual intercourse.[1] The three main factors influencing the likelihood of spontaneous conception are age of the female factor, time of unwanted nonconception, and other disease-related infertility. Similarly, the American Society of Reproductive Medicine (ASRM) defines

infertility as a disease (an interruption, cessation, or disorder of body functions, systems, or organs) of the male or female reproductive tract that prevents the conception of a child or the ability to carry to delivery.[2] While the accepted duration of regular unprotected intercourse with failure to conceive is about 12 months before an infertility evaluation is undertaken, fertility in females is known to decline steadily with age, and in 2008 the ASRM advocated a duration of trying to conceive of 6 months for females aged over 35 years to encourage earlier evaluation and treatment in this higher-risk group[3].

Around 15% of couples are labeled as infertile,[4] and the prevalence of infertility in reproductive-aged females has been estimated to be one in every seven couples in the western world and one in every four couples in developing countries.[5] Several epidemiological studies have reported that about half of all cases of infertility are related to female factors, while 20%–30% can be attributed to male factors, with the remainder due to causes in both partners.[5–7] According to the latest WHO statistics, around 50 to 80 million people worldwide suffer from infertility.[8] It is important to consider the significant heterogeneity of available data due to the varying duration of abstinence, couple demographic characteristics, methods of reporting, and quality assurance of semen analysis, as well as uncertainty about the comparability of the study populations across different periods.[9]

Male infertility is a heterogeneous and complex problem related to three broad categories: (1) pretesticular conditions (such as hypothalamic-pituitary conditions causing secondary hypogonadism); (2) testicular dysfunction (which may be associated with primary hypogonadism); and (3) posttesticular conditions (such as obstruction of seminal outflow, which is usually termed obstructive azoospermia).[10] The presence of abnormal semen parameters is synonymous with male infertility and contributes to 50% of all cases of infertility.[1,2] A recent systematic review showed a decline in total sperm counts by 59.3% since the 1970s across North America, Europe, and Australasia,[11] and the male infertility rate is likely higher in developing countries.[12] While the distribution of male causes of infertility has not been well defined and it is not possible to make accurate estimates because of the low quality of scientific evidence, the large geographical differences in sperm counts could be attributable to various factors such as fertility awareness, changes in lifestyles, control of sexually transmitted diseases, environmental pollutants, and the growing availability of effective assisted reproductive technology.[13–16]. Nonetheless, it is thought that up to half of cases of male infertility are classified as idiopathic or unexplained.[17]

EPIDEMIOLOGY OF MALE INFERTILITY

Male infertility is a global health concern, with global rates of male infertility ranging from 2.5%–12% (Fig. 1.1).[18] It is estimated that around 6%–8% of males in North America, 8% in Australia, and 8%–10% in Europe are infertile.[19–21] In contrast, infertility rates are higher in North Africa, Sub-Saharan Africa, Eastern Europe, and the Middle East compared to Western countries, and the true incidence of male infertility is likely underreported (and underdiagnosed) owing to cultural beliefs, especially among patriarchal societies.[22–24]

An evaluation of trends in infertility by sex in 195 countries and territories from 1990 to 2017 based on the Global Burden of Disease Study 2017[25] showed that the age-standardized prevalence of male infertility increased by 8.224% from 710.19 per 100,000 (95% uncertainty interval [UI]: 586.08, 848.94) in 1990 to 768.59 per 100,000 (95% UI: 623.20, 929.91) in 2017 globally, with an increasing rate of 0.291% per year (95% confidence interval [CI]: 0.241, 0.341) and an increasing trend in all sociodemographic index (SDI) countries, especially in low-SDI countries. Similarly, age-standardized, disability-adjusted life-years of male infertility increased by 8.843% from 4.20 per 100,000 (95% UI: 1.75, 8.75) in 1990 to 4.57 per 100,000 (95% UI: 1.89, 9.45) in 2017, at 0.293% per year (95% CI: 0.237, 0.349) during the observational period. A trend toward a negative association was observed between these estimates and SDI levels, perhaps related to the gradual improvement in national economies and the placement of greater emphasis on population growth, although the global disease burden of infertility increased from 1990 to 2017.

Unlike female infertility, the actual prevalence of male infertility in the general population often difficult to estimate, and male infertility is likely underdiagnosed.[26] Patient demographics, epidemiological definitions of infertility, type of presentation (normal vs. infertility clinics), and assessment approach (male vs. couple) vary in clinical studies.[18] Accurate statistics may not be available for many regions of the world, especially in patriarchal societies where sociocultural differences mean that the female partner is often blamed for infertility, and males often do not attend formal fertility evaluation due to stigma about masculine identity and low rates of health-seeking behavior.[1,6] Furthermore, male infertility is not defined as a disease in many societies, which could contribute to the sparse statistics.[18]

The WHO has stated that availability, access, and quality of interventions to address infertility remain a significant challenge in most countries, and that diagnosis and treatment of infertility are often not prioritized in many national populations.[27] Furthermore, the development and subsequent enactment of public policies and reproductive health strategies are rarely funded

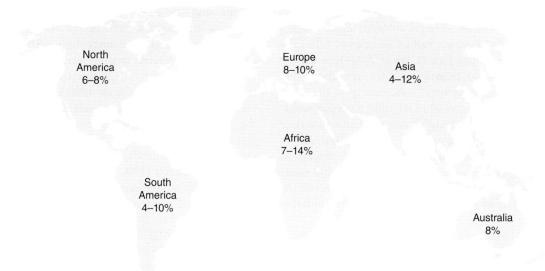

Fig. 1.1 Estimated Percentages of Male Infertility Worldwide. (Estimates of male infertility data obtained from the World Health Organization website; Agarwal A, Mulgund A, Hamada A, Chyatte MR. A unique view on male infertility around the globe. *Reprod Biol Endocrinol.* 2015;13:37; Kumar N, Singh AK. Trends of male factor infertility, an important cause of infertility: a review of the literature. *J Hum Reprod Sci.* 2015;8:191-196; Levine H, Jørgensen N, Martino-Andrade A, et al. Temporal trends in sperm count: a systematic review and meta-regression analysis. *Hum Reprod Update.* 2017;23:646-659; Mascarenhas MN, Flaxman SR, Boerma T, Vanderpoel S, Stevens GA. National, regional, and global trends in infertility prevalence since 1990: a systematic analysis of 277 health surveys. *PLoS Med.* 2012;9:e1001356; Australian Institute of Health and Welfare 2012. The health of Australia's males: a focus on five population groups. Cat. no. PHE 160. Canberra: AIHW; Martinez G, Daniels K, Chandra A. Fertility of males and females aged 15-44 years in the United States: National Survey of Family Growth, 2006-2010. *Natl Health Stat Report.* 2012;(51):1-28; Sun H, Gong TT, Jiang YT, Zhang S, Zhao YH, Wu QJ. Global, regional, and national prevalence and disability-adjusted life-years for infertility in 195 countries and territories, 1990-2017: results from a global burden of disease study, 2017. *Aging.* 2019;11:10952-10991; Infertility. Fact sheet. World Health Organization website, April 3, 2023. https://www.who.int/news-room/fact-sheets/detail/infertility.)

when insufficient public health financing is available because of inadequate infrastructure and the current high costs of treatment, especially assisted reproduction technologies, resulting in significant barriers even in countries that are actively addressing the needs of people with infertility. Government policies need to be implemented that provide comprehensive policies and programmatic interventions incorporating fertility awareness into national sexuality education programs; promoting healthy lifestyles to reduce specific behavioral risks, including prevention, diagnosis, and early treatment of sexually transmitted infections; preventing complications of unsafe abortion, postpartum sepsis, and abdominal/pelvic surgery; and addressing environmental toxins associated with infertility.[1,27]

HEALTH IMPLICATIONS OF MALE INFERTILITY

While reproductive health has always carried a special significance to females, particularly during their reproductive years, the general health of males is less affected by their reproductive health. Although male infertility is not deemed a reportable disease, the manifestations of male infertility can signify a future health concern.[28–31] As such, male infertility has been proposed as an independent risk factor for poor health status and early mortality, although the exact etiology of this relationship remains unclear, as studies that examine the prevalence of comorbidities, morbidity, and mortality among infertile males are often heterogeneous and contain a low level of evidence.[32,33]

Given that worldwide sperm counts appear to be falling over time,[18] coupled with an increase in the prevalence of male factor infertility,[25] the question arises of whether male infertility can serve as an important biomarker for future health and mortality.[34,35] Moreover, recent literature has identified lower sperm counts as an independent predictor of comorbidity and mortality.[11,29,36] In a study of males who underwent fertility testing, those with varicocele, which is associated with primary infertility in up to 35% of males, were shown to have a higher incidence of heart disease than males without varicocele (hazard ratio [HR], 1.22; 95% CI: 1.03, 1.45).[37]

Published literature suggests that semen parameters and overall testicular function may be important markers of general health.[38] Serum testosterone levels decline gradually with age in most males, and several epidemiological studies have demonstrated that low testosterone and male factor infertility are associated with increased cardiovascular health risk, including the incidence of cardiovascular diseases and overall mortality related to cardiovascular events.[39–41] The direct or indirect relationship between male infertility and future cardiovascular risk may involve hormonal dysregulation or perhaps male infertility could be considered, and male infertility as an independent risk factor for the subsequent development of chronic medical conditions is an intriguing possibility.[42] One study found that, compared with fertile males, infertile males had an increased incidence of hypertension, peripheral vascular disease, and heart disease (HR, 1.09; 95% CI: 1.02, 1.17; HR, 1.52; 95% CI: 1.12, 2.07; and HR, 1.20; 95% CI: 1.09, 1.32, respectively). In a 2021 study,[43] males with low sperm count (<39 million/ejaculate) were shown to be at a significantly higher risk of hypogonadism (odds ratio, 12.2; 95% CI: 10.2, 14.6) and were overall at higher risk for chronic metabolic and cardiovascular disorders. Similarly, a study of 136,416 males with infertility included in the Optum Clinformatics Data Mart Database demonstrated that infertile males were at higher risk of developing hypertension (HR, 1.15; 95% CI: 1.13, 1.18) and heart disease (HR, 1.34; 95% CI: 1.25, 1.45) than fertile controls.[44]

Social factors such as smoking, increased body mass index, consumption of alcohol, drug abuse, and psychological stress have been associated with an increased incidence of chronic diseases such as metabolic syndrome and organ dysfunction.[45,46] These same factors have been implicated in the development of male infertility and decreased semen parameters.[32,47]

While many cancers and cancer-related treatments are known to negatively impact male fertility, male infertility may also be associated with a future risk of developing cancer.[48,49] The underlying mechanism behind this potential link is largely unknown, although it is hypothesized that a complex interaction among genetics and epigenetics, developmental factors, and lifestyle or environmental factors can put males with infertility at risk of developing cancer(s) in the future.[50] At least 1500 genes are known to contribute to spermatogenesis, and any defect in these genes may also potentially lead to the development of infertility, male genitourinary cancer, and cancer in other organs.[51] Furthermore, at least 25 tumor suppressor genes or oncogenes could have a pleomorphic effect contributing to both male infertility and the development of malignancy.[52] An older study that used linkage data from the Danish Cancer Registry reported that males with abnormal semen characteristics had a small increase (standardized incidence ratio [SIR], 1.1; 95% CI: 1.0, 1.2) in the incidence of any type of cancer (36 cases per 32,442 males) compared with males with normal semen characteristics.[53] Another study found that infertile males were at a higher overall risk of developing cancer than fertile males (SIR, 1.7; 95% CI: 1.2, 2.5), with azoospermic males showing the highest risk of cancer (SIR, 2.9; 95% CI: 1.4, 5.4).[54] It is believed that male infertility, per se, may be a risk factor for the development of genitourinary cancers in males.[55] Males diagnosed with infertility or who have abnormal semen parameters are at significantly increased risk of developing male-specific malignancies such as testicular cancer and prostate cancer.[56–58]

SUMMARY

Current literature suggests an association between male infertility and the risk of chronic disease, comorbidity, cardiovascular disease, and cancer development. However, the volume of literature remains relatively small, with heterogeneous study populations and a lack of well-designed studies making it challenging to reach a definitive conclusion about a potential causal relationship. As infertile males are often evaluated early in life, there is an opportunity for a proper health assessment to allow for more adequate medical counseling, treatment, and behavioral and lifestyle modifications, as well as disease prevention, management, and follow-up.

REFERENCES

1. World Health Organization (WHO). *International Classification of Diseases, 11th Revision (ICD-11)*. Geneva: WHO; 2018.
2. Practice Committee of the American Society of Reproductive Medicine. Definitions of infertility and recurrent pregnancy loss: a committee opinion. *Fertil Steril.* 2020; 113(3):533-535.
3. Practice Committee of the American Society of Reproductive Medicine. Definitions of infertility and recurrent pregnancy loss. *Fertil Steril.* 2008;90(suppl 5):S60.
4. Thoma ME, McLain AC, Louis JF, et al. Prevalence of infertility in the United States as estimated by the current duration approach and a traditional constructed approach. *Fertil Steril.* 2013;99:1324-1331.
5. Vander Borght M, Wyns C. Fertility and infertility: definition and epidemiology. *Clin Biochem.* 2018;62:2-10.
6. Agarwal A, Mulgund A, Hamada A, Chyatte MR. A unique view on male infertility around the globe. *Reprod Biol Endocrinol.* 2015;13(1):37.
7. de La Rochebrochard E, Thonneau P. Paternal age >or= 40 years: an important risk factor for infertility. *Am J Obstet Gynecol.* 2003;189:901-905.
8. Kumar N, Singh AK. Trends of male factor infertility, an important cause of infertility: a review of the literature. *J Hum Reprod Sci.* 2015;8(4):191-196.
9. te Velde ER, Bonde JP. Misconceptions about falling sperm counts and fertility in Europe. *Asian J Androl.* 2013;15:195-198.
10. Krausz C. Male infertility: pathogenesis and clinical diagnosis. *Best Pract Res Clin Endocrinol Metab.* 2011;25(2): 271-285.
11. Levine H, Jørgensen N, Martino-Andrade A, et al. Temporal trends in sperm count: a systematic review and meta-regression analysis. *Hum Reprod Update.* 2017;23(6):646-659.
12. Barratt CLR, Björndahl L, De Jonge CJ, et al. The diagnosis of male infertility: an analysis of the evidence to support the development of global WHO guidance challenges and future research opportunities. *Hum Reprod Update.* 2017;23(6):660-680.
13. Sartorius GA, Nieschlag E. Paternal age and reproduction. *Hum Reprod Update.* 2009;16:65-79.
14. Homan GF, Davies M, Norman R. The impact of lifestyle factors on reproductive performance in the general population and those undergoing infertility treatment: a review. *Hum Reprod Update.* 2007;13:209-223.
15. Lesthaege R. The unfolding story of the second demographic transition. *Popul Dev Rev.* 2010;36:211-251.
16. Burdorf A, Figa-Talamanca I, Jensen TK, Thulstrup AM. Effects of occupational exposure on the reproductive system: core evidence and practical implications. *Occup Med (Lond).* 2006;56:516-520.
17. Hanson BM, Eisenberg ML, Hotaling JM. Male infertility: a biomarker of individual and familial cancer risk. *Fertil Steril.* 2018;109(1):6-19.
18. Mascarenhas MN, Flaxman SR, Boerma T, Vanderpoel S, Stevens GA. National, regional, and global trends in infertility prevalence since 1990: a systematic analysis of 277 health surveys. *PLoS Med.* 2012;9(12):e1001356.
19. Australian Institute of Health and Welfare. *The Health of Australia's Males: A Focus on Five Population Groups. Cat. no. PHE 160.* Canberra: AIHW; 2012.
20. Jungwirth A, Giwercman A, Tournaye H et al. European Association of Urology guidelines on male infertility: the 2012 update. *Eur Urol.* 2012;62:324-332.
21. Martinez G, Daniels K, Chandra A. Fertility of men and women aged 15-44 years in the United States: National Survey of Family Growth, 2006-2010. *Natl Health Stat Report.* 2012;(51):1-28.
22. Cooper TG, Noonan E, von Eckardstein S, et al. World Health Organization reference values for human semen characteristics. *Hum Reprod Update.* 2010;16:231-245.
23. Rutstein SO, Shah IH. *Infecundity, Infertility and Childlessness in Developing Countries. DHS Comparative Reports No. 9.* Calverton: ORC Macro and the World Health Organization; 2004.
24. Cates W, Farley TM, Rowe PJ. Worldwide patterns of infertility: is Africa different? *Lancet.* 1985;326:596-598.
25. Sun H, Gong TT, Jiang YT, Zhang S, Zhao YH, Wu QJ. Global, regional, and national prevalence and disability-adjusted life-years for infertility in 195 countries and territories, 1990-2017: results from a global burden of disease study, 2017. *Aging.* 2019;11(23):10952-10991.
26. Winters BR, Walsh TJ. The epidemiology of male infertility. *Urol Clin North Am.* 2014;41:195-204.
27. *Infertility. Fact sheet.* World Health Organization; April 3, 2023. Available at: https://www.who.int/news-room/fact-sheets/detail/infertility.
28. Rogers MJ, Walsh TJ. Male infertility and risk of cancer. *Semin Reprod Med.* 2017;35(3):298-303.
29. Glazer CH, Bonde JP, Eisenberg ML, et al. Male infertility and risk of nonmalignant chronic diseases: a systematic review of the epidemiological evidence. *Semin Reprod Med.* 2017;35(3):282-290.
30. Kasman AM, Del Giudice F, Eisenberg ML. New insights to guide patient care: the bidirectional relationship between male infertility and male health. *Fertil Steril.* 2020; 113(3):469-477.
31. Behboudi-Gandevani S, Bidhendi Yarandi R, Rostami Dovom M, Azizi F, Ramezani Tehrani F. The association between male infertility and cardiometabolic disturbances:

a population-based study. *Int J Endocrinol Metab.* 2021; 19(2):e107418.

32. Del Giudice F, Kasman AM, Ferro M, et al. Clinical correlation among male infertility and overall male health: a systematic review of the literature. *Investig Clin Urol.* 2020:61(4):355-371.

33. Glazer CH, Eisenberg ML, Tøttenborg SS, et al. Male factor infertility and risk of death: a nationwide record-linkage study. *Hum Reprod.* 2019;34:2266-2273.

34. Merzenich H, Zeeb H, Blettner M. Decreasing sperm quality: a global problem? *BMC Public Health.* 2010;10:24.

35. Chung E, Arafa M, Boitrelle F, et al. The new 6th edition of the WHO Laboratory manual for examination and processing of human semen: is it a step toward better standard operating procedure? *Asian J Androl.* 2022; 24(2):123-124.

36. Batty GD, Mortensen LH, Shipley MJ. Semen quality and risk factors for mortality. *Epidemiology.* 2019;30:e19-e21.

37. Wang NN, Dallas K, Li S, Baker L, Eisenberg ML. The association between varicoceles and vascular disease: an analysis of U.S. claims data. *Andrology.* 2018;6:99-103.

38. Kasman AM, Del Giudice F, Eisenberg ML. New insights to guide patient care: the bidirectional relationship between male infertility and male health. *Fertil Steril.* 2020;113:469-477.

39. Kloner RA, Carson C III, Dobs A, Kopecky S, Mohler ER III. Testosterone and cardiovascular disease. *J Am Coll Cardiol.* 2016;67:545-557.

40. Ponce OJ, Spencer-Bonilla G, Alvarez-Villalobos N, et al. The efficacy and adverse events of testosterone replacement therapy in hypogonadal men: a systematic review and meta-analysis of randomized, placebo-controlled trials. *J Clin Endocrinol Metab.* 2018;103:1745-1754.

41. Corona G, Rastrelli G, Di Pasquale G, Sforza A, Mannucci E, Maggi M. Endogenous testosterone levels and cardiovascular risk: meta-analysis of observational studies. *J Sex Med.* 2018;15:1260-1271.

42. Eisenberg ML, Li S, Cullen MR, Baker LC. Increased risk of incident chronic medical conditions in infertile men: analysis of United States claims data. *Fertil Steril.* 2016; 105:629-636.

43. Ferlin A, Garolla A, Ghezzi M, et al. Sperm count and hypogonadism as markers of general male health. *Eur Urol Focus.* 2021;7(1):205-213.

44. Kasman AM, Li S, Luke B, Sutcliffe AG, Pacey AA, Eisenberg ML. Male infertility and future cardiometabolic health: does the association vary by sociodemographic factors? *Urology.* 2019;133:121-128.

45. Sermondade N, Faure C, Fezeu L, et al. BMI in relation to sperm count: an updated systematic review and

46. Busetto GM, Del Giudice F, Virmani A, et al. Body mass index and age correlate with antioxidant supplementation effects on sperm quality: post hoc analyses from a double-blind placebo-controlled trial. *Andrologia.* 2020; 52:e13523.

47. Guerri G, Maniscalchi T, Barati S, et al. Syndromic infertility. *Acta Biomed.* 2019;90(10-S):75-82.

48. Behboudi-Gandevani S, Bidhendi-Yarandi R, Paahi MH, Vaismoradi M. A systematic review and meta-analysis of male infertility and the subsequent risk of cancer. *Front Oncol.* 2022;11:696702.

49. Matzuk MM, Lamb DJ. The biology of infertility: research advances and clinical challenges. *Nat Med.* 2008; 14:1197-1213.

50. Kasman AM, Del Giudice F, Eisenberg ML. New insights to guide patient care: the bidirectional relationship between male infertility and male health. *Fertil Steril.* 2020; 113(3):469-477.

51. Aston KI, Conrad DF. A review of genome-wide approaches to study the genetic basis for spermatogenic defects. *Methods Mol Biol.* 2013;927:397-410.

52. Nagirnaja L, Aston KI, Conrad DF. Genetic intersection of male infertility and cancer. *Fertil Steril.* 2018;109(1): 20-26.

53. Jacobsen R, Bostofte E, Engholm G, et al. Risk of testicular cancer in men with abnormal semen characteristics: cohort study. *BMJ.* 2000;321:789-792.

54. Eisenberg ML, Li S, Brooks JD, Cullen MR, Baker LC. Increased risk of cancer in infertile men: analysis of U.S. claims data. *J Urol.* 2015;193:1596-1601.

55. Del Giudice F, Kasman AM, De Berardinis E, Busetto GM, Belladelli F, Eisenberg ML. Association between male infertility and male-specific malignancies: systematic review and meta-analysis of population-based retrospective cohort studies. *Fertil Steril.* 2020;114(5):984-996.

56. Raman JD, Nobert CF, Goldstein M. Increased incidence of testicular cancer in men presenting with infertility and abnormal semen analysis. *J Urol.* 2005;174:1819-1822; discussion 1822.

57. Al-Jebari Y, Elenkov A, Wirestrand E, Schütz I, Giwercman A, Lundberg Giwercman Y. Risk of prostate cancer for men fathering through assisted reproduction: nationwide population based register study. *BMJ.* 2019;366:l5214.

58. Elenkov A, Giwercman A, Zhang H, Nilsson PM, Giwercman YL. Increased risk for prostate cancer related mortality among childless men in a population-based cohort followed for up to 40 years. *Scand J Urol.* 2021: 55(2):125-128.

Causes of Male Infertility

Pretesticular Causes of Male Infertility

Osvaldo Rajmil and Lluís Bassas

KEY POINTS

- This chapter revisits the pretesticular causes of male infertility and recalls the need to perform a thorough clinical evaluation of the male before the application of assisted reproductive techniques. The omission of a clinical evaluation can potentially result in both incorrect management decisions and loss of opportunities to diagnose and treat reversible causes of couple infertility in a timely fashion.
- Assisted reproductive techniques and fertility preservation procedures can be used as adjuvant therapies to improve the reproductive outcome in patients receiving medical treatment for hypogonadotropic hypogonadism.

INTRODUCTION

Males and females can both exhibit infertility. The initial approach to infertility screening begins with a careful medical history and a thorough physical examination, followed by hormone studies and semen testing. Currently, there is no routine comprehensive clinical evaluation of males.[1] This failure is largely attributable to the success and widespread availability of assisted reproductive techniques (ARTs), as well as to the desire of couples to achieve fast results.

Since the advent of laboratory techniques, intracytoplasmatic sperm injection (ICSI)[2-4] has progressively became the predominant treatment for couple infertility. The consequence of this attitude is a parallel decay of the clinical approach, focusing attention on retrieving oocytes and spermatozoa rather than identifying and resolving the etiology of male infertility.

Several causes of male infertility are recognized and can be summarized as pretesticular, testicular, or posttesticular (Table 2.1).

Improved knowledge of the infertile male and his treatment can lead to natural conception and prevent pathologies in the newborn and the father. This chapter provides an overview of the main principles of male infertility,[5] with special consideration given to investigation and management of pretesticular causes.[6]

PHYSIOPATHOLOGY OF THE HYPOTHALAMIC-PITUITARY-GONADAL AXIS

Regulation of the hypothalamic-pituitary-gonadal (HPG) axis occurs via feedback. Endogenous testosterone and other hormones or neurotransmitters act and regulate gonadotropin-releasing hormone (GnRH) and luteinizing hormone (LH) release at the hypothalamus and pituitary levels.

Endocrine regulation of the male reproductive system is part of this classic feedback loop. Gonadotropin, LH, and follicle-stimulating hormone (FSH) are released from the pituitary gland in response to GnRH secreted by the hypothalamus and act on the testicles respectively (Fig. 2.1).

TABLE 2.1	Pretesticular Causes of Male Hypogonadism	
Disease, Condition		**Level of Alteration**
Kallmann syndrome, idiopathic hypogonadotropic hypogonadism		H
Congenital syndromes (Prader-Willi, cerebellar ataxia, others)		H/P
Drugs (opiates, alcohol, androgenic steroids)		PreH/H/P
Central nervous system tumors		PreH/H
Prolactinoma, hyperprolactinemia, pituitary tumors		P
Stress, critical illness, hypercortisolism		PreH
Hemochromatosis, iron overload		PreH
Sarcoidosis, histiocytosis, and other granulomatous diseases		PreH/H/P
Empty sella syndrome, pituitary malformations		P
Traumatic brain injury		PreH
Aging, obesity		PreH/H
Environmental toxins and pollutants, radiotherapy		PreH/H/P

H, Hypothalamic; P, pituitary; PreH, prehypothalamic.

Various neurotransmitters are involved in controlling GnRH-secreting neurons and thus modulate GnRH pulses.[7]

Genes involved in controlling the onset of puberty including neurokinin B (*TAC3*), its related receptor (*TACR3*), and dynorphin.[8] Considered as a whole, the secretory activity of GnRH neurons represents the integrated response to many hormones, neurotransmitters, and environmental influences. Other input signals include sex steroids, glucocorticoids, leptin, insulin, IGF-1, ghrelin, FGF21, orexigenic peptides, and anorexigenic peptides, with the net effect of signal integration to govern pubertal maturation and ongoing reproductive function. It is clear that sudden or chronic imbalance of these axis-regulating elements would alter sexual or reproductive function.[9] The effect of LH and FSH on germ cell development is mediated by both androgen receptors and FSH receptors, which are present on Leydig and Sertoli cells, respectively. While FSH acts directly on the germinal epithelium, LH causes Leydig cells to secrete testosterone. Testosterone increases sperm production and virilization, provides feedback to

the hypothalamus, and regulates GnRH secretion by the pituitary gland. FSH stimulates Sertoli cells to secrete activin B, which supports spermatogenesis and negatively regulates FSH secretion. GnRH impulse generators are the major regulators of puberty, and production begins early in fetal development.[10]

At puberty, intratesticular testosterone acts on Sertoli cells in concert with FSH, inducing spermatogenesis and ending Sertoli cell proliferation. Each Sertoli cell supports several germ cells that are necessary to achieve high sperm counts and fertility. Estradiol produces negative feedback on LH pulse amplitude by reducing pituitary gonadotroph sensitivity to GnRH.[11]

CLINICAL PICTURE AND DIAGNOSIS

Physical Features

At first glance, the general appearance of a male patient may indicate his endocrine status. Hypogonadism can be suspected in patients with reduced facial hair, gynecomastia, long legs, and obesity. Symptoms and signs of hypogonadism, along with other features, define a eunuchoid pattern that is often associated with the prepubertal or pubertal onset of congenital hypogonadism.

In contrast, symptoms prevail over signs in hypogonadotropic hypogonadism (HH) with late onset.

A genital examination is mandatory. Testis palpation gives a rough idea of spermatogenic function.[12] The consistency and size of the testes offer valuable information before carrying out further laboratory testing. The epididymides and the vasa deferentia at the spermatic cord provide additional information on possible comorbidities. Features of late-onset HH and associated symptoms are less likely to be clinically significant at the examination.

The need for semen analysis, hormonal diagnosis, and other laboratory tests should be decided on in a step-by-step approach. Additionally, imaging of the hypothalamic and pituitary region is paradigmatic when searching for the cause of male infertility.

An additional benefit of the interview and clinical examination is the identification of relevant underlying medical conditions; for example, testicular cancer and pituitary tumors that can possibly manifest as subfertility.[13]

Endocrine Diagnostics

The basic diagnosis, with LH, FSH and total testosterone (TT) determination, clarifies whether a normal

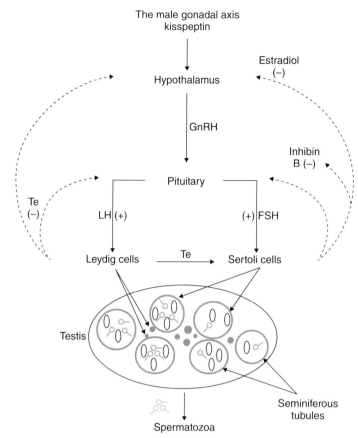

Fig. 2.1 Schematic Representation of the Human Male Hypothalamic-Pituitary-Gonadal Axis. The stimulatory effects of the hormones are indicated by solid lines and the inhibitory actions by dashed lines. The hypothalamus secretes gonadotropin-releasing hormone *(GnRH)*, which stimulates the production of luteinizing hormone *(LH)* and follicle-stimulating hormone *(FSH)* in the pituitary gland. LH stimulates the synthesis of testosterone in Leydig cells, while FSH activates mediators in Sertoli cells that are responsible for directing the entire process of spermatogenesis. Testosterone also acts on the germinal epithelium and on other peritubular cells not represented here. Testosterone passes into the general circulation and reaches target tissues, where it binds to specific receptors directly or through its metabolite dihydrotestosterone (DHT). Inhibitory control is carried out by inhibin B, produced in Sertoli cells, and also by testosterone and another of its metabolites, estradiol. (Modified and redrawn from Fraietta R, Zylberstejn DS, Esteves SC. Hypogonadotropic hypogonadism revisited. *Clinics.* 2013;68:81-88.)

pituitary-gonadal control loop is present and functional. Hormone levels vary from laboratory to laboratory, depending on the method and units used to express results. The reference values of each laboratory must be carefully observed before diagnosis.

In general, values of LH range from 2 to 10 IU/L, FSH 1.5 and 12.5 IU /L, and TT 9 to 27 nmol/L. Determining these values may be enough to assess Leydig cell function, which, in the case of some deviation from the normal values, can be confirmed by determination of free testosterone (fT) levels. The fT value can be obtained by Vermeulen's equation,[14] using the concentrations of TT, sex hormone binding globulin, and albumin. Furthermore, dihydrotestosterone levels can be determined in rare cases if there is a suspicion of a 5α-reductase deficiency. Determination of estradiol levels should be added if, for example, gynecomastia is clinically noticeable. Caution must be taken with borderline low testosterone concentrations because reported face values may differ from one laboratory to another.

Blood samples should be taken and analyzed in the morning, preferably before 10 a.m., with previous overnight fasting. Distinctions between hypergonadotropic (testicular responsibility) and hypogonadotropic (pretesticular responsibility) hypogonadism can be made using the concentrations of the gonadotropins LH and FSH.

Low or even undetectable gonadotropins (LH, FSH) indicate a hypothalamic or pituitary failure. These findings must be further clarified through a differential diagnosis. The main advisable explorations, in this case, are prolactin (PRL) measurement, determination of thyroid-stimulating hormone, evaluation of the corticotropic and somatotropic axis, a GnRH test,[15] and magnetic resonance imaging (MRI) of the pituitary region.[16]

Altogether, clinical and hormonal parameters and radiology can lead to a diagnosis of HH, which, in terms of infertility, can be successfully treated.

It should be noted that normal gonadotropin and TT levels, along with normal testicular volume, indicate a normal functional hypothalamic-hypophyseal-gonadal axis.

ETIOLOGIES OF HYPOGONADOTROPIC HYPOGONADISM

HH can be congenital or acquired. Congenital HH is divided into two main groups, depending on the presence of an intact sense of smell: anosmic (Kallmann syndrome [KS]) and normosmic (idiopathic). The incidence of congenital HH is approximately 1:100,000 to 10:100,000 live births, with approximately two-thirds and one-third of cases being KS and idiopathic HH, respectively.[10,17]

Genetic Causes

The progressive increase in new genetic factors associated with pretesticular etiologies is due to the development of sequencing techniques. A genetic basis of isolated HH can be found in almost 50% of cases. Other newly discovered gene mutations seem to be responsible for another small percentage of total patient cases.

Multiple genes have been identified as playing a role in the pathogenesis of KS, including *KAL1*. In KS, GnRH-secreting neurons fail to migrate to the hypothalamus, resulting in an absence of GnRH secretion and in hypogonadism.[18] The inheritance of KS can be X-linked (*KAL1*), meaning that the affected father will

transmit the mutation to his daughter, who will have a 50% probability of producing a son with KS, while all other listed genes are autosomal, and the transmission of the disease may be transmitted in an autosomal dominant manner (*FGFR1*). According to Mendelian laws, the chance of producing an affected child will be 50% with X-linked transmission, while the probability of disease occurrence in a child in the case of a recessive inheritance pattern depends on the genetic background of the partner, showing a higher risk in cases of consanguinity.[19] Patients affected by the syndrome not only present with hypogonadism and anosmia but can also suffer from additional nervous system anomalies, impaired hearing (including deafness), oral anomalies such as cleft lip or high arched palate, synkinesis of the extremities, and so on. X-linked KS is associated with unilateral renal aplasia in about 30% of individuals. This anatomical anomaly must be ruled out with abdominal/pelvic ultrasound of all affected patients.[20]

HH can be present with an intact sense of smell due to mutations in genes like *GnRH-R* and *GPR54/KiSS1*, as well as a few mutations affecting the beta subunits of LH and FSH that have been described in patients with selective gonadotropin deficiency.[21]

Drug-Induced Hypogonadotropic Hypogonadism

It is estimated that up to 2% of cases of male infertility can be explained by androgenic anabolic steroid abuse.[22–26] Exogenous androgens, which have a similar mechanism to endogenous androgens, exert an inhibitory effect at the hypothalamic and hypophyseal level, leading to an HH state characterized by a low level of serum testosterone, FSH, and LH. This induces a paradoxical decrease in intratesticular testosterone, blunting FSH production and resulting in a diminution, or complete cessation, of spermatogenesis.[27]

Clinically, the presentation is a male with diminished testicular volume and well-developed musculature that can be accompanied by gynecomastia and acne. Those patients often exhibit azoospermia or oligospermia, reduced sperm motility, and/or abnormal sperm morphology. Additionally, some users of anabolic substances are also taking human chorionic gonadotropin (hCG), growth hormone, and other combinations of drugs, a common behavior among bodybuilders, leading to a serious state of hypogonadism as well as low-quality semen parameters and infertility.[28]

Additional Nongenetic Causes

Central nervous system and pituitary tumors, hyperprolactinemia, cranial trauma, surgery, radiation, and infiltrative and systemic diseases can also cause HH.

Hyperprolactinemia

Hyperprolactinemia is an endocrine disorder that can influence male fertility. It is a common medical condition that affects 1% of the general population worldwide.[29]

High circulating levels of PRL cause hypogonadism by inhibiting GnRH pulsatile secretion and, consequently, FSH, LH, and testosterone secretion. As a result, central and peripheral inhibition produces spermatogenic arrest. Depending on how long this situation takes to develop, impaired sperm mobility, low sperm quality, and even a morphologic alteration of the testes and hypotrophic glands may be observed.[30,31]

Symptoms suggesting hyperprolactinemia are gynecomastia, erectile dysfunction, and loss of libido, with occasional galactorrhea seen in some males.[32]

In a large population of infertile males, the prevalence of prolactinoma was 35-fold higher than the prevalence in the general population.[33] Other causes of hyperprolactinemia include medical conditions such as renal failure, hypothyroidism, cirrhosis, systemic lupus erythematosus, and systemic sclerosis.

Frequently, the anamnesis should review the intake of drugs that produce elevated PRL levels, especially those that block the inhibitory effects of dopamine, such as antipsychotics and antidepressants showing serotoninergic activity.[34,35]

Stress and Other Causes

The induction of male reproductive dysfunction by acute and chronic conditions producing mental stress has been convincingly reported in the literature.[36,37] The HPG is controlled and influenced by the hypothalamic-pituitary-adrenal (HPA) axis, which is involved in the control of social behavior and reproduction.[38] Glucocorticosteroids have been shown to inhibit the release of GnRH into the pituitary portal system and in the hypothalamic median eminence.[39] The underlying mechanism of the impact of the HPA axis on GnRH activity is complex, and it is accepted that neuropeptides can directly and indirectly affect the HPG axis. The role of corticotropin-releasing hormone varies under physiological and stress conditions. When overproduced,

it may induce a decrease in gonadal secretion of steroid hormones. Additionally, long-term disease-induced elevation of pro-inflammatory cytokines that can negatively affect the HPA and HPG axis, and may lead to hypogonadism.[40]

Hemochromatosis. Hereditary haemochromatosis is a common genetic disorder (prevalence 1:200), characterized by an accumulation of iron that causes damage to multiple tissues.[41] As many as five types have been reported, all of which are related to mutations in the hepcidin–ferroportin axis. The most common is type 1, caused by mutations in the *HFE* gene, located on chromosome 6, with an autosomal recessive inheritance pattern. Depending on the type of mutation, signs range from laboratory abnormalities alone to multiple-organ disease in which liver damage, arthritis, cardiomyopathy, and endocrine abnormalities may develop. The clinical findings of tissue damage can include cirrhosis, pancreatic endocrine and exocrine insufficiency, polyarthritis, skin hyperpigmentation, hypogonadism, adrenal insufficiency, hypothyroidism, and heart failure.[42]

Sarcoidosis and tuberculosis. These granulomatous diseases are capable of compromising the hypothalamus and the pituitary gland, causing central hypogonadism.[43] Hypopituitarism can be the initial manifestation of neurosarcoidosis, which has an estimated prevalence of 1:100,000.[44] MRI shows sharp enhancement of the meninges with or without hypothalamic and pituitary abnormalities.[45]

Other tumors. They also arise in the hypothalamus and pituitary, including germinomas and lymphomas. Carcinomas can metastasize to the pituitary, primarily to the stalk.

Craniopharyngiomas and central system tumors thought to arise from squamous epithelial cells can be associated with acquired hypopituitarism. They are nonmalignant tumors involving the sellar and parasellar region. Although benign, they can infiltrate the hypothalamus area, the optic chiasm, and the local vascular structures. There are two different subtypes of craniopharyngiomas: adamantinomatous and papillary.[46] The differential diagnosis must be made by noting secondary metastasis, the infiltrative diseases mentioned previously, and cranial irradiation.

Empty sella syndrome (ESS). It is characterized by arachnoid herniation into the sellar fossa, which leads to flattening of the pituitary gland against the sellar floor.[47] Besides endocrine disturbances, patients with ESS may also have neuropsychiatric symptoms such as headache, dizziness, seizures, or schizophrenia. ESS was first described as a condition in which the sella is only partially filled by the pituitary gland. ESS is not considered to be an inherited condition; however, due to the advent of new methods of brain imaging and molecular genetics, this perspective on its origin may change in the future.

Although some patients remain asymptomatic, others (up to 20%–50%) may develop symptoms of hypopituitarism. An inferior displacement of the optic tracts with concomitant visual disturbance may be observed, as well as rhinorrhea and clinical signs of elevated intracranial pressure. Males may develop ESS secondary to pituitary surgery or radiotherapy[48,49] for adenomas or medical therapy for macroadenomas, spontaneous pituitary apoplexy, trauma, infection, or autoimmune disease.

Traumatic brain injury. Hypopituitarism is associated with traumatic brain injury, a common risk in patients under 35 years of age. The cause of posttraumatic hypopituitarism is believed to be infarction due to compression of the pituitary gland secondary to changes in the intracranial pressure as a consequence of cerebral edema, hemorrhage, or skull fracture.[50,51]

Partial Hypogonadism and Age-Related Conditions

Aging is associated with increased genetic and epigenetic abnormalities that may have repercussions for offspring. Changes in social behavior have tended to postpone the age at which males address fertility issues, thus delaying the possible diagnosis of health problems and potentially increasing the severity of infertility itself.

Aging is a consequence of a multiple intrinsic and extrinsic factors that are often difficult to unravel, but partial hypogonadism can be a contributory cause in some males. The mechanisms can be both pretesticular and testicular, first through the HPA and second due to a lower response of Leydig cells to gonadotropin stimulus.[52] In addition, a higher frequency of point mutations, presumably linked to sperm DNA strand breaks, genetic imprinting errors, and chromosomal anomalies, are responsible for age-associated reproductive failure in males.[53–55] In most retrospective studies, advanced paternal age was associated with poor embryo quality as well as a reduction in fertilization and implantation rates.[56,57]

Toxins and Lifestyle

A wide variety of risk factors, such as alcohol intake, may negatively influence sperm production.[58]

Obesity and Associated Conditions

Comorbidities such as metabolic disorders and cardiovascular disease are also associated with diminished spermatogenesis, highlighting the close relationship between male reproductive health and overall health.[59]

Metabolic syndrome explains a group of abnormalities, including obesity, dyslipidemia, hypertension, and insulin resistance, that are increasingly seen as contributory factors that impair normal testicular function.[60] Excessive adipose tissue might inhibit testicular function via insulin resistance.[61] The primary mechanism of hypogonadism in obesity plus subfertility might be due to the suppression of LH and FSH and the increased aromatization of testosterone to estradiol in the periphery. Inhibition of LH secretion via the HPA may also be affected by leptin resistance in patients with obesity-induced HH.[62,63] Weight reduction measures are associated with improvements in sperm quality and in fertility.[64]

MEDICAL TREATMENT OF HYPOGONADOTROPIC HYPOGONADISM

Briefly, purified hCG or recombinant chorionic gonadotropin (rhCG) acts as an LH analog, boosting testosterone production by Leydig cells. Human menopausal gonadotropin (hMG) is extracted from human urine and contains both FSH and LH. hMG is available as a urinary derivative, as highly purified FSH, as synthetic recombinant human FSH (rhFSH), and as corifollitropin alfa.[65]

Synthetic rhFSH has a short half-life, which means that it must be injected three times a week. Corifollitropin alfa is an FSH analog with a similar pharmacodynamic profile as rhFSH that has a longer half-life, so injections can be administered once a week.

Treatment regimens: usually hCG alone is started first, followed by semen analysis after 3 to 6 months of treatment. If no sperm is detected on semen analysis at that moment, FSH or hMG is added. Pretreatment with FSH for 4 months (so-called FSH priming) followed by pulsatile GnRH treatment for 2 years is one option. FSH priming induces gonadal maturation and Sertoli cell proliferation and doubles testicular volume.

Pretreatment with recombinant FSH (rFSH), followed by HCG/rFSH, also seems to be a promising strategy for inducing fertility.[66]

In some cases of HH, long-term testosterone treatment has led to setbacks in normal reproductive function. In the future, gene mutations may be identified that have diagnostic and prognostic value for selecting treatment options and predicting treatment response.[67]

Patients suffering from HH can achieve spermatogenesis when treated with gonadotropins or pulsatile administration of GnRH, but treatment courses often must be continued for long periods of time. The reason for prolonging treatment is that many males do not achieve normal sperm results after treatment, although fertility can be achieved even with low sperm numbers, either naturally or with the help of ICSI. However, treatment is expensive and, even if successful, achieving a second or third pregnancy requires new courses of treatment while the chances of success are reduced due to the aging of the couple. For these reasons, hypogonadal males undergoing gonadotropic treatment can benefit from sperm cryopreservation.

Predictors of a good response to gonadotropin therapy include postpubertal onset of gonadotropin deficiency, testicular volume >8 mL, and a record of having received previous courses of gonadotropic treatment. In contrast, underlying cryptorchidism, prepubertal onset of hypogonadism and low Tanner stage at the time of diagnosis can all reduce the chances of achieving full spermatogenesis.[68]

In the most unfavorable situation, some patients can remain azoospermic even after prolonged treatment. However, this does not mean that spermatogenesis is not occurring within the seminiferous tubules. As stated previously, primary testicular damage due to cryptorchidism can impair sperm production, but obstruction can also be present, especially if the treatment has substantially normalized testosterone concentrations and testicular volume. Therefore, testicular biopsy and surgical sperm retrieval is recommended before discontinuing gonadotropic treatment in males with HH who remain azoospermic after 2 years of stimulatory therapy.[69] The outcomes of ART using either fresh or cryopreserved sperm from patients with HH are equivalent to those using sperm from subjects with other nonobstructive causes of infertility.[70,71]

CLINICAL CASE SCENARIOS

CASE A

1) Scenario
A 40-year-old male presented with a 3-year history of infertility. He had no sexually transmitted diseases, history of surgery, genital trauma, or medication intake. His female partner was 37 years old, without previous pregnancies or abnormal gynecological findings.

Examination showed a male 185 cm in height, 92 kg in weight, with an athletic appearance, androgenetic baldness, normal bearing, mild bilateral gynecomastia, and acne on his shoulders. Examination of the external genitalia showed a normally developed penis, testis volume of 15 mL (right) and 12 mL (left) by a Prader orchidometer, and diminished consistency at palpation. Both the epididymis and vas deferens were present, with normal palpable aspect and without scrotal venous reflux.

2) Diagnosis
Investigations performed included a semen analysis, showing a volume of 3 mL, pH 7.5, and a very low sperm concentration, with only one sperm cell per every two high-power fields (corresponding to less than 200,000 sperm per mL), most of them immotile, and 15% displaying nonprogressive (grade c) motility. Citrate and fructose levels were normal. Serum TT was 5.6 nmol/L (normal range for the laboratory 8–27 nmol/L), LH <1.0 IU/L, and FSH <1.0 IU/L.

At a second visit, the patient was questioned again, and he admitted that he had been using anabolic steroids for 6 years with the goal of increasing muscle mass.

3) Management and Progression
The patient was treated for 6 months with clomiphene citrate 50 mg/day. Semen analysis 6 months later yielded the following results: 100,000 sperm/mL, 100% immotile, LH <0.1 IU/L, FSH 0.13 IU/L, testosterone 21.5 nmol/L. Treatment was switched to chorionic gonadotropin alfa 2100 UI twice/week. One year later, the semen analysis showed a volume of 3.5 mL, sperm count 20 million/mL,

motility 8% grade c, 29% grade b. The couple was scheduled to undergo an in vitro fertilization (IVF) cycle, but the wife spontaneously became pregnant while she was waiting for the treatment.

4) Considerations

Anabolic steroids can induce azoospermia or severe oligoasthenozoospermia. Overuse of androgens must be suspected in individuals with strongly developed musculature, normal to high testosterone levels, low or undetectable gonadotropin levels, and unexplained erythrocytosis. A physical examination can show a diminished testis consistency and/or volume. Self-administration of anabolic steroids can be denied by some of these males, and psychological dependence hinders successful rehabilitation. Androgen users often engage in polypharmacy,

taking other hormones and drugs of abuse. The recovery time can vary from months to almost 2 years, probably related to the doses administered and duration of use.

Treatment can start with clomiphene citrate, which can restore partially the pulsatility of hypothalamic feedback. Nevertheless, these patients frequently require treatment with hCG, which has a powerful effect on spermatogenesis. The need for a long recovery period requires patience from patients and from the clinician, and is rewarded by a high rate of success.

Furthermore, besides the consequences to fertility, there are multiple side effects associated with the use of anabolic steroids, including acne, alopecia, erectile dysfunction, and loss of libido. Moreover, cardiovascular side effects such as hypertension, arrhythmia, erythrocytosis, and ventricular dysfunctions have been reported.[25,72]

CASE B

1) Scenario

A 35-year-old male presents complaining of 2 years of infertility. He had experienced decreased libido but not erectile dysfunction. He was not taking any prescription medications. His 32-year-old wife had a normal gynecological examination. The semen analysis showed severe oligozoospermia (2 million sperm/mL, total count 4.5 million, progressive motility 3%). The couple was admitted to an ICSI program.

Physical Examination

The patient had normal male secondary sexual characteristics. His height was 180 cm and weight 78 kg. Development of the penis was normal, and both testes measured 25 mL with normal consistency, palpable vas deferens, and no venous reflux in the spermatic cords.

2) Progression

The second semen analysis results were similar to initial one. His blood hormone evaluation revealed an FSH level of 1.3 IU/L, LH level of 1.1 IU/L, testosterone level of 6.7 nmol/L, and PRL level of 90 ng/mL (reference value <20 ng/mL).

With a diagnosis of mild hyperprolactinemia, magnetic resonance image (MRI) of the hypothalamus and pituitary

with pre- and postgadolinium was performed. A nodular process with well-defined limits, 3 × 5 mm, was noted, with no compression of the surrounding structures.

He was treated with cabergoline 0.5 mg two times weekly. Three months later, PRL and testosterone levels had normalized, but the sperm count remained low. After 6 months of treatment the sperm count rose to 15 million /mL, 5% grade a, 10% grade b, and 1 year later, the patient reported his wife's spontaneous pregnancy. Treatment was maintained with 0.5 mg of cabergoline weekly, and a new MRI showed disappearance of the microadenoma.

3) Considerations

PRL-secreting microadenomas are a common cause of hyperprolactinemia. Lower PRL levels and tumor shrinkage are reported in most cases after treatment with a dopamine agonist.[73,74] High serum PRL levels adversely affect reproductive function in males. The patient was diagnosed based on clinical evaluation, which fortunately enabled the benign hypophyseal tumor to be managed with oral treatment, avoiding its continued growth and the consequent more difficult and aggressive neurosurgery that can be associated with persistent complications.

CASE C

1) Scenario

A 28-year-old male under treatment with testosterone undecanoate 1000 mg every 12 weeks was referred for infertility treatment. He reported HH and anosmia, bilateral cryptorchidism, and orchidopexy in his childhood. A simple cleft lip was treated with surgery in early life, and no relatives were affected by hypogonadism, anosmia, or delayed puberty.

The initial physical examination showed a weight of 93 kg, a height of 178 cm, complete secondary sexual characteristics, mild hypoplastic external genitalia, no penile malformations, intrascrotal testes with low volume (right 2–3 mL, left 1 mL), normal spermatic cords, and no inguinal hernias or adenopathy. No other abnormalities were observed in other organs and systems except for anosmia.

The genetic study was performed from blood DNA by PCR amplification of the coding exons and adjacent intronic regions of the *FGFR1* (*KAL2*) gene located at chromosomal region 8p11.2-p12. The patient was heterozygous for the rare variant c.1934C>T, resulting in an amino acid change (p. Ala645Val). This change affects a highly evolutionarily conserved residue and changes the physical-chemical characteristics of the protein.

2) Progression

After stopping androgen replacement therapy for 6 months, treatment with gonadotropins was initiated. During the first few months, increasing doses of hCG were administered and then supplemented with FSH (Fig. 2.2A). Testosterone concentrations increased to normal (Fig. 2.2B), the right testicular volume increased to 6–8 mL, and the left testicular volume increased to 3 mL (Prader orchidometer).

Spermatozoa appeared in the semen after 9 months of treatment, although the maximum concentration was only reached after 2 years of combined treatment and was always below 100,000 sperm/ejaculate (Fig. 2.2C). At 29 months, relative motility of more than 50% was achieved. The goal of achieving good spermatogenesis was hampered by a history of bilateral cryptorchidism, which is a limiting factor in the efficacy of gonadotropins (Fig. 2.2).

A cycle of IVF-ICSI was performed. The sperm sample on the day of oocyte retrieval had a concentration of 60,000 sperm/mL, and motility percentages of 0-39-24-37 (a-b-c-d). After sperm selection, 6000 progressively motile gametes were recovered, enough to perform ICSI, resulting in six zygotes with normal fertilization (2PN) and five good-quality embryos at day 3. Transfer of two embryos was followed by a successful singleton pregnancy and the birth of a healthy female who was not affected by the father's genetic mutation.

Preventive cryopreservation of one of the seminal samples was performed as a fertility reserve for the future. Once this treatment was finished, substitution with testosterone was reestablished.

3) Considerations

The patient was diagnosed with KS at 16 years of age due to delayed puberty, complete anosmia, simple cleft lip, bilateral cryptorchidism, moderately hypoplastic external genitalia without penile malformations, markedly hypoplastic testes, and no abnormalities in the vas deferens and spermatic cords. The diagnosis of KS relies on physical examination, hormonal determinations, and MRI. It is a male infertility condition that can be treated rationally and with efficacy that justifies the therapeutic effort. Early gonadotropin treatment could be more effective at restarting spermatogenesis; however, the safety and efficacy of the early procedure in young patients have not been evaluated.[75] After months of hormonal treatment, stimulation of spermatogenesis in this patient ultimately led to successful gestation.

When there is a female factor in conjunction with low sperm concentrations, it is possible to carry out ART with a good prognosis, even in patients who remain azoospermic.

Preimplantation genetic diagnosis (PGD) of embryos generated through IVF-ICSI is indicated in various situations that imply a chromosomal or genetic risk to the embryos. Monogenic diseases are an indication for performing PGD, especially when they appear early, seriously affect the lives of affected individuals, and have no effective curative treatment. The patient described in this case raised the possibility of performing PGD on the embryos to look for the known mutation of the *KAL2* gene; however, a review of the data collected by the European Consortium regarding all PGD cycles performed in Europe since this technique first came into use showed that there are no records for its use with KS. This makes sense, given that it is not a disease that usually compromises life, and it has a highly variable presentation, even in different subjects with the same genotype.

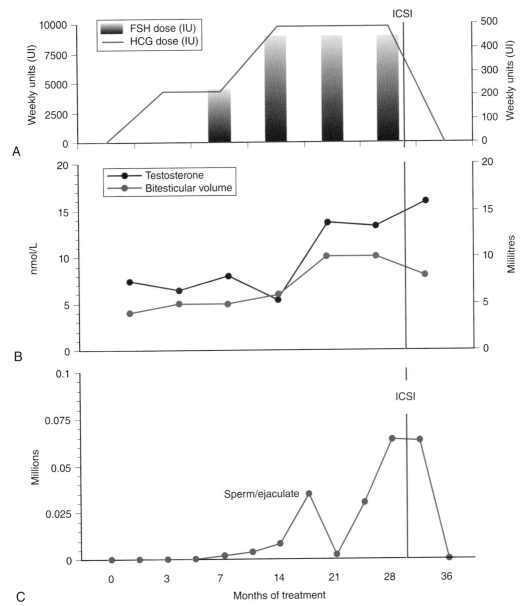

Fig. 2.2 Patient Progression During 29 Month-Period of Gonadotropic Treatment. (A) Weekly doses of human chorionic gonadotropin *(HCG; left axis, blue line)* and follicle-stimulating hormone *(FSH; right axis, red columns)* that were administered. (B) Changes in testosterone concentrations *(left axis, red line)* and bitesticular volume *(right axis, green line)*. (C) Total sperm per ejaculate during the course of treatment. *ICSI,* Intracytoplasmatic sperm injection.

SUMMARY

We have reviewed the more common entities associated with pretesticular male infertility that can be identified and successfully managed with a rational treatment. Some of the causes of HH are genetic in origin; therefore, andrologists should be aware of the clinical importance of the genetics of infertility to inform and give appropriate reproductive counseling to couples and warn of possible transmission of associated mutations to offspring.

The advent of ART has reinforced the idea that the male's contribution to fertility is to supply sperm to the couple. In this context, the female is considered the patient, and males are often not considered to be a possible cause of infertility.

Pretesticular causes of male infertility are good examples of why male diagnoses should be obtained without haste and before ART. This work-up can improve the chances of pregnancy as well as the quality of health for the males and the newborn.

Investigating comorbidities associated with impaired spermatogenesis through a comprehensive assessment, followed by a simple examination of genitalia and sexual characteristics, testicular size, and consistency, as well as systematic work-up by andrology-trained specialists, can significantly improve fertility potential. In some cases, deficiencies can be corrected, providing a less invasive and less costly treatment for infertility.[76] The gynecologist is the main point of contact for childless couples, and the gynecologist's task is to initiate parallel andrological examinations to obtain the earliest possible diagnosis and treatment. In addition, examining both members of the couple would result in a more accurate diagnosis and faster evaluation of treatment options.

REFERENCES

1. Ravitsky V, Kimmins S. The forgotten men: rising rates of male infertility urgently require new approaches for its prevention, diagnosis and treatment. *Biol Reprod.* 2019; 101(5)872-874.
2. Steptoe PC, Edwards RG. Birth after the reimplantation of a human embryo. *Lancet.* 1978;2(8085):366.
3. Palermo G, Joris H, Devroey P, Van Steirteghem AC. Pregnancies after intracytoplasmic injection of single spermatozoon into an oocyte. *Lancet.* 1992;340(8810): 17-18.
4. Schoysman R, Vanderzwalmen P, Nijs M, et al. Pregnancy after fertilisation with human testicular spermatozoa. *Lancet.* 1993;342(8881):1237.
5. Kumar N, Singh AK. Trends of male factor infertility, an important cause of infertility: a review of literature. *J Hum Reprod Sci.* 2015;8(4):191.
6. Practice Committee of the American Society for Reproductive Medicine. Diagnostic evaluation of the infertile male: a committee opinion. *Fertil Steril.* 2015;103(3):e18-e25.
7. Oduwole OO, Huhtaniemi IT, Misrahi M. The roles of luteinizing hormone, follicle-stimulating hormone and testosterone in spermatogenesis and folliculogenesis revisited. *Int J Mol Sci.* 2021;22(23):12735.
8. Oleari R, Massa V, Cariboni A, Lettieri A. The differential roles for neurodevelopmental and neuroendocrine genes in shaping GnRH neuron physiology and deficiency. *Int J Mol Sci.* 2021;22(17):9425.
9. Huhtaniemi I, Alevizaki M. Mutations along the hypothalamic–pituitary–gonadal axis affecting male reproduction. *Reprod Biomed Online.* 2007;15(6):622-632.
10. Fraietta R, Zylbersztejn DS, Esteves SC. Hypogonadotropic hypogonadism revisited. *Clinics.* 2013;68:81-88.
11. Russell N, Grossmann M. Mechanisms in endocrinology: estradiol as a male hormone. *Eur J Endocrinol.* 2019; 181(1):R23-R43.
12. Ruiz-Olvera SF, Rajmil O, Sanchez-Curbelo JR, Vinay J, Rodriguez-Espinosa J, Ruiz-Castane E. Association of serum testosterone levels and testicular volume in adult patients. *Andrologia.* 2018;50(3):e12933.
13. Hanson BM, Eisenberg ML, Hotaling JM. Male infertility: a biomarker of individual and familial cancer risk. *Fertil Steril.* 2018;109(1):6-19.
14. Vermeulen A, Verdonck L, Kaufman JM. A critical evaluation of simple methods for the estimation of free testosterone in serum. *J Clin Endocrinol Metab.* 1999;84(10): 3666-3672.
15. Besser GM, McNeilly AS, Anderson DC, et al. Hormonal responses to synthetic luteinizing hormone and follicle stimulating hormone-releasing hormone in man. *BMJ.* 1972;3:267-271.
16. Kirsch CFE. Imaging of sella and parasellar region. *Neuroimaging Clin N Am.* 2021;31(4):541-552.
17. Dodé C, Hardelin JP. Kallmann syndrome. *Eur J Hum Genet.* 2009;17:139-146.
18. Millar AC, Faghfoury H, Bieniek JM. Genetics of hypogonadotropic hypogonadism. *Transl Androl Urol.* 2021; 10(3):1401.
19. Young J, Xu C, Papadakis GE, et al. Clinical management of congenital hypogonadotropic hypogonadism. *Endocr Rev.* 2019;40(2):669-710.
20. Kim SH. Congenital hypogonadotropic hypogonadism and Kallmann syndrome: past, present, and future. *Endocrinol Metab (Seoul).* 2015;30(4):456-466.
21. Cangiano B, Swee DS, Quinton R, Bonomi M. Genetics of congenital hypogonadotropic hypogonadism: peculiarities and phenotype of an oligogenic disease. *Hum Genet.* 2021;140(1):77-111.
22. Dohle GR, Smit M, Weber RF. Androgens and male fertility. *World J Urol.* 2003;21(5):341-345.
23. El Osta R, Almont T, Diligent C, Hubert N, Eschwège P, Hubert J. Anabolic steroids abuse and male infertility. *Basic Clin Androl.* 2016;26:2. doi:10.1186/s12610-016-0029-4.
24. Schilling K, Toth B, Rösner S, Strowitzki T, Wischmann T. Prevalence of behaviour-related fertility disorders in a clinical sample: results of a pilot study. *Arch Gynecol Obstet.* 2012;286(5):1307-1314.

25. Horwitz H, Andersen JT, Dalhoff KP. Health consequences of androgenic anabolic steroid use. *J Intern Med.* 2019; 285:333-340.

26. Yates WR, Holman TL, Ellingrod VL, Scott SD. Testosterone suppression of the HPT axis. *J Investig Med.* 1997; 45(8):441-447.

27. MacIndoe JH, Perry PJ, Yates WR, Holman TL, Ellingrod VL, Scott SD. Testosterone suppression of the HPT axis. *J Investig Med.* 1997;45(8):441-447.

28. Karila T, Hovatta O, Seppälä T. Concomitant abuse of anabolic androgenic steroids and human chorionic gonadotrophin impairs spermatogenesis in power athletes. *Int J Sports Med.* 2004;25(4):257-263.

29. Salonia A, Rastrelli G, Hackett G, et al. Paediatric and adult-onset male hypogonadism. *Nat Rev Dis Primers.* 2019;5(1):38.

30. Biller BM, Luciano A, Crosignani PG, et al. Guidelines for the diagnosis and treatment of hyperprolactinemia. *J Reprod Med.* 1999;44(suppl 12):1075.

31. De Rosa M, Zarrilli S, Di Sarno A, et al. Hyperprolactinemia in men. *Endocrine.* 2003;20(1):75-82.

32. Singh P, Singh M, Cugati G, Singh AK. Hyperprolactinemia: an often missed cause of male infertility. *J Hum Reprod Sci.* 2011;4(2):102-103.

33. Ambulkar SS, Darves-Bornoz AL, Fantus RJ, et al. Prevalence of hyperprolactinemia and clinically apparent prolactinomas in men undergoing fertility evaluation. *Urology.* 2022;159:114-119.

34. Patel SS, Bamigboye V. Hyperprolactinaemia. *J Obstet Gynaecol.* 2007;27(5):455-459.

35. La Torre D, Falorni A. Pharmacological causes of hyperprolactinemia. *Ther Clin Risk Manag.* 2007;3(5):929.

36. Tian P, Lv P, Shi W, Zhu M, Cong B, Wen B. Chronic stress reduces spermatogenic cell proliferation in rat testis. *Int J Clin Exp Pathol.* 2019;12(5):1921-1931.

37. Lotti F, Maggi M. Sexual dysfunction and male infertility. *Nat Rev Urol.* 2018;15(5):287-307.

38. Gołyszny M, Obuchowicz E, Zieliński M. Neuropeptides as regulators of the hypothalamus-pituitary-gonadal (HPG) axis activity and their putative roles in stress-induced fertility disorders. *Neuropeptides.* 2022;91:102216. doi:10.1016/j.npep.2021.102216.

39. Calogero AE, Burrello N, Bosboom AMJ, et al. Glucocorticoids inhibit gonadotropin-releasing hormone by acting directly at the hypothalamic level. *J Endocrinol Invest.* 1999;22:666-670.

40. Parhar IS, Ogawa S, Ubuka T. Reproductive neuroendocrine pathways of social behavior. *Front Endocrinol (Lausanne).* 2016;7:28.

41. Angelopoulos NG, Goula A, Dimitriou F, Tolis G. Reversibility of hypogonadotropic hypogonadism in a patient with the juvenile form of hemochromatosis. *Fertil Steril.* 2005;84(6):1744. doi:10.1016/j.fertnstert.2005.05.070.

42. El Osta R, Grandpre N, Monnin N, et al. Hypogonadotropic hypogonadism in men with hereditary hemochromatosis. *Basic Clin Androl.* 2017;27:13.

43. Mageshkumar S, Patil DV, Philo AJ, Madhavan K. Hypopituitarism as unusual sequelae to central nervous system tuberculosis. *Indian J Endocrinol Metab.* 2011;15: 259-262.

44. Anthony J, Esper GJ, Ioachimescu A. Hypothalamic–pituitary sarcoidosis with vision loss and hypopituitarism: case series and literature review. *Pituitary.* 2016; 19:19-29.

45. Freda PU, Silverberg SJ, Post KD, Wardlaw SL. Hypothalamic-pituitary sarcoidosis. *Trends Endocrinol Metab.* 1992;3(9):321-325.

46. Gupta S, Bi WL, Giantini Larsen A, Al-Abdulmohsen S, Abedalthagafi M, Dunn IF. Craniopharyngioma: a roadmap for scientific translation. *Neurosurg Focus.* 2018; 44(6):E12.

47. De Marinis L, Bonadonna S, Bianchi A, Maira G, Giustina A. Primary empty sella. *J Clin Endocrinol Metab.* 2005;90(9):5471-5477.

48. Partoune E, Virzi M, Vander Veken L, Renard L, Maiter D. Occurrence of pituitary hormone deficits in relation to both pituitary and hypothalamic doses after radiotherapy for skull base meningioma. *Clin Endocrinol (Oxf).* 2021;95(3):460-468.

49. Kyriakakis N, Lynch J, Orme SM, et al. Pituitary dysfunction following cranial radiotherapy for adult-onset non-pituitary brain tumours. *Clin Endocrinol (Oxf).* 2016; 84(3):372-379.

50. Kelly DF, Gonzalo ITG, Cohan P, Berman N, Swerdloff R, Wang C. Hypopituitarism following traumatic brain injury and aneurysmal subarachnoid hemorrhage: a preliminary report. *J Neurosurg.* 2000;93(5):743-752.

51. Bondanelli M, Ambrosio MR, Zatelli MC, De Marinis L, degli Uberti EC. Hypopituitarism after traumatic brain injury. *Eur J Endocrinol.* 2005;152(5):679-691.

52. Camacho EM, Huhtaniemi IT, O'Neill TW, et al. Age-associated changes in hypothalamic–pituitary–testicular function in middle-aged and older men are modified by weight change and lifestyle factors: longitudinal results from the European Male Ageing Study. *Eur J Endocrinol.* 2013;168(3):445-455.

53. Sartorius GA, Nieschlag E. Paternal age and reproduction. *Hum Reprod Update.* 2010;16(1):65-79.

54. Robinson L, Gallos ID, Conner SJ, et al. The effect of sperm DNA fragmentation on miscarriage rates: a systematic review and meta-analysis. *Hum Reprod.* 2012; 27(10):2908-2917.

55. Kobayashi N, Miyauchi N, Tatsuta N, et al. Factors associated with aberrant imprint methylation and oligozoospermia. *Sci Rep.* 2017;7(1):1-9.

56. Frattarelli JL, Miller KA, Miller BT, Elkind-Hirsch K, Scott Jr RT. Male age negatively impacts embryo development and reproductive outcome in donor oocyte assisted reproductive technology cycles. *Fertil Steril.* 2008;90(1):97-103.

57. Luna M, Finkler E, Barritt J, et al. Paternal age and assisted reproductive technology outcome in ovum recipients. *Fertil Steril.* 2009;92(5):1772-1775.

58. Durairajanayagam D. Lifestyle causes of male infertility. *Arab J Urol.* 2018;16(1):10-20.

59. Bungum AB, Glazer CH, Bonde JP, Nilsson PM, Giwercman A, Søgaard Tøttenborg S. Risk of metabolic disorders in childless men: a population-based cohort study. *BMJ Open.* 2018;8(8):e020293.

60. Sermondade N, Faure C, Fezeu L, et al. BMI in relation to sperm count: an updated systematic review and collaborative meta-analysis. *Hum Reprod Update.* 2013; 19(3):221-231.

61. Teerds KJ, de Rooij DG, Keijer J. Functional relationship between obesity and male reproduction: from humans to animal models. 2011. *Hum Reprod Update.* 2011;17:667-683.

62. Liu Y, Ding Z. Obesity, a serious etiologic factor for male subfertility in modern society. *Reproduction.* 2017;154:R123-R131.

63. Hofstra J, Loves S, van Wageningen B, Ruinemans-Koerts J, Jansen I, de Boer H. High prevalence of hypogonadotropic hypogonadism in men referred for obesity treatment. *Neth J Med.* 2008;66:103-109.

64. Faure C, Dupont C, Baraibar MA, et al. In subfertile couple, abdominal fat loss in men is associated with improvement of sperm quality and pregnancy: a case-series. *PLoS One.* 2014;9(2):e86300.

65. Nieschlag E, Bouloux PG, Stegmann BJ, et al. An open-label clinical trial to investigate the efficacy and safety of corifollitropin alfa combined with hCG in adult men with hypogonadotropic hypogonadism. *Reprod Biol Endocrinol.* 2017;15(1):17.

66. Pitteloud N, Dwyer A. Hormonal control of spermatogenesis in men: therapeutic aspects in hypogonadotropic hypogonadism. *Ann Endocrinol (Paris).* 2014;75(2):98-100.

67. Raivio T, Falardeau J, Dwyer A, et al. Reversal of idiopathic hypogonadotropic hypogonadism. *N Engl J Med.* 2007;357(9):863-873.

68. Warne DW, Decosterd G, Okada H, Yano Y, Koide N, Howles CM. A combined analysis of data to identify predictive factors for spermatogenesis in men with hypogonadotropic hypogonadism treated with recombinant human follicle-stimulating hormone and human chorionic gonadotropin. *Fertil Steril.* 2009;92(2):594-604.

69. Meseguer M, Garrido N, Remohí J, Pellicer A, Gil-Salom M. Testicular sperm extraction (TESE) and intracytoplasmic sperm injection (ICSI) in hypogonadotropic hypogonadism with persistent azoospermia after hormonal therapy. *J Assist Reprod Genet.* 2004;21(3):91-94.

70. Karacan M, Alwaeely F, Erkan S, et al. Outcome of intracytoplasmic sperm injection cycles with fresh testicular spermatozoa obtained on the day of or the day before oocyte collection and with cryopreserved testicular sperm in patients with azoospermia. *Fertil Steril.* 2013;100(4):975-980.

71. Gao Y, Yu B, Mao J, Wang X, Nie M, Wu X. Assisted reproductive techniques with congenital hypogonadotropic hypogonadism patients: a systematic review and meta-analysis. *BMC Endocr Disord.* 2018;18(1):85.

72. Kolettis PN, Purcell ML, Parker W, Poston T, Nangia AK. Medical testosterone: an iatrogenic cause of male infertility and a growing problem. *Urology.* 2015;85(5):1068-1073.

73. Verhelst J, Abs R, Maiter D, et al. Cabergoline in the treatment of hyperprolactinemia: a study in 455 patients. *J Clin Endocrinol Metab.* 1999;84(7):2518-2522.

74. Chanson P, Maiter D. The epidemiology, diagnosis and treatment of prolactinomas: the old and the new. *Best Pract Res Clin Endocrinol Metab.* 2019;33(2):101290.

75. Gong C, Liu Y, Qin M, Wu D, Wang X. Pulsatile GnRH is superior to hCG in therapeutic efficacy in adolescent boys with hypogonadotropic hypogonadodism. *J Clin Endocrinol Metab.* 2015;100(7):2793-2799.

76. Eisenberg ML, Li S, Behr B, et al. Semen quality, infertility, and mortality in the USA. *Hum Reprod.* 2014;29:1567-1574.

3

Testicular Causes of Male Infertility

Raghavender Kosgi and Vineet Malhotra

KEY POINTS

- Testicular disorders are one of the most common causes of male infertility. These can be primary or secondary.
- Cryptorchidism should be diagnosed early, and orchiopexy is advised between 6 months and 18 months for better fertility preservation.
- Klinefelter syndrome is the most common genetic cause of male infertility.
- Genetic counseling is mandatory for individuals with genetic abnormalities.

- Varicocele is the most common correctable cause of male infertility.
- Basic semen analysis, hormone profile, karyotyping, and Yq microdeletion analysis are needed for the evaluation of nonobstructive azoospermia.
- Microtesticular sperm extraction gives the best possible sperm retrieval rates in patients with nonobstructive azoospermia with small testes.

INTRODUCTION

Across the globe, for various reasons, many couples are facing infertility problems. Males are significantly contributing to infertility, either alone or in combination with female factors. Proper evaluation and timely management of treatable causes of male infertility and in time referral to female reproductive specialists for untreatable causes will enhance the heterosexual couple's chances of natural conception or assisted reproductive technique (ART) outcomes. Causes of male infertility are broadly classified into pretesticular, testicular, and posttesticular. Testicular diseases are the most common cause of male infertility, accounting for 49% to 93% of males with azoospermia.[1] This chapter gives an overview of various testicular causes and their management. It also highlights the importance of practical clinical case scenarios to help the clinicians in day-to-day practice.

Testicular causes of male infertility may be primarily related to testicular disorders or secondary effects of other disorders (Table 3.1).

CONGENITAL CAUSES OF MALE INFERTILITY

Cryptorchidism

Cryptorchidism is a condition in which a testis may be arrested somewhere along the descent pathway. It is the most common congenital abnormality of male external genitalia.[2] Approximately 1% of male infants suffer from cryptorchidism by the age of 1 year. Based on its location, an undescended testis (UDT) can be categorized as intraabdominal, inguinal, and ectopic. Undescended testis can be unilateral or bilateral. It is an important risk factor for infertility and testicular tumors. Bilateral UDTs have a more severe impact on fertility than the unilateral. Patients with unilateral UDTs may have a lower fertility rate, but they have a paternity rate like the normal population. Unfortunately, many males either are not aware of this condition since birth or conceal the disease condition before marriage and face difficulties after marriage, especially those with bilateral UDTs with small gonads, leading to unnecessary relationship

TABLE 3.1   Testicular Causes of Male Infertility

Primary Testicular Causes	Secondary Testicular Causes
1. **Congenital:** Anorchia Cryptorchidism Disorders of sexual differentiation Vanishing testes syndrome 2. **Genetic:** Klinefelter syndrome Y chromosome microdeletions XX male XYY male Translocations/ inversions 3. **Infective:** Bacterial orchitis Viral orchitis 4. **Disorders of spermatogenesis** Spermatogenic arrest Germ cell aplasia (Sertoli cell–only syndrome) Structural defects of sperm: a. Globozoospermia b. Immotile cilia syndrome 5. **Testicular tumors** 6. **Testicular trauma** 7. **Testicular microcalcifications**	1. **Secondary testicular failure** 2. **Varicocele** 3. **Gonadotoxins:** a. Chemotherapy b. Radiotherapy c. Drugs 4. **Systemic causes:** a. Chronic renal failure b. Chronic liver failure c. Obesity 5. **Idiopathic**

distress at personal, marital, and family levels. In our clinical practice, we see many patients with UDTs not operated on during childhood between 6 months to 18 months, even with advancement of medical care and guidance in the current era.

Pathophysiology

During pregnancy, gonads develop intraabdominally in the retroperitoneum of the fetus and descend to an extraabdominal, intrascrotal position for optimal function. Testicular descent occurs in two phases, namely the transabdominal phase and the inguinoscrotal phase, under the influence of hormones and growth processes. Disruption of the hormonal pathways due to various environmental and genetic factors leads to testicular maldescent. The unfavorable environment of a cryptorchid testis impairs fetal gonocyte differentiation and apoptosis of undifferentiated gonocytes. Mutations in the insulin-like growth factor 3 (*INSL3*) and leucine-rich repeat containing G protein-coupled receptor 8 (*LGR8*) genes are associated with cryptorchid testis. UDT is associated with degeneration of germ cells, with subsequent spermatogenic dysfunction leading to subfertility.[3]

GENETIC CAUSES

Genetic causes of male infertility are transmissible to the next generation. There has been a growing interest in the research of a genetic basis of male infertility in the past two decades. A majority of times, an unidentifiable cause of male infertility is a frustrating situation for the patient as well as the treating physician. Identifying an etiological agent helps in better prognostication and counseling of the patient.

There is increased concern over transmitting genetic abnormalities to offspring due to widespread use of intracytoplasmic sperm injection (ICSI) for fertilization, as it bypasses the process of natural selection of healthy sperm. Now it is important to identify genetic etiology to avoid unwanted birth defects. Genetic causes are grossly divided into chromosomal numerical or structural aberrations, specific gene mutations, and Y-chromosome microdeletions.[4,5]

Klinefelter Syndrome

Klinefelter syndrome is the most common chromosomal disorder, which accounts for two-thirds of karyotypic abnormalities in males with infertility.[6] It is characterized as a classical form with 47,XXY (an extra X chromosome) or mosaic form with 46,XY/47,XXY. Incidence of this syndrome is 1 in 660 males, but it will contribute to up to 3.1% of the infertile male population and 10% of nonobstructive azoospermia (NOA) patients.[7,8] Most males with Klinefelter syndrome may present with small, firm testes with elevated follicle-stimulating hormone (FSH), luteinizing hormone (LH), estradiol, and low or low-normal testosterone. Classical phenotypic features of tall, eunuchoid body habitus with gynecomastia may not be present in many patients. A high index of clinical suspicion is needed to order karyotyping testing.

XX Male Syndrome

This rare syndrome occurs in 1 in 10,000 to 20,000 of newborns.[9] In the majority, this syndrome is caused by sex-determining region of the Y chromosome (SRY) translocation to the X chromosome. Clinical features of these males are similar to Klinefelter males (small, firm testes; hypogonadism; and azoospermia). As azoospermia in these patients is due to complete absence of azoospermia factor (AZF) genes, there is no possibility of sperm retrieval.[4]

47,XYY Syndrome

This is a syndrome of an extra Y chromosome. These patients may present with macrocephaly, macroorchidism, and hypotonia. In general, these patients are fertile, but some patients may have sperm aneuploidy.[10]

Translocations and Inversions

These are autosomal structural karyotypic abnormalities. Chromosomal rearrangements and crossover may happen in some individuals. Robertsonian translocations, reciprocal translocations, paracentric inversions, and marker chromosomes are the most common autosomal structural abnormalities. These are associated with increased risk of aneuploidy.

Patients with Robertsonian translocations may have 45 chromosomes. This is one of the most common structural autosomal abnormalities. Patients with these abnormalities may require preimplantation genetic diagnosis or amniocentesis to prevent genetic aberrations in future offspring.

Y-Chromosome Microdeletions

The Y chromosome is the smallest human chromosome and consists of a long arm (q) and a short arm (p). The SRY gene of short arm is responsible for male differentiation. The long arm consists of genes responsible for spermatogenesis. Microdeletions of the long arm of the Y chromosome are responsible for many cases of NOA. Y chromosome deletions are too small to be detected on routine karyotyping, and hence are called microdeletions.[11] Three areas are identified, namely AZFa, AZFb, and AZFc. Males with complete deletion of AZFa, AZFb, AZFb/c, and AZFabc will be azoospermic, and the chance

of getting sperm with sperm retrieval procedures (microsurgical testicular sperm extraction [micro-TESE]/ testicular mapping) is almost negligible. These patients show poor sperm retrieval prognostic histopathology patterns like Sertoli cell–only syndrome or maturation arrest.[12] Partial deletions of these AZF regions are also reported to negatively affect spermatogenesis.

Gene Mutations

About 2000 genes on autosomes are involved in spermatogenesis.[13] Polymorphisms and mutations of these genes are involved in the majority of the cases of idiopathic male infertility. Point mutations in the androgen receptor gene are associated with spermatogenic failure. The androgen receptor gene is situated on the long arm of the X chromosome.[14] Complete androgen insensitivity or testicular feminization syndrome may result from severe mutations of androgen receptor gene. It is characterized by a 46,XY karyotype and female phenotype with cryptorchid testes. Moderate mutations may lead to partial androgen insensitivity (Reifenstein syndrome), which manifests in the form of ambiguous external genitalia and lack of virilization. Milder forms of mutations may lead to infertility, gynecomastia, and lack of virilization.

INFECTIVE CAUSES

Orchitis

Orchitis is an inflammatory lesion of the testes, which is associated with exudates of leukocytes inside and outside of the seminiferous tubules, causing tubular damage. It can cause intratesticular obstruction in about 15% of cases of azoospermia due to obstructive causes.[15] Genital infections are potentially curable causes of male infertility. They may be caused by various bacteria, viruses, fungi, and protozoa. Infective etiology is more common in underdeveloped and developing countries. It may be acute in onset or chronic in nature. The majority of genital infections are asymptomatic. As per the World Health Organization (WHO), urethritis, prostatitis, orchitis, and epididymitis are considered as male accessory gland infections (MAGIs).[16] Most of the time, orchitis is associated with an epididymitis due to retrograde ascending infections of close proximity structures. The prevalence of isolated orchitis is very rare (0.42%), as found in a large study.[17]

There is contradictory evidence regarding the deleterious effects of symptomatic or asymptomatic infections on semen parameters.[18] Infections may cause spermatogenic dysfunction due to direct damage to the testis, oxidative stress, and high DNA fragmentation. Infections may affect sperm development, maturation, and transportation. Sexually transmitted infection due to *Chlamydia trachomatis* and *Neisseria gonorrhoeae* are responsible for acute infections in younger males less than 35 years of age, and *Escherichia coli* is the causative agent in older males.[19] The mumps virus may cause orchitis in 20% to 30% of patients due to hematogenous spread, and 13% unilateral and 30% to 87% bilateral orchitis patients may suffer from infertility.

Genital tuberculosis may cause granulomatous orchitis. It is more common in low socioeconomic groups, immunocompromised patients, and countries with high prevalence of tuberculosis. It may cause obstruction of excurrent duct system leading to obstructive azoospermia. As a delayed complication, testicular atrophy may occur. In the Indian subcontinent, we encounter many patients with clinical features suspicious for genital tuberculosis (beaded vas, craggy epididymis, and thick spermatic cord), but it is difficult to prove diagnostically due to high false-negative rates of available tests.

DISORDERS OF SPERMATOGENESIS

The process of production of spermatozoa is called spermatogenesis. Complete spermatogenesis requires 72 to 74 days, with an optimum temperature of 34°C. Disruptions of spermatogenesis may lead to oligoasthenoteratozoospermia. These disorders are evaluated by testicular biopsy.

Germ Cell Aplasia (Sertoli Cell–Only Syndrome)

Sertoli cells reside along the seminiferous tubules and support various stages of germ cell development. They contain FSH receptors, which help in binding of FSH, and produce activin and inhibin hormones, which are regulators of the hypothalamic-pituitary-gonadal (HPG) axis. Histologically, it is characterized by complete absence of the germ cells, and only Sertoli cells are present.

Structural Sperm Defects
Globozoospermia

It is an autosomal recessive disorder characterized by round-headed sperm due to absence of acrosome, with inability to fertilize oocytes. ICSI is the only option for these patients when it has low success rates due to lack of acrosomal enzymes necessary for activation of oocytes and high incidence of sperm aneuploidy.[20]

Primary Ciliary Dyskinesia

It is also known as immotile cilia syndrome. Almost 50% of the cases of primary ciliary dyskinesia are due to Kartagener syndrome, characterized by immotile sperm, chronic sinusitis, bronchiectasis, and situs inversus.[21] Sperm motility disorder is due to sperm tail cytoskeleton defects, like absence of dynein arms, radial spokes, or the central doublet. Light microscopy only shows asthenozoospermia. It is only identified by electron microscopy. ICSI is successful for these patients.

TESTICULAR TUMORS

Testicular germ cell tumors (TGCTs) are the most common malignancy in western White males aged 15 to 40 years, and affecting approximately 1% of infertile males.[22] Patients having TGCT may have decreased semen parameters before starting cancer therapy. Azoospermia has been noted in 5% to 8% of males with TGCTs,[23] and oligospermia in 50%.[24] Patients with TGCT also suffer from Leydig cell dysfunction, even in the opposite testis, in addition to the spermatogenic dysfunction.[25] The risk of hypogonadism is higher in males treated for TGCT. It is better to measure pretreatment baseline serum levels of testosterone, sex hormone–binding globulin, LH, and estradiol to identify patients at increased risk of hypogonadism.

TRAUMA TO THE TESTIS

Direct trauma to the testis may cause loss of testicular volume and obstruction due to scarring. Indirect damage to the testis may be because of infection or inflammatory conditions of the testis. Trauma breaches the blood testicular barrier and may cause formation of antisperm antibodies (ASAs).

TORSION OF THE TESTIS

Testicular torsion is more common in adolescents and younger males. It is more common than testicular tumors. About half of the males who had a previous history of torsion may suffer from spermatogenic defects. As it disrupts the testicular architecture and blood–testis barrier, 11% of males develop ASAs after testicular torsion.

TESTICULAR MICROCALCIFICATIONS

Testicular microcalcifications (TMs) have been found on scrotal ultrasound with greater prevalence in patients with testicular tumors, UDTs, infertility, torsion and atrophy of testis, Klinefelter syndrome, hypogonadism, and varicocele.[26] TMs in infertile males have an 18 times higher prevalence of testicular cancer as indicated by recent systematic review and metaanalysis of case-control studies.[27] The premalignant nature of TM is controversial; however, it is better to counsel the patients and keep high-risk patients (infertility, UDTs, bilateral testicular microcalcifications) under regular testicular self-examination and annual follow-up with scrotal sonography. Routine testicular biopsy is not indicated to identify germ cell neoplasia in situ due to its very low incidence.

CELL PHONE RADIATION

With the advent of the communication revolution in the current digital world, human beings are excessively dependent on smartphones. Commonly, cell phones are kept in the pockets of pants, near the gonads, which may cause higher radiation exposure. Experimental evidence suggests that radiofrequency electromagnetic waves produced by mobile phones reduce the activity of superoxide dismutase 1 and increase the malondialdehyde levels.[28]

HEAT EXPOSURE

A lower temperature is necessary for optimal spermatogenesis. Various scrotal adaptations are there to maintain lower temperatures in the scrotum. Scrotal temperature is 1 to 2°C cooler than the core body temperature (37°C). Countercurrent heat exchange reduces the testicular inflow temperature. The corrugated scrotal skin surface dissipates heat to cool the testes. Animal studies have clearly proven that exposure to heat causes spermatogenic dysfunction.[29] Varicocele, cryptorchidism, lifestyle changes, and occupations like driving, cooking, furnace operation, and welding may cause scrotal hyperthermia, which leads to poor sperm parameters.[30] Hot baths, sauna use, excessive exercise, and tight underclothing may raise scrotal temperatures.

SECONDARY TESTICULAR CAUSES OF MALE INFERTILITY

Varicocele

Varicocele is an abnormal dilatation of the pampiniform plexus of veins, with reflux of blood. It is one of the most common correctable causes of male infertility. It is a progressive condition, with possible spermatogenic dysfunction present in 35% to 40% of infertile males.[31,32] However, 15% of the normal population may be seen with varicocele without fertility problems. Varicoceles disrupt the countercurrent heat exchange mechanism in the scrotum, which leads to scrotal hyperthermia, oxidative stress, and a raised DNA fragmentation index. Reflux of blood causes venous hypertension, hypoxia, and renal and adrenal exposure to toxins. Varicocele is associated with abnormal semen parameters and reduction of the testicular volume and may cause chronic orchialgia in some patients. Clinically palpable varicoceles impair the sperm parameters significantly. Larger varicoceles have a more significant impact on spermatogenesis. Subclinical varicoceles (diagnosed only by scrotal Doppler but not clinically palpable) may not have much impact on spermatogenesis. The majority of varicoceles are left-sided due to a long gonadal vein and the right-angle entry of the gonadal vein into the left renal vein.

Gonadotoxins

Drugs

Various drugs are implicated in testicular dysfunction. Side effects of these drugs may range from impaired spermatogenesis to antiandrogenic effects and sexual dysfunction.

Recreational drugs are detrimental to male fertility and sexual function. Marijuana decreases spermatogenesis.[33] Alkylating agents like cyclophosphamide and immunosuppressive drugs are toxic to the testes. Sperm cryopreservation is recommended before initiating chemotherapy. Contraception is advised during the course of treatment to avoid unwanted teratogenic effects on the progeny.

Radiotherapy

Radiation exposure has become inevitable for patients as well as for healthcare staff in our clinical practice. Radiological imaging and radiotherapy are the sources of radiation. Human testes are sensitive to radiation-induced damage. This damage may be dependent on the dose and duration of exposure to radiation. Exposure of the testes to ionizing radiation causes germ cell damage and Leydig cell dysfunction. Pelvic irradiation for various cancers has maximal toxic effects on the gonads. Proper gonadal shielding and limiting the collateral damage with accurate radiotherapy to the target is needed with image guidance.

MANAGEMENT OF TESTICULAR CAUSES OF MALE INFERTILITY

Basic Clinical Evaluation of the Infertile Male

Basic evaluation of the infertile male should include a thorough medical and reproductive history, focused physical examination, and two semen analyses separated by at least 1 month. However, as infertility is a couples issue, both partners should be evaluated simultaneously to avoid wasting biological time. It is an opportunity to address the problems at the earliest.

History

Medical history and the physical examination are the aspects of utmost importance in the male infertility evaluation, which gives clinical clues and helps the treating clinician for diagnosis and guides for further testing. A complete history must be taken, covering all the factors that may impact the fertility potential of an individual.

Developmental History

Inquire about the congenital anomalies of the urogenital system. These anomalies may have an impact on future reproductive potential. Prune belly syndrome and bladder exstrophy are associated with cryptorchidism. Bilateral cryptorchidism has a more profound fertility impact than unilateral.

Sexual History

Sexual history should focus on a heterosexual couple's current attempts at conception, duration of sexual relationship without contraception, coital frequency, timing of intercourse around ovulation, and use of any lubricants.

Arousal, libido, erection, and ejaculation problems should be noted. Patients with sexual dysfunction and/or symptoms and signs of hypogonadism may require hormonal evaluation. Semen volume should be checked, as hypogonadism patients may have less volume due to reduced accessory gland function.

Past Medical History

Male genital tract infections such as epididymoorchitis, seminal vesiculitis, prostatitis, urethritis, and tuberculosis can cause scarring in the genital tract, decrease sperm quality, and increase oxidative stress and DNA fragmentation. History of exposure to gonadotoxins such as chemotherapy, radiotherapy, and systemic diseases like obesity, chronic renal disease, and chronic liver disease should also be noted. Genital trauma history should be noted, as it may cause ASAs, obstructions of the reproductive tract, and atrophy of the testicles.

Past Surgical History

Surgeries performed in the past, especially orchiopexy for UDTs, inguinal hernia repair, hydrocele repair, varicocele fixation, and orchidectomy for testicular tumors/pyocele/torsion should be documented. Inguinal and scrotal surgeries may cause iatrogenic damage to the testicular vessels, vas deferens, and epididymis.

Personal and Social History

Chronic alcoholism, excessive smoking, recreational drug abuse, and occupational exposure to gonadotoxins and heat should be inquired.

Family History

A family history of birth defects, miscarriages, genetic anomalies, and infertility problems should also be inquired (see sexual history section). It may give a clinical clue to a genetic etiology.

Physical Examination

The examination should be done in a quiet, comfortable, and warm room, with adequate privacy.

In the general physical examination, secondary sexual characteristics (hair distribution, gynecomastia, body habitus) and possible thyroid enlargement should be noted.

Genital Examination

The size of the penis, location of urethral meatus, any active urethral discharge, and scrotal sac development should be noted. Epididymal size, consistency, and spermatic cord thickness should be noted. The examination is done in the standing and supine positions to rule out the presence of varicocele. Varicocele is a clinical diagnosis. Dubin and Amelar clinical grading is widely adopted in clinical practice:[34] Grade I:

palpable on Valsalva, grade II: palpable without Valsalva, grade III: visible varicocele.

The vas deferens is palpated as a firm, round, distinct cordlike structure that slips between the examiner's fingers in the posterior aspect of spermatic cord.

Examination can reveal location, size, and consistency of both the testes. Testicular volume is measured by a Prader orchidometer or by using a pachymeter or a caliper. The normal adult testis is about 18 to 20 mL in volume, with firm consistency. Eighty-five percent of testicular volume is made up of seminiferous tubules involved in spermatogenesis. Patients with soft and low-volume testes may suffer from spermatogenic dysfunction; however, it may not rule out presence of sperms on sperm retrieval.

In patients with primary testicular failure like Klinefelter syndrome, the testes will be small. Large testicular tumors are palpable as hard, irregular masses. In patients with acute epididymoorchitis, the epididymis and testis will be tender to touch. In chronic epididymoorchitis, the epididymis and testes are irregular, firm to hard, and mildly tender. The inguinal and genital areas should be inspected for scars from previous surgeries like herniorrhaphy, hydrocele repair, and orchidopexy. They may cause damage to the testicular blood supply, vasal damage, or blockage due to fibrotic reaction of Prolene hernia mesh. Clinical examination should also include palpation of the spermatic cord and a digital rectal examination.

Semen Analysis

The semen analysis is an important basic laboratory evaluation, although it may not give information on functional aspects of sperm. This simple, noninvasive test gives information on the functional status of the male accessory glands like the seminal vesicles and prostate, presence or absence of sperm, and patency of the male reproductive tract. This test should be performed by well-trained lab personnel in a standard andrology lab with rigorous quality control measures, following WHO manual 5th or 6th edition guidelines.[35] In our clinical practice, we commonly encounter substandard reports, causing unnecessary apprehension to the patient. At least two semen analyses must be ordered one month apart due to wide biological variation in individuals. Klinefelter patients may present with azoospermia or severe oligozoospermia. Globozoospermia is identified by the absence of acrosome, showing round-headed sperm on morphological assessment.

Leukocytospermia Testing

More than five round cells per high-power field on basic semen analysis is an indication for leukocytospermia testing to differentiate leucocytes from immature germ cells or excessive residual cytoplasm. Endtz test (peroxidase staining test) is used to identify polymorphonuclear leukocytes that contain granules. Leukocytes greater than 1 million/mL (1×10^6) of semen is considered significant.

Semen Culture

Semen culture is indicated in patients with leukocytospermia and clinical features suggestive of MAGIs (thick, tender vas deferens and/or spermatic cord; enlarged/tender epididymis, testis, and/or prostate).

Antisperm Antibody Testing

ASA tests are indicated in patients with testicular trauma, genital infections, cryoptorchidism, testes biopsy, and torsion of the testes, and in vasectomized patients. Impaired motility and excessive sperm agglutination on semen analysis and abnormal postcoital tests are clues for ASA testing. Increased ASAs can impair sperm motility and affect sperm–oocyte interactions, leading to reduced fertilization rates. The immunobead test is commonly used to detect IgA and IgG ASAs.

Endocrine Evaluation

The HPG axis plays an important role in spermatogenesis. Dysfunction of HPG leads to hormonal dysregulation and may cause infertility. In patients with a sperm count of less than 10 million, erectile dysfunction, clinical features suggestive of endocrinopathy, and symptoms and signs of hypogonadism, an endocrine work-up is necessary. Basic hormone evaluation includes early morning fasting FSH and total testosterone levels. If testosterone is low, it should be confirmed with repeat testing, along with LH and prolactin measurement.

High FSH, LH, and low or low-normal testosterone levels are noted in primary testicular failure due to various causes (e.g., Klinefelter syndrome). Most of the patients with Klinefelter syndrome may have a reduced testosterone-to-estradiol ratio.[36] Isolated elevation of FSH may indicate severe spermatogenic dysfunction. A normal hormonal profile in patients with normal-sized gonads may indicate obstructive azoospermia; however, in patients with maturation arrest, FSH levels and gonadal size may be normal. In obese patients and in patients with gynecomastia (e.g., Klinefelter syndrome) serum estradiol should be measured.

Infertile males with a reduced testosterone-to-estradiol ratio (<10) may have significant but reversible seminal abnormalities.[35] Hyperestrogenism due to higher conversion of testosterone to estradiol in Klinefelter patients causes negative feedback and reduces testosterone synthesis. In these patients, overexpression of aromatase CYP19 in the testes is noted at molecular level.[37]

Genetic Evaluation

Patients with azoospermia, especially suspected NOA, severe oligoasthenoteratozoospermia (OAT) of less than 5 million sperm count (especially <1 million sperm count), clinical features, and/or family history suggestive of genetic etiology may require genetic evaluation. The genetic tests most often performed initially are karyotyping and Y chromosome microdeletion analysis. However, many unknown genetic causes may not be identified by these tests.

Y chromosome microdeletion testing gives information on the genetic basis of the male infertility, and the type of microdeletion gives clues for chance of successful sperm retrieval. Only a male child will inherit these microdeletions, as they are passed on via the Y chromosome. After a positive genetic report, some patients may consider other options like donor sperm or adoption, as they do not want to transmit genetic anomalies to their offspring.

Imaging
Scrotal Ultrasound

It is a simple, noninvasive, and economic test that adds additional information about testes, epididymis, vas, spermatic cord, and vascular pathology. Scrotal ultrasound is useful in (1) measuring the testicular volume, (2) identifying scrotal content masses (e.g., testicular tumors), (3) identifying testicular parenchymal non-homogeneous architecture (microcalcifications), and (4) detecting indirect signs of obstruction (dilatation of rete testis, enlarged epididymis, absent vas deferens).[38] It is also used to diagnose varicocele in cases of inconclusive physical examination like obesity, hydrocele, hernia, high-riding testis, ticklish scrotum, and previous scrotal or inguinal surgeries, to document the presence of clinically diagnosed varicocele before surgical intervention and to reevaluate recurrent or persistent varicocele.[37] Varicocele that is impalpable on clinical

examination but diagnosed only on scrotal ultrasound is called subclinical varicocele. Scrotal color Doppler ultrasound criteria for varicocele (i.e., maximum vein diameter ≥3 mm with reflux of venous blood) has a 50% sensitivity and 90% specificity compared to clinical examination.[39,40] A high-frequency (7.5–9 Mhz) handheld pencil probe Doppler aids in the identification of reflux of venous blood with audible sound with or without performing Valsalva, depending on the severity of varicocele.

Magnetic Resonance Imaging

Magnetic resonance imaging (MRI) of the pituitary is helpful in suspected cases (patients with headache, visual symptoms, hyperprolactinemia) of pituitary adenomas. An MRI of the abdomen and pelvis is ordered to look for an intraabdominal testis.

Testicular Biopsy

In current practice, testicular biopsy is done during the course of testicular sperm extraction for the purpose of ICSI. Testicular biopsy is helpful in equivocal cases of azoospermia to differentiate obstructive versus non obstructive azoospermia. These include cases with normal volume testes with normal FSH, LH, and total testosterone, presence of at least one vas, and normal volume on semen analysis. The testicular biopsy specimen should be transported in Bouin, Zenker, or glutaraldehyde solutions. Formalin should not be used as fixative solution as it may cause testicular architectural distortion. Testicular histopathology may reveal normal spermatogenesis, hypospermatogenesis, early or late maturation arrest, Sertoli cell—only syndrome (germ cell aplasia), tubular sclerosis, or a combination of these patterns. It will help in prognosis of future sperm retrieval but may not be absolutely accurate due to the heterogeneous nature of spermatogenesis in the testes, and a limited number of biopsy specimen may not reflect actual spermatogenesis.

TREATMENT

The principles of management of above-mentioned causes of male infertility will follow the same measures that guide treatment for all male infertility.

The factors affecting outcomes after treatment include:

- Duration of infertility
- Severity of male factor

- Female age
- Reproductive potential of partner

The treatment methods can be broadly divided into the following categories:

- Preventive measures
- Medical treatment
- Surgical treatment
- Surgical sperm retrieval for ICSI

Preventive Measures

These include obesity, heat exposure, exposure to toxins, smoking, use of recreational drugs, exogenous use of testosterone or anabolic steroids, and excessive exposure to cell phone radiation. Adherence to a healthy diet, lifestyle changes, and regular exercise are recommended for preventing poor sperm quality. Infertile males are also counseled about all habits that may be deleterious to sperm quality and function.[41] It can take greater than a year for semen to improve after cessation of exogenous androgen use.[42] It has been shown that excessive weight loss or high-intensity exercise may be detrimental to sperm quality, and a moderation of these lifestyle changes are to be followed.

Medical Treatment

Medical therapy for male infertility is only recommended for hypogonadotropic hypogonadism. All other medical therapies are considered empirical. These include the use of gonadotropins, selective estrogen receptor modulators, aromatase inhibitors, and antioxidants.[43]

Gonadotropin therapy in the form of human chorionic gonadotropin (HCG) alone or in combination with FSH has been used empirically in males with idiopathic azoospermia and NOA secondary to Klinefelter syndrome. Highly purified FSH or recombinant FSH has also been used as monotherapy to allow testicular stimulation and initiation of spermatogenesis. These are used in males with NOA or severe oligoasthenoteratozoospermia with contradictory outcomes and are not part of the current guidelines.[44–46]

Orchitis secondary to bacterial or tubercular etiology is managed by appropriate medical therapy.

Surgical Intervention

Varicocele is the commonest surgically correctable cause of male infertility. It is also the most debated issue, as there is lack of consensus between urologists and gynecologists relating to the effect of varicocele on male fertility. The current American Urological Association (AUA) guidelines[47] and other guidelines, including the European Association of Urology (EAU)[48] and the American Society for Reproductive Medicine (ASRM)[47] have stated the following indications for a varicocele repair:

- Infertility of greater than 1 year's duration
- Female factor is normal or correctable
- Clinical varicocele
- At least one abnormal parameter in the semen analysis

Based on current evidence, varicocele repair for subclinical varicocele is not recommended, and varicocele repair for grade I varicoceles may be considered after discussing the lower likelihood of significant benefit.[49] Varicocele repair in case of NOA is more challenging as the outcomes are less favorable and difficult to predict. Several studies have shown sperm in the ejaculate of males undergoing varicocele repair for NOA.[50] Currently, it is preferred to operate on males with large clinical varicoceles and NOA. The sperm retrieval rates are also higher in the males undergoing repair as compared with untreated males.

Microsurgical subinguinal varicocelectomy is the preferred method of varicocele repair, with the lowest incidence of complications and recurrence.

Cryptorchid or undescended testes are best operated on before 1 year of age to protect fertility. They should be operated on at diagnosis if that happens after 1 year of age. The longer the history of maldescent, the poorer the outcome. The germ cell damage is higher in a testis located further away from the scrotum. Normal sperm counts were observed in 75% of males who underwent an orchiopexy between 10 months and 4 years of age compared with 26% of males who underwent orchiopexy between 4 and 14 years of age. Surgical sperm retrieval maybe attempted in azoospermic males 6 months after an orchiopexy procedure.

Surgical Sperm Retrieval

Nonobstructive azoospermia secondary to primary testicular failure is a common testicular etiology that requires a sperm retrieval procedure for assisted reproduction. There are focal areas of spermatogenesis in these conditions allowing the possibility of surgical sperm retrieval. This may be performed by a needle testicular sperm aspiration, conventional testicular sperm extraction, testicular mapping, or micro-TESE. A needle biopsy may occasionally also be performed for severe OATS and in cases of recurrent failures of ICSI or recurrent pregnancy loss due to a high sperm DNA fragmentation index.

The sperm retrieval rates vary depending on the etiology of the defect.

Sperm retrieval rates vary from 25% to 50% in males with Klinefelter syndrome, and there is usually no transmission of the genetic trait in the offspring. *AZFa* and *AZFb* microdeletions of the long arm of the Y chromosome are associated with no chance of sperm retrieval and are contraindicated for a retrieval procedure. Predictability of sperm retrieval is poorly suggested by prior lab tests but may be possible if prior histopathology from the testes is known. Late maturation arrest and hypospermatogenesis are associated with higher retrieval rates compared to conditions such as Sertoli cell–only syndrome.

Early maturation arrest on histopathology precludes the finding of sperms and is contraindicated for a retrieval procedure.

CLINICAL CASE SCENARIOS

CASE 1

Scenario

A 34-year-old male, married to a 31-year-old female for 4 years, reported that he was unable to impregnate his partner in the last 4 years. Medical and reproductive history was otherwise unremarkable. Physical examination revealed mild obesity with tall stature and bilateral gynecomastia. Focused genital examination had shown bilateral small testes (4 cc, Prader orchidometer). Vas deferens was palpable.

How to approach this couple for management of infertility?

Management

Based on the available history and physical examination findings, it looks like a case of primary testicular failure (dysgenetic testes). Basic laboratory evaluation was done. Patient laboratory values are shown in Table 3.2.

Basic semen analysis and hormone profile (FSH/LH/total testosterone/obesity) revealed nonobstructive azoospermia and elevated gonadotropins with low normal testosterone and low testosterone-to-estradiol ratio (4.22 [ng/dL/pg/ml]). Genetic work-up with karyotyping and Y chromosome microdeletions were advised as it is a case

TABLE 3.2 Basic Laboratory Parameters of the Patient

Semen analysis	Volume 1.2 mL, azoospermia, fructose positive, alkaline pH
Follicle-stimulating hormone	25.2 mIU/mL
Luteinizing hormone	14 mIU/mL
Total testosterone	190 ng/dL
Estradiol	45 pg/mL

of NOA. Karyotype revealed 47,XXY (Fig. 3.1)(Klinefelter syndrome), and Y chromosome microdeletions were absent. Finally, it was diagnosed as a primary infertility with NOA in a primary testicular failure patient of Klinefelter origin. We had counseled the couple for various management options like donor insemination, adoption, testicular mapping, and micro-TESE. After genetic counseling, the couple opted for micro-TESE.

Preoperatively, the patient was empirically treated with anastrozole 1 mg once daily and injections of HCG 2000 IU twice weekly for 2 months. Microdissection TESE was done after 2 months of empirical treatment, and we could not find sperm. The couple proceeded with ICSI with donor sperm.

The patient is advised to have lifelong endocrine follow-up for possible hypogonadism sequelae identification and prompt management.

CASE 2

Scenario

A 28-year-old male married for 3 years to a 25-year-old female was suffering from primary infertility. Female evaluation was unremarkable. History was not significant. On physical examination, the male found to have clinically palpable left grade 3 and right grade 2 varicocele. Semen analysis revealed oligoasthenoteratozoospermia. Hormone profile was normal. Scrotal Doppler confirmed varicocele on both sides.

What are the best management options for the couple?

Management

It was a case of primary infertility in a young heterosexual couple with male factor revealing bilateral clinically palpable varicocele with oligoasthenoteratozoospermia and normal female evaluation.

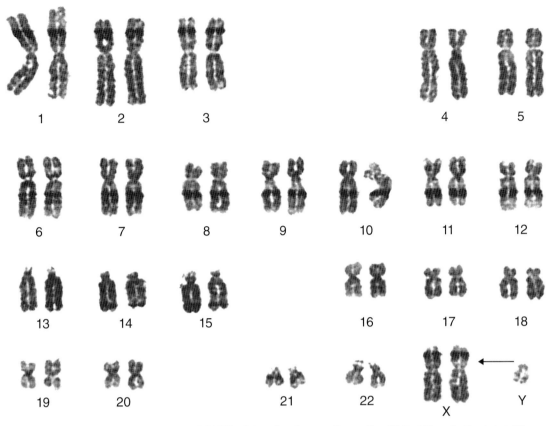

Fig. 3.1 Karyogram Showing 47,XXY Klinefelter Syndrome. (From: Baydilli N, Gökçe A, Karabulut SY, Ekmekcioglu O. Klinefelter's syndrome with unilateral absence of vas deferens. *Fertil Steril.* 2010;94(4):1529. e1-1529.e2.)

Based on the available literature and our clinical experience, the patient was advised varicocele repair. Other management options are empirical medical treatment and one of the ART procedures (intrauterine insemination/in vitro fertilization/ICSI). The couple opted for varicocele fixation after counseling. Patient underwent microsurgical varicocelectomy with intraoperative Doppler assistance. Postoperatively, the patient followed up at 3 months, and 6 months with semen analysis, total testosterone, and FSH. Sperm count and motility improved 20% from baseline at 6 months. The wife conceived naturally at the end of one year. In our clinical practice, 10-15% of couples conceive naturally post varicocelectomy within two years of varicocele fixation.

SUMMARY

Male infertility is commonly caused by diseases that primarily affect the testes or those that result in its dysfunction. They may present with obvious developmental history, as in the case of an undescended testis, or lack of androgenization, as in Klinefelter syndrome. Varicocele is the most common surgically correctable cause of male infertility and is detected on clinical examination. The spectrum of disorders due to these factors may range from minor variations in semen reports to azoospermia. There can be significant impact on sperm DNA fragmentation rate and oxidative stress that can independently affect fertility outcome. Treatment will depend on multiple factors, including duration of infertility and age of the couple, presence of additional factors in the partner, and previous treatment history. Medical therapy is favored for younger couples with minor affection of semen parameters. Surgical correction is indicated for clinical varicocele as per guidelines. Sperm retrieval can be ordered for males with NOA secondary to testicular causes.

REFERENCES

1. Jarvi K, Lo K, Fischer A, et al. CUA guideline: The workup of azoospermic males. *Can Urol Assoc J.* 2010;4(3):163-167.
2. Berkowitz GS, Lapinski RH, Dolgin SE, Gazella JG, Bodian CA, Holzman IR. Prevalence and natural history of cryptorchidism. *Pediatrics.* 1993;92:44.
3. Gracia J, Gonzelez N, Gomez ME, Plaza L, Sanchez J, Alba J. Clinical and anatomopathological study of 2000 cryptorchid testes. *Br J Urol.* 1995;75:697.
4. Krausz C, Riera-Escamilla A. Genetics of male infertility. *Nat Rev Urol.* 2018;15(6):369-384.
5. Jungwirth A, Giwercman A, Tournaye H, et al. European Association of Urology guidelines on male infertility: the 2012 update. *Eur Urol.* 2012;62:324-332.
6. Male Infertility Best Practice Policy Committee of the American Urological Association, Practice Committee of the American Society for Reproductive Medicine. Report on optimal evaluation of the infertile male. *Fertil Steril.* 2006;86:S202-S209.
7. Ramasamy R, Ricci JA, Palermo GD, Gosden LV, Rosenwaks Z, Schlegel PN. Successful fertility treatment for Klinefelter's syndrome. *J Urol.* 2009;182:1108-1113.
8. Bojesen A, Gravholt C. Klinefelter syndrome in clinical practice. *Nat Clin Pract Urol.* 2007;4:192-204.
9. Tuttelmann F, Ropke A. Genetics of male infertility. In: Simoni M, Huhtaniemi I, eds. *Endocrinology of the Testis and Male Reproduction.* Cham, Switzerland: Springer; 2017.
10. Han TH, Ford JH, Flaherty SP, Webb GC, Matthews CD. A fluorescent in situ hybridization analysis of the chromosome constitution of ejaculated sperm in a 47, XYY male. *Clin Genet.* 1994;45:67-70.
11. Tiepolo L, Zuffardi O. localization of factors controlling spermatogenesis in the nonfluorescent in portion of the human Y-chromosome long arm. *Hum Genet.* 1976; 34:119-124.
12. Hopps CV, Mienik A, Goldstein M, Palermo GD, Rosenwaks Z, Schlegel PN. Detection of sperm in men with Y-chromosome microdeletions of the AZFa, AZFb and AZFc regions. *Hum Reprod.* 2003;18:1660-1665.
13. Krausz C, Escamilla AR, Chianese C. Genetics of male infertility: from research to clinic. *Reproduction.* 2015;150:R159-R174.
14. Ferlin A, Vinanzi C, Garolla A, et al. Male infertility and androgen receptor gene mutations: clinical features and identification of seven novel mutations. *Clin Endocrinol (Oxf).* 2006;65:606-610.
15. Weidner W, Colpi GM, Hargreave TB, et al. EAU guidelines on male infertility. *Eur Urol.* 2002;42:313-322.
16. WHO. *WHO Manual for the Standardized Investigation, Diagnosis and Management of the Infertile Male.* Cambridge: Cambridge University Press; 2000.
17. Nistal M, Paniaqua R. Gomez-Alvarez RP. *Testicular and Epididymal Pathology.* New York: Thieme; 1984.
18. Gimenes F, Souza RP, Bento JC, et al. Male infertility: a public health issue caused by sexually transmitted pathogens. *Nat Rev Urol.* 2014;11:672.
19. Schuppe HC, Meinhardt A, Allam JP, et al. chronic orchitis: a neglected cause of male infertility? *Andrologia.* 2008;40:84-91.
20. Ray PF, Toure A, Metzler- Guillemain C, et al. Genetic abnormalities leading to qualitative defects of sperm morphology or function. *Clin Genet.* 2017;91:217-232.
21. Ortega HA, Vega Nde A, Santos BQ, et al. Primary ciliary dyskinesia: Considerations regarding six cases of Kartagener syndrome. *J Bras Pneumol.* 2007;33(5)602-608.
22. Peng, X, Zeng X, Peng S, et al. The association risk of male subfertility and testicular cancer: a systematic review. *PLoS One.* 2009;4:e5591.
23. Petersen PM, Skakkebaek NE, Vistisen K, Rorth M, Giwercman A. Semen quality and reproductive hormones before orchiectomy in men with testicular cancer. *J Clin Oncol.* 1999;17:941.
24. Moody JA, Ahmed K, Yap T, Minhas S, Shabbir M. Fertility managment in testicular cancer: the need to establish a standardized and evidence-based patient-centric pathway. *BJU Int.* 2019;123:160.
25. Willemse PH, Sleijfer DT, Sluiter WJ, Schraffordt Koops H, Doorenbos H. Altered Leydig cell function in patients with testicular cancer: evidence for bilateral testicular defect. *Acta Endocrinol (Copenh).* 1983;102:616.
26. Zhang L, Wang XH, Zheng XM, et al. Maternal gestational smoking, diabetes, alcohol drinking, pre-pregnancy obesity and the risk of cryptorchidism: a systematic review and meta-analysis of observational studies. *PLoS One.* 2015;10:e0119006.
27. Barbonetti A, Martorella A, Minaldi E, et al. Testicular cancer in infertile men with and without testicular microlithiasis: a systematic review and meta-analysis of case-control studies. *Front Endocrinol (Lausanne).* 2019;10:164.
28. Stopczyk D, Gnitecki W, Buczynski A, Kowalski W, Buczynska M, Kroc A. Effect of electromagnetic field produced by mobile phones on the activity of superoxide dismutase (SOD-1)—in vitro researches. *Ann Acad Med Stetin.* 2005;51(suppl 1):125-128.

29. Jung A, Schuppe HC. Influence of genital heat stress on semen quality in humans. *Andrologia.* 2007;39(6):203-215.

30. Thonneau P, Bujan L, Multigner L, Mieusset R. Occupational heat exposure and male infertility: a review. *Human Reprod.* 1998;13(8):2122-2125.

31. Khera M, Lipshultz LI. Evolving approach to the varicocele. *Urol Clin North Am.* 2008;35:183.

32. Esteves SC, Glina S. Recovery of spermatogenesis after microsurgical subinguinal varicocele repair in azoospermic men based on testicular histology. *Int Braz J Urol.* 2005;31:541-548.

33. Buffum J. Pharmacosexology update: prescription drugs and sexual function. *J Psychoactive Drugs.* 1986;18(2):97-106.

34. Dubin L, Amelar RD. Varicocele size and results of varicocelectomy in selected sub-fertile men with varicocele. *Fertil Steril.* 1970;21(8):606-609.

35. Esteves SC, Miyaoka R, Agarwal A. An update on the clinical assessment of the infertile male. *Clinics (Sao Paulo).* 2011;66(4):691-700.

36. Raman JD, Schlegel PN. Aromatase inhibitors for male infertility. *J Urol.* 2002;167:624-629.

37. Vaucher L, Carreras E, Mielnik A, Schlegel PN, Paduch D. Over expression of aromatase CYP19 in human testis is most likely reason for hypogonadism in men with Klinefelter syndrome. *J Urol.* 2009;181:681-681.

38. Lotti F, Maggi M. Ultrasound of the male genital tract in relation to male reproductive health. *Hum Reprod Update.* 2015;21:56.

39. Chiou RK, Anderson JC, Wobig RK, et al. Color Doppler ultrasound criteria to diagnose varicoceles: correlation of a new scoring system with physical examination. *Urology.* 1997;50(6):953-956.

40. Vaamonde D, Da Silva-Grigoletto ME, Garcia-Manso JM, Barrera N, Vaamonde-Lemos R. Physically active men show better semen parameters and hormone values than sedentary men. *Eur J Appl Physiol.* 2012;112(9):3267-3273.

41. Shankara-Narayana N, Yu C, Savkovic S, et al. Rate and extent of recovery from reproductive and cardiac dysfunction due to androgen abuse in men. *J Clin Endocrinol Metab.* 2020;105(6):1827-1839.

42. Ko EY, Siddiqi K, Brannigan RE, Sabanegh ES. Empirical medical therapy for idiopathic male infertility: a survey of the American Urological Association. *J Urol.* 2012;187(3):973-978.

43. Hussein A, Ozgok Y, Ross L, Rao P, Niederberger C. Optimization of spermatogenesis-regulating hormones in patients with non-obstructive azoospermia and its impact on sperm retrieval: a multicentre study. *BJU Int.* 2013;111(3 Pt B):E110-E114.

44. Santi D, Granata AR, Simoni M. FSH treatment of male idiopathic infertility improves pregnancy rate: a meta-analysis. *Endocr Connect.* 2015;4(3):R46-R58.

45. Cavallini G, Biagiotti G, Bolzon E. Multivariate analysis to predict letrozole efficacy in improving sperm count of non-obstructive azoospermic and cryptozoospermic patients: a pilot study. *Asian J Androl.* 2013;15(6):806-811.

46. Schlegel PN, Sigman M, Collura B, et al. Diagnosis and treatment of infertility in men. AUA/ASRM guideline part II. *J Urol.* 2021;205(1):44-51.

47. Minhas S, Bettocchi C, Boeri L, et al. European Association of Urology guidelines on male sexual and reproductive health: 2021 update on male infertility. *Eur Urol.* 2021;80(5):603-620.

48. Shah R, Agarwal A, Kavoussi P, et al. Consensus and diversity in the management of varicocele for male infertility: results of a global practice survey and comparison with guidelines and recommendations. *World J Mens Health.* 2023;41(1):164-197.

49. Weedin JW, Khera M, Lipshultz LI. Varicocele repair in patients with nonobstructive azoospermia: a meta-analysis. *J Urol.* 2010;183(6):2309-2315.

50. Corona G, Pizzocaro A, Lanfranco F, et al. Sperm recovery and ICSI outcomes in Klinefelter's syndrome: a systematic review and meta-analysis. *Hum Reprod Update.* 2017;23(3):265-275.

4

Posttesticular Causes of Male Infertility

Marlon Pedrozo Martinez and Ranjith Ramasamy

KEY POINTS

- Infertile males with posttesticular etiologies often have normal spermatogenesis. The causes of infertility are mainly due to obstruction in the flow of the seminal fluid or dysfunctions in erection and ejaculation.
- Failure in emission and expulsion can lead to ejaculatory dysfunction. Any imbalance in the integration of the central nervous system, peripheral nerves, and penile erectile tissues can precipitate abnormalities in the erection process. Failure in emission or expulsion will result in infertility.
- Sperm retrieval with assisted reproduction or microsurgical reconstruction are valuable treatment

options in males with obstruction along the reproductive tract.
- A thorough preoperative evaluation is of utmost importance before any microsurgical reconstruction is considered. Detailed focused history, meticulous physical examination, hormonal evaluation, and imaging may anticipate any technical difficulty that may affect a successful surgical outcome.
- Shared decision making between the infertile couples and the reproductive specialists will result to a more favorable fertility outcome.

INTRODUCTION

Infertility affects 8% to 12% of reproductive-aged couples globally.[1] Male factor infertility (MFI) is solely responsible for 20% to 30% of cases and contributory in another 50%. Compared to other countries, MFI rates were highly observed in Africa and Central/Eastern Europe.[2] MFI is often related to problems in spermatogenesis, which is significantly regulated by the hypothalamic-pituitary-gonadal axis.[3] Any disruptions in the secretion of the gonadotropins, formation of spermatozoa within the testis, and its passage along the reproductive tract can result to infertility. There are several etiologies of male poor reproductive potential stratified as pretesticular, testicular, and posttesticular causes.[4] These causes can be congenital, acquired, or idiopathic.[5]

This chapter focuses on the posttesticular causes (Fig. 4.1) of inability of males to have their own biological children. Clinical presentation, diagnosis, and treatment options are discussed.

POSTTESTICULAR CAUSES OF MALE INFERTILITY

After spermatozoa are formed within the testis, they travel to the epididymis, vas deferens (VD), ejaculatory duct, and penile urethra during antegrade ejaculation.[6] This is in coordination with the normal functions of the muscles involved in the emission and expulsion phases of ejaculation, controlled by the autonomic and somatic divisions of the nervous system.[7] In addition, penile erection also contributes to this complex process of passage of seminal fluid along the reproductive tract.[8]

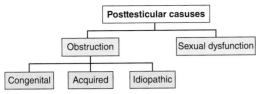

Fig. 4.1 Posttesticular Causes of Male Infertility.

Infertile males with posttesticular etiologies often have normal sperm production.[9] Causes of infertility in these cases are mainly due to blockade in the flow of the seminal fluid or sexual dysfunctions. Treatment options (Table 4.1) depend on the different clinical scenarios and couples' factors.

Obstruction of the Male Reproductive Tract

Etiologies of obstruction of the male reproductive tract can be due to congenital, acquired, or idiopathic causes. Males with obstructions usually present with azoospermia, which occurs in 1% of the general population and 10% to 15% of infertile males.[10] Males with absent sperm in their ejaculate should be assessed in order to distinguish blockade along the reproductive tract from impaired spermatogenesis. Semen volume, physical examination, and follicle-stimulating hormone (FSH) level can be used to differentiate the type of azoospermia.[11]

Obstructive azoospermia (OA) comprises 40% of all cases of azoospermia.[10] Males with OA have a blockage in the conduit of sperm, rather than abnormality in spermatogenesis.[12] They can be offered surgery to allow passage of sperm, which can translate to natural conception or sperm retrieval followed by assisted reproductive technologies (ART) such as in vitro fertilization (IVF) and intracytoplasmic sperm injection (ICSI).[9] Sperm can be harvested from either the testis or epididymis in males who opt for sperm retrieval.[13]

Congenital Causes

Congenital posttesticular etiologies of infertile males include cystic fibrosis transmembrane conductance regulator (*CFTR*) gene mutation, Wolffian duct developmental defect, and unknown genetic origin.[14] Some of these can be corrected surgically, while others are nonreconstructible and would require ART.

Congenital bilateral absence of vas deferens. (CBAVD) is seen in 1% to 2% of infertile males and can be found in 6% of males with OA.[15] Males with CBAVD can present with infertility due either to an isolated OA or atypical manifestations of cystic fibrosis (CF), which

Posttesticular Causes	Treatment Options
Obstruction	
Congenital	
CBAVD	Sperm retrieval + IVF/ICSI
CUAVD	Transeptal vasoepididymostomy
	Sperm retrieval + IVF/ICSI
Young syndrome	Sperm retrieval + IVF/ICSI
EDO	TURED
	Transurethral vesiculoscopy
	Balloon dilation
	Sperm retrieval + IVF/ICSI
Acquired	
Vasectomy	Surgical reconstruction (Vasovasostomy/vasoepididymostomy)
	Sperm retrieval + IVF/ICSI
Infection	Surgical reconstruction (Vasovasostomy/vasoepididymostomy)
	Sperm retrieval + IVF/ICSI
Iatrogenic	Surgical reconstruction (Vasovasostomy-robot-assisted/ laparoscopy-assisted)
	Sperm retrieval + IVF/ICSI
Idiopathic	
	Surgical reconstruction
	Sperm retrieval + IVF/ICSI
Sexual Dysfunction	
Erectile dysfunction	Phosphodiesterase inhibitors
	Vacuum erection device
	Topical
	Intraurethral/intracavernosal injection
	Low-intensity shockwave therapy
	Penile prosthesis implantation
	Vascular surgery
	Sperm retrieval + IVF/ICSI
Retrograde ejaculation	Sympathomimetics
	Alkalinization of urine with or without urethral catheterization
	Induced ejaculation
	Sperm retrieval + IVF/ICSI

TABLE 4.1 Treatment Options for the Different Etiologies From Posttesticular Origin

CBAVD, Congenital bilateral absence of vas deferens; EDO, ejaculatory duct obstruction; ICSI, intracytoplasmic sperm injection; IVF, in vitro fertilization; TURED, transurethral resection of ejaculatory duct.

is an autosomal recessive disorder.[16] As 98% of males with clinical CF also have CBAVD, researchers believe that there is a common genetic origin.[14] Mutation in CFTR, a protein regulator of chloride levels across the epithelial membrane, can cause CBAVD, pancreatic insufficiency, and respiratory diseases.[17] Approximately 12% of males with the *CFTR* mutation carry two mild alleles, while 88% carry both mild and severe alleles. *CFTR* mutation carrier testing for 5T allele assessment is recommended in males with vasal agenesis since it is the most common mild *CFTR* mutation.[13] On the other hand, F508del is considered a severe mutation, which should also be assessed along with the *CFTR* mutation analysis. Genetic evaluation of the female partner in heterosexual couples is recommended if the male partner has a *CFTR* mutation.[13] In a systematic review and metaanalysis of *CFTR* mutations in males with CBAVD, 78% of patients had at least one CFTR mutation, and 46% of them had two. A higher frequency of F508del and lower frequency of 5T was observed in White patients compared with non-White patients.[16] More than 2000 CF-causing *CFTR* mutations have been determined.[18] Males with CBAVD who are *CFTR* mutation–negative should be evaluated for mutations in *ADGRG2*.[19] This can account for 10% to 15% of males with CBAVD who are *CFTR* mutation–negative.

Males with CBAVD can present with renal agenesis in 5% to 10% of cases and seminal vesicle (SV) atresia or agenesis in 50%. Males with CBAVD also present with a typical semen phenotype, which includes an acidic (pH <7) and low-volume (<1 mL) azoospermia.[20] Other manifestations include normal-sized or slightly small testis, atrophic or absent cauda epididymis, and normal FSH level.[18] Imaging can be adjunct in the diagnosis of CBAVD. Scrotal ultrasound can differentiate VD from the other cordlike structures in the spermatic cord.[21] This might be helpful in demonstrating unique features of epididymal abnormalities, including cystic and tubular dilatation.[22] In a study of 36 males with CBAVD, normal testicular volume, dilatation of the epididymis and absence of the VD were observed. In addition, 21% of the heads of the epididymis were identified, while in 67% both the heads and bodies of epididymis were seen. These findings showed the atresia of the distal portion of the epididymis.

ART is the cornerstone of management for males with CBAVD, since surgical reconstruction is not a viable option. The treatment of choice is to perform sperm retrieval followed by IVF/ICSI.[23] Sperm can be retrieved by microsurgical epididymal sperm aspiration (MESA), percutaneous epididymal sperm aspiration, testicular sperm aspiration, or testicular sperm extraction (TESE). Males with CBAVD without CF have superior outcomes compared to those with CF. In a comparative study of males with CF with CBAVD (n = 10) or CBAVD (n = 28) alone, the former had poorer reproductive outcomes.[24] Compared to males with CBAVD alone, males who also had CF exhibited a significantly lower sperm concentration (61.4 M/mL vs. 14.8 M/mL, p = 0.02), lower total motile sperm count (11.4 M vs. 2.9 M, p = 0.01), higher rescue TESE rate (27.6% vs. 70.0%, p < 0.03), and lower fertilization rate with ICSI (68.9% vs. 32.5%, p < 0.01).

Congenital unilateral absence of vas deferens. (CUAVD) is a sequela of the Wolffian duct developmental defect that occurs in 1% of males.[25] This can be incidentally encountered during physical evaluation or surgical procedure of the scrotal area.[26] In 23,013 White males seeking vasectomy, 82 demonstrated CUAVD.[25] Approximately 30% to 50% of males with CUAVD carry at least one *CFTR* mutation, particularly in males with renal genesis.[14] As a result, *CFTR* testing is recommended for males with CUAVD as well due to this increased risk. The association between CUAVD and *CFTR* mutation was confirmed in a systematic review and metaanalysis of 23 studies, where 46% of males with CUAVD had at least one *CFTR* variant.[27] Males with CUAVD were 5.79 times more susceptible to 5T allele mutation than fertile males. In males with CUAVD, the overall incidence of renal abnormalities was 22%, and unilateral renal genesis could be seen in 26%.[28] Renal ultrasound is recommended in males with vasal agenesis to determine abnormalities in the kidneys.[11] A high percentage of males with CUAVD can present with hypoplastic or absent SV.[29] Palpation of the VD and scrotal and transrectal ultrasound (TRUS) constitute the standard means for diagnosis of CUAVD.[30]

In a retrospective, cross-sectional, case-control study of CUAVD (n = 69) cases and controls (n = 78), independent predictors for the diagnosis of CUAVD were identified.[30] Compared to controls, males with CUAVD had significantly lower semen volume (50% less than 1.5 mL), higher proportion of azoospermia, and lower epididymal biomarkers such as free L-carnitine and glycerophosphocholine. The probability of diagnosis of CUAVD increased with the presence of history of unilateral cryptorchidism (5.84×) and seminal fructose

<13 mmol/ejaculate (4.95×). The presence of seminal alpha-1,4 glucosidase can decrease this probability. TRUS is recommended if these predictors are present to confirm the diagnosis.

Males with CUAVD often present with primary infertility due to OA. However, males with CUAVD can still be fertile. In a study of 63 males, 33.3% presented with normozoospermia, while 27% had oligozoospermia.[28] Only 39.7% displayed absence of sperm in their ejaculate. Natural conception was achieved in 42% of males. Males with CUAVD who present with OA will require ART or reconstruction, depending on the clinical scenario.

Young syndrome. A relatively rare condition described initially by Dr. Donald Young in 1950, this demonstrates a combination of male infertility due to OA secondary to bilateral epididymal obstruction with bronchiectasis and sinusitis.[31] It is now believed that Young syndrome is caused by *CFTR* gene mutations.[32] As a result, CF screening and genetic counseling should be offered in the management of Young syndrome. Young syndrome is differentiated from primary ciliary dyskinesia (PCD), which is an autosomal recessive disease resulting from ciliary and flagellar dysfunctions demonstrating immotility, by the absence of sperm in the ejaculate, and the finding of motile sperm on retrieval.[33] On the other hand, Young syndrome may resemble Kartagener syndrome, a subset of PCD characterized by immotile spermatozoa; however, it is not definitive if ciliary dysfunction is the main culprit of the former.[34] OA in males with Young syndrome resulted from the accumulation of impacted sperm, particularly in the head of the epididymis, due to functional obstruction where sperm is found in viscous, lipid-rich mucus.[31] As a consequence of the obstruction, there is a blockade of sperm transport from the epididymis down to the genital tract.[34] Sperm retrieval with IVF/ICSI is the best treatment option since surgical reconstruction, although technically feasible, resulted in unfavorable outcomes.

Ejaculatory duct obstruction. (EDO). Ejaculatory ducts are tubular structures formed from the confluence of the VD and SV. Blockage within these paired and collagenous structures can result in EDO. This accounts for 1% to 5% of MFI cases.[35] There are varied clinical presentations of males with EDO, aside from poor reproductive potential due to OA.[36] Some patients may complain of hematospermia, decreased volume of ejaculated seminal fluid, painful ejaculation, scrotal pain, perineal pain, or dysuria. Other males may experience epididymitis and prostatitis.

History, physical evaluation, semen analysis, and imaging establish the diagnosis of EDO.[13] The hallmark findings in a semen analysis, particularly in males with complete EDO, are azoospermia, low semen volume (<1.5 mL), acidic pH (<7.2), and low or absent fructose (<13 μmol/ejaculate). In addition, appreciation of palpable VD and SV can contribute to the diagnosis.[37]

There are several diagnostic methods for EDO. These include vasography, TRUS, SV aspiration, SV chromotubation, seminal vesiculography, magnetic resonance imaging, and manometry.[13] TRUS is recommended in azoospermic males with acidic pH, semen volume less than 1.5 mL, normal serum testosterone level, and present VD.[11] EDO should be increasingly suspected in males with an enlarged SV with a diameter more than 1.5 cm and ejaculatory duct greater than 2.3 mm.[13] Other diagnostic techniques increase the diagnosis of EDO. In a prospective study involving males with suspected EDO based on clinical findings and TRUS evaluation showed that chromotubation confirmed the diagnosis of EDO using ultrasound in 52% of cases. This was higher than the diagnostic ability of vesiculography (36%) and SV aspiration (48%).[38,39]

Treatment options for males with EDO are transurethral resection of ejaculatory duct (TURED), transutricular seminal vesiculoscopy, balloon dilation, midline prostatic cyst aspiration, and sperm retrieval followed by IVF/ICSI.[13] There are integral components for an effective TURED for males with EDO.[40] Instillation of methylene blue into the SV will allow identification of ejaculatory ducts without difficulty. At the end of TURED, vesiculography will identify any newly opened ejaculatory ducts. In addition, this will allow passive drainage from the SV. TURED can deliver improvement of the semen parameters postoperatively. In a systematic review of 29 studies comprising of 634 patients, TURED resulted in improvement in semen volume, motility, and concentration in 83%, 63%, and 62.5% of patients, respectively.[41] The median natural pregnancy rate was 25%.

There are also acquired etiologies of EDO which include SV calculi, urethral trauma, indwelling catheter use, inflammation, and scarring as a result from transurethral bladder neck incision and resection of the prostate.[42] Compared to congenital EDO, males with acquired EDO experienced lower improvement in semen parameters after TURED. In addition, a lower pregnancy rate was achieved.[43]

Acquired Causes

Other etiologies of obstruction along the reproductive tract are acquired in nature. These are mainly surgical procedures in the scrotal, inguinal, and pelvic areas.[44,45] Iatrogenic injuries to these sites are also contributory.[42] Inflammatory reactions, particularly those caused by sexually transmitted infections (STIs), can result in scarring and fibrosis leading to obstruction.[46] Some obstructions have unknown etiologies.[47] All these causes can precipitate OA, leading to infertility.

Vasectomy.   This is one of the most widely used surgical male contraception procedures.[44] Approximately 20% of males who undergo vasectomy will express their desire to reestablish their fertility potential, and about 6% of them will undergo vasectomy reversal (VR).[37] A thorough preoperative evaluation is warranted before any microsurgical reconstruction in order to ensure that it is the best-suited treatment option for restoration of the fertility potential of a male patient. A detailed focused history, meticulous physical examination, and hormonal evaluation may anticipate technical and functional difficulties that may affect the success of the surgery.[48]

Sperm retrieval with IVF-ICSI or VR is a plausible treatment option for heterosexual couples desiring to have biological offspring after vasectomy.[49] It is of utmost importance for reproductive urologists and reproductive endocrinologists to be familiar with recent advances in the treatment options for infertile heterosexual couples in order to provide optimal guidance in their decision making.[50] There are several factors to take into account before undergoing fertility treatment after vasectomy. Advanced paternal and maternal age, presence of female factor infertility, longer obstructive interval (OI), and treatment cost might suggest sperm retrieval with IVF/ICSI rather than VR.[49] In a study of 175 heterosexual couples, age of the male and female partners and status of the ovarian reserve did not contribute significantly in choosing the preferred treatment option after vasectomy. However, longer OI was a factor towards choosing sperm retrieval with IVF/ICSI. Microsurgical VR is considered the most cost-effective treatment option for infertile heterosexual couples who desire to restore their fertility following vasectomy.[51] There are several prognostic factors for a successful VR (Fig. 4.2). These include surgeon's skill, OI, previous

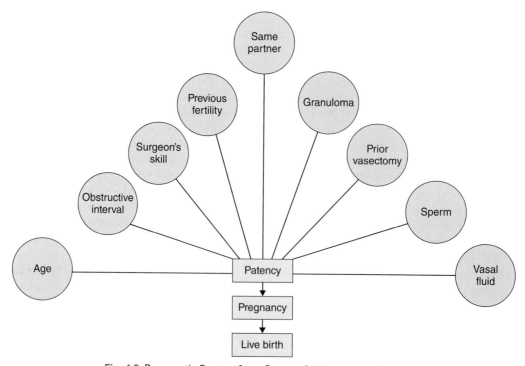

Fig. 4.2 Prognostic Factors for a Successful Vasectomy Reversal.

partner fertility, same partner, age of female partner, presence of granuloma, and prior VR.[52,53] Reproductive outcomes are superior in males who underwent VR who had the same partners as before the vasectomy. In a prospective study of 258 males who underwent VR while with the same partner, they had a significantly higher clinical natural pregnancy rate compared to the general VR population (83% vs. 60%, p < 0.0001).[54] Advanced age is not an independent predictor of achieving pregnancy after VR.[55] In a comparative study of males less than 50 years (n = 2700) and males greater than 50 years (n = 353), the latter had a lower pregnancy rate (26.1% vs. 33.4%, p = 0.007), although this finding did not reach statistical significance. In a multi-institutional analysis of 171 males, OI (odds ratio [OR] = 1.01), age (OR = 0.96), presence of motile sperm (OR = 0.81), and characteristic of epididymal fluid did not predict a successful bilateral vasoepididymostomy (VE).[56] Reproductive urologists should determine which microsurgical technique must be performed, depending on the characteristics of the vasal fluid and, more importantly, the absence or presence of sperm (Fig. 4.3). Vasovasostomy (VV) is warranted if spermatozoa are present from the expressed fluid from transected VS, while VE should be performed if there is no sperm, which indicates an epididymal obstruction.[57]

Infection. In the most recent systematic review on the long-term sequelae of STIs on male reproduction functions, bacterial, viral, and protozoan pathogens were found to cause testicular damage and formation of antisperm antibodies.[46] Epithelial inflammatory reactions from these infections can lead to scarring of the epididymis, VD, and ejaculatory duct, and subsequent obstruction in the of the flow of the seminal fluid. Infection can also cause impairment of the secretory capacity of the epididymis, SV, and prostate.[58] The prevalence of infection leading to inflammatory response within the male reproductive tract is 6% to 10%.[59] Males with history of acute epididymitis, such as that caused by STIs, can develop persistent azoospermia in 10% of cases, while 30% of males can experience oligozoospermia. Inflammatory genitourinary conditions like epididymitis and orchitis can also result in epididymal and vasal obstruction.[60]

Several infectious pathogens have been reported to cause inflammatory OA.[61] Gonorrhea is one of the bacterial infections caused by a gram-negative diplococcus, *Neisseria gonorrhea*.[62] In a study of 133 male patients with a single cause of OA, infections accounted for 47% of those causes.[63] Gonorrheal infections were seen in 7.5% of cases. In a recent systematic review and meta-analysis of 147 prevalence studies from 56 countries, the pooled mean prevalence of infection with gonorrheal infection in the infertile population was 2.2%.[64] Compared to males in the developed countries, a higher incidence of postinfectious OA is observed in developing countries.[65]

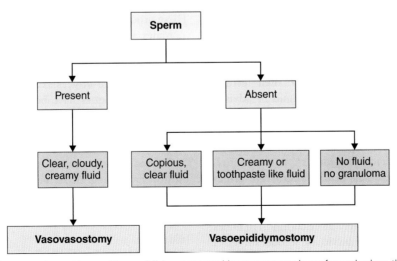

Fig. 4.3 Vasovasostomy Versus Vasoepididymostomy. Vasovasostomy is performed when there is the presence of sperm regardless of the characteristic of the vasal fluid, while vasoepididymostomy is performed when sperm is absent.

In cases of tuberculous OA, granulomas can impede the flow of the seminal fluid along the VD, or the VD can be disfigured by extensive scarring and fibrosis from the surrounding tissues.[66] Involvement of the prostate and SV can cause low-volume azoospermia. Most of the cases of male infertility complicated by genitourinary tuberculosis are not amenable to microsurgical reconstruction due to scarring at multiple levels along the reproductive tract and will require ART.

In a prospective, single-center study of 198 males with suspected epididymal OA due to infection, 149 experienced orchitis, epididymitis, or urethritis.[65] Eighty percent underwent scrotal exploration and VE (bilateral = 132; unilateral = 27). Sperm was present in the epididymal fluid in 159 males, particularly in those with netlike ectasia or tubular ectasia of the epididymal tubules. VE was not performed in 31 patients because there were obstructions of the VD in the pelvic region or multiple vasal obstructions. Ten out of 37 males with a history of gonorrheal infections did not proceed with VE due to multiple levels of vasal obstructions. Patency rate was 72% after VE. Natural pregnancy and live birth rates were 38.7% and 32.7%, respectively.

Males with infectious OA are amenable to microsurgical reconstructive surgery. However, those with multiple obstructions along the reproductive tract are candidates for sperm retrieval with ART.

Iatrogenic. Any injury, especially from surgical procedures, can impede the flow of the semen along the reproductive tract, leading to ejaculatory dysfunction and OA. This impairment can be irreversible or surgically reconstructed.[42] In cancer patients who will be undergoing radical surgeries, adequate informed counseling should be offered regarding the possibility of negative impact of these procedures to their fertility potential.[67] Sperm cryopreservation should be advised before surgery, especially for those males who plan to have children.

Inguinal herniorrhaphy is one of the most commonly performed surgical procedures.[68] A higher incidence of OA was observed in a pediatric age group (0.8%–2.0%) compared to an older population (0.3%) following surgical repair of hernia.[69] However, iatrogenic vasal injuries (7.2%) were more common in males with a history of inguinal, pelvic, or scrotal surgeries other than vasectomy.[70] Use of mesh during herniorrhaphy can be a culprit of MFI.[71] Upon placement of mesh, a dense fibroblastic inflammatory reaction may ensue around the surrounding tissues. This can result to scar formation causing vasal obstruction.[72] In addition, transection, crushing, or overstretching of the VD can be contributory. In an earlier study, inguinal herniorrhaphy without mesh had no effect on male fertility potential.[45] OA was demonstrated in males who underwent open (0.03%) and laparoscopic (2.5%) hernia repair with mesh use. In contrast, in a systematic review comprising 29 clinical studies, which included seven randomized controlled trials on the mesh hernia repair, both open and laparoscopic surgeries had no significant impact on male fertility potential.[73] Compared with heavyweight mesh, use of lightweight mesh is associated with decreased sperm motility after 1 year of follow-up, but no change was observed after 3 years. Correction of vasal obstruction following childhood herniorrhaphy demonstrated positive impact in the improvement of semen parameters and reproductive outcomes. In a study of 56 males with OA due to hernia repair, overall patency and pregnancy rates were 87.5% and 42%, respectively.[69] The abdominal side of the vasal remnants were not identified in 11 patients; hence laparoscopy-assisted VV was performed.

Surgical reconstruction for iatrogenic vasal injury is technically more challenging than VR due to the possibility of long segment loss of the VD, failure to locate the distal end of the VD, and the presence of secondary epididymal obstruction.[74] Several case reports presented intraabdominal robot-assisted VV to address vasal obstruction due to bilateral inguinal herniorrhaphy.[75] These procedure showed promising results.

Males who underwent radical prostatectomy and radical cystectomy reported a negative impact on quality of life.[76] Transection of VD and removal of SV in both these radical surgeries can result in OA. As a result, modified techniques have been developed to preserve the continuity of the reproductive tract.[67] Despite these improvements, sperm cryopreservation should be offered before any definitive treatment.

The management of iatrogenic vasal injuries is technically challenging. Meticulous dissection and careful identification of the different surgical anatomical structures are extremely important.

Idiopathic

The exact etiologies of MFI remain undetermined in 30% to 50% of cases; hence they are classified as idiopathic.[77] Some causes of obstruction are without discernible origin. Idiopathic obstruction is the most common etiology of epididymal obstruction of males from Asian countries compared to males from western countries. In a study of 134 Chinese males with suspected epididymal obstruction who underwent scrotal exploration, the causes of obstruction were surgery (1.2%), infection (9.9%), or idiopathic (88.9%).[57] In contrast, in a study of 72 American males, the most common cause of epididymal obstruction was vasectomy (69%), while idiopathic cause was only 3%.[78] In another study of 23 Indian males with idiopathic OA, 48% achieved patency with a mean of 6.6 months after surgery.[79] Presence of motile sperm and bilateral anastomosis were predictors of a successful reconstruction.

Failure to achieve clinical pregnancy with a female partner can be a sign of male genitourinary tuberculosis, for which is sometimes difficult to establish a definitive diagnosis. Screening for tuberculosis is not warranted in the evaluation of males with idiopathic OA because it has low yield and no impact on clinical management.[80] One hundred males with idiopathic OA were screened for tuberculosis using a semen polymerase chain reaction (PCR) test. Only 7% had positive results, and none had additional examinations that were positive for tuberculosis. All of them had a previous history of tuberculosis. Of the males with positive PCR, four had clinical findings suggestive of genitourinary tuberculosis. All of them had low-volume azoospermia with nodular VD, and two had epididymis.

Microsurgical VE is a technically challenging procedure for idiopathic epididymal obstruction. However, it will obviate the need for sperm retrieval and subsequent ART.

Sexual Dysfunction

Normal sexual function is a fundamental element of reproduction. The integration of the ejaculation and erection processes occurs in the central nervous system and peripheral nerves. This is in coordination with the seminal tract, pelvic floor muscles, and penile erectile tissues. Ejaculation, accompanied by sexual orgasm, happens with forcible ejection of seminal fluid out of the urethral meatus.[81] Emission and expulsion are the two main phases of a normal antegrade ejaculation.[82] Failure of these two vital steps can lead to ejaculatory dysfunction, resulting in MFI. In addition, any imbalance in the integration of psychologic, neurologic, endocrine, or vasoactive factors and trabecular smooth muscles can precipitate problems with the control of tumescence and detumescence, leading to dysfunction in the erection process.[8]

Sexual dysfunction is more prevalent in infertile males compared to fertile males. In a comparative study between 200 infertile and 200 fertile males, the infertile males had a lower Sexual Health Inventory for Males (SHIM) erectile score (19 vs. 22, p = 0.001).[83] In another study of 3280 males aged between 18 and 52 years referred to an andrology unit, the prevalence of ejaculatory dysfunctions in infertile males was 1.8%.[84] In addition, radical cancer surgeries, which include retroperitoneal lymph node dissection (RPLND), pelvic colon procedures, and anterior spine surgeries, can result in ejaculatory dysfunction.[67]

Healthcare providers who are evaluating infertile males should thoroughly assess for the presence of any sexual dysfunctions.[85] In the setting of poor reproductive potential, these can add to the burden of the couple trying to conceive.

Erectile Dysfunction

Erectile dysfunction (ED) is the persistent inability to sustain penile erection sufficient to reach orgasm and sexual satisfaction.[86] Some patients can be managed solely on the basis of medical and sexual history, while others need specific diagnostic tests like the nocturnal penile tumescence and rigidity test, intracavernous injection test, dynamic duplex ultrasound of the penis, arteriography, and cavernosography. There are several validated tools, such as the International Index of Erectile Function (IIEF), SHIM, and Erectile Hardness Score, that can aid in the assessment of different sexual function domains and penile rigidity.[87] Different treatment modalities[86] for males with ED are listed in Table 4.1.

In infertile heterosexual couples, ED has been reported in 9% to 62% of male partners.[88] ED can be associated with feelings of loss of masculinity and psychological pressure on failure to conceive. In addition, ED can be linked mainly with depressive symptoms.[89] It is more prevalent in males with secondary infertility than in males with primary infertility.[90] In a study of 448 males in infertile heterosexual couples, a higher prevalence of ED was observed compared to a control group (18.3% vs. 0%, p = 0.006).[91] The prevalence of ED in this group increased as the semen quality deteriorated (p < 0.0001). Azoospermia was associated with the worst erectile function and psychopathological disturbances.

Male sexual dysfunction can be associated with abnormal semen parameters. In a study of 183 infertile males and their partners, there were positive correlations between sperm count, motility, morphology, testosterone level, and IIEF score.[92] Males were divided into three groups (group 1: males with azoospermia; group 2: males with sperm concentration <15 million/mL; group 3: males with sperm concentration >15 million/mL). Mean IIEF score was lowest in group 1 (18.78 vs. 22.64 vs. 26.45). Likewise, group 1 had the lowest mean testosterone level (2.66 nmol/L vs. 3.46 nmol/L vs. 5.21 nmol/L). Lower mean IIEF scores were observed in males with low sperm morphology and motility. Medical treatment for males with ED not only enhances erection but also helps in the improvement of semen parameters.[93]

Clinicians should pay careful attention during early diagnosis of males with ED to select appropriate interventions. This will help them to improve their quality of life and achieve good reproductive outcome.

Retrograde Ejaculation

Aspermia, or dry ejaculate, is characterized as a complete absence of expulsion of seminal fluid out of the urethral meatus.[94] This is further categorized as lack of emission, called anejaculation or ejaculation failure in an antegrade direction, called retrograde ejaculation (RE). Several neurotransmitters play an important role in the physiology of ejaculation; however, exact mechanisms have yet to be studied. RE accounts for 0.4% to 2.0% of causes of MFI.[95] There are varied etiologies of males with RE. These include idiopathic causes, congenital abnormalities, diabetes mellitus, spinal cord injury, bladder neck surgeries, and RPLND.[96]

The diagnosis of RE is established when 10 to 15 sperm per high-power field are present in the postejaculatory urine (PEU) after centrifugation.[96] Infertile males with RE may be managed with sympathomimetics, alkalinization of urine with or without urethral catheterization, induced ejaculation, and sperm retrieval.[13] Several well-known medical therapies are used for males with RE; however, there is still no clear consensus on their use and efficacy. In a study of 20 males medically treated with pseudoephedrine 60 mg every

6 hours on the day before the semen collection and 2 × 60 mg on the day of semen collection, sperm were recovered in an antegrade ejaculation in 58.3% of patients, in which 10 males (50%) achieved an antegrade total sperm count of more than 39 million.[97]

There are several techniques for sperm retrieval in males with RE.[98] These include ejaculation on a full bladder, Hotchkiss technique, and centrifugation and resuspension of PEU samples. Using a modified Hotchkiss technique wherein a sterile culture medium is instilled into the urinary bladder via catheterization while sperm retrieval is achieved by masturbation, 63 males with RE were able to bank their sperm, which were used for ICSI cycles.[99] Nine clinical pregnancies were achieved in six couples, resulting in an average live birth rate of 28% per transfer.

CLINICAL SCENARIOS

CASE 1

A 39-year-old male came to the clinic due to azoospermia. He has a new 25-year-old female partner with a normal evaluation. He had a vasectomy 9 years ago. Sperm granuloma was noted on the right side, and an indurated epididymis was palpated on the left. He underwent microsurgical VR. Intraoperatively, upon transection of the right VD, expressed fluid showed multiple motile sperm, and VV was performed. Toothpaste like vasal fluid was appreciated from the left VD that revealed absence of sperm; subsequently, VE was performed. This resulted in a natural conception 8 months after the surgery, and a healthy baby boy was safely delivered.

CASE 2

A 34-year-old male was referred by a colleague due to azoospermia. History revealed recurrent chest symptoms. Physical examination revealed no palpable VD on either side, with only epididymal heads appreciated. *CFTR* testing showed positive for mutation. He underwent MESA. They were able to retrieve multiple motile sperm. This was followed by IVF/ICSI, which resulted in conception and delivery of healthy offspring.

CASE 3

A 36-year-old diabetic male presented in the clinic due to anejaculation. Both testes were normal in size, with palpable bilateral VD and epididymis. Total testosterone and FSH were at normal levels. TRUS was likewise unremarkable. PEU showed presence of 15 sperm per high-power field. Pharmacologic treatment was unsuccessful in extruding seminal fluid after ejaculation. The Hotchkiss method was done. The semen sample retrieved was centrifuged and resuspended and was used for IVF/ICSI.

SUMMARY

Several etiologies of MFI are posttesticular in origin. These causes are mainly due to obstruction along the reproductive tract or sexual dysfunctions such as RE and erectile dysfunction. Obstruction can precipitate from congenital, acquired, or idiopathic causes. Gene mutations and Wolffian duct malformations constitute the congenital causes, while vasectomy, infection, and iatrogenic injuries are the known acquired causes. Some causes remain idiopathic. In general, males with posttesticular causes of infertility have normal spermatogenesis. For males who are infertile due to seminal tract obstruction, sperm retrieval with ART or microsurgical reconstruction are valuable treatment options. Technically challenging surgeries such as VV and VE can translate into natural conception if done correctly. Sperm harvest during surgical reconstruction is a reasonable option as well. Surgical procedures for obstruction due to iatrogenic injuries and infections are technically challenging due to extensive scarring and fibrosis. The surgeon's skill and patient factors should be considered as predictors that can affect successful outcomes such as patency, pregnancy, and live birth. An extensive preoperative evaluation is warranted to help ensure that the patient has the best chance of restoring his reproductive capacity. Males with sexual dysfunction can be initially managed with medications, while others need to undergo assisted reproduction. Reproductive specialists who are familiar with recent advances of obstruction management will be best able to provide guidance in the shared decision making of these infertile patients.

REFERENCES

1. Vander Borght M, Wyns C. Fertility and infertility: definition and epidemiology. *Clin Biochem.* 2018;62:2-10.
2. Agarwal A, Mulgund A, Hamada A, et al. A unique view on male infertility around the globe. *Reprod Biol Endocrinol.* 2015;13:37.
3. Neto FT, Bach PV, Najari BB, et al. Spermatogenesis in humans and its affecting factors. *Semin Cell Dev Biol.* 2016;59:10-26.
4. Dimitriadis F, Adonakis G, Kaponis A, et al. Pre-testicular, testicular, and post-testicular causes of male infertility. In: Simoni M, Huhtaniemi I, eds. *Endocrinology of the Testis and Male Reproduction. Endocrinology.* Cham: Springer; 2017:981-1027.
5. Agarwal A, Baskaran S, Parekh N, et al. Male infertility. *Lancet.* 2021;397(10271):319-333.
6. Puppo V, Puppo G. Comprehensive review of the anatomy and physiology of male ejaculation: premature ejaculation is not a disease. *Clin Anat.* 2016;29(1):111-119.
7. Clement P, Giuliano F. Physiology and pharmacology of ejaculation. *Basic Clin Pharmacol Toxicol.* 2016;119 (suppl 3):18-25.
8. MacDonald SM, Burnett AL. Physiology of erection and pathophysiology of erectile dysfunction. *Urol Clin North Am.* 2021;48(4):513-525.
9. Practice Committee of the American Society for Reproductive Medicine in collaboration with the Society for Male Reproduction and Urology. The management of obstructive azoospermia: a committee opinion. *Fertil Steril.* 2019;111(5):873-880.
10. Jarow JP, Espeland MA, Lipshultz LI. Evaluation of the azoospermic patient. *J Urol.* 1989;142(1):62-65.
11. Schlegel PN, Sigman M, Collura B, et al. Diagnosis and treatment of infertility in men: AUA/ASRM guideline part I. *Fertil Steril.* 2021;115(1):54-61.
12. Minhas S, Bettocchi C, Boeri L, et al. European Association of Urology Guidelines on male sexual and reproductive health: 2021 update on male infertility. *Eur Urol.* 2021;80(5):603-620.
13. Schlegel PN, Sigman M, Collura B, et al. Diagnosis and treatment of infertility in men: AUA/ASRM guideline part II. *Fertil Steril.* 2021;115(1):62-69.
14. Bieth E, Hamdi SM, Mieusset R. Genetics of the congenital absence of the vas deferens. *Hum Genet.* 2021;140(1): 59-76.
15. de Souza DAS, Faucz FR, Pereira-Ferrari L, Sotomaior VS, Raskin S. Congenital bilateral absence of the vas deferens as an atypical form of cystic fibrosis: reproductive implications and genetic counseling. *Andrology.* 2018; 6(1):127-135.

16. Yu J, Chen Z, Ni Y, et al. CFTR mutations in men with congenital bilateral absence of the vas deferens (CBAVD): a systemic review and meta-analysis. *Hum Reprod.* 2012; 27(1):25-35.

17. Wong R, Gu K, Ko Y, et al. Congenital absence of the vas deferens: cystic fibrosis transmembrane regulatory gene mutations. *Best Pract Res Clin Endocrinol Metab.* 2020; 34(6):101476.

18. Cui X, Wu X, Li Q, et al. Mutations of the cystic fibrosis transmembrane conductance regulator gene in males with congenital bilateral absence of the vas deferens: reproductive implications and genetic counseling (Review). *Mol Med Rep.* 2020;22(5):3587-3596.

19. Ferlin A, Stuppia L. Diagnostics of CFTR-negative patients with congenital bilateral absence of vas deferens: which mutations are of most interest? *Expert Rev Mol Diagn.* 2020;20(3):265-267.

20. Cioppi F, Rosta V, Krausz C. Genetics of azoospermia. *Int J Mol Sci.* 2021;22(6):3264.

21. Li L, Liang C. Ultrasonography in diagnosis of congenital absence of the vas deferens. *Med Sci Monit.* 2016;22:2643-2647.

22. Liu J, Wang Z, Zhou M, et al. Scrotal ultrasonic features of congenital bilateral absence of vas deferens. *Ultrasound Q.* 2017;33(2):153-156.

23. Persily JB, Vijay V, Najari BB. How do we counsel men with obstructive azoospermia due to CF mutations?-a review of treatment options and outcomes. *Transl Androl Urol.* 2021;10(3):1467-1478.

24. McBride JA, Kohn TP, Mazur DJ, et al. Sperm retrieval and intracytoplasmic sperm injection outcomes in men with cystic fibrosis disease versus congenital bilateral absence of the vas deferens. *Asian J Androl.* 2021;23(2):140-145.

25. Miller S, Couture S, James G, et al. Unilateral absence of vas deferens: prevalence among 23.013 men seeking vasectomy. *Int Braz J Urol.* 2016;42(5):1010-1017.

26. Weiske WH, Sälzler N, Schroeder-Printzen I, et al. Clinical findings in congenital absence of the vasa deferentia. *Andrologia.* 2000;32(1):13-18.

27. Cai H, Qing X, Niringiyumukiza JD, et al. CFTR variants and renal abnormalities in males with congenital unilateral absence of the vas deferens (CUAVD): a systematic review and meta-analysis of observational studies. *Genet Med.* 2019;21(4):826-836.

28. Mieusset R, Fauquet I, Chauveau D, et al. The spectrum of renal involvement in male patients with infertility related to excretory-system abnormalities: phenotypes, genotypes, and genetic counseling. *J Nephrol.* 2017;30(2): 211-218.

29. Raviv G, Mor Y, Levron J, et al. Role of transrectal ultrasonography in the evaluation of azoospermic men with low-volume ejaculate. *J Ultrasound Med.* 2006;25(7):825-829.

30. Brusq C, Mieusset R, Hamdi SM. Development of a multivariable prediction model for congenital unilateral absence of the vas deferens in male partners of infertile couples. *Andrology.* 2022;10(2):262-269.

31. Arya AK, Beer HL, Benton J, et al. Does Young's syndrome exist? *J Laryngol Otol.* 2009;123(5):477-481.

32. Goeminne PC, Dupont LJ. The sinusitis-infertility syndrome: Young's saint, old devil. *Eur Respir J.* 2010;35(3):698.

33. Sangeeta A, Karande S, Limaye C, et al. Young syndrome. *Bombay Hosp J.* 2011;53(3):672-673.

34. Mohammed SK, Jan A. Young syndrome. In: *StatPearls.* Treasure Island, FL: StatPearls Publishing; December 22, 2020.

35. Modgil V, Rai S, Ralph DJ, et al. An update on the diagnosis and management of ejaculatory duct obstruction. *Nat Rev Urol.* 2016;13(1):13-20.

36. Avellino GJ, Lipshultz LI, Sigman M, et al. Transurethral resection of the ejaculatory ducts: etiology of obstruction and surgical treatment options. *Fertil Steril.* 2019; 111(3):427-443.

37. Sharma V, Le BV, Sheth KR, et al. Vasectomy demographics and postvasectomy desire for future children: results from a contemporary national survey. *Fertil Steril.* 2013; 99(7):1880-1885.

38. Pryor JP, Hendry WF. Ejaculatory duct obstruction in subfertile males: analysis of 87 patients. *Fertil Steril.* 1991;56(4):725-730.

39. Purohit RS, Wu DS, Shinohara K, et al. A prospective comparison of 3 diagnostic methods to evaluate ejaculatory duct obstruction. *J Urol.* 2004;171(1):232-235; discussion 235-236.

40. Sávio LF, Palmer J, Prakash NS, et al. Transurethral resection of ejaculatory ducts: a step-by-step guide. *Fertil Steril.* 2017;107(6):e20.

41. Mekhaimar A, Goble M, Brunckhorst O, et al. A systematic review of transurethral resection of ejaculatory ducts for the management of ejaculatory duct obstruction. *Turk J Urol.* 2020;46(5):335-347.

42. Sigman M. Iatrogenic male infertility: medical and surgical treatments that impair male fertility. *Fertil Steril.* 2021; 116(3):609-610.

43. Kadioglu A, Cayan S, Tefekli A, et al. Does response to treatment of ejaculatory duct obstruction in infertile men vary with pathology? *Fertil Steril.* 2001;76(1):138-142.

44. Eisenberg ML, Lipshultz LI. Estimating the number of vasectomies performed annually in the United States: data from the National Survey of Family Growth. *J Urol.* 2010;184(5):2068-2072.

45. Kordzadeh A, Liu MO, Jayanthi NV. Male infertility following inguinal hernia repair: a systematic review and pooled analysis. *Hernia.* 2017;21(1):1-7.

46. Henkel R. Long-term consequences of sexually transmitted infections on men's sexual function: a systematic review. *Arab J Urol.* 2021;19(3):411-418.

47. Peng J, Yuan Y, Cui W, et al. Causes of suspected epididymal obstruction in Chinese men. *Urology.* 2012;80(6):1258-1261.

48. Andino JJ, Gonzalez DC, Dupree JM, et al. Challenges in completing a successful vasectomy reversal. *Andrologia.* 2021;53(6):e14066.

49. Dubin JM, White J, Ory J, et al. Vasectomy reversal vs. sperm retrieval with in vitro fertilization: a contemporary, comparative analysis. *Fertil Steril.* 2021;115(6):1377-1383.

50. Brannigan RE. Vasectomy and vasectomy reversal: a comprehensive approach to the evolving spectrum of care. *Fertil Steril.* 2021;115(6):1363-1364.

51. Cheng PJ, Kim J, Craig JR, et al. "The back-up vasectomy reversal." Simultaneous sperm retrieval and vasectomy reversal in the couple with advanced maternal age: a cost-effectiveness analysis. *Urology.* 2021;153:175-180.

52. Patel AP, Smith RP. Vasectomy reversal: a clinical update. *Asian J Androl.* 2016;18(3):365-371.

53. Elzanaty S, Dohle GR. Vasovasostomy and predictors of vasal patency: a systematic review. *Scand J Urol Nephrol.* 2012;46(4):241-246.

54. Ostrowski KA, Polackwich AS, Kent J, et al. Higher outcomes of vasectomy reversal in men with the same female partner as before vasectomy. *J Urol.* 2015;193(1):245-247.

55. Nusbaum DJ, Marks SF, Marks MBF, et al. The effect of male age over 50 years on vasectomy reversal outcomes. *Urology.* 2020;145:134-140.

56. Ory J, Nackeeran S, Blankstein U, et al. Predictors of success after bilateral epididymovasostomy performed during vasectomy reversal: a multi-institutional analysis *Can Urol Assoc J.* 2022;16(3):E132-E136.

57. Fantus RJ, Halpern JA. Vasovasostomy and vasoepididymostomy: indications, operative technique, and outcomes. *Fertil Steril.* 2021;115(6):1384-1392.

58. Marconi M, Pilatz A, Wagenlehner F, et al. Impact of infection on the secretory capacity of the male accessory glands. *Int Braz J Urol.* 2009;35(3):299-309.

59. Schuppe HC, Pilatz A, Hossain H, et al. Urogenital infection as a risk factor for male infertility. *Dtsch Arztebl Int.* 2017;114(19):339-346.

60. Berardinucci D, Zini A, Jarvi K. Outcome of microsurgical reconstruction in men with suspected epididymal obstruction. *J Urol.* 1998;159(3):831-834.

61. Marshall FF, Chang T, Vindivich D. Microsurgical vasoepididymostomy to corpus epididymidis in treatment of inflammatory obstructive azoospermia. *Urology.* 1987;30(6):565-567.

62. Hill SA, Masters TL, Wachter J. Gonorrhea - an evolving disease of the new millennium. *Microb Cell.* 2016;3(9):371-389.

63. Han H, Liu S, Zhou XG, et al. Aetiology of obstructive azoospermia in Chinese infertility patients. *Andrologia.* 2016;48(7):761-764.

64. Chemaitelly H, Majed A, Abu-Hijleh F, et al. Global epidemiology of *Neisseria gonorrhoeae* in infertile populations: systematic review, meta-analysis and metaregression. *Sex Transm Infect.* 2021;97(2):157-169.

65. Chen XF, Chen B, Liu W, et al. Microsurgical vasoepididymostomy for patients with infectious obstructive azoospermia: cause, outcome, and associated factors. *Asian J Androl.* 2016;18(5):759-762.

66. Moon SY, Kim SH, Jee BC, et al. The outcome of sperm retrieval and intracytoplasmic sperm injection in patients with obstructive azoospermia: impact of previous tuberculous epididymitis. *J Assist Reprod Genet.* 1999;16(8):431-435.

67. Huang Z, Berg WT. Iatrogenic effects of radical cancer surgery on male fertility. *Fertil Steril.* 2021;116(3):625-629.

68. Rutkow IM. Surgical operations in the United States. Then (1983) and now (1994). *Arch Surg.* 1997;132(9):983-990.

69. Wang J, Liu Q, Zhang Y, et al. Treatment for vas deferens obstruction following childhood herniorrhaphy. *Urology.* 2018;112:80-84.

70. Sheynkin YR, Hendin BN, Schlegel PN, et al. Microsurgical repair of iatrogenic injury to the vas deferens. *J Urol.* 1998;159(1):139-141.

71. Shin D, Lipshultz LI, Goldstein M, et al. Herniorrhaphy with polypropylene mesh causing inguinal vasal obstruction: a preventable cause of obstructive azoospermia. *Ann Surg.* 2005;241(4):553-558.

72. Bouchot O, Branchereau J, Perrouin-Verbe MA. Influence of inguinal hernia repair on male fertility. *J Visc Surg.* 2018;155(suppl 1):S37-S40.

73. Dong Z, Kujawa SA, Wang C, et al. Does the use of hernia mesh in surgical inguinal hernia repairs cause male infertility? A systematic review and descriptive analysis. *Reprod Health.* 2018;15(1):69.

74. Jiang HT, Yuan Q, Liu Y, et al. Multiple advanced surgical techniques to treat acquired seminal duct obstruction. *Asian J Androl.* 2014;16(6):912-916.

75. Wang T, Yu Z, Liu Z, et al. Intra-abdominal robot-assisted vasovasostomy of obstructive azoospermia in an Asian population following multiple bilateral inguinal herniorrhaphy in childhood: a case report and literature review. *Transl Androl Urol.* 2021;10(6):2521-2527.

76. Lardas M, Liew M, van den Bergh RC, et al. Quality of life outcomes after primary treatment for clinically localised prostate cancer: a systematic review. *Eur Urol.* 2017;72(6):869-885.

77. Chehab M, Madala A, Trussell JC. On-label and off-label drugs used in the treatment of male infertility. *Fertil Steril.* 2015;103(3):595-604.

78. Chan PT, Lee R, Li PS, et al. Six years of experience with microsurgical longitudinal intussusception vasoepididy-mostomy (LIVE): a prospective analysis. *J Urol.* 2008; 179(4):591-592.

79. Kumar R, Mukherjee S, Gupta NP. Intussusception vaso-epididymostomy with longitudinal suture placement for idiopathic obstructive azoospermia. *J Urol.* 2010;183(4):1489-1492.

80. Gupta R, Singh P, Kumar R. Should men with idiopathic obstructive azoospermia be screened for genitourinary tuberculosis? *J Hum Reprod Sci.* 2015;8(1):43-47.

81. Revenig L, Leung A, Hsiao W. Ejaculatory physiology and pathophysiology: assessment and treatment in male infertility. *Transl Androl Urol.* 2014;3(1):41-49.

82. Giuliano F, Clément P. Physiology of ejaculation: emphasis on serotonergic control. *Eur Urol.* 2005; 48(3):408-417.

83. Gabr AA, Omran EF, Abdallah AA, et al. Prevalence of sexual dysfunction in infertile versus fertile couples. *Eur J Obstet Gynecol Reprod Biol.* 2017;217:38-43.

84. Mazzilli R, Defeudis G, Olana S, et al. The role of ejaculatory dysfunction on male infertility. *Clin Ter.* 2020; 171(6):e523-e527.

85. Practice Committee of the American Society for Reproductive Medicine in Collaboration with the Society for Male Reproduction and Urology. Diagnostic evaluation of sexual dysfunction in the male partner in the setting of infertility: a committee opinion. *Fertil Steril.* 2018; 110(5):833-837.

86. Salonia A, Bettocchi C, Boeri L, et al. European Association of Urology Guidelines on sexual and reproductive health-2021 update: male sexual dysfunction. *Eur Urol.* 2021;80(3):333-357.

87. Mulhall JP, Goldstein I, Bushmakin AG, et al. Validation of the erection hardness score. *J Sex Med.* 2007;4(6): 1626-1634.

88. Capogrosso P, Jensen CFS, Rastrelli G, et al. Male sexual dysfunctions in the infertile couple-recommendations from the European Society of Sexual Medicine (ESSM). *Sex Med.* 2021;9(3):100377.

89. Lotti F, Maggi M. Sexual dysfunction and male infertility. *Nat Rev Urol.* 2018;15(5):287-307.

90. Ma J, Zhang Y, Bao B, et al. Prevalence and associated factors of erectile dysfunction, psychological disorders, and sexual performance in primary vs. secondary infertility men. *Reprod Biol Endocrinol.* 2021;19(1):43.

91. Lotti F, Corona G, Castellini G, et al. Semen quality impairment is associated with sexual dysfunction according to its severity. *Hum Reprod.* 2016;31(12):2668-2680.

92. Kızılay F, Şahin M, Altay B. Do sperm parameters and infertility affect sexuality of couples? *Andrologia.* 2018; 50(2):e12879. doi:10.1111/and.12879.

93. Dong L, Zhang X, Yan X, et al. Effect of phosphodiesterase-5 inhibitors on the treatment of male infertility: a systematic review and meta-analysis. *World J Mens Health.* 2021;39(4):776-796.

94. Mehta A, Sigman M. Management of the dry ejaculate: a systematic review of aspermia and retrograde ejaculation. *Fertil Steril.* 2015;104(5):1074-1081.

95. Yavetz H, Yogev L, Hauser R, et al. Retrograde ejaculation. *Hum Reprod.* 1994;9(3):381-386.

96. Jefferys A, Siassakos D, Wardle P. The management of retrograde ejaculation: a systematic review and update. *Fertil Steril.* 2012;97(2):306-312.

97. Shoshany O, Abhyankar N, Elyaguov J, et al. Efficacy of treatment with pseudoephedrine in men with retrograde ejaculation. *Andrology.* 2017;5(4):744-748.

98. Gupta S, Sharma R, Agarwal A, et al. A comprehensive guide to sperm recovery in infertile men with retrograde ejaculation. *World J Mens Health.* 2021;39:e29.

99. Philippon M, Karsenty G, Bernuz B, et al. Successful pregnancies and healthy live births using frozen-thawed sperm retrieved by a new modified Hotchkiss procedure in males with retrograde ejaculation: first case series. *Basic Clin Androl.* 2015;25:5.

5

Environmental/Lifestyle Factors and Male Infertility

Pallav Sengupta, Sulagna Dutta,
Damayanthi Durairajanayagam, and Ashok Agarwal

KEY POINTS

- Exposure to xenobiotics, including phthalates, bisphenol A, and polychlorinated biphenyls, contributes to aberrant spermatogenesis and diminished male fertility.
- Cumulative detriments of smoking, alcohol consumption, and recreational drug use induce oxidative stress and perturb semen parameters.
- Excessive adiposity, strenuous physical exercise, and elevated scrotal temperatures elicit deleterious effects on sperm parameters, including reduced sperm concentration and compromised sperm quality.

- Chronic psychological stress and advanced paternal age engender telomere attrition, DNA fragmentation, and epigenetic modifications, culminating in male infertility.
- Imbalanced dietary habits, excessive caffeine intake, and inadequate micronutrient consumption impinge on semen quality and sperm function.

INTRODUCTION

Infertility, defined as the inability to achieve conception after 1 year of regular, unprotected intercourse, is a pervasive issue that affects 8% to 12% of couples globally.[1,2] Male infertility contributes to approximately 50% of these cases, with diverse etiological factors, including genetic, environmental, and lifestyle factors.[3–5] These factors can be categorized as modifiable or nonmodifiable, and their effects can be influenced by the time of exposure during the lifecycle of a male. Understanding these factors and their potential impact is essential for developing effective strategies to prevent or manage male infertility.[3,5] The modifiable risk factors for male infertility (Fig. 5.1) include lifestyle and environmental factors such as smoking, alcohol consumption, drug abuse, obesity, and exposure to environmental toxins such as pesticides and heavy metals.[6] These factors can disrupt spermatogenesis, impair sperm function and quality, and increase the risk of DNA damage.[7,8] Nonmodifiable risk factors include genetics, age, and medical conditions such as varicocele, cryptorchidism, and testicular cancer.[9] These factors can also impact the production and quality of sperm and affect male fertility.[6,10]

Duration of exposure to environmental or lifestyle risk factors is crucial and can have varying effects on male fertility. Exposure during the gestational period can lead to structural abnormalities of the fetal reproductive system and cause impaired spermatogenesis in adulthood.[11,12] Prepubertal exposure can affect the onset of puberty and subsequently reduce fertility potential, while exposure as an adult can cause direct damage to sperm and affect their motility, morphology, and DNA integrity.[13]

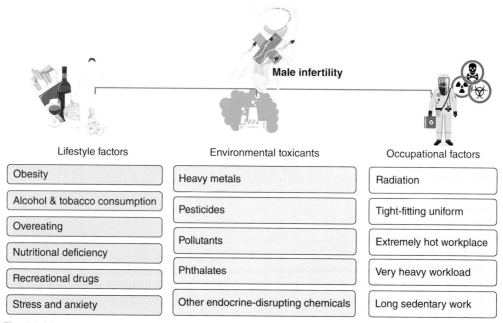

Fig. 5.1 Major lifestyle, environmental, and occupational factors with the potential to cause male infertility.

This chapter aims to provide an updated understanding of the impact of environmental and lifestyle factors on male infertility. The chapter will explore the effects of various modifiable and nonmodifiable risk factors and their potential impact on male fertility. Additionally, it will discuss the current clinical utility of data and provide an overview of the latest research on the prevention and management of male infertility. Overall, this chapter provides a comprehensive review of the current understanding of male infertility risk factors, their effects, and the potential implications of exposure to these factors at different stages of the male lifecycle. This information is crucial for developing effective strategies to prevent or manage male infertility and improve male reproductive health.

ENVIRONMENTAL/OCCUPATIONAL FACTORS AND MALE INFERTILITY

Potential Exposure Routes for Environmental/Occupational Factors

In recent years, male infertility has become a significant public health issue globally.[3] Lifestyle and occupational exposures have been identified as significant contributors to male infertility.[6,8] Exposure to environmental toxins through oral, inhalation, and dermal routes can affect male fertility by damaging the testes, disrupting hormone levels, and reducing sperm quality.[8]

Oral exposure to environmental toxins is a significant risk factor for male infertility. The consumption of contaminated food and water sources is one of the most common ways that these toxins enter the body.[14] The toxins can be derived from several sources, including pesticides, herbicides, heavy metals, and plasticizers.[15] Pesticides and herbicides, for example, can cause damage to the testes and reduce sperm count and motility.[8,16] Exposure to heavy metals, such as lead (Pb), cadmium (Cd), and mercury (Hg), can also cause significant damage to the testes and disrupt hormone levels in the body.[8,17] Plasticizers, such as phthalates, can mimic the action of estrogen in the body, leading to hormonal imbalances and reducing sperm quality. Inhalation exposure is another significant route of exposure to environmental toxins that can affect male fertility. Air pollution is a major contributor to inhalation exposure, with industrial emissions, vehicular exhaust, and indoor air pollution being the most common sources. Exposure to air pollutants can lead to oxidative stress (OS), inflammation, and hormonal imbalances, which

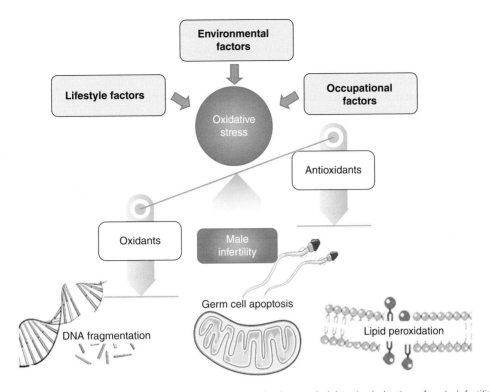

Fig. 5.2 Oxidative stress plays a central role in the mechanism underlying the induction of male infertility through lifestyle, environmental, and occupational factors.

can affect male fertility (Fig. 5.2). Polycyclic aromatic hydrocarbons (PAHs), for example, are a group of air pollutants that can reduce sperm count and motility. Exposure to nitrogen oxides (NOx) and particulate matter (PM) can also affect sperm quality and reduce fertility. Dermal exposure to environmental toxins is another route of exposure that can affect male fertility. Skin contact with contaminated soil, water, and consumer products can lead to the absorption of toxic chemicals into the body. Exposure to chemicals such as pesticides, solvents, and heavy metals can cause damage to the testes and reduce sperm quality. Certain consumer products, such as cosmetics, personal care products, and cleaning agents, can also contain chemicals that can disrupt hormone levels and reduce fertility.

Occupational exposure is a significant risk factor for male infertility. Males working in industries such as agriculture, manufacturing, construction, and transportation are at increased risk of exposure to environmental toxins. Pesticides and herbicides, heavy metals, solvents, and diesel exhaust are common occupational exposures

that can affect male fertility. Exposure to pesticides and herbicides has been associated with reduced sperm count and motility, while exposure to Pb, Cd, and Hg can damage the testes and disrupt hormone levels. Solvents, such as benzene and toluene, can also reduce sperm count and motility. Diesel exhaust contains a complex mixture of chemicals, including PAHs and NOx, which can reduce fertility.

Strategies to reduce exposure to these toxins, such as improving air quality, regulating pesticide use, and reducing occupational exposures, are essential to address this growing health concern. Additionally, further research is needed to better understand the mechanisms by which environmental toxins affect male fertility and to develop effective interventions to mitigate these effects.

Organochlorine Compounds

In recent years, a growing body of evidence has implicated organochlorine compounds (OCs) as potential contributors to male infertility.[18–20] These lipophilic, recalcitrant compounds, found in a variety of industrial and agricultural settings, pose significant health risks due to their persistence and bioaccumulation in the environment. OCs encompass a broad range of anthropogenic chemicals, including polychlorinated biphenyls (PCBs), dichlorodiphenyltrichloroethane (DDT), and hexachlorobenzene, among others.[15] These environmental pollutants have been linked to an array of detrimental health consequences, including endocrine disruption, neurotoxicity, and carcinogenicity.[21] The impact of OCs on male fertility has gained particular attention due to their potential endocrine-disrupting properties, which have been associated with decreased semen quality, impaired sperm function, and altered hormone levels in males.[19,22,23]

Epidemiological studies have revealed a significant association between OC exposure and reduced semen quality, including diminished sperm concentration, motility, and morphology.[20,24] A metaanalysis conducted by Toft et al. (2006) demonstrated a significant negative correlation between serum concentrations of DDT and its metabolites and sperm motility and morphology.[25] Similarly, Hauser et al. (2003) observed an inverse relationship between PCB exposure and sperm motility in a cohort of males from a fishing community.[26] This decline in semen quality could be attributed to various mechanisms, including OS, DNA damage, and perturbation of spermatogenesis.

OCs can induce the generation of reactive oxygen species (ROS) in spermatozoa, leading to OS. OS is characterized by an imbalance between ROS production and antioxidant defense mechanisms, which can result in lipid peroxidation, protein oxidation, and DNA damage.[5,27] The high polyunsaturated fatty acid content in the sperm plasma membrane renders spermatozoa particularly susceptible to oxidative damage. Excessive ROS production has been linked to impaired sperm function, including reduced motility, compromised membrane integrity, and impaired fertilizing capacity.[5] In addition, DNA damage is another critical factor that can compromise male fertility.[7] OCs have been shown to induce DNA damage in spermatozoa through direct interaction with DNA molecules or indirectly via the production of ROS.[24] Studies have revealed that males with higher serum concentrations of PCBs and DDT display increased levels of sperm DNA damage, as assessed by the Comet assay.[28,29] Moreover, DNA damage in spermatozoa has been associated with reduced fertilization

rates, impaired embryo development, and an increased risk of miscarriage and congenital anomalies.[30,31]

OCs also exert their endocrine-disrupting effects via a panoply of mechanisms, including agonism or antagonism of steroid hormone receptors, modulation of steroid biosynthesis and metabolism, and perturbation of the hypothalamic-pituitary-gonadal (HPG) axis.[32,33] Accumulating evidence delineates the association between organochlorine exposure and male reproductive pathologies such as cryptorchidism, hypospadias, and testicular dysgenesis syndrome.[34] Furthermore, a spate of epidemiological studies indicates the potential for transgenerational epigenetic inheritance, whereby paternal exposure to organochlorines may propagate adverse effects to subsequent generations.[34] Given the gravity of the situation, elucidating the molecular pathways and epigenetic mechanisms underpinning organochlorine-induced endocrine disruption remains a high-priority research area. Additionally, regulatory measures to curtail the production and dissemination of OCs, as well as the development of efficacious remediation strategies, are imperative to mitigate the ramifications of these insidious environmental contaminants on human health and ecosystems.

Organophosphorus Compounds

The detrimental influence of organophosphorus compounds (OPs) on male fertility has garnered significant attention in recent years. These organic compounds, primarily utilized as pesticides, are often associated with neurological and physiological disorders.[35] OPs comprise a broad class of organophosphates and organothiophosphates characterized by the presence of a phosphorus atom bonded to one or more carbon atoms.[36] The ubiquity of OPs, particularly as insecticides, herbicides, and fungicides in agricultural practices, raises concerns over their potential impact on human health.[35] There is accumulating evidence suggesting that exposure to OPs may adversely affect male fertility, contributing to a growing global health issue.[37]

The pathophysiological mechanisms of OP-induced male infertility are complex and multifaceted, involving OS, endocrine disruption, and interference with spermatogenesis.[38] OPs exert their toxic effects by inhibiting acetylcholinesterase (AChE), an enzyme responsible for the hydrolysis of the neurotransmitter acetylcholine (ACh).[39] Inhibition of AChE leads to the accumulation of ACh in the synaptic cleft, overstimulating the cholinergic receptors and resulting in neurotoxicity.[39] Furthermore, OPs have been shown to induce OS in testicular tissue by generating ROS and impairing the antioxidant defense system.[40] The excessive production of ROS can cause lipid peroxidation, DNA damage, and protein oxidation, ultimately affecting sperm function and viability (Fig. 5.3).[5]

OPs are known to possess endocrine-disrupting properties, as they can interfere with the HPG axis, thereby disrupting the hormonal milieu necessary for normal testicular function.[40] OPs can modulate the synthesis, secretion, and metabolism of key hormones, such as gonadotropin-releasing hormone (GnRH), luteinizing hormone (LH), follicle-stimulating hormone (FSH), and testosterone.[41] Disruption of the HPG axis can result in impaired spermatogenesis and altered sperm parameters, including reduced sperm count, motility, and morphology.[41]

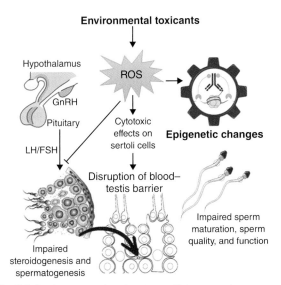

Fig. 5.3 Environmental toxicants mediate excessive generation of reactive oxygen species (ROS) and subsequent endocrine, molecular, and epigenetic disruption of reproductive tissues. ROS can interfere with the reproductive regulations of the hypothalamo-pituitary-testicular axis, thereby hindering the release of gonadotropin-releasing hormone (GnRH) as well as luteinizing hormone (LH) and follicle-stimulating hormone (FSH). These in turn impair normal steroidogenesis and spermatogenesis in the Leydig cells and Sertoli cells, respectively. Environmental toxicants may also disrupt the blood-brain barrier via the cytotoxic effects of ROS upon the Sertoli cells. Moreover, ROS may induce genetic and epigenetic changes in the sperm, thereby altering sperm quality and function.

OPs can directly affect germ cells and Sertoli cells, which play crucial roles in the process of spermatogenesis.[42] OP exposure can lead to germ cell apoptosis, disruption of the blood–testis barrier (BTB), and alterations in the expression of genes involved in spermatogenesis, such as protamine and transition protein genes. These molecular perturbations can manifest as decreased sperm production, impaired sperm maturation, and increased sperm DNA fragmentation.[42]

Carbamates

Carbamates, a class of organic compounds, have attracted significant attention due to their widespread application as pesticides in agriculture. Recent studies have elucidated the potential association between carbamate exposure and male infertility, raising concerns about their impact on human reproductive health.[43] Carbamates are a group of organic compounds derived from carbamic acid, characterized by the presence of a carbamate functional group (R-O-C(=O)-NR'-R").[44] They have been extensively used as insecticides, fungicides, and herbicides due to their ability to inhibit AChE activity in pests. However, growing evidence suggests that these compounds may also adversely affect human health, particularly by contributing to male infertility.[43,44]

The potential impact of carbamates on male fertility has become a significant area of concern, necessitating a thorough examination of the molecular mechanisms underlying this relationship.[43] Carbamate exposure has been shown to impair spermatozoa function, which is crucial for successful fertilization. Multiple *in vitro* and *in vivo* studies have reported a dose-dependent reduction in sperm motility, viability, and count upon exposure to carbamates.[45,46] The impairment of spermatozoa function can be attributed to (1) *AChE inhibition:* carbamates target AChE, an enzyme that hydrolyzes ACh, a neurotransmitter involved in the regulation of sperm motility. Inhibition of AChE results in the accumulation of ACh, leading to aberrant activation of cholinergic receptors and subsequent disruption of sperm motility[39]; (2) *disruption of sperm membrane integrity:* carbamates can interact with the phospholipid bilayer of the sperm plasma membrane, altering its structural integrity and fluidity. This interaction may compromise the membrane's selective permeability, leading to an influx of ions and water, which can ultimately cause osmotic imbalance and spermatozoa dysfunction;[46] and (3) *interference with sperm metabolism:* carbamates have been reported to interfere with sperm energy metabolism by inhibiting enzymes involved in glycolysis and oxidative phosphorylation. The resulting energy deficit impairs the sperm's ability to generate the adenosine triphosphate required for motility and other vital processes.[47]

Carbamates have also been identified as potential endocrine-disrupting chemicals (EDCs), which can interfere with the body's hormonal balance and impair reproductive function.[43,45] These compounds may disrupt the HPG axis, which plays a critical role in regulating male fertility by controlling the production and secretion of key reproductive hormones.[43]

Xenoestrogens (Bisphenol A)

Xenoestrogens are a group of EDCs that mimic or modulate the actions of endogenous estrogens, exerting disruptive effects on the endocrine system.[5,16] Bisphenol A (BPA) is a ubiquitous xenoestrogen, commonly found in polycarbonate plastics, epoxy resins, and thermal paper receipts.[16] Despite its widespread use, a growing body of evidence has implicated BPA in various adverse health outcomes, with a significant focus on its role in male infertility.[48]

BPA exhibits estrogenic activity by binding to estrogen receptors (ERs), namely ERα, ERβ, and the G protein-coupled estrogen receptor.[49] Upon binding, BPA alters the transcription of estrogen-responsive genes, resulting in dysregulated hormone synthesis and signaling. In males, this disruption can lead to reduced testosterone levels and increased estradiol production, contributing to an altered hormonal milieu detrimental to spermatogenesis.[49]

BPA exposure has also been linked to increased production of ROS, leading to OS in the male reproductive system.[50] This oxidative damage impairs sperm membrane integrity, alters sperm motility, and induces DNA fragmentation which, in turn, can compromise fertilization capacity and embryo development.[48] BPA can interfere with the epigenetic machinery, affecting DNA methylation, histone modifications, and noncoding RNA expression. These epigenetic alterations can impact the expression of genes crucial for spermatogenesis, resulting in impaired germ cell development and function.[51]

BPA can directly impair spermatogenesis by interfering with Sertoli and Leydig cell function.[52] Sertoli cells are essential for germ cell support and nourishment, while Leydig cells are responsible for testosterone production. BPA-induced dysfunction of these cells can lead to reduced sperm production and compromised sperm quality.[49,52] Numerous in vitro studies have demonstrated the detrimental effects of BPA on sperm parameters, including reduced sperm motility, increased DNA fragmentation, and impaired fertilization capacity.[53,54] Animal models have corroborated these findings, with BPA exposure linked to reduced sperm count, altered sperm morphology, and impaired fertility in rodents.[49,52,54] Epidemiological studies have provided further evidence of the association between BPA exposure and male infertility. Several cross-sectional studies have reported significant negative correlations between urinary BPA levels and sperm count, motility, and morphology in humans.[53,55]

Polychlorinated Biphenyls

PCBs are a class of persistent organic pollutants (POPs) that have been implicated in various deleterious health effects, including male infertility.[56] These are synthetic organic chemicals consisting of 209 congeners, which are characterized by their varying degrees of chlorine substitution on biphenyl rings.[57] Despite their ban in the late 20th century due to their persistent and toxic nature, PCBs continue to pervade ecosystems and bioaccumulate in the food chain, posing significant risks to human health.[57] Epidemiological and experimental studies have suggested a link between PCB exposure and male infertility, a burgeoning public health issue that has seen a decline in sperm quality and increased rates of subfertility among the male population.[58]

PCBs are well known for their endocrine-disrupting potential, primarily through their capacity to interfere with hormone synthesis, secretion, transport, and receptor binding.[59,60] The HPG axis plays a pivotal role in regulating male reproductive function, and PCB exposure has been shown to perturb hormonal homeostasis at multiple levels of this axis.[61] PCBs can disrupt the HPG axis by modulating the release of GnRH from the hypothalamus and consequently, altering the synthesis and secretion of LH and FSH from the pituitary gland. These gonadotropins are integral to the regulation of spermatogenesis and steroidogenesis, and their aberrant secretion may culminate in male infertility.[61] PCBs have been implicated in perturbations of testicular steroidogenesis, primarily through the inhibition of key enzymes involved in testosterone synthesis, such as cytochrome P450 side-chain cleavage enzyme (P450scc) and 17α-hydroxylase/17,20-lyase.[62] Reductions in testosterone levels can adversely impact spermatogenesis and disrupt the hormonal milieu, ultimately contributing to male infertility.

PCBs have been demonstrated to induce OS, both directly and indirectly.[63] Direct mechanisms include the generation of ROS due to the redox cycling of PCB metabolites, and indirect mechanisms involve the upregulation of cytochrome P450 enzymes, which can result in the production of ROS as by products.[63] In addition to OS, exposure to PCBs has been shown to induce apoptosis in germ cells, reducing the number of viable spermatozoa and potentially contributing to male infertility. PCB-mediated apoptosis may occur through intrinsic and extrinsic pathways, involving the activation of caspases and the modulation of proapoptotic and antiapoptotic proteins.[64]

Recent evidence suggests that PCB exposure may have transgenerational effects on male fertility through epigenetic modifications.[65] Epigenetic changes induced by PCBs may persist across generations, with potential implications for the heritability of male infertility.[66]

Phthalates

Phthalates, a diverse family of synthetic organic chemicals ubiquitously employed as plasticizers in various consumer products, have recently garnered attention for their deleterious effects on human health.[67] The ubiquitous nature of these compounds has led to widespread exposure and subsequent bioaccumulation in both humans and wildlife.[67] Consequently, the implications of phthalate exposure on male infertility have become a pressing concern in reproductive toxicology.[68] The insidious effects of phthalates on male fertility are largely attributed to their endocrine-disrupting properties.[16] Phthalates function as antiandrogens, eliciting their detrimental impact through perturbation of the HPG axis.[69] Specifically, phthalates interfere with testosterone synthesis by inhibiting the activity of key enzymes involved in steroidogenesis, such as P450scc and 17β-hydroxysteroid dehydrogenase (17β-HSD). Consequently, the resulting decline in circulating testosterone levels culminates in disrupted spermatogenesis, contributing to male infertility.[69]

Phthalate exposure has been linked to the generation of ROS in the testicular milieu, resulting in OS-induced

cellular damage.[70] Elevated ROS levels have the propensity to induce lipid peroxidation, protein oxidation, and DNA damage, compromising the structural integrity and functional capacity of spermatozoa. Moreover, OS impairs the antioxidant defense system, resulting in further exacerbation of cellular damage and apoptosis in germ cells.[68] Collectively, these events precipitate a decline in sperm quality, motility, and viability, ultimately manifesting as male infertility.[68]

The sustentacular Sertoli cells, integral constituents of the seminiferous tubules, play a pivotal role in maintaining the structural and functional integrity of the testicular microenvironment.[71] Phthalate-induced Sertoli cell dysfunction, characterized by altered tight junction dynamics and impaired cell-cell communication, has been implicated as a key factor in compromised spermatogenesis.[72] Furthermore, phthalate exposure can induce apoptosis and autophagy in Sertoli cells, exacerbating the disruption of the BTB and impairing the nourishment and support of developing germ cells.[73]

Recent evidence implicates phthalate-induced epigenetic modifications as a major contributor to male infertility.[66] These alterations, including DNA methylation, histone modifications, and noncoding RNA–mediated regulation, can exert lasting effects on gene expression and cellular function. Specifically, phthalates have been demonstrated to dysregulate the expression of genes associated with germ cell development, steroidogenesis, and OS response, collectively contributing to impaired spermatogenesis and male infertility.[68] Intriguingly, the consequences of phthalate exposure transcend the directly affected individual, with ramifications extending to subsequent generations. Studies in animal models have demonstrated that paternal phthalate exposure can induce epigenetic modifications in spermatozoa which are subsequently carried forward to the next generations.[66,74]

Polycyclic Aromatic Hydrocarbons

PAHs are a class of organic compounds comprising two or more fused aromatic rings, which are primarily formed as byproducts of incomplete combustion of fossil fuels, tobacco, and other organic materials.[75] Ubiquitously present in the environment, these lipophilic molecules bioaccumulate in human tissues, potentially leading to a multitude of adverse health effects, including carcinogenicity, mutagenicity, and teratogenicity.[76] Recent studies have highlighted the detrimental impact of PAHs on male fertility, prompting an in-depth investigation into the associated molecular mechanisms.[77] A plethora of studies have reported a strong association between PAH exposure and decreased semen quality parameters, such as sperm concentration, motility, and morphology.[77,78] Investigations conducted on occupationally exposed individuals and general populations have consistently demonstrated a reduction in sperm parameters, thereby corroborating the negative impact of PAHs on male fertility.[79] Moreover, research has also revealed disruptions in the hormonal milieu, including altered levels of testosterone, LH, and FSH, suggesting a potential endocrine-disrupting role for these xenobiotics.[80]

PAHs have been identified as potent inducers of OS, a critical factor in the pathophysiology of male infertility.[81] PAHs, as well as their metabolites, can interact with cellular macromolecules, generating ROS that overwhelm the intrinsic antioxidant defense mechanisms.[70] This imbalance leads to oxidative damage to cellular components, including lipids, proteins, and nucleic acids. In the context of male fertility, OS can result in lipid peroxidation of sperm membranes, compromising sperm motility and increasing susceptibility to DNA damage, ultimately impairing fertilization capacity.[5,70]

The genotoxic potential of PAHs and their metabolites has been well established, with studies demonstrating their capacity to form DNA adducts and induce DNA strand breaks.[79] The presence of bulky DNA adducts can impede DNA replication and transcription, leading to errors and mutations that adversely affect sperm function. Additionally, PAHs can promote the formation of DNA crosslinks, further compromising genomic integrity.[79] Collectively, these DNA lesions can contribute to reduced sperm quality and impaired fertilization, as well as an increased risk of transmitting genetic defects to the offspring.[7] In addition to direct genotoxic effects, PAHs have been implicated in the modulation of epigenetic processes, such as DNA methylation, histone modifications, and noncoding RNA expression.[74] Aberrant epigenetic patterns have been observed in spermatozoa exposed to PAHs, potentially altering gene expression profiles crucial for male fertility. Furthermore, these epigenetic alterations can be transmitted to the offspring, leading to intergenerational effects and increased susceptibility to disease.[74]

Dioxins

Dioxins, a heterogeneous group of environmental pollutants, are formed as byproducts of industrial and combustion processes, including waste incineration and chlorine bleaching.[82] They are lipophilic and persistent, leading to bioaccumulation in the food chain and human exposure through diet. Epidemiological and experimental evidence has linked dioxin exposure to multiple adverse health outcomes, including reproductive dysfunction and male infertility.[83]

The androgen receptor (AR) plays a pivotal role in regulating spermatogenesis, and its dysregulation is a well-established factor contributing to male infertility.[84] Dioxins exert their effects primarily through the activation of the aryl hydrocarbon receptor (AhR), a ligand-activated transcription factor.[83] The AhR-dioxin complex translocates to the nucleus, where it modulates the transcription of numerous target genes. Accumulating evidence suggests that dioxin-mediated AhR activation interferes with AR signaling, disrupting the hormonal milieu necessary for normal spermatogenesis.[85] Dioxins can also impede the production of testosterone, the principal androgen responsible for maintaining spermatogenesis. The inhibition of testosterone synthesis occurs via the downregulation of key steroidogenic enzymes, such as cytochrome P450 11A1 and 17A1, ultimately leading to diminished spermatogenesis and testicular atrophy.[86]

Dioxins can induce OS through multiple pathways, such as the induction of cytochrome P450 enzymes, which generate ROS as byproducts during their catalytic activities.[87] Additionally, dioxins have been shown to disrupt the cellular redox balance by impairing the expression and activity of antioxidant enzymes, including catalase, superoxide dismutase, and glutathione peroxidase. Consequently, dioxin-induced OS can lead to lipid peroxidation, DNA damage, and apoptosis in spermatogenic cells, culminating in compromised sperm quality and male infertility.[70]

At the epigenetic level, dioxin exposure elicits aberrant DNA methylation patterns, histone modifications, and noncoding RNA expression, collectively referred to as epigenetic alterations.[83] These alterations can be transmitted across generations through the germline, thereby propagating the deleterious effects of dioxins on male reproductive health.[66] Studies have demonstrated that in utero and early life dioxin exposure can result in transgenerational epigenetic alterations, culminating in diminished sperm quality, reduced sperm count, and impaired fertility in subsequent generations.[87] Despite the mounting evidence, the intricate nexus among dioxin exposure, epigenetic alterations, and male infertility remains enigmatic. Elucidating the precise mechanisms by which dioxins induce transgenerational epigenetic changes holds immense promise for mitigating the impact of these ubiquitous pollutants on human reproductive health.[83] Furthermore, the development of targeted epigenetic therapies may pave the way for novel treatment modalities to counteract the pernicious effects of dioxins on male fertility.

Heavy Metals

Heavy metals such as Cd, Pb, and Hg are ubiquitously present in the environment and can be found in air, soil, and water. Human exposure occurs through various routes, including inhalation, ingestion, and dermal contact, resulting in the bioaccumulation of these metals in tissues and organs.[8,16] The deleterious effects of heavy metals on male reproductive function are mediated through a complex interplay of multiple molecular pathways.[88] Heavy metals, particularly Cd, Pb, and Hg, are known to induce OS by generating ROS, which subsequently overwhelms the cellular antioxidant defense systems.[89] The resultant OS adversely affects spermatogenesis by disrupting the mitochondrial membrane potential, leading to apoptosis of germ cells.[5] Moreover, the increase in lipid peroxidation and protein oxidation compromises sperm membrane integrity, thereby impairing sperm motility and reducing fertilization potential.[5]

Heavy metals have been demonstrated to interfere with the HPG axis, disrupting the secretion and action of gonadotropins and sex steroids.[8,84] For instance, Cd exposure has been implicated in the downregulation of LH receptor and FSH receptor expression in Leydig and Sertoli cells, respectively. Furthermore, Cd and Pb have been shown to directly inhibit testosterone biosynthesis by interfering with steroidogenic enzymes, including 17β-HSD and P450scc.[90]

Recent studies have highlighted the potential of heavy metals to induce epigenetic modifications, including DNA methylation, histone modifications, and noncoding RNA regulation.[91] These epigenetic alterations could potentially disrupt the expression of genes critical for spermatogenesis and sperm function, further exacerbating the negative impact on male fertility.[74]

Organic Solvents

The rapid proliferation of industrial and chemical applications has led to an increased prevalence of organic solvents in occupational and environmental settings.[16] Concurrently, male infertility has emerged as a pressing public health issue, with studies implicating organic solvents as one of its potential causative agents.[92] Organic solvents are volatile organic compounds characterized by their lipophilic properties, rendering them capable of diffusing across biological membranes and exerting detrimental effects on the male reproductive system.[92,93] These solvents encompass a diverse range of chemical classes, including aliphatic hydrocarbons, aromatic hydrocarbons, and halogenated hydrocarbons.[16] The lipophilic nature of these solvents facilitates their diffusion across the BTB, culminating in the disruption of the intricate cellular interactions and signaling pathways governing spermatogenesis.[94] Organic solvents may impair the mitotic and meiotic divisions of spermatogonia and spermatocytes, respectively, leading to aberrant chromosomal segregation and aneuploidy.[94] Additionally, solvents may interfere with the differentiation of spermatids into mature spermatozoa, thereby compromising sperm morphology and function. Aliphatic hydrocarbons, such as hexane, have been demonstrated to induce testicular atrophy and disrupt Sertoli cell function, thereby impairing spermatogenesis.[95] Aromatic hydrocarbons, including benzene and toluene, may cause germ cell apoptosis, germinal epithelial degeneration, and reduced sperm count.[95] Halogenated hydrocarbons, exemplified by trichloroethylene, have been associated with diminished sperm motility and impaired sperm–oocyte interaction, compromising fertilization potential.[92]

Organic solvents also exert deleterious effects on sperm function, including motility, capacitation, acrosome reaction, and sperm–oocyte fusion.[94] These processes are critical for successful fertilization and are modulated by intricate signaling pathways and ion channel activity.[96,97] Organic solvents may alter sperm membrane fluidity and permeability, impeding intracellular signaling and compromising the aforementioned functions.[94] Furthermore, solvents may induce OS, generating ROSs that damage sperm membrane integrity and impair mitochondrial function, ultimately reducing sperm motility and viability.[94] Organic solvents have also been reported to disrupt the HPG axis at multiple levels, causing hormonal imbalances that adversely affect spermatogenesis and male fertility.[98] For example, the disruption of Leydig cell function by organic solvents results in reduced testosterone synthesis, which in turn, impairs spermatogenesis and Sertoli cell function.[98]

Heat Stress

Spermatogenesis is a highly organized and temperature-sensitive physiological process that occurs within the seminiferous tubules of the testes, resulting in the production of mature spermatozoa.[84] The optimal temperature for human spermatogenesis is approximately 2°C to 4°C below core body temperature (35°C–36°C).[84,99] This temperature regulation is maintained by the intricate structure of the scrotum, which facilitates heat exchange through the pampiniform plexus—a countercurrent heat exchange mechanism—and the cremasteric reflex.[99]

The testicular microenvironment is critical for the maintenance of spermatogenesis. Prolonged exposure to elevated temperatures disrupts this delicate balance, leading to a condition known as heat-induced testicular hyperthermia.[99] This rise in scrotal temperature is compounded by factors such as extended periods of sitting, tight clothing, and occupational heat exposure.[100] The resultant hyperthermia is associated with a myriad of deleterious effects on male fertility, including alterations in the BTB, testicular atrophy, and OS. The BTB, constituted by tight junctions between adjacent Sertoli cells, plays a pivotal role in maintaining the immunoprivileged environment of the seminiferous tubules.[100,101] Heat-induced testicular hyperthermia disrupts the integrity of the BTB, allowing the infiltration of immunological factors and subsequent activation of the immune response.[100] This immune-mediated attack on developing germ cells compromises the process of spermatogenesis and adversely affects male fertility.[101,102] Heat-induced testicular hyperthermia can result in testicular atrophy, characterized by a reduction in the size and weight of the testes.[100,103] Prolonged thermal exposure triggers apoptotic pathways in germ cells, primarily via the intrinsic mitochondrial pathway, leading to cellular degradation and the eventual cessation of spermatogenesis. This decline in germ cell production manifests as a reduced sperm count and impaired fertility.[103]

Elevated testicular temperature induces OS, characterized by an imbalance between the production and detoxification of ROS.[103] Excessive ROS generation damages cellular components, such as lipids, proteins, and DNA, which in turn, compromises sperm function and integrity. Moreover, the resultant OS disrupts the antioxidant defense system within the testicular microenvironment, further exacerbating the negative impact on male fertility.[100,103]

Seminal fluid, produced by accessory glands, plays a crucial role in supporting sperm function and protecting against oxidative damage.[104] Heat-induced testicular hyperthermia has been implicated in altering the composition and function of seminal fluid, thus compromising its protective role. These alterations include a reduction in the seminal plasma volume, decreased fructose levels, and diminished antioxidant capacity. Collectively, these changes undermine sperm viability and motility, ultimately impairing male fertility.[6,103]

Lifestyle Factors and Male Infertility
Smoking/Tobacco Use

Tobacco smoke contains a multitude of toxicants, including PAHs, heavy metals, and ROSs, which are known to elicit a panoply of deleterious effects on male reproductive function.[105] The increased generation of ROS in the seminal plasma of smokers engenders OS, which compromises sperm function by inducing lipid peroxidation, DNA fragmentation, and protein oxidation.[10] These oxidative insults adversely impact sperm viability, motility, and the acrosome reaction, a cascade of events culminating in sperm-oocyte fusion.[5] Moreover, the seminal plasma of tobacco users exhibits diminished antioxidant capacity, exacerbating the deleterious effects of OS on spermatozoa.[106] Concomitantly, the dysregulation of endocrine function, characterized by perturbations in gonadotropin and testosterone levels, has been documented in tobacco users.[105] These hormonal imbalances can precipitate spermatogenic dysfunction, impairing the production and maturation of spermatozoa.[105]

Nicotine and its metabolites, such as cotinine, have been detected in seminal fluid, testicular tissue, and spermatozoa of tobacco users, implicating their direct contribution to the pathogenesis of male infertility.[107] In vitro studies have revealed the inhibitory effects of nicotine on testicular steroidogenesis, spermatogenesis, and sperm capacitation. Additionally, tobacco-induced alterations in sperm epigenetic signatures, such as DNA methylation and histone modifications, may potentially affect male fertility through the disruption of gene expression and chromatin architecture.[108]

Epidemiological studies have corroborated the aforementioned mechanistic insights, demonstrating a strong association between tobacco consumption and suboptimal semen parameters.[106,109] Cumulative evidence suggests that the magnitude of the detrimental impact on male fertility is dose dependent, with a higher prevalence of oligozoospermia, asthenozoospermia, and teratozoospermia observed in habitual smokers.[105]

Alcohol Consumption

Alcohol consumption has been extensively investigated for its potential to disrupt male fertility, with numerous studies highlighting a correlative relationship between ethanol intake and diminished reproductive capabilities.[110–112] Ethanol has been demonstrated to induce aberrations in sperm quality, including sperm motility, morphology, and concentration.[112] Ethanol metabolism results in the generation of acetaldehyde and ROS, which can inflict damage to sperm cell membranes and impair their functionality.[110] The excess of ROS culminates in lipid peroxidation, protein oxidation, and DNA fragmentation, ultimately leading to compromised spermatozoa integrity.[110,112] Furthermore, ethanol-induced alterations in the expression of protamines, the proteins responsible for DNA condensation within the sperm nucleus, exacerbate chromatin abnormalities and reduce fertilization potential.[112] This oxidative damage also manifests as reduced seminiferous tubule diameter, disrupted spermatogenic cell maturation, and decreased Sertoli cell functionality, all of which are crucial for sperm development and maturation.

Ethanol consumption has been implicated in the dysregulation of the HPG axis, a central regulatory system for male reproductive function.[111] Chronic alcohol exposure perturbs the secretion of GnRH from the hypothalamus and LH and FSH from the anterior pituitary gland.[111] The suppression of these crucial hormones culminates in diminished testosterone production by Leydig cells in the testes, negatively impacting spermatogenesis and libido.

Recreational Drug Use

Recreational drug use has emerged as a pressing public health concern due to its multifarious detrimental effects on various physiological systems, including the male reproductive system.[113] Recreational drugs, encompassing cannabinoids, opioids, and psychostimulants such as amphetamines and cocaine, have been implicated in perturbing the homeostasis of the HPG axis, a pivotal neuroendocrine system regulating male reproductive function.[111] The HPG axis modulates spermatogenesis, the complex process through which spermatogonia differentiate into mature spermatozoa, via the orchestration of hormonal signaling cascades involving GnRH, LH, and FSH, as well as testosterone.[111]

Cannabinoid exposure, for instance, has been demonstrated to attenuate GnRH secretion, culminating in the downregulation of LH and FSH synthesis and release.[114] This subsequently impairs testicular Leydig and Sertoli cells, which are responsible for testosterone production and the nourishment of developing germ cells, respectively, thereby compromising the structural and functional integrity of spermatozoa.[111] Opioids, on the other hand, primarily exert their deleterious effects on male fertility via the activation of μ-opioid receptors, which are expressed in various regions of the HPG axis.[115] The stimulation of these receptors has been associated with the suppression of GnRH and LH secretion, culminating in hypogonadotropic hypogonadism and a concomitant decline in sperm quality.[111] Psychostimulants, such as amphetamines and cocaine, have been shown to disrupt the dopaminergic neurotransmission system, which plays a critical role in modulating the HPG axis.[111,115] By dysregulating dopamine levels, these substances can indirectly contribute to an imbalance in GnRH and downstream hormone release, culminating in impaired spermatogenesis.[111]

Moreover, OS, a state of disequilibrium between the production of ROS and the antioxidant defense system, has been posited as a key mechanistic link between recreational drug use and male infertility.[6,10] A surfeit of ROS generation, induced by the metabolic byproducts of recreational drugs, can inflict oxidative damage upon spermatozoa, thereby compromising their motility, viability, and DNA integrity.[10]

Physical Exercise

In recent years, the effects of physical exercise on male fertility has garnered significant attention within the scientific community, with studies elucidating the complex interplay between physical activity and spermatogenesis, endocrine homeostasis, and OS.[116,117] Physical exercise has been demonstrated to modulate spermatogenesis, the intricate process of spermatozoa production within the seminiferous tubules of the testes.[117] Exercise-induced alterations in testicular blood flow, temperature, and hormonal milieu can directly influence germ cell development and function.[100] Interestingly, the impact of exercise on spermatogenesis appears to be contingent on the intensity and duration of physical activity.[118] Moderate exercise has been linked to improved semen quality, whereas excessive or high-intensity exercise may elicit deleterious effects, such as reduced sperm concentration and motility, through the induction of local and systemic inflammatory responses.[118] Physical exercise also exerts modulatory effects on the HPG axis, a crucial regulatory system that governs hormone production and secretion.[118] While moderate exercise can bolster testosterone levels and improve fertility outcomes, excessive exercise may disrupt the HPG axis, culminating in reduced gonadotropin secretion and testosterone production, which can consequently impair spermatogenesis and contribute to male infertility.[117]

Strenuous exercise can exacerbate OS by augmenting ROS production, leading to cellular damage and sperm DNA fragmentation.[119] Conversely, moderate exercise has been shown to bolster antioxidant defense mechanisms, ameliorating OS and mitigating the detrimental effects of ROS on sperm function.[118,119]

Obesity

Obesity, defined as an excessive accumulation of adipose tissue resulting in a body mass index of 30 or above, has reached epidemic proportions worldwide. An often-overlooked consequence of this malady is its deleterious impact on male reproductive health, as corroborated by a burgeoning body of evidence.[120] The intricate mechanisms underlying obesity-induced male infertility are manifold, encompassing hormonal perturbations, OS, and epigenetic modifications.[121] One primary contributor to the nexus between obesity and male infertility is the disruption of the HPG axis.[122] In obese males, increased adiposity leads to the overproduction of leptin, a hormone that modulates energy homeostasis and appetite.[122–124] This hyperleptinemia engenders a state of leptin resistance, consequently impairing the secretion of GnRH and downstream gonadotropins, such as LH and FSH.[122,123] The attendant decrease in testosterone biosynthesis and spermatogenesis, compounded by the elevated levels of aromatase

enzyme that converts testosterone to estradiol, culminates in hypogonadotropic hypogonadism and suboptimal sperm parameters.[122]

Obesity is also inextricably linked to systemic inflammation and OS, which exert detrimental effects on sperm quality.[120,121] Excess adipose tissue generates ROS, which in turn, damage sperm DNA, impair sperm motility, and compromise sperm membrane integrity. Additionally, elevated ROS levels can induce apoptosis in germ cells, further exacerbating the decline in sperm production.[120] Emerging evidence implicates epigenetic alterations in the etiology of obesity-related male infertility. Obesity has been shown to modulate sperm DNA methylation patterns, histone modifications, and small non-coding RNA expression.[125] These epigenetic aberrations may not only adversely affect sperm function but also have potential transgenerational repercussions, thereby amplifying the deleterious impact of obesity on male reproductive health.[125]

Psychological Stress

Increasing body of evidence implicates psychological stress as a significant determinant of male infertility.[126] The intricate nature of this association necessitates a multidisciplinary approach, integrating molecular, physiological, and psychological perspectives. Psychological stress triggers the activation of the hypothalamic-pituitary-adrenal axis, resulting in the increased secretion of cortisol, a potent glucocorticoid hormone.[127] Prolonged cortisol elevation instigates OS, which impairs spermatogenesis by inducing DNA damage, lipid peroxidation, and protein oxidation. Concomitantly, cortisol mediates a decrease in testosterone production, further compromising sperm quality and quantity.[4,5]

Chronic stress negatively impacts key physiological parameters essential for male fertility, such as erectile function and ejaculatory reflexes.[128] Stress-induced dysregulation of the autonomic nervous system, characterized by heightened sympathetic activity, engenders vasoconstriction, deterring optimal penile blood flow and precipitating erectile dysfunction.[128] Additionally, stress impairs ejaculatory control, potentially exacerbating fertility challenges.[128] Psychological stress can perpetuate a vicious cycle of infertility, perpetuating further stress and anxiety.[127] Stress-induced performance anxiety, depression, and relationship discord can hamper sexual intimacy and further reduce the likelihood of conception.[126,127] Moreover, the societal stigmatization of male infertility amplifies the psychological burden on affected individuals, exacerbating the adverse impact of stress on fertility.

Radiation

In high doses, radiation can cause severe damage to the reproductive system and result in male infertility.[129] The male reproductive system is particularly vulnerable to the damaging effects of radiation due to its high sensitivity to OS.[5] Radiation exposure can result in damage to the DNA of germ cells, leading to cell death, decreased sperm production, and impaired sperm function.[130] Ionizing radiation, which includes X-rays and gamma rays, is particularly damaging to the reproductive system.[129,130] It has been shown that exposure to ionizing radiation at levels as low as 10 cGy can cause damage to the testes and impair fertility.[130] Furthermore, radiation-induced OS can result in the production of ROS, which can damage DNA and other cellular structures.[130]

The mechanism by which radiation causes male infertility is complex and not fully understood. However, it is believed that radiation-induced DNA damage can lead to the activation of apoptotic pathways, resulting in the death of germ cells.[129] In addition, radiation-induced damage to the DNA can result in mutations that can be passed on to offspring, leading to genetic abnormalities and increased risk of infertility and other health problems.[131] Studies have shown that the effects of radiation on male fertility are dose dependent, with higher doses resulting in more severe damage.[131,132] However, even low doses of radiation can have long-term effects on fertility, as the damage to germ cells may not be immediately apparent.[129] Furthermore, the effects of radiation on fertility may be influenced by other factors such as age, genetic susceptibility, and lifestyle factors such as smoking and exposure to other environmental toxins.[129–131]

Advanced Paternal Age

Advanced paternal age, defined as the father's age exceeding 35 years at the time of conception, has been increasingly recognized as a risk factor for male infertility.[133] The phenomenon of advanced paternal age and its impact on male fertility has been the subject of numerous studies, with evidence suggesting that as males age, their sperm quality and quantity decline.[134] This decline in sperm quality can lead to a reduction in fertility, with older males having a higher risk of infertility and genetic abnormalities in their offspring.[135]

The decline in sperm quality associated with advanced paternal age is due to a number of factors, including OS, DNA damage, and changes in sperm epigenetics.[133] OS, caused by the production of ROS, can cause damage to sperm DNA and other cellular components, leading to infertility and genetic abnormalities in the offspring.[5] DNA damage, such as single- and double-stranded breaks, can also accumulate with age, leading to an increased risk of infertility and genetic abnormalities.[7] In addition to these direct effects on sperm quality, advanced paternal age has been associated with changes in sperm epigenetics, including alterations in DNA methylation patterns and histone modifications.[136] These changes in sperm epigenetics can have long-lasting effects on gene expression and can contribute to the increased risk of infertility and genetic abnormalities in offspring.[133,136]

The decline in sperm quality associated with advanced paternal age can also lead to an increased risk of infertility and decreased success with assisted reproductive technologies (ARTs), such as in vitro fertilization and intracytoplasmic sperm injection.[137] In these ARTs, sperm quality is a critical factor in determining the success of the procedure, and older males may have decreased success rates due to their declining sperm quality.[137] Despite the evidence linking advanced paternal age to male infertility and decreased success with ARTs, it is important to note that not all older males will experience infertility.[134] However, males over the age of 40 years have been shown to have a significantly higher risk of infertility and decreased success with ARTs compared to younger males.[133,134]

Dietary Habits

Dietary habits have emerged as a significant determinant in the multifaceted etiology of male infertility, which encompasses diminished sperm quality, impaired motility, and aberrant morphology.[116] The complex interplay between dietary factors and reproductive health warrants a rigorous investigation of the intricate pathways through which nutrition modulates spermatogenesis, OS, and endocrine homeostasis.[116] Recent studies elucidate the deleterious consequences of a Western dietary pattern, characterized by excessive intake of saturated fats, processed meats, refined carbohydrates, and sugar-sweetened beverages, on spermatogenic function.[138,139]

These dietary components engender a state of systemic inflammation, exacerbating OS and perturbing the HPG axis, ultimately culminating in suboptimal sperm parameters.[116,138] Conversely, adherence to a Mediterranean diet, replete with whole grains, fruits, vegetables, legumes, and healthy fats, has been positively correlated with improved sperm quality.[140] Antioxidant-rich foods, which mitigate OS and curtail sperm DNA fragmentation, are particularly efficacious in ameliorating male infertility.[141] Omega-3 fatty acids, derived from fish and plant sources, have demonstrated the ability to enhance sperm motility and morphology through modulation of the prostaglandin metabolism and membrane fluidity.[140,141] Thus the indisputable role of dietary habits in male infertility necessitates a paradigm shift towards the adoption of a balanced, nutrient-dense diet to bolster reproductive health.[116] Future research endeavors should focus on elucidating the molecular underpinnings of nutrition-induced alterations in spermatogenesis and developing targeted dietary interventions to combat male infertility.

Caffeine Intake

Caffeine is a central nervous system stimulant commonly found in beverages such as coffee, tea, and energy drinks.[142] Despite its widespread use, recent studies have suggested that excessive caffeine intake may have negative effects on male fertility.[143] The mechanisms by which caffeine affects male fertility are not fully understood; however, several studies have demonstrated that caffeine intake can lead to decreased sperm count, motility, and morphology.[142,143] This can be due to caffeine's ability to interfere with the process of spermatogenesis, the production of sperm in the testes, as well as its impact on testosterone levels.[10] Additionally, caffeine has been shown to increase OS in the testes, which can lead to cellular damage and decreased fertility.[143] It is important to note that the impact of caffeine on male fertility may be dose dependent.[143] While moderate caffeine intake is unlikely to have a significant effect on fertility, excessive caffeine intake has been associated with decreased sperm parameters.[142,143] The American Society for Reproductive Medicine recommends that males limit their caffeine intake to less than 200 mg per day, which is equivalent to approximately one cup of coffee.[144] Thus excessive caffeine intake has been linked to decreased male fertility, potentially through its effects on spermatogenesis and testosterone levels, as well as

OS.[142,143] As such, it is recommended that males limit their caffeine intake to reduce the potential negative impact on their fertility.[142,143] Further research is needed to fully understand the mechanisms by which caffeine affects male fertility and to determine the optimal intake levels for maximizing fertility.

SUMMARY

Environmental and lifestyle factors are increasingly recognized as significant determinants of male fertility. Gynecologists, andrologists, and reproductive scientists must remain vigilant in elucidating the interplay of these factors, implementing preventative measures, and advocating for public health initiatives to mitigate their deleterious effects on spermatogenesis, sperm function, and overall reproductive capacity. Epigenetic, endocrine, and OS pathways serve as primary conduits through which environmental and lifestyle factors exert their influence. Exposure to EDCs, POPs, and heavy metals are implicated in the disruption of the HPG axis, resulting in impaired spermatogenesis and compromised sperm quality. Additionally, the ubiquity of phthalates, BPA, and other EDCs in consumer products raises concern for their deleterious impact on male fertility via epigenetic mechanisms, necessitating further exploration into transgenerational effects. Lifestyle factors, including diet, exercise, stress, and sleep, critically modulate sperm health. Obesity, characterized by hyperinsulinemia and a proinflammatory state, potentiates OS, thus contributing to sperm DNA damage, lipid peroxidation, and alterations in sperm epigenetic marks. Furthermore, dietary patterns replete with antioxidants and antiinflammatory compounds may foster improved sperm function and resilience to environmental toxins. Tobacco, alcohol, and illicit drug consumption have well-established associations with diminished sperm parameters, warranting a multifaceted approach to promote cessation and minimize exposure. Lastly, clinicians should remain informed about emerging evidence surrounding the impact of electromagnetic radiation from electronic devices on male fertility. As multidisciplinary professionals in the field of reproductive health, it is incumbent upon us to actively engage in research, patient education, and advocacy efforts to address the complex interrelationship between environmental and lifestyle factors and male infertility.

REFERENCES

1. Tamrakar SR, Bastakoti R. Determinants of infertility in couples. *J Nepal Heal Res Coun*. 2019;17(1):85-89.

2. Esteves SC, Schattman GL, Agarwal A. Definitions and relevance of unexplained infertility in reproductive medicine. In: Schattman GL, Esteves SC, Agarwal A, eds. *Unexplained Infertility: Pathophysiology, Evaluation and Treatment*. New York: Springer; 2015:3-5.

3. Agarwal A, Baskaran S, Parekh N, et al. Male infertility. *Lancet*. 2021;397(10271):319-333.

4. Agarwal A, Leisegang K, Sengupta P. *Oxidative Stress in Pathologies of Male Reproductive Disorders. Pathology*. Cambridge, Massachusetts, United States: Academic Press, Elsevier; 2020:15-27.

5. Agarwal A, Sengupta P. Chapter 6: Oxidative stress and its association with male infertility. In: Parekattil SJ, Agarwal A, eds. *Male Infertility: Contemporary Clinical Approaches, Andrology, ART and Antioxidants*. Springer, Cham; 2020:57-68.

6. Durairajanayagam D. Lifestyle causes of male infertility. *Arab J Urol*. 2018;16(1):10-20.

7. Agarwal A, Majzoub A, Baskaran S, et al. Sperm DNA fragmentation: a new guideline for clinicians. *World J Men's Health*. 2020;38(4):412.

8. Sengupta P. Environmental and occupational exposure of metals and their role in male reproductive functions. *Drug Chem Toxicol*. 2013;36(3):353-368.

9. Povey A, Clyma JA, McNamee R, et al. Modifiable and non-modifiable risk factors for poor semen quality: a case-referent study. *Hum Reprod*. 2012;27(9):2799-2806.

10. Leisegang K, Dutta S. Do lifestyle practices impede male fertility? *Andrologia*. 2021;53(1):e13595.

11. Almeida DL, Pavanello A, Saavedra LP, Pereira TS, de Castro-Prado MAA, de Freitas Mathias PC. Environmental monitoring and the developmental origins of health and disease. *J Dev Origins Health Dis*. 2019;10(6):608-615.

12. Yahaya TO, Oladele EO, Anyebe D, et al. Chromosomal abnormalities predisposing to infertility, testing, and management: a narrative review. *Bull Nat Res Cent*. 2021;45(1):1-15.

13. Wei C, Crowne E. The impact of childhood cancer and its treatment on puberty and subsequent hypothalamic pituitary and gonadal function, in both boys and girls. *Best Pract Res Clin Endocrinol Metab*. 2019;33(3):101291.

14. Mudgal V, Madaan N, Mudgal A, Singh R, Mishra S. Effect of toxic metals on human health. *Open Nutraceut J*. 2010;3(1):94-99.

15. Brusseau M, Artiola J. Chemical contaminants. In: Brusseau ML, Pepper IL, Gerba CP, eds. *Environmental and Pollution Science*. Cambridge, Massachusetts, United States: Academic Press, Elsevier; 2019:175-190.

16. Sengupta P, Banerjee R. Environmental toxins: alarming impacts of pesticides on male fertility. *Hum Exp Toxicol*. 2014;33(10):1017-1039.

17. Rana S. Perspectives in endocrine toxicity of heavy metals—a review. *Biol Trace Elem Res*. 2014;160(1):1-14.

18. Wirth JJ. *Effects of Organochlorine Compounds and Heavy Metals on Male Reproductive Health*. Michigan State University; 2001.

19. Cook MB, Trabert B, McGlynn KA. Organochlorine compounds and testicular dysgenesis syndrome: human data. *Int J Androl*. 2011;34(4 Pt 2):e68-e85.

20. Abou Ghayda R, Sergeyev O, Burns JS, et al. Peripubertal serum concentrations of organochlorine pesticides and semen parameters in Russian young men. *Env Int*. 2020;144:106085.

21. Choi SM, Yoo SD, Lee BM. Toxicological characteristics of endocrine-disrupting chemicals: developmental toxicity, carcinogenicity, and mutagenicity. *J Toxicol Env Heal*. 2004;7(1):1-23.

22. Bastos AM, Souza Mdo C, Almeida Filho GL, Krauss TM, Pavesi T, Silva LE. Organochlorine compound lev-els in fertile and infertile women from Rio de Janeiro, Brazil. Arq Bras Endocrinol Metab. 2013;57:346-353.

23. Amir S, Tzatzarakis M, Mamoulakis C, et al. Impact of organochlorine pollutants on semen parameters of infertile men in Pakistan. *Env Res*. 2021;195:110832.

24. Dallinga JW, Moonen EJ, Dumoulin JC, Evers JL, Geraedts JP, Kleinjans JC. Decreased human semen quality and organochlorine compounds in blood. *Hum Reprod*. 2002;17(8):1973-1979.

25. Toft G, Rignell-Hydbom A, Tyrkiel E, et al. Semen quality and exposure to persistent organochlorine pollutants. *Epidemiology*. 2006;17:450-458.

26. Hauser R, Chen Z, Pothier L, Ryan L, Altshul L. The relationship between human semen parameters and environmental exposure to polychlorinated biphenyls and p, p′-DDE. *Env Health Perspect*. 2003;111(12):1505-1511.

27. Dutta S, Sengupta P, Slama P, Roychoudhury S. Oxidative stress, testicular inflammatory pathways, and male reproduction. *Int J Mol Sci*. 2021;22(18):10043.

28. Meeker J, Ryan L, Barr D, Herrick R, Bennett D, Hauser R. Contemporary use insecticides and human semen quality. *Epidemiology*. 2004;15(4):S190.

29. Franken C, Koppen G, Lambrechts N, et al. Environmental exposure to human carcinogens in teenagers and the association with DNA damage. *Env Res*. 2017;152:165-174.

30. Casanovas A, Ribas-Maynou J, Lara-Cerrillo S, et al. Double-stranded sperm DNA damage is a cause of delay in embryo development and can impair implantation rates. *Fertil Steril*. 2019;111(4):699-707.e1.

31. Gualtieri R, Kalthur G, Barbato V, et al. Sperm oxidative stress during in vitro manipulation and its effects on

sperm function and embryo development. *Antioxidants.* 2021;10(7):1025.

32. Martyniuk CJ, Mehinto AC, Denslow ND. Organochlorine pesticides: agrochemicals with potent endocrine-disrupting properties in fish. *Mol Cell Endocrinol.* 2020;507:110764.

33. Freire C, Koifman RJ, Sarcinelli PN, Rosa ACS, Clapauch R, Koifman S. Association between serum levels of organochlorine pesticides and sex hormones in adults living in a heavily contaminated area in Brazil. *Int J Hygiene Env Heal.* 2014;217(2-3):370-378.

34. Cano-Sancho G, Ploteau S, Matta K, et al. Human epidemiological evidence about the associations between exposure to organochlorine chemicals and endometriosis: systematic review and meta-analysis. *Env Int.* 2019;123:209-223.

35. Karalliedde L, Feldman S, Henry J, Marrs T. *Organophosphates and health.* London: Imperial College Press; 2001.

36. De Silva H, Samarawickrema N, Wickremasinghe A. Toxicity due to organophosphorus compounds: what about chronic exposure? *Transac Royal Soc Trop Med Hygiene.* 2006;100(9):803-806.

37. Aamer A, Mahran Z, Ismaiel A, Elsaied MH, Shukri M. Chronic organophosphorus exposure and male fertility of agriculture workers. *Al-Azhar Assiut Med J.* 2015;13(4):95.

38. Ray A, Chatterjee S, Ghosh S, Bhattacharya K, Pakrashi A, Deb C. Quinalphos-induced suppression of spermatogenesis, plasma gonadotrophins, testicular testosterone production, and secretion in adult rats. *Env Res.* 1992; 57(2):181-189.

39. Dhull V, Gahlaut A, Dilbaghi N, Hooda V. Acetylcholinesterase biosensors for electrochemical detection of organophosphorus compounds: a review. *Biochem Res Int.* 2013;2013:731501.

40. Gumusay U, Sebe A, Satar DA, Ay MO, Yilmaz M, Mete UO. Effects of antidotal therapy on testis tissue in organophosphate poisoning. *Acta Med.* 2014;30:435.

41. Moreira S, Pereira SC, Seco-Rovira V, Oliveira PF, Alves MG, Pereira MdL. Pesticides and male fertility: a dangerous crosstalk. *Metabolites.* 2021;11(12):799.

42. Degraeve N, Chollet MC, Moutschen J. Cytogenetic effects induced by organophosphorus pesticides in mouse spermatocytes. *Toxicol Lett.* 1984;21(3):315-319.

43. Moreira S, Silva R, Carrageta DF, et al. Carbamate pesticides: shedding light on their impact on the male reproductive system. *Int J Mol Sci.* 2022;23(15):8206.

44. Gupta RC, Milatovic D. Toxicity of organophosphates and carbamates. In: Marrs T, ed. *Mammalian Toxicology of Insecticides.* The Royal Society of Chemistry, Cambridge, UK: 2012:104-136.

45. Sikka SC, Gurbuz N. Reproductive toxicity of organophosphate and carbamate pesticides. In: Gupta RC, ed. *Toxicology of Organophosphate & Carbamate Compounds.*

Cambridge, Massachusetts, United States: Academic Press, Elsevier; 2006:447-462.

46. Kimaro W. Morphological changes in the sperm storage tubules of the Japanese quail exposed to methy-2-benz-imidazole carbamate. *Anat J Afr.* 2016;5(2):713-720.

47. Menezes E, Velho A, Santos F, et al. Uncovering sperm metabolome to discover biomarkers for bull fertility. *BMC Genom.* 2019;20:1-16.

48. Cariati F, D'Uonno N, Borrillo F, Iervolino S, Galdiero G, Tomaiuolo R. Bisphenol A: an emerging threat to male fertility. *Reprod Biol Endocrinol.* 2019;17:1-8.

49. Cao LY, Ren XM, Li CH, et al. Bisphenol AF and bisphenol B exert higher estrogenic effects than bisphenol A via G protein-coupled estrogen receptor pathway. *Env Sci Technol.* 2017;51(19):11423-11430.

50. Gassman NR. Induction of oxidative stress by bisphenol A and its pleiotropic effects. *Env Mol Mut.* 2017;58(2):60-71.

51. Mileva G, Baker SL, Konkle AT, Bielajew C. Bisphenol-A: epigenetic reprogramming and effects on reproduction and behavior. *Int J Env Res Pub Heal.* 2014;11(7):7537-7561.

52. Zhang GL, Zhang XF, Feng YM, et al. Exposure to bisphenol A results in a decline in mouse spermatogenesis. *Reprod Fertil Dev.* 2013;25(6):847-859.

53. Kiwitt-Cárdenas J, Adoamnei E, Arense-Gonzalo JJ, et al. Associations between urinary concentrations of bisphenol A and sperm DNA fragmentation in young men. *Env Res.* 2021;199:111289.

54. Özlem ÇA, Hatice P. Effects of bisphenol A on the embryonic development of sea urchin (Paracentrotus lividus). *Env Toxicol.* 2008;23(3):387-392.

55. Mantzouki C, Bliatka D, Iliadou PK, et al. Serum bisphenol A concentrations in men with idiopathic infertility. *Food Chem Toxicol.* 2019;125:562-565.

56. Meeker JD, Hauser R. Exposure to polychlorinated biphenyls (PCBs) and male reproduction. *Syst Biol Reprod Med.* 2010;56(2):122-131.

57. Te B, Yiming L, Tianwei L, et al. Polychlorinated biphenyls in a grassland food network: concentrations, biomagnification, and transmission of toxicity. *Sci Total Env.* 2020;709:135781.

58. Montano L, Pironti C, Pinto G, et al. Polychlorinated biphenyls (PCBs) in the environment: occupational and exposure events, effects on human health and fertility. *Toxics.* 2022;10(7):365.

59. Zhang CQ, Qiao HL. Effect of polychlorinated biphenyls on spermatogenesis and testosterone secretion in adult cocks. *J Zhejiang Univ Sci.* 2004;5(2):193-197.

60. Ruiz P, Ingale K, Wheeler JS, Mumtaz M. 3D QSAR studies of hydroxylated polychlorinated biphenyls as potential xenoestrogens. *Chemosphere.* 2016;144:2238-2246.

61. Bell MR. Endocrine-disrupting actions of PCBs on brain development and social and reproductive behaviors. *Curr Opinion Pharmacol.* 2014;19:134-144.

62. Supornsilchai V. *Effects of Endocrine Disruptors on Adreno-Cortical and Leydig Cell Steroidogenesis*. Norrbacka/Rehabsalen: Institutionen för kvinnors och barns hälsa; 2007.

63. Liu J, Tan Y, Song E, Song Y. A critical review of polychlorinated biphenyls metabolism, metabolites, and their correlation with oxidative stress. *Chem Res Toxicol*. 2020;33(8):2022-2242.

64. Pocar P, Nestler D, Risch M, Fischer B. Apoptosis in bovine cumulus–oocyte complexes after exposure to polychlorinated biphenyl mixtures during in vitro maturation. *Reproduction*. 2005;130(6):857-688.

65. Mennigen JA, Thompson LM, Bell M, Tellez Santos M, Gore AC. Transgenerational effects of polychlorinated biphenyls: 1. Development and physiology across 3 generations of rats. *Env Heal*. 2018;17(1):1-12.

66. Guerrero-Bosagna CM, Skinner MK. Epigenetic transgenerational effects of endocrine disruptors on male reproduction. *Semin Reprod Med*. 2009;27(5):403-408.

67. Ventrice P, Ventrice D, Russo E, De Sarro G. Phthalates: European regulation, chemistry, pharmacokinetic and related toxicity. *Env Toxicol Pharmacol*. 2013;36(1):88-96.

68. Martino-Andrade AJ, Chahoud I. Reproductive toxicity of phthalate esters. *Mol Nutr Food Res*. 2010;54(1):148-157.

69. Hlisníková H, Petrovičová I, Kolena B, Šidlovská M, Sirotkin A. Effects and mechanisms of phthalates' action on reproductive processes and reproductive health: a literature review. *Int J Env Res Pub Heal*. 2020;17(18):6811.

70. Virant-Klun I, Imamovic-Kumalic S, Pinter B. From oxidative stress to male infertility: review of the associations of endocrine-disrupting chemicals (bisphenols, phthalates, and parabens) with human semen quality. *Antioxidants*. 2022;11(8):1617.

71. Zhao Y, Li XN, Zhang H, et al. Phthalate-induced testosterone/androgen receptor pathway disorder on spermatogenesis and antagonism of lycopene. *J Hazard Mat*. 2022;439:129689.

72. Jenardhanan P, Panneerselvam M, Mathur PP, eds. Effect of environmental contaminants on spermatogenesis. *Semin Cell Dev Biol*. 2016;59:126-140.

73. Erkekoglu P, Zeybek ND, Giray B, Asan E, Hincal F. The effects of di (2-ethylhexyl) phthalate exposure and selenium nutrition on sertoli cell vimentin structure and germ-cell apoptosis in rat testis. *Arch Env Contam Toxicol*. 2012;62:539-547.

74. Van Cauwenbergh O, Di Serafino A, Tytgat J, Soubry A. Transgenerational epigenetic effects from male exposure to endocrine-disrupting compounds: a systematic review on research in mammals. *Clin Epigenet*. 2020;12(1):1-23.

75. Lawal AT. Polycyclic aromatic hydrocarbons. A review. *Cogent Env Sci*. 2017;3(1):1339841.

76. Kim K-H, Jahan SA, Kabir E, Brown RJ. A review of airborne polycyclic aromatic hydrocarbons (PAHs) and their human health effects. *Env Int*. 2013;60:71-80.

77. Kakavandi B, Rafiemanesh H, Giannakis S, et al. Establishing the relationship between polycyclic aromatic hydrocarbons (PAHs) exposure and male infertility: a systematic review. *Ecotoxicol Env Safety*. 2023;250:114485.

78. Saad AA, Hussein T, El-Sikaily A, et al. Effect of polycyclic aromatic hydrocarbons exposure on sperm DNA in idiopathic male infertility. *J Heal Pollut*. 2019;9(21):190309.

79. Gaspari L, Chang SS, Santella RM, Garte S, Pedotti P, Taioli E. Polycyclic aromatic hydrocarbon-DNA adducts in human sperm as a marker of DNA damage and infertility. *Mut Res*. 2003;535(2):155-160.

80. Zhang Y, Dong S, Wang H, Tao S, Kiyama R. Biological impact of environmental polycyclic aromatic hydrocarbons (ePAHs) as endocrine disruptors. *Env Poll*. 2016;213:809-824.

81. Ramesh A, Harris KJ, Archibong AE. Reproductive toxicity of polycyclic aromatic hydrocarbons. In: Gupta RC, ed. *Reproductive and Developmental Toxicology*. Cambridge, Massachusetts, United States: Academic Press, Elsevier; 2022:759-778.

82. Patrizi B, Siciliani de Cumis M. TCDD toxicity mediated by epigenetic mechanisms. *Int J Mol Sci*. 2018;19(12):4101.

83. Pilsner JR, Parker M, Sergeyev O, Suvorov A. Spermatogenesis disruption by dioxins: epigenetic reprograming and windows of susceptibility. *Reprod Toxicol*. 2017;69:221-229.

84. Sengupta P, Arafa M, Elbardisi H. Hormonal regulation of spermatogenesis. In: Singh R, ed. *Molecular Signaling in Spermatogenesis and Male Infertility*. New Delhi: CRC Press; 2019:41-49.

85. Li S, Pei X, Zhang W, Xie HQ, Zhao B. Functional analysis of the dioxin response elements (DREs) of the murine CYP1A1 gene promoter: beyond the core DRE sequence. *Int J Mol Sci*. 2014;15(4):6475-6487.

86. Sun XL, Kido T, Honma S, et al. Influence of dioxin exposure upon levels of prostate-specific antigen and steroid hormones in Vietnamese men. *Envl Sci Poll Res*. 2016;23:7807-7813.

87. Galimova E, Amirova Z, Galimov SN. Dioxins in the semen of men with infertility. *Env Sci Poll Res*. 2015;22:14566-14569.

88. Choudhury BP, Roychoudhury S, Sengupta P, Toman R, Dutta S, Kesari KK. Arsenic-induced sex hormone disruption: an insight into male infertility. In: Roychoudhury S, Kesari KK, eds. *Oxidative Stress and Toxicity in Reproductive Biology and Medicine. A Comprehensive Update on Male Infertility Volume II*. Springer Cham; 2022:83-95.

89. Paithankar JG, Saini S, Dwivedi S, Sharma A, Chowdhuri DK. Heavy metal associated health hazards: an interplay of oxidative stress and signal transduction. *Chemosphere*. 2021;262:128350.

90. Bhardwaj JK, Paliwal A, Saraf P. Effects of heavy metals on reproduction owing to infertility. *J Biochem Mol Toxicol*. 2021;35(8):e22823.

91. Vecoli C, Montano L, Andreassi MG. Environmental pollutants: genetic damage and epigenetic changes in male germ cells. *Env Sci Poll Res*. 2016;23:23339-23348.

92. Cherry N, Labreche F, Collins J, Tulandi T. Occupational exposure to solvents and male infertility. *Occup Env Med*. 2001;58(10):635-640.

93. David E, Niculescu VC. Volatile organic compounds (VOCs) as environmental pollutants: occurrence and mitigation using nanomaterials. *Intl J Env Res Pub Heal*. 2021;18(24):13147.

94. Yoo DC, Choi DW. Effects of organic solvents on mucus penetration distance, motility and survival rate of human sperm in vitro. *Env Ana Heal Toxicol*. 2004;19(2):177-182.

95. Le Cornet C, Fervers B, Pukkala E, et al. Parental occupational exposure to organic solvents and testicular germ cell tumors in their offspring: NORD-TEST study. *Env Heal Perspect*. 2017;125(6):067023.

96. Dutta S, Henkel R, Sengupta P, Agarwal A. Physiological role of ROS in sperm function. In: Parekattil SJ, Esteves SC, Agarwal A, eds. *Male Infertility: Contemporary Clinical Approaches, Andrology, ART and Antioxidants*. Springer, Cham; 2020:337-345.

97. Darbandi S, Darbandi M, Khorshid HRK, Sengupta P. Electrophysiology of human gametes: a systematic review. *World J Men's Heal*. 2022;40(3):442.

98. Arabi H, Yazdi MT, Faramarzi M. Influence of whole microalgal cell immobilization and organic solvent on the bioconversion of androst-4-en-3, 17-dione to testosterone by Nostoc muscorum. *J Mol Catal*. 2010; 62(3-4):213-217.

99. Liu YX. Temperature control of spermatogenesis and prospect of male contraception. *Front Biosci Schol*. 2010;2(2):730-755.

100. Gao Y, Wang C, Wang K, He C, Hu K, Liang M. The effects and molecular mechanism of heat stress on spermatogenesis and the mitigation measures. *Syst Biol Reprod Med*. 2022;68(5-6):331-347.

101. Dutta S, Sandhu N, Sengupta P, Alves MG, Henkel R, Agarwal A. Somatic-immune cells crosstalk in-the-making of testicular immune privilege. *Reprod Sci*. 2022;29(10):2707-2718.

102. Dutta S, Sengupta P, Chhikara BS. Reproductive inflammatory mediators and male infertility. *Chem Biol Lett*. 2020;7(2):73-74.

103. Durairajanayagam D, Sharma RK, du Plessis SS, Agarwal A. Testicular heat stress and sperm quality. In: du Plessis SS, Agarwal A, Sabanegh ES, eds. *Male Infertility: A Complete Guide to Lifestyle and Environmental Factors*. New York: Springer; 2014:105-125.

104. Nishimura H, L'Hernault SW. Spermatogenesis. *Curr Biol*. 2017;27(18):R988-R994.

105. Bundhun PK, Janoo G, Bhurtu A, et al. Tobacco smoking and semen quality in infertile males: a systematic review and meta-analysis. *BMC Pub Heal*. 2019;19(1):1-11.

106. Saleh RA, Agarwal A, Sharma RK, Nelson DR, Thomas Jr AJ. Effect of cigarette smoking on levels of seminal oxidative stress in infertile men: a prospective study. *Fertil Steril*. 2002;78(3):491-499.

107. Dai JB, Wang ZX, Qiao ZD. The hazardous effects of tobacco smoking on male fertility. *Asian J Androl*. 2015; 17(6):954.

108. Zhang W, Li M, Sun F, et al. Association of sperm methylation at LINE-1, four candidate genes, and nicotine/alcohol exposure with the risk of infertility. *Front Genet*. 2019;10:1001.

109. Mostafa T. Cigarette smoking and male infertility. *J Adv Res*. 2010;1(3):179-186.

110. Ramgir SS, Abilash V. Impact of smoking and alcohol consumption on oxidative status in male infertility and sperm quality. *Indian J Pharm Sci*. 2019;81(5): 933-945.

111. Pasqualotto FF, Lucon AM, Sobreiro BP, Pasqualotto EB, Arap S. Effects of medical therapy, alcohol, smoking, and endocrine disruptors on male infertility. *Revis Hosp Clín*. 2004;59:375-382.

112. Akang E, Oremosu A, Osinubi A, et al. Alcohol-induced male infertility: is sperm DNA fragmentation a causative? *J Exp Clin Anat*. 2017;16(1):53.

113. Schifano N, Chiappini S, Mosca A, et al. Recreational drug misuse and its potential contribution to male fertility levels' decline: a narrative review. *Brain Sci*. 2022; 12(11):1582.

114. Rajanahally S, Raheem O, Rogers M, et al. The relationship between cannabis and male infertility, sexual health, and neoplasm: a systematic review. *Andrology*. 2019;7(2):139-147.

115. Fronczak CM, Kim ED, Barqawi AB. The insults of illicit drug use on male fertility. *J Androl*. 2012;33(4): 515-528.

116. Hayden RP, Flannigan R, Schlegel PN. The role of lifestyle in male infertility: diet, physical activity, and body habitus. *Curr Urol Reports*. 2018;19:1-10.

117. Arce JC, De Souza MJ. Exercise and male factor infertility. *Sports Med*. 1993;15:146-169.

118. du Plessis SS, Kashou A, Vaamonde D, Agarwal A. Is there a link between exercise and male factor infertility? *Open Reprod Sci J*. 2011;3(1):105-113.

119. Hajizadeh Maleki B, Tartibian B, Chehrazi M. Effectiveness of exercise training on male factor infertility: a systematic review and network meta-analysis. *Sports Heal*. 2022;14(4):508-517.

120. Leisegang K, Sengupta P, Agarwal A, Henkel R. Obesity and male infertility: mechanisms and management. *Andrologia*. 2021;53(1):e13617.
121. Chaudhuri GR, Das A, Kesh SB, et al. Obesity and male infertility: multifaceted reproductive disruption. *Middle East Fertil Soc J*. 2022;27(1):8.
122. Dutta S, Biswas A, Sengupta P. Obesity, endocrine disruption and male infertility. *Asian Pac J Reprod*. 2019;8(5):195.
123. Bhattacharya K, Sengupta P, Dutta S, Bhattacharya S. Pathophysiology of obesity: endocrine, inflammatory and neural regulators. *Res J Pharm Technol*. 2020;13(9):4469-4478.
124. Sengupta P, Bhattacharya K, Dutta S. Leptin and male reproduction. *Asian Pac J Reprod*. 2019;8(5):220.
125. Craig JR, Jenkins TG, Carrell DT, Hotaling JM. Obesity, male infertility, and the sperm epigenome. *Fertil Steril*. 2017;107(4):848-859.
126. Nargund VH. Effects of psychological stress on male fertility. *Nat Rev Urol*. 2015;12(7):373-382.
127. McGrady A. Effects of psychological stress on male reproduction: a review. *Arch Androl*. 1984;13(1):1-7.
128. Fode M, Krogh-Jespersen S, Brackett NL, Ohl DA, Lynne CM, Sønksen J. Male sexual dysfunction and infertility associated with neurological disorders. *Asian J Androl*. 2012;14(1):61.
129. Kesari KK, Agarwal A, Henkel R. Radiations and male fertility. *Reprod Biol Endocrinol*. 2018;16(1):1-16.
130. Ahmad G, Agarwal A. Ionizing radiation and male fertility. In: Gunasekaran K, Pandiyan N, eds. *Male Infertility: A Clinical Approach*. New Delhi: Springer; 2017:185-196.
131. De Felice F, Marchetti C, Marampon F, Cascialli G, Muzii L, Tombolini V. Radiation effects on male fertility. *Andrology*. 2019;7(1):2-7.
132. Wdowiak A, Skrzypek M, Stec M, Panasiuk L. Effect of ionizing radiation on the male reproductive system. *Ann Agr Env Med*. 2019;26(2):210-216.
133. Kovac JR, Addai J, Smith RP, Coward RM, Lamb DJ, Lipshultz LI. The effects of advanced paternal age on fertility. *Asian J Androl*. 2013;15(6):723.
134. Brandt JS, Cruz Ithier MA, Rosen T, Ashkinadze E. Advanced paternal age, infertility, and reproductive risks: a review of the literature. *Prenat Diag*. 2019;39(2):81-87.
135. de La Rochebrochard E, Mcelreavey K, Thonneau P. Paternal age over 40 years: the "amber light" in the reproductive life of men? *J Androl*. 2003;24(4):459-465.
136. Sharma R, Agarwal A, Rohra VK, Assidi M, Abu-Elmagd M, Turki RF. Effects of increased paternal age on sperm quality, reproductive outcome and associated epigenetic risks to offspring. *Reprod Biol Endocrinol*. 2015;13:1-20.
137. McPherson NO, Zander-Fox D, Vincent AD, Lane M. Combined advanced parental age has an additive negative effect on live birth rates—data from 4057 first IVF/ICSI cycles. *J Assist Reprod Genet*. 2018;35:279-287.
138. Ricci E, Al-Beitawi S, Cipriani S, et al. Dietary habits and semen parameters: a systematic narrative review. *Andrology*. 2018;6(1):104-116.
139. Nazni P. Association of western diet & lifestyle with decreased fertility. *Indian J Med Res*. 2014;140(suppl 1):S78.
140. Montano L, Maugeri A, Volpe MG, et al. Mediterranean diet as a shield against male infertility and cancer risk induced by environmental pollutants: a focus on flavonoids. *Int J Mol Sci*. 2022;23(3):1568.
141. Muffone ARM, de Oliveira Lübke PD, Rabito EI. Mediterranean diet and infertility: a systematic review with meta-analysis of cohort studies. *Nutr Rev*. 2022:nuac087. doi:10.1093/nutrit/nuac087.
142. Ricci E, Viganò P, Cipriani S, et al. Coffee and caffeine intake and male infertility: a systematic review. *Nutr J*. 2017;16:1-14.
143. Bu FL, Feng X, Yang XY, Ren J, Cao HJ. Relationship between caffeine intake and infertility: a systematic review of controlled clinical studies. *BMC Womens Health*. 2020;20(1):1-9.
144. Kim HH. Selecting the optimal gestational carrier: medical, reproductive, and ethical considerations. *Fertil Steril*. 2020;113(5):892-896.

6

Idiopathic Male Infertility

Mohit Butaney and Amarnath Rambhatla

KEY POINTS

- Male infertility is a complex, multifactorial disorder, and a better understanding of the underlying causes remains a high priority, given the epidemiological trends.
- Research into newer diagnostics tools that can be used to understand these trends is crucial to develop more personalized treatments for males dealing with this.
- The mainstay of current treatment for idiopathic infertility focuses on lifestyle modification, empiric medical therapy, antioxidant therapy, and assisted reproduction.

INTRODUCTION

Definitions–Idiopathic Versus Unexplained Male Infertility

The World Health Organization defines infertility as the inability to achieve pregnancy after 12 months of regular, unprotected sexual intercourse. Several known congenital and acquired causes of infertility exist, including but not limited to congenital urogenital abnormalities, malignancies and their associated treatments, infections, hormonal abnormalities, varicoceles, immunological factors, and genetic aberrations. Although infertility is often recognized as a complex process likely affected by multiple known variables, the underlying causes remain elusive in 30% to 50% of patients. Idiopathic male infertility is diagnosed in the presence of altered sperm parameters without an identifiable cause and the absence of female factor infertility. This is in contrast to unexplained infertility, where sperm parameters and evaluation for the couple are normal. This distinction might be crucial to general comparable research data and, consequently, better understanding the underlying etiology.

Epidemiology of Idiopathic Male Infertility

In the United States, approximately 15% of heterosexual couples report infertility, with a male component contributing to this in up to 50% of cases.[1] Approximately 30% to 50% of males are diagnosed with unexplained or idiopathic infertility.[2] Male infertility has been rising and multiple studies have shown the decreasing trend of sperm counts over the last century, making our understanding of the etiology of male infertility a crucial issue to address.[3] The reasons for this decline are still unclear; however, several causes have been postulated, including environmental pollutants and endocrine-disrupting chemicals (EDCs). Male infertility may be associated with reduced longevity and also a risk factor for certain malignancies and medical comorbidities. There is also a significant psychological and marital strain that the diagnosis of infertility creates. An important consideration in present-day society is that the average age when patients are seeking fertility has increased, and age certainly plays a role in fertility potential for a couple. While the effect of maternal age is well known, increasing paternal age has also more recently been shown to increase likelihood of disorders such as autism, bipolar disorder, cancers, and other genetic disorders, highlighting the need for counseling based on the age of the prospective father as well. Our understanding of the pathophysiology is crucial to developing targeted treatments in the future.

ETIOLOGY AND PREVAILING THEORIES

Given the multifactorial nature of male infertility, it is challenging to definitively place a number of patients who are dealing with idiopathic infertility into a single category of potential causes. However, a number of theories have been proposed that play a role in these patients with an otherwise unknown cause, and eventually, better diagnostics are likely the key to being able to better characterize these patients. Idiopathic male infertility is likely due to previously unidentified pathological factors. Advancements in male infertility research are identifying potential causes such as elevated sperm DNA fragmentation (SDF), reactive oxygen species (ROS), genetic and epigenetic factors, and EDCs impacting the reproductive axis.[4] The more recognized and known causes of infertility are not considered to be idiopathic infertility and are outside the scope of this chapter. The theories below are rapidly evolving to ideally transition patients out of the category of idiopathic infertility.

Immunologic Causes

While sperm are "immunologically privileged" and protected by the blood–testis barrier, the barrier can be destroyed due to reasons such as trauma, surgery, and infection, or may not be present in early stages of spermatic development. Antisperm antibodies (ASAs) are immunoglobulins directed against sperm surface antigens. These antibodies have been postulated to form due to these reasons and discussed for many decades; their presence does not always lead to an effect of sperm parameters and infertility with significant limitations to draw clear conclusions using available literature.[5] The use of ASA testing and steroids in treatment has limited evidence but continues to be used in practice by a significant proportion of urologists and thus continues to be an important area of further research.[6] Prior genitourinary infections may cause direct damage to sperm function, cause damage due to inflammation or immunologic response in male reproductive organs, or even have anatomical consequences such as in the case of

an infection-associated stricture.[7] While classic viral orchitis is associated with a mumps infection causing direct damage to testicular germ cells, it can be caused by a number of other viral or bacterial pathogens as well.[8] Sexually transmitted infections, such as human papillomavirus infection, have been shown to impair sperm quality and induce development of ASAs.[9] More recently, the sequelae of COVID-19 in the male reproductive system needs to be better understood.[10] Given the role of leukocyte-induced oxidative stress and the direct effect of bacteria and viruses, these infections are potentially an important piece of the puzzle.[11]

Noninfectious causes of inflammation also need to be considered, such as those potentially caused by autoimmune or systemic inflammatory diseases. Interestingly, data from an insurance claims database has been used to show that infertile males have a higher risk of having certain autoimmune disorders in the years following an infertility evaluation. This includes rheumatoid arthritis, multiple sclerosis, psoriasis, thyroiditis, and Graves disease, further hinting at a link between fertility and immunity.[12] Clinically, these events present as a history of urethritis, prostatitis, epididymitis, and orchitis; however, a considerable portion of the patient population might be unaware of previous episodes of genitourinary infection or inflammation. These infections have the potential to affect fertility irreversibly on various levels.[13] Interestingly, ASAs have been reported to be more common in cases of chronic prostatitis; however, this mechanism is not completely understood.[14] Additionally, while knowledge about their role in the reproductive axis is still being completely understood, the above-described sources of inflammation and infection can lead to deregulation of cytokines, eventually leading to infertility.[15]

Endocrine Disruption

The male endocrine system, specifically the hypothalamic-pituitary-gonadal (HPG) axis, plays a significant role in reproductive function and spermatogenesis, and can be disrupted by several different mechanisms. Sertoli and Leydig cells in the testis play a key role in spermatogenesis and testicular steroidogenesis. They are heavily regulated by pituitary hormones such as the follicle-stimulating hormone (FSH) and luteinizing hormone (LH). Hypogonadotropic hypogonadism, characterized by decreased LH and FSH, leads to low serum testosterone, as well as severe oligospermia or azoospermia. On the other hand, elevated gonadotropin levels indicate hypergonado-trophic hypogonadism or failure at the testicular level. A high FSH level is indicative of abnormal spermato-genesis. While several causes of hypogonadotrophic hypogonadism are known, the causes for idiopathic or isolated hypogonadotrophic hypogonadism are still not completely understood.[16] Additionally, the HPG axis works closely with the immune system, leading to additional dysregulation from an immunological per-spective. For example, testosterone has been identified to play a key role in mediating inflammation and cytokines.[17]

There is an interdependence of various male body systems and pathophysiology leading to endocrine dysfunction, which may also affect infertility. Both hypo- and hyperthyroidism can lead to sperm and sexual dysfunction. Given the growing obesity pan-demic, the hormonal dysregulation caused by the additional adiposity is important to understand. The abnormal estrogen-to-testosterone ratios due to in-creased aromatase activity are well known, but it is also important to continue to understand the effect of other adipokines, hormones produced by adipose tis-sue, such as leptin, adiponectin, resistin, and visfatin, that have been shown to affect the reproductive axis.[15] Additionally, studies have often discussed the impact of vitamin D on semen quality; however, these results continue to be inconclusive.

Our understanding of hormonal physiology and its effect on fertility continues to evolve to provide us with better markers of and insights into idiopathic infertility. While much is known about some of the neuropeptides involved in the HPG axis, such as gonadotropin-releas-ing hormone, more recently, kisspeptin has been identi-fied as yet another neuropeptide that potentially plays an important role in this axis and its impact on fertil-ity.[18] Even hormones that have been studied for many years, such as the anti-Mullerian hormone, which is known to cause regression of Mullerian structures dur-ing male development, has been shown to be a potential marker for dysfunction and guide treatment decisions.[19] More recently, several other biomarkers have been stud-ied to better understand the intratesticular hormonal state, including 17-hydroxyprogesterone (17-OHP) and insulin-like factor 3 (INSL3).[20,21] Serum 17-OHP is an intermediate in the production of testosterone from cholesterol. Serum INSL3 is secreted by Leydig cells and,

while it is still not totally understood, it seems to be involved in bone metabolism and in spermatogenesis. It has been shown that serum INSL3 levels appear to re-flect the number of functional Leydig cells in males.[21] These serum biomarkers can potentially provide us with a deeper insight into the intratesticular endocrinologi-cal state without the need for invasive sampling and provide us with a better proxy than serum testosterone. An enhanced understanding of the endocrinological mechanisms of infertility can aid in the development of medical therapy for male infertility.

Role of the Environment and Lifestyle Factors

Environmental exposure to chemicals and lifestyle fac-tors are risks for male infertility. Specifically, smoking, alcohol, drugs, obesity, and psychological stress have all been linked to infertility. The increasing incidence of obesity has been correlated with infertility in several studies and further contributes both directly and indi-rectly.[22] Obesity can act to impair fertility potential through a few different routes. As discussed previously, it can lead to endocrinological derangements but also a higher risk of other comorbidities, and even directly due to increased DNA fragmentation.[23,24] Specifically, it is well known that obese males may have a high degree of peripheral conversion of testosterone to estrogen in adipose tissue, leading to a high estradiol state. Other comorbidities such as diabetes, which has been associ-ated with low testosterone, higher SDF, and impaired sperm parameters, can further exacerbate sperm dys-function. EDCs are a heterogeneous group of chemicals that can interfere with endogenous hormones and lead to adverse physiological effects.[25] Despite several de-cades of research, the data about their effects on fertility are controversial; however, early exposure in utero to EDCs has been linked to testicular dysgenesis syn-drome, which includes cryptorchidism, hypospadias, testicular malignancy, and infertility.[25] While animal studies have helped drive knowledge in this field, there are still many unknowns regarding mechanisms and the true clinical impact in humans.

Lifestyle factors are crucial to understand on a per-sonalized basis, as they contribute to a significant por-tion of the initial approach to idiopathic infertility. Hyperthermia is a known factor that affects sperm production and can be due to several lifestyle choices or activities such as use of specific underwear, seden-tary lifestyle, or biking. A study has even correlated decreased semen quality with the use of cell phones, which is an increasing issue in today's modern world.[26] While we know that several toxins and drugs can affect sperm parameters, it will be important to make a conscious effort to investigate and consider their effect on sperm parameters, as well as for patterns of change in alcohol, tobacco, and drug usage. This is particularly important considering major changes such as marijuana legalization, the opioid crisis, and the growing use of e-cigarettes and vaping, with limited long-term data. A superficial discussion of a patient's lifestyle can often lead to an underappreciation of the effect of a patient's lifestyle on their fertility potential.

While the external environment clearly has an impact on fertility potential, there is growing evidence that other, more recently understood intrinsic environmental factors play a role as well. Sperm dysfunction can be due to the environment in which the spermatozoa mature due to defects in semen viscosity, volume, or acidity. The microbiome refers to the genetic material compromising the unique microbes residing within the human body that play a critical role in normal physiology and, as we have learned more recently, in pathogenesis. Recent work investigating the relationship between the genitourinary and gastrointestinal microbiomes and male reproduction in a small subset of males found several important bacterial and metabolic pathway differences, with potential to aid in diagnosis and management of male infertility in the future.[27] They had several other interesting findings such as the different expression of the S-adenosyl-L-methionine cycle between fertile and infertile males in semen, which has several potential ways it could affect spermatogenesis, and identified differences in pathway expression when comparing patients who had a varicocele. While these are early proof-of-concept studies, this is certainly an area that needs to be explored further, particularly due to the potential avenues of management available.

Molecular Underpinnings of Idiopathic Male Infertility (i.e., Genetics and Epigenetics)

Genetic factors account for at least 15% of male infertility. Spermatogenesis is a complex, intricate process involving several proteins and genes. Mutations in any of these genes may lead to male infertility. Several forms of infertility cannot be passed on genetically; however, mutations can still be passed in a recessive or X-linked pattern. Given the de novo nature of several of these

mutations, their characterization has been challenging. Several genetic variants have been detected rapidly over the past decade with the use of advancing technologies such as next-generation sequencing and genome-wide association studies, as well as decreasing costs associated with these methods.[28,29] With the advent of high-throughput technologies such as whole-genome sequencing and more insight into methods to test genetic hypotheses, several efforts have been made to better understand the underlying genomic disruptions leading to infertility, but their translation and utility in clinical medicine has not been fully realized.

The primary known genetic causes of male infertility include Y chromosome microdeletions, Klinefelter syndrome, cystic fibrosis transmembrane receptor (*CFTR*) gene mutations in males with congenital bilateral absence of the vas deferens (CBAVD), Kallmann syndrome, Robertsonian translocations, and other chromosomal abnormalities leading to deterioration of testicular function. Events leading to chromosomal abnormalities can have effects on fertility potential and are the most commonly found genetic abnormalities in males, including events such as chromosomal translocations, inversions, and deletions. As previously discussed, the endocrinological environment plays a significant role in fertility. Molecular alterations in the hypothalamic-pituitary axis can disrupt sperm development at multiple levels. For example, while Kallmann syndrome might account for a significant number of congenital hypogonadotropic hypogonadism, a significant number of cases do not have a cause identified despite discovery of a few candidate genes. Further downstream, there have been genetic changes directly associated with spermatic development in patients who have previously been found to be diagnosed with idiopathic infertility. Several of these genes have been identified to alter specific parameters such as quantitative production of sperm, morphology, or motility. For example, the cause of nonobstructive azoospermia (NOA) is often unknown. Given the diversity of phenotypes from a Sertoli cell–only syndrome leading to a complete lack of germ cells to various forms of maturation arrest or hypospermatogenesis, a significant number of candidate genes have been discovered, but replicating studies and quantifying their role remains challenging. Even further downstream, CBAVD is typically associated with *CFTR* mutations. However, mutations or loss of other genes can also lead to absence of the vas deferens, and a cohort of patients who have CBAVD may have non-*CFTR* mutations that remain to be discovered.[30]

While some of these findings, such as those associated with certain Yq microdeletions, are helpful in prognostication of the utility of assisted reproductive technologies (ARTs), many of the findings will need functional and clinical validation of the gene–disease relationships.[31] Without this, there is the significant potential of misdiagnosis and mismanagement—guidelines regarding genetic testing in this patient population are appropriately lagging as we assimilate all this information. While mouse spermatogonial stem cell cultures have been performed, the in vitro culture of human cells has yet to materialize and is likely a key to truly unlocking the potential shown by these high-throughput technologies. Apart from functional validation, in vitro human spermatogenesis and the ability to culture testicular tissue can potentially lead to genetic technologies to restore spermatogenesis in a number of cases.[32] The CRISPR/Cas9 system catapulted over other gene editing technologies and, since its discovery, has been used in several different ways. Several animal studies have reported success in using this technology as a therapeutic intervention to edit spermatogonial stem cells in preclinical models and to model infertility driven by genetic causes.[33] There are certainly ethical and safety considerations, with a significant degree of refinement still needed via preclinical studies and trials; however, this remains an extremely promising area of research. Given the growing rise of technology and data, it is likely that interpretation rather than diagnosis will be a more prominent issue than detection in the near future.

Simultaneously, numerous proteomic studies have been performed on this population as well, particularly in patients in whom it is possible to obtain sufficient proteins to analyze.[34] More recently, with the development of the field of metabolomics, studies have been able to demonstrate differences in sperm metabolism when evaluating patients with altered sperm parameters, but this field is still in its early phases.[35] Finally, damage to DNA integrity has been increasingly discussed in recent literature, and measures of DNA integrity have been shown to be associated with outcomes of ART. However, its use in the clinical setting is still controversial, and further research is needed to better understand its utility. A number of extrinsic and intrinsic environmental factors discussed previously can lead to DNA damage. Additionally, several recent studies have

suggested a role for epigenetic modifications affecting male infertility.[36] Epigenetics is the study of processes that might alter gene expression. This includes histone modification and hypomethylation of specific DNA regions. Another aspect being researched is DNA packaging into chromatin, which includes protamine packaging. More recently, RNA expression and regulation have been found to be a potential useful marker for male infertility.[37] Additionally, abnormal centrioles can affect ability of sperm to fertilize.[37] In addition to all the above, natural aging, the environment, and other lifestyle factors can influence the genome and consequently, spermatogenesis and pregnancy.

As the era of "big data" is ushered in, technologies to better analyze these vast amounts of data, ideally associated with the decreasing costs, and collaboration between institutions will be paramount to understand this sector effectively. An essential aspect of these efforts would be the correlation to a complete phenotype associated with these patients. Without this integration of data, truly establishing causality and moving towards clinical utility is challenging.[38] Given all the rapidly growing genetic data and a golden era associated with technology investigating genomics, there is a growing belief that there is a genetic basis in a significant proportion of cases of idiopathic severe male infertility.

Male Oxidative Stress Infertility

Oxidative stress is an increasingly recognized and understood cause of idiopathic infertility. Oxidative stress could result due to several extrinsic or intrinsic causes contributing to infertility. Endogenous sources of ROS include infections, autoimmune/inflammatory conditions, leukocytes, and even structural variations in anatomy such as varicoceles and cryptorchidism.[39] Exogenous sources can include radiation, smoking, alcohol, or other toxins.[39] While ROS are naturally produced through several pathophysiological mechanisms and small quantities are required to ensure normal cellular function including sperm development, studies have suggested elevated seminal oxidation-reduction potential in 30% to 80% of males with infertility.[40] The body attempts to use dietary or endogenously produced antioxidants to compensate for this imbalance; however, this oxidative stress can affect fertility through a few different routes.[41] Given the spermatic structure has a high–lipid content plasma membrane and a small amount of cytoplasm, it is vulnerable to oxidative stress.

This can be due to direct damage to sperm or an alteration of the process that eventually leads to fertilization.[42,43] Additionally, oxidative stress can have long-term effects on the health of the subsequent offspring.[44] Several diagnostic tests have focused on the quantification of DNA damage based on the premise that this would lead to a better understanding of male fertility potential and treatment decisions. The term male oxidative stress infertility (MOSI) has been proposed as a novel descriptor for infertile males with abnormal semen parameters and oxidative stress.[45]

Last, it is certainly possible that patients might not have a single clear etiology for their infertility, with multiple etiologies or generally poor overall health status contributing to their eventual idiopathic infertility.

DIAGNOSIS OF IDIOPATHIC MALE INFERTILITY

Beyond a Basic Semen Analysis

Investigation of male infertility begins with a detailed reproductive history, physical examination, and a semen analysis. Males presenting with idiopathic infertility have no obvious red flags in their history and physical examination, and this is a crucial first step in the initial management of a male patient where the etiology of infertility is unknown. Conditions such as varicoceles or issues in coital technique can be readily eliminated during a thorough initial visit. A thorough investigation of a female factor should also simultaneously occur. Assessment of semen analyses is based on evaluation of volume, sperm concentration, sperm motility, and sperm morphology. The most common abnormalities in routine semen analysis are azoospermia (absence of spermatozoa), oligozoospermia (low sperm concentration in the ejaculate), teratozoospermia (abnormal sperm morphology), and/or asthenozoospermia (abnormal sperm motility). Additionally, multiple sperm defects can occur in a single patient, and these are potentially underreported in the literature.

Given the multiple theories but often unclear etiology of infertility and the lack of actionable findings on these primary diagnostics, it is essential to look beyond the semen analysis to understanding the underlying etiology in the investigation of idiopathic infertility. Table 6.1 attempts to guide us in our growing ability to investigate idiopathic infertility beyond a semen analysis and highlights potential clues to direct us towards underlying etiologies. Current guidelines recommend two semen analyses separated by a period of up to 1 month. However, semen analyses continue to have issues with reproducibility, subjectivity, and eventually, poor prediction of fertility.[44] A basic semen analysis eventually only provides diagnostic clues with limited information about the underlying functional defects. This is a rapidly evolving field, and biomarkers to better direct patients to therapeutic interventions would certainly be helpful. In the future, a panel of tests including SDF, oxidative stress, and specialized structural and functional sperm tests will be included in the work-up of idiopathic male infertility.

Endocrine Evaluation

It is recommended by the American Urological Association (AUA)/American Society for Reproductive Medicine (ASRM) male infertility guideline to obtain an endocrine evaluation if there is oligospermia or azoospermia on semen analysis, a history of erectile dysfunction or reduced libido, or evidence of hormonal abnormality on physical exam.[45] Hormonal causes account for approximately 10% of infertility cases in males. However, a recent survey evaluating treatment of idiopathic infertility found that only 35% of respondents would perform a hormonal evaluation prior to recommending treatment.[46] A single-center study evaluating the utility of routine hormone evaluation in all males presenting for infertility found that hypoandrogenism is common among this population, and these findings are potentially helpful to optimize the endocrine function of patients attempting to conceive. This would be particularly helpful in identifying males who would potentially benefit from hormone modulators and potentially avoid attempts at using ART.[47] Per the AUA/ASRM guideline, an initial panel of testosterone, LH, and FSH can be utilized, followed by a repeat measurement of total and free testosterone, as well as determination of serum, LH, estradiol, and prolactin in patients whose the fasting total testosterone level is less than 300 ng/dL. Sex hormone–binding globulin (SHBG) can be checked if there is a concern for other medical conditions that may alter the SHBG level. While there is some controversy in the literature associated with this topic, a morning lab draw including total testosterone, LH, FSH, and estradiol would be a reasonable endocrine evaluation to begin with. Novel biomarkers such as

TABLE 6.1   **An Attempt to Investigate Idiopathic Infertility Based on Prevailing Etiologies**

Immunologic Cause
- History of prior genitourinary infections, autoimmune diseases, and testicular trauma/surgery
- Appropriate investigation, treatments, or referrals for infections or conditions as required including but not limited to urine or semen culture
- Considering role of inflammation and its mediators (cytokines, adipokines, etc.)

Endocrine Disruption
- History of other endocrine disorders, physiological symptoms or signs of hormonal anomalies, obesity
- Evaluation of reproductive hormones: testosterone, LH, FSH, prolactin, estradiol
- Evaluation of thyroid hormones
- Evaluation using experimental novel biomarkers such as 17-OHP and INSL3

Role of the Environment
- History of exposure to radiation, toxins/drugs, dietary factors, or environments with significant pollution
- History of smoking, alcohol use, or other drug use
- History of prior surgeries, trauma, or anatomic abnormality, such as cryptorchidism or varicocele, affecting the environment for sperm development
- History of or current occupation or lifestyle hazard leading to chronic heat exposure or stress
- Considering impact of endocrine disruptors during development

Molecular Underpinnings of Male Idiopathic Infertility
- Diagnosis or symptoms of Klinefelter, cystic fibrosis, idiopathic hypogonadotrophic hypogonadism
- Karyotyping, Y chromosome microdeletion testing, and *CFTR* testing when indicated
- DNA fragmentation testing: direct tests include terminal deoxynucleotidyl transferase dUTP nick end labeling and single-cell gel electrophoresis assay (Comet). Indirect tests include sperm chromatin structure assay and sperm chromatic dispersion
- Whole-exome and -genome sequencing
- Other experimental tests to further evaluate sperm components include evaluation of sperm RNA, sperm proteomics, or fluorescence-based ratiometric assessment of centrioles

Oxidative Stress
- History of factors leading to any other etiology could be contributing factors towards the rise of oxidative stress
- Multiple assays available currently: chemiluminescence for reactive oxidative stress, total antioxidant capacity for antioxidants, and for malondialdehyde assays for post hoc damage from lipid peroxidation, measurement of oxidation reduction potential using the male oxidative system

Infertility as a Marker of Overall Poorer Health Status and Comorbidities
- History of other systemic diseases or cancer
- Necessary treatment or referrals for optimization of other conditions as indicated

Other Investigations Beyond a Semen Analysis Based on History and Physical
- Semen analysis
- Postejaculatory urine analysis
- Ultrasonography (scrotal and transrectal)
- Antisperm antibodies (mixed antiglobulin reaction test, immunobead test, and enzyme-linked immunosorbent assay)
- Ensure parallel assessments of female partner

CFTR, Cystic fibrosis transmembrane receptor; *FSH*, follicle-stimulating hormone; *INSL3*, insulin-like factor 3; *LH*, luteinizing hormone; *17-OHP*, 17-hydroxyprogesterone .

17-OHP and INSL3 will certainly be worth keeping an eye on as data regarding this continues to evolve.[20,21] An evaluation of thyroid hormones can also be helpful. Depending on the way a practice is set up, the involvement of a reproductive urologist/andrologist is helpful to ensure a thorough evaluation from this perspective.

Measuring Oxidative Stress

There is no current consensus and validated method to measure oxidative stress. Interestingly, routine sperm analysis can also provide clues with regard to patients who have a high degree of oxidative stress, such as the presence of asthenozoospermia or seminal plasma hyperviscosity.[48] Although a few assays are now available to measure oxidative stress, including chemiluminescence for reactive oxidative stress, total antioxidant capacity for antioxidants, and malondialdehyde assays for post hoc damage from lipid peroxidation, their complexity and cost have slowed their translational use in the clinical setting.[49–51] The most recent test to enter the market, the male infertility oxidative system for the assessment of oxidative reduction potential, might have circumvented some of these issues.[52] A multicenter evaluation of this system was able to establish a cut-off of 1.34 mV/10^6 sperm/mL for oxidation-reduction potential to distinguish between abnormal and normal semen quality, using 2092 patients with male infertility.[53] The utility of this test in a randomized controlled trial (RCT) would help further cement its role in diagnostics for idiopathic infertility. Additionally, the population with oxidative stress but normal semen characteristics has still not been fully characterized; that will likely provide us further insight into the utility of oxidative stress.[40,54] The lack of studies and consensus on the utility of these tests is affecting the use of these tests in clinical practice.[55]

Molecular Genetics and Cytogenetic Analysis

Research on intracellular sperm analysis is scarce but has evolved rapidly more recently. Apart from quantification of male oxidative stress, research on several other aspects of understanding the molecular basis of infertility is ongoing, including SDF, defective centrioles, sperm aneuploidy, and abnormal RNA.[56] Current AUA/ASRM guidelines recommend karyotyping and Y chromosome microdeletion testing for males with primary infertility and azoospermia or severe oligozoospermia (<5 million/mL concentration) with elevated FSH, testicular atrophy, or a presumed diagnosis of NOA. Karyotyping detects any chromosomal defects and should be part of the primary genetic evaluation for azoospermic/severely oligospermic males. The azoospermia factor (AZF) region on the long arm of the Y chromosome encodes genes associates with spermatogenesis. While AZFa or AZFb microdeletions are not associated with successful sperm retrieval with a microscopic testicular sperm extraction, it is often successful in AZFc microdeletions, helping prognosticate treatment and counsel patients. Additionally, *CFTR* testing is recommended

in males with vasal agenesis (CBAVD) or idiopathic obstructive azoospermia. When indicated, these tests would be helpful to rule out any potential known causes of infertility. While research so far might have picked the "low-hanging fruit" of one gene–one phenotype infertility, it is certainly possible that deciphering the rest of this cohort of patients would require a more complex understanding of the numerous factors involved in eventually leading to their specific phenotype.

SDF is a well-studied mechanism potentially leading to male infertility; however, it is not yet recommended in the initial evaluation of the infertile couple as per the AUA/ASRM guidelines, given the limited prospective data to support it.[47,57–59] A number of assays to better understand DNA integrity have been proposed; however, they have not yet been widely adopted into clinical use. These include tests that can directly detect DNA breaks such as terminal deoxynucleotidyl transferase dUTP nick end labeling and single-cell gel electrophoresis assay (Comet). The sperm chromatin structure assay (SCSA) and sperm chromatic dispersion are indirect tools for assessment. The SCSA is the most well developed and widely used. A DNA fragment index of greater than 50% on this test has been associated with poor in vitro fertilization outcomes. The absence of standardization of measures and protocols as well as robust prospective data in this realm is currently a barrier to its widespread utility. The predictive capacity of these tests for pregnancy conception and live births after ART has been found to be limited and unreliable. However, given the limited amount of data available in the literature so far, DNA fragmentation can be useful in counseling certain patients, such as males in couples with repeated in vitro fertilization (IVF) failures or males with varicoceles and abnormal semen parameters.

The evolution of next-generation sequencing technologies such as whole-exome and -genome sequencing have sparked a wave of research in better understanding the molecular etiology of idiopathic infertility; however, the translation of such technology to clinical medicine remains to be seen. Studies such as the BabySeq project are under way to establish the utility of genomic sequencing in newborns to anticipate childhood- and adult-onset diseases, and the impact of this data on health care and science will be tremendous as this cohort of patients ages.[60] Additionally, this information has limited clinical implications currently, so an important piece of this puzzle would be the clinical and functional validation of findings through these technologies. Despite the discoveries of the past decade, the recommended diagnostic genetic tests associated with infertility have remained largely unchanged, given the relative infrequency of these genes and lack of clinical validation. In addition to analyzing DNA, novel methods to investigate intracellular sperm function further are being developed. For example, a fluorescence-based ratiometric assessment of centrioles (FRAC) was recently developed to better quantify centriole dysfunction.[61] Their findings suggested that FRAC was sensitive and that patient age and sperm morphology were both associated with centriole quality. Eventually, given the results so far, it appears that a multiparametric machine-based analysis to analyze all the various components of sperm structure and development is what is needed.

Other Testing

While several of the tests outlined below are not required for routine investigation, they may be indicated in certain circumstances, depending on the history and physical examination. Given that idiopathic infertility is a diagnosis of exclusion, it is essential to consider the utility of such tests when making the eventual diagnosis.

Postejaculatory Urine Analysis

Postejaculatory urine analysis for any patient who has low ejaculate volume can be helpful when considering the diagnosis of retrograde ejaculation. Diagnosis is often limited by technique of collection, so it is essential to ensure a complete collection with a reasonable abstinence period and centrifuging the sample for 10 minutes at a minimum of 300 × g and microscopically inspecting the pellet at 400× magnification. However, the definition of "significant number of sperm" in urine to make the diagnosis of retrograde ejaculation is unclear.

Ultrasonography

Ultrasound continues to be a commonly used tool in the evaluation of male infertility and can be offered to patients particularly due to its low cost and noninvasive nature. Findings of obstruction, testicular mass, or a reversible pathology such as a varicocele can help reduce the number of patients with an unknown etiology of male infertility.[62] Transrectal ultrasonography is indicated in azoospermic patients with palpable vasa

and low ejaculate volumes to determine if ejaculatory duct obstruction exists.[47] It can also be useful to diagnose other anomalies associated with obstruction, such as ejaculatory duct cysts or seminal vesicular anomalies. While scrotal pathology is palpable on physical examination, a scrotal ultrasound can be useful in patients where the physical examination is felt to be difficult or inadequate.[47] The advent of newer, higher-resolution microultrasound devices can further aid in visualization of anatomy for etiological diagnosis and also for treatment preparation. While in many cases a physical examination is often sufficient to make a diagnosis, imaging can be helpful in inconclusive or idiopathic cases.

Antisperm Antibodies

ASAs can usually be found in three different locations: serum, seminal plasma, or sperm bound. Additionally, these antibodies can also be found in cervical fluid. The sperm-bound ASAs are the most clinically relevant. ASAs can be detected by various methods, including the mixed antiglobulin reaction (MAR) test, the immunobead (IBT) test, and enzyme-linked immunosorbent assay (ELISA). The IBT test provides the most information about the type and presence of immunoglobulins and their localization in sperm. Current AUA/ASRM guidelines do not recommend these in the initial evaluation of male infertility, but this test can be considered as part of an advanced work-up.[47]

TREATMENT OF IDIOPATHIC MALE INFERTILITY
Lack of Guidelines

As the field rapidly grows to better understand the etiology of male infertility, there is an understandable lack of evidence-based guidelines on this front. While guidelines specifically discuss the limited use of selective estrogen receptor modulators (SERMs) relative to ART and consideration of an FSH analog, there is limited further evidence or discussion with regard to investigating and managing idiopathic infertility.[47]

Treatment Options

Among acquired factors, varicocele is the most common and correctable cause of infertility in males, with a prevalence of about 40%. Given our limited understanding of idiopathic infertility, targeted and evidence-based treatment is challenging. Table 6.2 highlights a number of

TABLE 6.2 **Treatment of Idiopathic Male Infertility**
Lifestyle Modifications
• Optimization of comorbidities and evaluation of medications being taken
• Weight loss if needed to achieve a healthy body composition through exercise and a balanced diet
• Critically evaluating occupational or environmental factors
• Cutting down smoking, alcohol, or other drugs
• Attempt at reduction in any psychological stress
• Timed intercourse
Selective Estrogen Receptor Modulators
• Clomiphene citrate
• Tamoxifen
Aromatase Inhibitors
• Anastrozole
• Letrozole
Gonadotropin Analogs
• FSH-based such as Gonal-F
• FSH and LH–based such as Menopur
• LH-based such as hCG
Vitamins and Antioxidants
• Arginine
• Carnitines
• Carotenoids
• Coenzyme Q10
• Cysteine
• Micronutrients (folate, selenium, zinc)
• Vitamin E
• Vitamin C
• Polyunsaturated fatty acids
• Vitamin B (complex)
• Vitamin D
• N-acetyl cysteine
• Combination products such as FH Pro for Males, Fertilix, and combinations of hormone-modulating drugs with antioxidants
Assisted Reproductive Technology
• Intrauterine insemination with or without ovarian stimulation
• In vitro fertilization
• Intracytoplasmic sperm injection

FSH, Follicle-stimulating hormone; *hCG*, human chorionic gonadotropin; *LH*, luteinizing hormone.

the options commonly used to treat idiopathic infertility. A greater understanding of the underlying biology can help in the development of future treatments that can potentiate sperm parameters and fertility. The challenge with current treatment strategy and diagnostics is the inability to stratify patients based on diagnostics to direct them to assisted reproduction or alternately, start them with more conservative, less expensive approaches first, while not being concerned about losing precious time while pursuing such treatments.

Lifestyle Modification

First-line therapy in patients diagnosed with idiopathic infertility should include behavioral and lifestyle modification. Given the rise of the pandemic and the multipronged effect on infertility, lifestyle modifications to counter obesity and increase physical activity have been shown to play a significant role in the management of its effect on semen quality and infertility.[63,64] Weight loss, with the goal of influencing infertility, can have several important peripheral effects as well, such as improved endocrine function and cardiovascular health. Some studies have demonstrated improved sperm parameters after bariatric surgery, but the data regarding this are still early and controversial.[65,66] A reduction of any known toxins is a crucial aspect of lifestyle modifications during this period. This includes but is not limited to tobacco, alcohol, and other drugs.

An understanding of the patient's occupation and lifestyle is helpful to counsel patients regarding changes in activities to support a healthy environment to promote spermatogenesis. Exposure to high temperatures has been shown to decrease sperm quality. This could include avoiding activities that increase scrotal or perineal pressure such as bike or horseback riding, and avoiding long exposures to wet heat, such as in saunas or hot tubs. Interestingly, devices such as Snowballs and Underdog that have been developed to aid in scrotal cooling and potentially affect sperm parameters have significant issues of patient compliance.[67] The development of pragmatic devices is necessary before further research in this field is done to truly understand the potential impact of such devices. Timed intercourse is often part of the initial recommendation for treatment of couples presenting with idiopathic infertility.[52]

A diagnosis of idiopathic infertility is frustrating for both the physician and the patient. A likely underappreciated concept associated with infertility is the fact that it causes substantial psychological and social distress on the patient that should be proactively managed if possible. In addition to the burden of pathology itself, the cost associated with treatment imposes a significant economic burden on patients as well. From a urological standpoint, this psychological distress can potentially contribute to sexual dysfunction, further adding to the frustration of this diagnosis.[68] Eventually a number of these lifestyle modifications are challenging to assess on an individual basis, but an effort to achieve these goals can contribute to an overall reduction in morbidity and mortality apart from increasing fertility potential, making an aggressive approach towards modification a key aspect of treating these patients.

Empiric Medical Therapy Including Hormone-Modulating Treatment and Associated Outcomes

Given the lack of an etiology, there is no standard rational empirical medical therapy for idiopathic infertility. However, the mainstay of hormonal medical therapy for idiopathic infertility involves SERMs and aromatase inhibitors (AIs). A 2012 survey of members of the AUA showed that a majority of respondents used empirical medical therapy to treat idiopathic male infertility, with a lack of consensus on optimal medication and no clear pattern to evaluate or identify patients who might benefit from such therapy.[75] While empirical medical therapy has been used for nearly half a century in this population, the results associated with its use have been largely inconclusive, and this remains an important area of research and standardization in an already vulnerable patient population.[70,71]

Current AUA/ASRM guidelines give clinicians an option to use AIs, human chorionic gonadotropin (hCG), SERMs, or a combination of these medical therapies for infertile males with low serum testosterone. SERMs work by augmenting LH and FSH to affect testosterone levels and spermatogenesis. This has also been shown to improve pregnancy rates. Although not approved by the US Food and Drug Administration (FDA) for use, drugs such as clomiphene citrate or tamoxifen are often prescribed in the setting of idiopathic infertility due to their estrogen-modulating effect. Based on the current evidence and per expert opinion in the AUA/ASRM guidelines, the use of SERMs has limited benefits relative to the results of ART. A systematic review published in 2019 looking to gather data on efficacy of SERMs for the treatment of male infertility showed an increase in sperm concentration, total count, motility, serum gonadotrophins, total testosterone, and pregnancy rates,

encouraging the use of SERMs; however, it also highlighted a paucity of high-quality data to draw any definitive conclusion.[72] The key in these situations is to better characterize patients who would benefit from these drugs and potentially avoid ART, along with its associated costs and invasive nature. A recent study found that FSH can be a potential marker to predict response to clomiphene and help better elucidate the mechanism for success associated with treatment involving clomiphene in these patients.[73] Interestingly, a recent systematic review has also highlighted that 20% of males may show paradoxically worsening sperm parameters with hormonal treatment and a large proportion of patients not recovering after discontinuation of therapy, highlighting the need to further understand this area.[74] AIs, such as anastrozole or letrozole, are used to block the peripheral conversion of testosterone to estrogen to normalize testosterone levels. A systematic review evaluating data on AIs found that either steroidal (testolactone) or nonsteroidal (anastrozole or letrozole) AIs positively affected hormonal and seminal outcomes, with a safe tolerability profile.[75] However, they also highlighted that future prospective RCTs are necessary to better define the efficacy of these drugs. hCG has found a role in treating males with hypogonadotrophic hypogonadism and those using steroids or testosterone replacement to recover or preserve spermatogenesis.[76] This works as a LH analog and, consequently, maintains intratesticular testosterone levels. hCG has also been shown to contribute to higher rates of sperm retrieval in males with infertility, such as in cases of NOA and nonmosaic Klinefelter. Similar to other hormone treatments, data associated with the use of hCG are limited.

While FSH is not FDA approved for use in males, AUA/ASRM guidelines state that a clinician may consider treatment using an FSH analog with the aim of improving sperm concentration, pregnancy rate, and live birth rate in males with idiopathic infertility.[53] FSH is primarily involved in initiation of spermatogenesis and testicular growth. While a metaanalysis of the data available so far suggests that FSH may improve pregnancy rates and sperm quality, the evidence associated with these studies is weak for a generalized FSH administration to all.[77] Hormonal therapies have a strong basis for males who are hypogonadal; however, there is very limited efficacy with treatment in males who are eugonadal.

Interestingly, the same 2012 survey of AUA members showed that 25% of respondents used exogeneous testosterone to treat infertility.[69] Exogenous testosterone should not be used for male infertility treatment because it inhibits spermatogenesis, and this highlighted the need for education among urologists but also potentially just a lack of treatment availability in this field. Given the growing usage of exogenous testosterone in general, this is an important and easily addressed public issue.[78] However, newer formulations of testosterone supplementation that do not suppress the HPG axis and spermatogenesis provide us with a unique opportunity to better investigate this relationship in this population of patients.[79]

Nutraceuticals, Vitamins, and Antioxidants

Given our growing understanding of the implications of oxidative stress in infertility, treatment of MOSI with antioxidants can theoretically improve fertility outcomes and is the focus of multiple ongoing research studies. These studies include antioxidants such as vitamin C, vitamin E, zinc, L-carnitine, coenzyme Q10, and many others.[80,81] This has led to the development of several combination supplements consisting of multiple antioxidants that have shown some success in studies based on semen parameters.[82] Additionally, studies have also shown that biomarkers based on protein analyses or gene polymorphisms are useful to monitor or predict the effect of antioxidant therapy in males with idiopathic infertility, which will be an active area of research in this field.[83,84] While a recent Cochrane review showed a positive effect on males with subfertility treated with antioxidants in regard to rates of live birth and clinical pregnancy, the study also highlighted the "low" to "very low" quality of the studies included on the topic, largely due to small sample sizes and significant heterogeneity in published studies.[85] A 2019 recent systematic review and metaanalysis evaluating empiric use of medical and nutritional supplements, such as pentoxifylline, coenzyme Q10, L-carnitine, FSH, tamoxifen, and kallikrein, in idiopathic infertility improved semen parameters but has limited data with regard to pregnancy and live birth rates. Overall, there continues to be limited evidence of the benefit of supplements, but this is clearly an area of promise, and further large-scale RCTs will be helpful to delineate the benefit of specific antioxidants in this setting.[86] The key to being able to understand the cohort of patients that could benefit from this is to better understand and quantify oxidative stress and its impact. Both will be essential in understanding factors such as the proper dosages and lengths of treatment necessary to have an impact on fertility potential and concurrently ensuring there are no negative consequences of this.[87] Given the availability of antioxidants over the counter and for a reasonable cost, there is concern that patients can overmedicate with antioxidants, leading to an increase in reductive stress, which can also have detrimental effects. A survey of reproductive specialists across the globe revealed that 85% of reproductive specialists would recommend antioxidant use for the treatment of male infertility.[55] The most common clinical conditions for which therapy was prescribed were based on risk factors for oxidative stress (obesity, age, smoking, etc.), idiopathic oligoasthenoteratozoospermia, isolated asthenozoospermia, and teratozoospermia.[55] The most commonly prescribed individual antioxidants were zinc, vitamin E, L-carnitine, and coenzyme Q10.[55] Current AUA/ASRM guidelines state that there are no clear, reliable data related to the variety of supplements available and while they likely are not harmful, it is questionable whether they will provide any tangible improvement in fertility potential.[51] More recently, as our understanding of the microbiome and its varied effects improved, the use of probiotics and prebiotics has also been shown to improve sperm parameters, leading us down yet another potential avenue for further research in the field.[96] Given the generally increasing understanding and effect of nutrition on various body systems, dietary modification promises to be an important aspect of fertility optimization over the next decade.

Assisted Reproductive Technologies

ARTs commonly used in the treatment of unexplained infertility, such as intrauterine insemination (IUI) and IVF, can overcome idiopathic male infertility as well. However, these techniques are expensive and invasive, creating a large need to further effective diagnostics and treatment options for idiopathic infertility. IUI is a form of assisted reproduction where sperm collected from a male partner are artificially instilled into a female partner's uterus, avoiding potential effects of the environment or cervical factor infertility. This can be offered in natural cycles or in combination with ovarian stimulation. IVF involves eggs retrieved transvaginally from ovaries before normal ovulation fertilized with washed sperm in vitro. Intracytoplasmic sperm injection (ICSI) involves the microscopic injection of a single sperm into the intracytoplasmic space of an egg. In both IVF and

ICSI, the embryo is placed back into the female uterus. While plenty of research has been done on success of these technologies, specific data for this population are scarce. However, the growing research in the field promises to enhance our understanding of the use of these technologies. The quality of sperm has been shown to influence ICSI, highlighting the need for selection prior to ICSI to prevent vertical transmission of genetic defects and facilitate appropriate counseling.[89] With our growing knowledge of DNA fragmentation, it is also clear that testicular sperm may have improved outcomes when compared to ejaculated sperm due to lower levels of DNA fragmentation and can be considered in certain situations.[90] Simultaneously, efforts to better understand augmentation of these using medical therapy can be helpful.

On the Horizon

Given the rapidly evolving technology associated with diagnostics and our growing understanding of the etiology of idiopathic infertility, the field is yearning for trials in this space and subsequent guidelines to help this patient population. Collaborative efforts between centers where the resources might be available to utilize these diagnostics and pool data are crucial in moving this field forward. The growing use of "-omic" technologies has already shown promise in identifying potential underlying etiologies. The use of artificial intelligence and machine-learning algorithms to help parse through a lot of this data and eventually even be used in clinical practice is a space that ideally needs to simultaneously evolve with our growing understanding of etiology.

Some of the most exciting potential developments for management of idiopathic infertility have already been seen in the laboratory over the last decade, but it remains to be seen if they will translate into the clinic. Basic science advances in the utility of stem cells and organ cultures for spermatogenesis to impact this population of patients has been highlighted over the past decade to better understand some of the genetic changes we are finding and to potentially move towards gene therapy as a management approach. Yet another growing area of research is the development of techniques to successfully autograft already-banked testicular tissue. While these areas of research certainly bring along with it several ethical questions, they also promise to better shed some light on the true etiology and treatment of idiopathic infertility as it currently stands.

SUMMARY

Male infertility is a complex, multifactorial disorder, and a better understanding of the underlying causes remains a high priority, given the current epidemiological trends. Research into novel technology and diagnostic tools can be used to reduce the uncertainty of cause in this population and can help us better target our efforts in this field towards personalized treatments for patients dealing with this.

REFERENCES

1. Thonneau P, Marchand S, Tallec A, et al. Incidence and main causes of infertility in a resident population (1,850,000) of three French regions (1988-1989). *Hum Reprod.* 1991;6(6):811-816.
2. Sigman M, Lipshultz L, Howards SS. Office evaluation of the subfertile male. *Infertil Male.* 2009;4:153-176.
3. Levine H, Jørgensen N, Martino-Andrade A, et al. Temporal trends in sperm count: a systematic review and meta-regression analysis. *Hum Reprod Update.* 2017;23(6):646-659.
4. European Association of Urology. Male Infertility, EAU Guidelines. Paper presented at the EAU Annual Congress Amsterdam, Arnhem, The Netherlands; 2022.
5. Cui D, Han G, Shang Y, et al. Antisperm antibodies in infertile men and their effect on semen parameters: a systematic review and meta-analysis. *Clin Chim Acta.* 2015;444:29-36.
6. Gupta S, Sharma R, Agarwal A, et al. Antisperm antibody testing: a comprehensive review of its role in the management of immunological male infertility and results of a global survey of clinical practices. *World J Mens Health.* 2022;40(3):380-398.
7. Kasturi S, Osterberg EC, Tannir J, Brannigan RE. The effect of genital tract infection and inflammation on male infertility. In: *Infertil Male.* Cambridge University Press; 2010:295-330.
8. Schuppe HC, Meinhardt A, Allam JP, Bergmann M, Weidner W, Haidl G. Chronic orchitis: a neglected cause of male infertility? *Andrologia.* 2008;40(2):84-91.
9. Muscianisi F, De Toni L, Giorato G, Carosso A, Foresta C, Garolla A. Is HPV the novel target in male idiopathic infertility? A systematic review of the literature. *Front Endocrinol (Lausanne).* 2021;12:643539.
10. Achua JK, Chu KY, Ibrahim E, et al. Histopathology and ultrastructural findings of fatal COVID-19 infections on testis. *World J Mens Health.* 2021;39(1):65-74.
11. Ho CLT, Vaughan-Constable DR, Ramsay J, et al. The relationship between genitourinary microorganisms and oxidative stress, sperm DNA fragmentation and semen

parameters in infertile men. *Andrologia.* 2022;54(2): e14322.

12. Brubaker WD, Li S, Baker LC, Eisenberg ML. Increased risk of autoimmune disorders in infertile men: analysis of US claims data. *Andrology.* 2018;6(1):94-98.

13. Schuppe HC, Pilatz A, Hossain H, Diemer T, Wagenlehner F, Weidner W. Urogenital infection as a risk factor for male infertility. *Dtsch Arztebl Int.* 2017;114(19):339-346.

14. Jiang Y, Cui D, Du Y, et al. Association of anti-sperm antibodies with chronic prostatitis: a systematic review and meta-analysis. *J Reprod Immunol.* 2016;118:85-91.

15. Syriou V, Papanikolaou D, Kozyraki A, Goulis DG. Cytokines and male infertility. *Eur Cytokine Netw.* 2018; 29(3):73-82.

16. Millar AC, Faghfoury H, Bieniek JM. Genetics of hypogonadotropic hypogonadism. *Transl Androl Urol.* 2021; 10(3):1401-1409.

17. Bianchi VE. The anti-inflammatory effects of testosterone. *J Endocr Soc.* 2019;3(1):91-107.

18. Sharma A, Thaventhiran T, Minhas S, Dhillo WS, Jayasena CN. Kisspeptin and testicular function-is it necessary? *Int J Mol Sci.* 2020;21(8):2958.

19. Benderradji H, Prasivoravong J, Marcelli F, et al. Contribution of serum anti-Mullerian hormone in the management of azoospermia and the prediction of testicular sperm retrieval outcomes: a study of 155 adult men. *Basic Clin Androl.* 2021;31(1):15.

20. Lima TFN, Patel P, Blachman-Braun R, Madhusoodanan V, Ramasamy R. Serum 17-hydroxyprogesterone is a potential biomarker for evaluating intratesticular testosterone. *J Urol.* 2020;204(3):551-556.

21. Albrethsen J, Johannsen TH, Jorgensen N, et al. Evaluation of serum insulin-like factor 3 quantification by LC-MS/MS as a biomarker of Leydig cell function. *J Clin Endocrinol Metab.* 2020;105(6):dgaa145.

22. Craig JR, Jenkins TG, Carrell DT, Hotaling JM. Obesity, male infertility, and the sperm epigenome. *Fertil Steril.* 2017;107(4):848-859.

23. Hammoud AO, Gibson M, Peterson CM, Meikle AW, Carrell DT. Impact of male obesity on infertility: a critical review of the current literature. *Fertil Steril.* 2008;90(4):897-904.

24. Dupont C, Faure C, Sermondade N, et al. Obesity leads to higher risk of sperm DNA damage in infertile patients. *Asian J Androl.* 2013;15(5):622-625.

25. Lymperi S, Giwercman A. Endocrine disruptors and testicular function. *Metabolism.* 2018;86:79-90.

26. Agarwal A, Deepinder F, Sharma RK, Ranga G, Li J. Effect of cell phone usage on semen analysis in men attending infertility clinic: an observational study. *Fertil Steril.* 2008;89(1):124-128.

27. Lundy SD, Sangwan N, Parekh NV, et al. Functional and taxonomic dysbiosis of the gut, urine, and semen microbiomes in male infertility. *Eur Urol.* 2021;79(6):826-836.

28. Ray PF, Toure A, Metzler-Guillemain C, Mitchell MJ, Arnoult C, Coutton C. Genetic abnormalities leading to qualitative defects of sperm morphology or function. *Clin Genet.* 2017;91(2):217-232.

29. Mitchell MJ, Metzler-Guillemain C, Toure A, Coutton C, Arnoult C, Ray PF. Single gene defects leading to sperm quantitative anomalies. *Clin Genet.* 2017;91(2):208-216.

30. McCallum T, Milunsky J, Munarriz R, Carson R, Sadeghi-Nejad H, Oates R. Unilateral renal agenesis associated with congenital bilateral absence of the vas deferens: phenotypic findings and genetic considerations. *Hum Reprod.* 2001;16(2):282-288.

31. Oud MS, Volozonoka L, Smits RM, Vissers L, Ramos L, Veltman JA. A systematic review and standardized clinical validity assessment of male infertility genes. *Hum Reprod.* 2019;34(5):932-941.

32. Komeya M, Sato T, Ogawa T. In vitro spermatogenesis: a century-long research journey, still half way around. *Reprod Med Biol.* 2018;17(4):407-420.

33. Wu Y, Zhou H, Fan X, et al. Correction of a genetic disease by CRISPR-Cas9-mediated gene editing in mouse spermatogonial stem cells. *Cell Res.* 2015;25(1):67-79.

34. Panner Selvam MK, Finelli R, Agarwal A, Henkel R. Proteomics and metabolomics—Current and future perspectives in clinical andrology. *Andrologia.* 2021;53(2):e13711.

35. Longo V, Forleo A, Provenzano SP, et al. HS-SPME-GC-MS metabolomics approach for sperm quality evaluation by semen volatile organic compounds (VOCs) analysis. *Biomed Phys Eng Exp.* 2018;5(1):015006.

36. Jenkins TG, Aston KI, James ER, Carrell DT. Sperm epigenetics in the study of male fertility, offspring health, and potential clinical applications. *Syst Biol Reprod Med.* 2017;63(2):69-76.

37. Pandruvada S, Royfman R, Shah TA, et al. Lack of trusted diagnostic tools for undetermined male infertility. *J Assist Reprod Genet.* 2021;38(2):265-276.

38. Patel DP, Jenkins TG, Aston KI, et al. Harnessing the full potential of reproductive genetics and epigenetics for male infertility in the era of "big data". *Fertil Steril.* 2020;113(3):478-488.

39. Agarwal A, Sengupta P. Oxidative stress and its association with male infertility. In: Parekattil S, Esteves S, Agarwal A, eds. *Male Infertility.* Cham, Switzerland: Springer; 2020:57-68.

40. Agarwal A, Parekh N, Selvam MKP, et al. Male oxidative stress infertility (MOSI): proposed terminology and clinical practice guidelines for management of idiopathic male infertility. *World J Mens Health.* 2019;37(3):296-312.

41. Walczak–Jedrzejowska R, Wolski JK, Slowikowska–Hilczer J. The role of oxidative stress and antioxidants in male fertility. *Cent European J Urol.* 2013;66(1):60.

42. Agarwal A, Saleh RA, Bedaiwy MA. Role of reactive oxygen species in the pathophysiology of human reproduction. *Fertil Steril.* 2003;79(4):829-843.

43. Aitken RJ. DNA damage in human spermatozoa; important contributor to mutagenesis in the offspring. *Transl Androl Urol.* 2017;6(suppl 4):S761.

44. Esteves SC, Sharma RK, Gosalvez J, Agarwal A. A translational medicine appraisal of specialized andrology testing in unexplained male infertility. *Int Urol Nephrol.* 2014;46(6):1037-1052.

45. Schlegel PN, Sigman M, Collura B, et al. Diagnosis and treatment of infertility in men: AUA/ASRM guideline part II. *J Urol.* 2021;205(1):44-51.

46. Patel V, Ginsberg K, Etnyre E, et al. Practice patterns for the treatment of idiopathic infertility: is there a role for advanced semen testing? *AME Med J.* 2019;4.

47. Schlegel PN, Sigman M, Collura B, et al. Diagnosis and treatment of infertility in men: AUA/ASRM guideline part I. *J Urol.* 2021;205(1):36-43.

48. Aydemir B, Onaran I, Kiziler AR, Alici B, Akyolcu MC. The influence of oxidative damage on viscosity of seminal fluid in infertile men. *J Androl.* 2008;29(1):41-46.

49. Agarwal A, Roychoudhury S, Bjugstad KB, Cho CL. Oxidation-reduction potential of semen: what is its role in the treatment of male infertility? *Ther Adv Urol.* 2016;8(5):302-318.

50. Vessey W, Perez-Miranda A, Macfarquhar R, Agarwal A, Homa S. Reactive oxygen species in human semen: validation and qualification of a chemiluminescence assay. *Fertil Steril.* 2014;102(6):1576-1583.e4.

51. Grotto D, Santa Maria L, Boeira S, et al. Rapid quantification of malondialdehyde in plasma by high performance liquid chromatography–visible detection. *J Pharm Biomed Anal.* 2007;43(2):619-624.

52. Agarwal A, Sharma R, Roychoudhury S, Du Plessis S, Sabanegh E. MiOXSYS: a novel method of measuring oxidation reduction potential in semen and seminal plasma. *Fertil Steril.* 2016;106(3):566-573.e10.

53. Agarwal A, Panner Selvam MK, Arafa M, et al. Multicenter evaluation of oxidation-reduction potential by the MiOXSYS in males with abnormal semen. *Asian J Androl.* 2019;21(6):565-569.

54. Pasqualotto F, Sharma R, Kobayashi H, Nelson D, Agarwal A. Oxidative stress in normospermic men undergoing infertility evaluation. *J Androl.* 2001;22(2):316-322.

55. Agarwal A, Finelli R, Selvam MKP, et al. A global survey of reproductive specialists to determine the clinical utility of oxidative stress testing and antioxidant use in male infertility. *World J Mens Health.* 2021;39(3):470-488.

56. Calogero AE, Burrello N, De Palma A, Barone N, D'Agata R, Vicari E. Sperm aneuploidy in infertile men. *Reprod Biomed Online.* 2003;6(3):310-317.

57. Oleszczuk K, Augustinsson L, Bayat N, Giwercman A, Bungum M. Prevalence of high DNA fragmentation index in male partners of unexplained infertile couples. *Andrology.* 2013;1(3):357-360.

58. Simon L, Proutski I, Stevenson M, et al. Sperm DNA damage has a negative association with live-birth rates after IVF. *Reprod Biomed Online.* 2013;26(1):68-78.

59. Tan J, Taskin O, Albert A, Bedaiwy MA. Association between sperm DNA fragmentation and idiopathic recurrent pregnancy loss: a systematic review and meta-analysis. *Reprod BioMed Online.* 2019;38(6):951-960.

60. Ceyhan-Birsoy O, Murry JB, Machini K, et al. Interpretation of genomic sequencing results in healthy and ill newborns: results from the babyseq project. *Am J Hum Genet.* 2019;104(1):76-93.

61. Turner KA, Fishman EL, Asadullah M, et al. Fluorescence-based ratiometric analysis of sperm centrioles (FRAC) finds patient age and sperm morphology are associated with centriole quality. *Front Cell Dev Biol.* 2021;9:658891.

62. Armstrong JM, Keihani S, Hotaling JM. Use of ultrasound in male infertility: appropriate selection of men for scrotal ultrasound. *Curr Urol Rep.* 2018;19(8):58.

63. Ibañez-Perez J, Santos-Zorrozua B, Lopez-Lopez E, Matorras R, Garcia-Orad A. An update on the implication of physical activity on semen quality: a systematic review and meta-analysis. *Arch Gynecol Obstet.* 2019;299(4):901-921.

64. Håkonsen LB, Thulstrup AM, Aggerholm AS, et al. Does weight loss improve semen quality and reproductive hormones? Results from a cohort of severely obese men. *Reprod Health.* 2011;8(1):1-8.

65. El Bardisi H, Majzoub A, Arafa M, et al. Effect of bariatric surgery on semen parameters and sex hormone concentrations: a prospective study. *Reprod Biomed Online.* 2016;33(5):606-611.

66. Calderón B, Huerta L, Galindo J, et al. Lack of improvement of sperm characteristics in obese males after obesity surgery despite the beneficial changes observed in reproductive hormones. *Obes Surg.* 2019;29(7):2045-2050.

67. Benidir T, Remondini T, Lau S, Jarvi KA. Evaluation of patient compliance with the use of scrotal cooling devices. *F S Rep.* 2021;2(3):289-295.

68. Lotti F, Maggi M. Sexual dysfunction and male infertility. *Nat Rev Urol.* 2018;15(5):287-307.

69. Ko EY, Siddiqi K, Brannigan RE, Sabanegh Jr ES. Empirical medical therapy for idiopathic male infertility: a survey of the American Urological Association. *J Urol.* 2012;187(3):973-978.

70. Tadros NN, Sabanegh ES. Empiric medical therapy with hormonal agents for idiopathic male infertility. *Indian J Urol.* 2017;33(3):194-198.

71. Chehab M, Madala A, Trussell J. On-label and off-label drugs used in the treatment of male infertility. *Fertil Steril.* 2015;103(3):595-604.

72. Cannarella R, Condorelli RA, Mongioì LM, Barbagallo F, Calogero AE, La Vignera S. Effects of the selective estrogen

receptor modulators for the treatment of male infertility: a systematic review and meta-analysis. *Expert Opin Pharmacother.* 2019;20(12):1517-1525.

73. Lundy SD, Doolittle J, Farber NJ, Njemanze S, Munoz-Lopez C, Vij SC. Follicle-stimulating hormone modestly predicts improvement in semen parameters in men with infertility treated with clomiphene citrate. *Andrologia.* 2022;54(6):e14399.

74. Gundewar T, Kuchakulla M, Ramasamy R. A paradoxical decline in semen parameters in men treated with clomiphene citrate: a systematic review. *Andrologia.* 2021;53(1):e13848.

75. Del Giudice F, Busetto GM, De Berardinis E, et al. A systematic review and meta-analysis of clinical trials implementing aromatase inhibitors to treat male infertility. *Asian J Androl.* 2020;22(4):360-367.

76. Lee JA, Ramasamy R. Indications for the use of human chorionic gonadotropic hormone for the management of infertility in hypogonadal men. *Trans Androl Urol.* 2018;7(suppl 3):S348.

77. Santi D, Granata AR, Simoni M. FSH treatment of male idiopathic infertility improves pregnancy rate: a meta-analysis. *Endocr Connect.* 2015;4(3):R46-R58.

78. Kolettis PN, Purcell ML, Parker W, Poston T, Nangia AK. Medical testosterone: an iatrogenic cause of male infertility and a growing problem. *Urology.* 2015;85(5):1068-1073.

79. Ramasamy R, Masterson TA, Best JC, et al. Effect of Natesto on reproductive hormones, semen parameters and hypogonadal symptoms: a single center, open label, single arm trial. *J Urol.* 2020;204(3):557-563.

80. Kobori Y, Ota S, Sato R, et al. Antioxidant cosupplementation therapy with vitamin C, vitamin E, and coenzyme Q10 in patients with oligoasthenozoospermia. *Arch Ital Urol Androl.* 2014;86(1):1-4.

81. Alahmar AT, Sengupta P. Impact of coenzyme Q10 and selenium on seminal fluid parameters and antioxidant status in men with idiopathic infertility. *Biol Trace Elem Res.* 2021;199(4):1246-1252.

82. Arafa M, Agarwal A, Majzoub A, et al. Efficacy of antioxidant supplementation on conventional and advanced sperm function tests in patients with idiopathic male infertility. *Antioxidants.* 2020;9(3):219.

83. Agarwal A, Panner Selvam MK, Samanta L, et al. Effect of antioxidant supplementation on the sperm proteome of idiopathic infertile men. *Antioxidants (Basel).* 2019;8(10):488.

84. Zhang HY, Mu Y, Chen P, et al. Metabolic enzyme gene polymorphisms predict the effects of antioxidant treatment on idiopathic male infertility. *Asian J Androl.* 2022;24(4):430-435.

85. Smits RM, Mackenzie-Proctor R, Yazdani A, Stankiewicz MT, Jordan V, Showell MG. Antioxidants for male subfertility. *Cochrane Database Syst Rev.* 2019;3(3):CD007411.

86. Omar MI, Pal RP, Kelly BD, et al. Benefits of empiric nutritional and medical therapy for semen parameters and pregnancy and live birth rates in couples with idiopathic infertility: a systematic review and meta-analysis. *Eur Urol.* 2019;75(4):615-625.

87. Henkel R, Sandhu IS, Agarwal A. The excessive use of antioxidant therapy: a possible cause of male infertility? *Andrologia.* 2019;51(1):e13162.

88. Abbasi B, Abbasi H, Niroumand H. Synbiotic (FamiLact) administration in idiopathic male infertility enhances sperm quality, DNA integrity, and chromatin status: a triple-blinded randomized clinical trial. *Int J Reprod Biomed.* 2021;19(3):235.

89. Lee SH, Song H, Park YS, Koong MK, Song IO, Jun JH. Poor sperm quality affects clinical outcomes of intracytoplasmic sperm injection in fresh and subsequent frozen-thawed cycles: potential paternal effects on pregnancy outcomes. *Fertil Steril.* 2009;91(3):798-804.

90. Esteves SC, Roque M, Bradley CK, Garrido N. Reproductive outcomes of testicular versus ejaculated sperm for intracytoplasmic sperm injection among men with high levels of DNA fragmentation in semen: systematic review and meta-analysis. *Fertil Steril.* 2017;108(3):456-467.e1.

Diagnosis of Male Infertility

7

Medical History and Physical Examination of Infertile Males

Kareim Khalafalla and Mohamed Arafa

KEY POINTS

- Evaluation of male infertility almost always starts by an accurate history and a thorough physical examination.
- A physician should always have all relevant clinical information related to infertility ready during the history taking.

- Obtaining a history could be challenging and complicated in certain scenarios.
- A proper physical examination could identify crucial causes of male infertility.

INTRODUCTION

Infertility is a broad term that is usually misdefined. Its agreed-upon definition is the inability of a heterosexual couple to conceive after at least 1 year of unprotected intercourse. Due to the current increased awareness for fertility globally, its prevalence among couples is estimated to be around 8% to 12% worldwide, where the male factor contributes to 50% of the etiology.[1] Initial assessment of an infertile couple should include history taking, physical examination, and diagnostic testing. Physicians focus during the assessment on identifying the predisposing factors that could have affected fertility and on investigating all possible etiologies that could contribute to the complaint. These give valuable information to guide the future management of male infertility, including the request for the relevant investigations and choosing the appropriate line of therapy.

HISTORY

Objectives

The aim of this section is to emphasize the different aspects of history taking for a heterosexual couple presenting for fertility evaluation and annotating its relevance to the different causes of infertility in males (Fig. 7.1).

Fertility Evaluation History List

- Type and duration of the complaint
  - Past medical history
  - Past surgical history
  - Social and lifestyle history
  - Family history
  - Sexual history
  - Spouse/partner history

Type and Duration of Complaint

Primary infertility is defined as heterosexual couples who have not become pregnant at all after 1 year of continuous, unprotected intercourse, while secondary infertility is defined as the couple's inability to have further pregnancies after being able to get pregnant at least once.[2] Differentiating between primary and secondary infertility helps to guide the physician on the possible causes of their complaint. Congenital etiologies, as an example, could be found in primary infertility, while they are highly unlikely to contribute

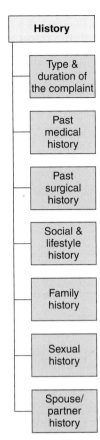

Fig. 7.1 Flowchart summarizing different history points during assessment of the male partner of an infertile heterosexual couple.

to infertility in a couple who had a previous natural pregnancy. Moreover, inquiring about the number of children in cases of secondary infertility and the age of the youngest child is also important so that a physician can sequence the events that started after having their last child and try to identify possible causes that could have affected the patient's fertility status, like a recent history of infections or recent scrotal surgeries that could affect the testicular hormonal and reproductive functions.

Identifying the time period of infertility is important. In some cases, couples may present with only a few months' history of trying to conceive, thus not fulfilling the 12-month period recommended in the definition of infertility. Infertility duration may also guide the management, as couples with long infertility duration may be counseled to go for assisted reproductive technology.

Another point to consider is the presence of both partners together during the 1-year trial of conceiving. One of the partners may be consistently traveling for many months and thus the actual period that the couple spent together is much shorter, which by itself may affect fertility.

Last, asking about unprotected sex is important, as couples' knowledge of safe sex and contraception varies, and our role as fertility specialists as to clarify and confirm such methods to ensure the couple had enough opportunity to naturally conceive before proceeding with further diagnostic and treatment measures.

Past medical history. Males's past medical history includes multiple categories, in which each should be questioned in detail due to its significant importance. This includes a history of previous infections; trauma; iatrogenic, chronic comorbidities; scrotal trauma; medications; previous history of infertility treatment; and pubertal history. We will discuss each below in brief with its medical significance to fertility.

Infections

Epididymoorchitis. A history of previous epididymoorchitis (EDO), laterality, and recurrence is one of the causes of male infertility via deterioration of semen parameters' being affected and presence of white blood cells in the seminal fluid.[3] In the acute phase of EDO, pathogens and their produced inflammatory molecules affect sperm via oxidative reduction potential and sperm DNA integrity. On the other hand, chronic recurrent EDO causes an element of testicular scarring and atrophy, with possible epididymal obstruction, which affects the process of sperm maturity.[4,5]

Sexually transmitted infections. The association of sexually transmitted infections (STIs) in general and chlamydia in particular with male infertility has been extensively reported over the past decade. Seminal parameters were affected by reactive oxygen species production, increased oxidative stress, and DNA fragmentation.[6] Chronic recurrent STIs, especially in untreated patients, could be complicated, with epididymal canal disfigurement and obstruction leading to a picture of oligozoospermia or even azoospermia in bilateral cases.[7,8]

Mumps infection. The incidence of mumps infection has decreased over the years with childhood vaccinations, but questioning the history of its infection during childhood is considered one of the essential questions.

Mumps orchitis was reported to cause testicular atrophy, deterioration of sperm parameters, and formation of antisperm antibodies, all of which can lead to infertility.[9]

COVID-19 and vaccination. With the current era of the COVID-19 pandemic, medical history included a new category to the fertility evaluation, which is a history of COVID-19 infection and vaccination status. Studies published early in the pandemic reported the detection of the virus in the semen of infected patients, which subsequently means reaching the testicles.[10–12] Moreover, multiple authors described different variability of sperm counts, motility, and morphology in infected patients.[13,14] The association of COVID-19 infection with high fever is believed to affect male semen parameters[15] and can even impact pregnant couples.[16] Patients being treated with antivirals, antiretrovirals, and steroid medications are susceptible to testicular being affected and semen derangements.[17] Hajizadeh Maleki and Tartibian, in their prospective longitudinal cohort study that included 84 COVID-19 infected patients and 105 controls, studied semen samples of both groups. They reported an inverse correlation with sperm DNA fragmentation, oxidative stress, inflammatory cytokine production, and sperm cell apoptosis induction in the COVID-19–positive group compared with controls, thus explaining possible further etiologies for associated infertility with SARS-COV-2 virus.[18]

On the other hand, vaccination was proven safe and does not affect semen parameters from a fertility standpoint. This information should be included during counseling because it is a frequent concern for infertile couples.[19]

Urinary tract infections. The presence of uropathogens, their components, or even associated inflammatory markers causes direct sperm quality being affected, accessory gland dysfunction, and inflammatory-related obstruction, and triggers cellular and humoral immune responses, all of which can cause infertility in males.[5]

Iatrogenic

Exogenous testosterone and anabolic steroids. The use of anabolic androgenic steroids (testosterone derivatives) is one of the important causes of male infertility nowadays, especially with the widespread and easy accessibility to adolescents/young males. The suppression and shutdown of the hypothalamic-pituitary-adrenal axis is the main mechanism behind the dysfunction caused.[20] Although this effect is mostly reversible, however, spermatogenesis in some males may not recover completely, resulting in defective semen parameters that may be severe enough to present with nonobstructive azoospermia.[21] Therefore asking about the doses and duration of anabolic steroids intake is important.

Medication history. There are multiple medications that could cause male fertility problems via various mechanisms, so part of the history taking is knowing the patient's medication cabinet; this includes all supplements and prescribed medications. Unfortunately, misuse of some supplements could have negative effects on semen, while other over-the-counter supplements that are not approved by the US Food and Drug Administration may contain different elements of testosterone, which has deleterious effects on spermatogenesis.[20] Here are examples of medications and their transient effect on fertility: some antibiotics (tetracycline and erythromycin) affect sperm motility via calcium chelation, other fluoroquinolones may have a direct effect on sperm quality, spironolactone has antiandrogen effects, sulfasalazine and colchicine affect sperm count, antifungals (ketoconazole and fluconazole) decrease testosterone production, 5-alpha-reductase inhibitors (finasteride and dutasteride) decrease sperm concentration, and alpha blockers (silodosin, tamsulosin, alfuzosin, terazosin, doxazosin) decrease seminal emission and cause retrograde ejaculation.[22–24]

Chemotherapy. Despite the high rate of cancer detection nowadays due to increased awareness, advancements in diagnostics, and availability of new treatments, the quality of life in general and fertility preservation specifically post survival remain a challenge. The hazardous effect of chemotherapeutic agents on semen depends on the type and dose of the chemotherapeutic agent, which cells are being affected, and the exact disruption of the spermatogenesis cycle. The effect could be transient or permanent, as the gonadotoxic effect strikes the rapidly proliferating cells in the body, whether they are cancerous or normal tissues like testicular cells. Howell et al. reported that 50% of cancer survivors post chemotherapy had recovered spermatogenesis in 2 years and up to 80% in 5 years.[25]

Some agents such as platinum analogs (cisplatin and carboplatin) can cross the blood–testis barrier and directly affect testicular cells through interstitial cell fibrosis, while other alkylating agents (cyclophosphamide and melphalan) can alter DNA integrity by adding alkyl groups to it.[26] Therefore detailed information on the chemotherapy treatment is essential in the history taking for proper counseling and management of male infertility and for fertility preservation.

Radiotherapy. As the testes are considered one of the radiosensitive organs in the body, radiation can permanently cause dysfunction. The extent of damage depends on multiple factors, including the dose of radiation, fractions received, and location of irradiation (whether direct to the testes, nearby, or scattered radiation), direct being the worst, but scattered radiation could have poorer effects according to the organ site targeted. With current improvements in gonadal shielding techniques, scattered radiation effect has decreased to some extent.[27] One important point to mention is that radiation doses as low as 0.1 to 1.2 Gy disrupt the process of sperm production, while doses reaching 4 Gy may have a permanent effect. Leydig cells in particular are considered the most radioresistant, as they can withstand up to 30 Gy without being injured.[28,29]

Radiation causes apoptosis of rapidly dividing cells (e.g., germ cells in the testes), leading to germ cell dysfunction and loss.[30] A detailed history of the treatment and whether fertility preservation was done prior to it is of vast importance for male infertility management. Spermatogenesis recovery was described as being radiotherapy dose–dependent, with up to 18 months for 1-Gy doses, 30 months in 2- to 3-Gy doses, and 5 years in 4-Gy doses.[25]

The combination of both chemotherapy and radiotherapy had more dreadful and gonadotoxic effects than each therapy type alone. Fertilization rates were reported in post combined-treatment patients to be affected despite sperm recovery due to DNA fragmentation impairment, which could extend a further 2 years after the return of sperm.[28,31]

Chronic diseases/comorbidities. A history of a patient's chronic comorbidities is a necessity during history taking. The presence of an illness should be followed by its duration, treatments received, and whether it was controlled or not. Each comorbidity could have a different effect on the fertility potential. Diabetes causes male sexual dysfunction in the form of erection problems or ejaculatory disorders (retrograde ejaculation and anejaculation). Hormonal regulation of spermatogenesis and sperm DNA integrity have also been reported to be affected in diabetic patients, which plays a role in infertility.[32] Liver diseases could cause decrease in reproductive hormones, as well as alterations in sperm count and motility,[33] while renal failure impairs spermatogenesis

directly through a sperm toxic effect and indirectly through hormonal imbalance and sexual dysfunction.[34] Respiratory diseases could be directly related to male infertility. Primary ciliary dyskinesia is usually associated with sperm tail defects and severe being affected of sperm motility.[35] Similarly, cystic fibrosis is usually associated with congenital absence of the vas deferens.[36]

Another important segment of chronic comorbidity inquiry is the presence of endocrine disorders, like hypo- and hyperthyroidism. Many authors have studied the effects of thyroid disease on fertility. They reported that hypothyroidism decreases the sex hormone binding globulin levels, which in turn decreases testosterone; other articles showed sperm concentration, motility, and morphology alterations. On the other hand, hyperthyroidism is believed to affect semen parameters through changing sex steroid levels.[37]

Malignancy. Testicular tumors are associated with reduced testicular functions, both spermatogenic and endocrine. This may lead to severe decrease in semen parameters, even before orchidectomy and chemo- or radiotherapy.[38] Nonseminomatous germ cell tumors were found to have more deleterious effects on semen.[39] Therefore a detailed history of testicular tumors, including side, type, date of diagnosis, and treatment should be documented during history taking.

Additionally, malignancy has various effects on fertility, depending on the type of cancer, its location, treatments received, and whether sperm cryopreservation had been established before treatment or not. Cancer could exert a direct toxic effect on sperm motility through cytokine release. It could affect testosterone production via imbalance of the hypothalamic-pituitary-gonadal (HPG) axis, especially if present in the central nervous system, or exert its effects through associated malnutrition and cachexia affecting testicular function.[40]

Trauma. Scrotal trauma may play a part in infertility, depending on the location and extent of trauma. Testicular rupture with loss of testicular tissue, for example, could affect the basic function of testosterone production and spermatogenesis.[41] Moreover, antisperm antibodies are formed with any disruption of the blood–testis barrier that could be a contributing factor.[42,43] This should be asked in the history taking in detail: the date of incident, laterality, consequences including hematoma, scrotal swelling, hospitalization, operative intervention, and outcome.

Spinal cord injury leads to being affected of male fertility through different pathophysiologies. It may lead to erectile dysfunction and anejaculation, therefore affecting semen deposition in the vagina. Also, it may lead to being affected of semen parameters with severe deterioration of sperm vitality and morphology.[44]

Pubertal history. Documenting the age of puberty for males presenting with infertility and associated secondary sexual characteristic development could point out some unseen disorders. With delayed puberty and incomplete secondary sexual characters, testosterone is reported usually lower than normal which, in turn, affects sperm production. It could also unmask underlying congenital endocrine disorders like Kallmann syndrome and Klinefelter syndrome.[45]

Childhood urological disorders. We must ask the patient about important urological disorders that may affect fertility. Cryptorchidism can cause subfertility/infertility due to being affected of testicular germ cell number and maturation, absence or delay of luteinizing hormone surge, and testosterone hormonal imbalance. Therefore early detection and surgical intervention in such patients during infancy is crucial to preserve fertility and decrease the risk of malignant transformation.[46,47] Other disorders of importance are urethral abnormalities, hypospadias, or epispadias that may lead to abnormal deposition of semen and may be associated with cryptorchidism.[48]

Previous infertility treatments. This includes inquiring about past medical and surgical treatment of infertility, along with assisted reproductive techniques like intrauterine insemination, in vitro fertilization, and intracytoplasmic sperm injection. Obtaining the details of such interventions could emphasize the cause of infertility and guide us on the proper investigations to be ordered next and treatment plans.

Past surgical history. A patient's surgical history could give us more insight on his past medical conditions that might have been missed or not mentioned, especially if related to fertility. This can be divided into inguinal surgeries (hernia repair, varicocelectomy, spermatic cord denervation), scrotal surgeries (hydrocele, testicular biopsy, spermatocelectomy, vasectomy), and pelvic and abdominal surgeries (prostatic surgeries, retroperitoneal lymph node dissections, orchiopexy for undescended testis).[49]

The surgery itself can have a role in infertility in cases of vas deferens injury, occurrence of testicular atrophy post arterial injury, presence of anejaculation post prostate surgeries and retroperitoneal lymph node dissection, and testicular dysfunction due to undescended testes and late orchiopexy.[49]

Social and lifestyle history. Social habits including smoking, alcohol intake, and recreational drug usage may affect fertility and therefore must be investigated in detail during history taking, including duration and amount used.

Many studies have reported the detrimental effects of smoking on sperm motility and morphology through the production of reactive oxygen species and increased oxidative stress.[50] Other articles annotated the harmful effect of heavy/binge drinking on semen parameters that has been mainly attributed to decreased testosterone levels.[51,52]

With regard to recreational drug intake, depending on the type of drug used, different side effects could affect the patient's fertility potential via various mechanisms that include hormonal axis, testicular structure, and sperm production.[53]

One of the commonly forgotten questions is "What is your occupation?" It aids us in excluding exposure to chemicals, radiation, pesticides, heat, and heavy metals in a patient's workplace that could have a hazardous effect on testicular hormonal function and sperm manufacturing.[54,55] Frequent exposure to heat, whether for leisure in the form of a sauna, jacuzzi, or hot bath, or occupational exposure like iron welders or truck drivers, poses a risk to fertility through increased oxidative stress mechanisms. Therefore looking into these risks should be included in the initial evaluation of males.[56]

Family history. Besides asking about a patient's family history of chronic diseases, from an infertility standpoint, we inquire about a family history of infertility in siblings and relatives. This could shed light on the presence of unknown or undiagnosed family conditions that are important in our assessment. Also, genetic conditions related to fertility should be included, as up to 8% of infertility causes are linked to genetics, and this increases up to 19% in special conditions like nonobstructive azoospermia.[57] For instance, cystic fibrosis, which is an autosomal recessive disorder, may lead to congenital bilateral absence of the vas deferens, with consequent obstructive azoospermia.[58] Moreover, inbreeding or the presence of consanguinity between the couple or their parents, which is common in certain parts of the world, may play a role in the etiology of infertility.[59]

Sexual history. This involves asking about the patient's sexual desire, presence of adequate erections, and ejaculation concerns. Sexual dysfunction is not an uncommon cause for infertility. It may be the main cause for infertility due to failure of semen deposition into the vagina secondary to erectile or ejaculatory disorders, or it may cast a shadow over hormonal imbalance, which in turn could lead to infertility.[60]

In addition, information about the sexual intercourse patterns of the couple is important, including frequency of intercourse, the use of lubricants, and intravaginal ejaculation. The spermicidal effects of different lubricants used during intercourse has been studied, compared, and reported between couples. The main mechanisms found were being affected of sperm motility and alteration of sperm chromatin integrity.[61] On top of that, addressing the male patient's pattern and frequency of intercourse during his female partner's ovulation period is paramount for increasing the chance of natural conception.[62]

Female partner. Part of completing the history taking of a couple is the female partner/spouse's condition, which includes age, regularity of menstrual cycles, evaluation by a reproductive endocrinologist, comorbidities, medical and surgical history, and family history. This adds up to the final image and whether it is solely a male infertility issue or a combined etiology for both.

PHYSICAL EXAMINATION

Objectives

A systematic, meticulous physical examination is necessary to evaluate infertile patients. Correlation of the patient's complaint and history with physical examination is a cornerstone of reaching accurate causes of infertility (Fig. 7.2).

General Examination

The main target of performing a general examination in infertile males is excluding hypogonadal signs, which could be in the form of increased central obesity or underdeveloped secondary sexual characters like scarce body, facial, and pubic hair; eunuchoid body proportions; and the presence of gynecomastia. All these hypogonadal signs could be correlated with imbalance in the hormonal profile in such patients, which in turn affects their fertility capabilities.

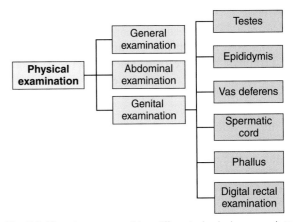

Fig. 7.2 Flowchart summarizing different physical exam points during assessment of the male partner of an infertile heterosexual couple.

Obesity, described as increased body fat and adipose tissue accumulation, precipitates the peripheral conversion of testosterone to estrogen, disrupting the HPO hormonal axis, steroidogenesis, and spermatogenesis. It also dysregulates the induction of apoptosis, which affects testicular germ cells.[63] Multiple reports have linked deranged sperm parameters in obese males or males with a high body mass index.[64–66] Besides, other studies described abnormal DNA integrity with obesity as a factor in male infertility.[67,68] Last, clinical pregnancy and live birth outcomes in assisted reproductive techniques were reported to be inversely associated with obesity.[69,70]

Abdominal Examination

This includes inspection for scars of previous surgeries, especially hernia repairs, pelvic trauma, and assessment of hernial orifices.

Genital Examination

There are a few considerations to facilitating the genital examination. They includes preparing a private room for patient tranquility at a warm temperature to allow cremasteric muscle relaxation and remembering to wear gloves and warm the hands as well. The examination should be done in standing and recumbent positions with proper exposure from the waist all the way down to ease the inspection and palpation process.

Scrotal examination involves evaluating both testes, epididymis, spermatic cords, and penis, and performing a digital rectal examination.

Testis

By inspection and then palpation, we assess the presence of both testes in the scrotum. Then we examine and compare their size, consistency, tenderness (associated with orchitis), and presence of cysts or masses. Testicular size could be estimated by measuring its volume using a Prader orchidometer (Fig. 7.3) or measuring its length and width using a caliper (Seager) orchidometer. It has been reported that the average volume of the testes differs according to body habitus as well as regional and racial background.[71] Normal testicular volume range is 12 to 30 cm,[3] with an average of 18 cm^3 per testis.[72] The presence of testicular size discrepancy could indicate existence of a unilateral varicocele causing decrease of the testicular volume or aid in the detection of a mass or cyst on the contralateral, abnormally increased side.[73,74] Testicular consistency could provide additional information that guides the clinician to search for the cause if abnormal. The uniform consistency of the testes is firm and rubbery, while softness could indicate a process of degeneration and effect of a varicocele. On the other hand, if you encounter hard texture, then suspect a testicular mass until proved otherwise.[75]

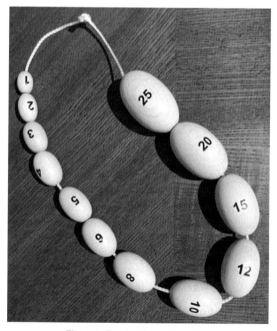

Fig. 7.3 Prader Orchidometer.

Epididymis

Careful bimanual examination while holding the testicle is preferred to assess unilateral or bilateral agenesis (which relates to Wolffian duct malformation),[76] a sense epididymal fullness (in cases of obstructive azoospermia),[77] identify cysts or masses, and finally, determine tenderness (which could indicate the presence of epididymitis).[78]

Vas Deferens

The aim is to detect the presence or absence of one or both vas deferens (which could indicate presence of congenital diseases like cystic fibrosis with *CFTR* gene mutation and unilateral renal agenesis with abnormal mesonephric duct development),[79,80] and also detect irregularities along its length (a beaded vas deferens could be a sign of tuberculosis).[81]

Spermatic Cord

The main goal is identifying varicocele presence and its laterality and grade. Proper examination of varicocele is in a standing position at first, then repeated while recumbent. The spermatic cord is felt at the neck of the scrotum between the index and thumb, while the veins are assessed in a relaxed state and then during a Valsalva maneuver if they were not discovered initially. A large varicocele could be detected by inspection and by palpation, where a sense of a bag of worms is felt. On the other hand, smaller varicoceles are usually detected during Valsalva, where the retrograde blood flow is felt like an impulse/reflux.

The Dubin and Amelar classification[82] is one of the clinically commonly used grading systems and divides varicocele into:
- Grade 1: varicocele is felt with Valsalva only
- Grade 2: varicocele is felt with palpation in a relaxed state and cannot be seen through the scrotal skin
- Grade 3: varicocele is seen through the scrotal skin without Valsalva, known as the bag of worms appearance

Phallus

Check whether it is circumcised or not. The prepuce is inspected for skin lesions and retracted to inspect for any penile lesions involved in the glans. The meatus is examined for its location (hypospadias or epispadias), presence of stricture, and urethral discharge. Finally, penile palpation is performed to detect plaques or chordee that cause penile curvature, which could contribute to sexual dysfunction or failure of proper semen deposition in the vagina.[83]

Digital Rectal Examination

The goal is to assess anal tone initially, then prostate size (benign prostatic hyperplasia), tenderness (sign of prostatitis), nodules or masses (sign of prostate cancer), seminal vesicle induration, masses, and cysts.

The patient's position could be lateral decubitus with flexed hip and knees or standing position with spread legs and a 90-degree waist bend. Examination is done with a well-lubricated, gloved dominant hand, while the nondominant hand is used for fixation, spreading the gluteal folds, and exposing the anus.[84,85]

TELEHEALTH AND MALE INFERTILITY ASSESSMENT

Telehealth is defined as the administration of healthcare services via telehealth communication technologies and electronic information.[86] Over the past 2 years, during the COVID-19 pandemic, the healthcare system has reshaped and transformed. Physicians were rushed to utilize telehealth without proper assessment or feasibility studies of its utilization for different specialties. An increase in the different forms of telehealth has occurred in all medical specialties, including urology. Despite current data scarcity in literature, emerging studies investigating this effect have been established.

There are definite benefits for the patients for this implementation, including cost effectiveness, convenience, easier accessibility to health care if living in rural areas or having mobility restrictions, and most importantly, limiting the potential of infection and spread of the virus from accessing healthcare facilities. However, the long-term effects of such modalities are still not properly investigated, given the short period of widespread telehealth usage.[87] On the other hand, some difficulties are met with telehealth. Patients still need to access healthcare facilities physically to perform diagnostic tests and imaging studies and to have physical examinations performed. Another drawback is the security risk for electronic record transfer and the potential breach of confidentiality with the usage of virtual communication programs. Finally, insurance companies might not cover all service costs related to telehealth for both patients and physician reimbursements.[88]

The male infertility clinic has a specific nature due to sensitivity of the topics dealt with in the clinic and the need for extreme confidentiality in some cases. However, a pilot study by Zu et al. (2020) on 56 male infertility patients who underwent 70 video virtual consultations showed that telehealth was feasible, convenient, and cost effective for male infertility patients.[89] However, more studies from male infertility centers from different areas of the world are needed to prove the effectiveness of such a method and to identify the patient groups suitable for telehealth.

SUMMARY

History taking and physical examination are fundamental components of male infertility assessment. The main objectives are to identify possible causes and risk factors of male infertility and thus guide further management, including appropriate laboratory and radiological tests and lines of treatment.

REFERENCES

1. Agarwal A, Baskaran S, Parekh N, et al. Male infertility. *Lancet.* 2021;397(10271):319-333. doi:10.1016/S0140-6736(20)32667-2.
2. World Health Organization, *Infertility.* World health Organization; April 3, 2023. https://www.who.int/news-room/fact-sheets/detail/infertility.
3. Rusz A, Pilatz A, Wagenlehner F, et al. Influence of urogenital infections and inflammation on semen quality and male fertility. *World J Urol.* 2012;30(1):23-30. doi:10.1007/s00345-011-0726-8.
4. Haidl G, Allam JP, Schuppe HC. Chronic epididymitis: impact on semen parameters and therapeutic options. *Andrologia.* 2008;40(2):92-96. doi:10.1111/j.1439-0272.2007.00819.x.
5. Schuppe HC, Pilatz A, Hossain H, Diemer T, Wagenlehner F, Weidner W. Urogenital infection as a risk factor for male infertility. *Dtsch Arztebl Int.* 2017;114(19):339-346. doi:10.3238/arztebl.2017.0339.
6. Henkel R. Infection in infertility. In: Parekattil SJ, Agarwal A, eds. *Male Infertility: Contemporary Clinical Approaches, Andrology, ART & Antioxidants.* New York: Springer; 2012: 261-272.
7. Harkness AH. The pathology of gonorrhoea. *Br J Vener Dis.* 1948;24(4):137-147.
8. Brookings C, Goldmeier D, Sadeghi-Nejad H. Sexually transmitted infections and sexual function in relation to male fertility. *Korean J Urol.* 2013;54(3):149-156. doi:10.4111/kju.2013.54.3.149.

9. Masarani M, Wazait H, Dinneen M. Mumps orchitis. *J R Soc Med*. 2006;99(11):573-575. doi:10.1258/jrsm. 99.11.573.

10. Machado B, Barcelos Barra G, Scherzer N, et al. Presence of SARS-CoV-2 RNA in Semen-cohort study in the United States COVID-19 positive patients. *Infect Dis Rep*. 2021;13(1):96-101. doi:10.3390/idr13010012.

11. Holtmann N, Edimiris P, Andree M, et al. Assessment of SARS-CoV-2 in human semen-a cohort study. *Fertil Steril*. 2020;114(2):233-238. doi:10.1016/j.fertnstert. 2020.05.028.

12. Li D, Jin M, Bao P, Zhao W, Zhang S. Clinical characteristics and results of semen tests among men with coronavirus disease 2019. *JAMA Netw Open*. 2020;3(5):e208292. doi:10.1001/jamanetworkopen.2020.8292.

13. Temiz MZ, Dincer MM, Hacibey I, et al. Investigation of SARS-CoV-2 in semen samples and the effects of COVID-19 on male sexual health by using semen analysis and serum male hormone profile: a cross-sectional, pilot study. *Andrologia*. 2021;53(2):e13912. doi:10.1111/and. 13912.

14. Gacci M, Coppi M, Baldi E, et al. Semen impairment and occurrence of SARS-CoV-2 virus in semen after recovery from COVID-19. *Hum Reprod*. 2021;36(6):1520-1529. doi:10.1093/humrep/deab026.

15. Kharbach Y, Khallouk A. Male genital damage in COVID-19 patients: Are available data relevant? *Asian J Urol*. 2021;8(3):324-326. doi:10.1016/j.ajur.2020.06.005.

16. Delahoy MJ, Whitaker M, O'Halloran A, et al. Characteristics and maternal and birth outcomes of hospitalized pregnant women with laboratory-confirmed COVID-19 - COVID-NET, 13 States, March 1-August 22, 2020. *MMWR Morb Mortal Wkly Rep*. 2020;69(38):1347-1354. doi:10.15585/mmwr.mm6938e1.

17. Lorusso F, Palmisano M, Chironna M, et al. Impact of chronic viral diseases on semen parameters. *Andrologia*. 2010;42:121-126.

18. Hajizadeh Maleki B, Tartibian B. COVID-19 and male reproductive function: a prospective, longitudinal cohort study. *Reproduction*. 2021;161(3):319-331. doi:10.1530/ REP-20-0382.

19. Gonzalez DC, Nassau DE, Khodamoradi K, et al. Sperm parameters before and after COVID-19 mRNA vaccination. *JAMA*. 2021;326(3):273-274. doi:10.1001/jama.2021.9976.

20. Esposito M, Salerno M, Calvano G, et al. Impact of anabolic androgenic steroids on male sexual and reproductive function: a systematic review. *Panminerva Med*. 2023;65(1): 43-50. doi:10.23736/s0031-0808.22.04677-8.

21. McBride JA, Coward RM. Recovery of spermatogenesis following testosterone replacement therapy or anabolic-androgenic steroid use. *Asian J Androl*. 2016;18(3):373-380. doi:10.4103/1008-682x.173938.

22. Ding J, Shang X, Zhang Z, et al. FDA-approved medications that impair human spermatogenesis. *Oncotarget*. 2017;8(6):10714-10725. doi:10.18632/oncotarget.12956.

23. Brezina PR, Yunus FN, Zhao Y. Effects of pharmaceutical medications on male fertility. *J Reprod Infertil*. 2012; 13(1):3-11.

24. Schlegel PN, Chang TS, Marshall FF. Antibiotics: potential hazards to male fertility. *Fertil Steril*. 1991;55(2): 235-242. doi:10.1016/s0015-0282(16)54108-9.

25. Howell SJ, Shalet SM. Spermatogenesis after cancer treatment: damage and recovery. *J Natl Cancer Inst Monogr*. 2005;(34):12-17. doi:10.1093/jncimonographs/lgi003.

26. Vakalopoulos I, Dimou P, Anagnostou I, Zeginiadou T. Impact of cancer and cancer treatment on male fertility. *Hormones (Athens)*. 2015;14(4):579-589. doi:10.14310/ horm.2002.1620.

27. Nalesnik JG, Sabanegh Jr ES, Eng TY, Buchholz TA. Fertility in men after treatment for stage 1 and 2A seminoma. *Am J Clin Oncol*. 2004;27(6):584-588. doi:10.1097/01.coc.0000135736.18493.dd.

28. Ståhl O, Eberhard J, Jepson K, et al. Sperm DNA integrity in testicular cancer patients. *Hum Reprod*. 2006;21(12):3199-3205. doi:10.1093/humrep/del292.

29. Shalet SM, Tsatsoulis A, Whitehead E, Read G. Vulnerability of the human Leydig cell to radiation damage is dependent upon age. *J Endocrinol*. 1989;120(1):161-165. doi:10.1677/joe.0.1200161.

30. Okada K, Fujisawa M. Recovery of spermatogenesis following cancer treatment with cytotoxic chemotherapy and radiotherapy. *World J Mens Health*. 2019;37(2): 166-174. doi:10.5534/wjmh.180043.

31. Barrass BJ, Jones R, Graham JD, Persad RA. Practical management issues in bilateral testicular cancer. *BJU Int*. 2004;93(9):1183-1187. doi:10.1111/j.1464-410X.2003.04837.x.

32. Agbaje IM, Rogers DA, McVicar CM, et al. Insulin dependant diabetes mellitus: implications for male reproductive function. *Hum Reprod*. 2007;22(7):1871-1877. doi:10.1093/humrep/dem077.

33. Li Y, Liu L, Wang B, Chen D, Wang J. Nonalcoholic fatty liver disease and alteration in semen quality and reproductive hormones. *Eur J Gastroenterol Hepatol*. 2015; 27(9):1069-1073. doi:10.1097/meg.0000000000000408.

34. Lundy SD, Vij SC. Male infertility in renal failure and transplantation. *Transl Androl Urol*. 2019;8(2):173-181. doi:10.21037/tau.2018.07.16.

35. Sironen A, Shoemark A, Patel M, Loebinger MR, Mitchison HM. Sperm defects in primary ciliary dyskinesia and related causes of male infertility. *Cell Mol Life Sci*. 2020;77(11): 2029-2048. doi:10.1007/s00018-019-03389-7.

36. Ahmad A, Ahmed A, Patrizio P. Cystic fibrosis and fertility. *Curr Opin Obstet Gynecol*. 2013;25(3):167-172. doi:10.1097/GCO.0b013e32835f1745.

37. Krajewska-Kulak E, Sengupta P. Thyroid function in male infertility. *Front Endocrinol (Lausanne).* 2013;4:174. doi:10.3389/fendo.2013.00174.

38. Petersen PM, Skakkebaek NE, Vistisen K, Rørth M, Giwercman A. Semen quality and reproductive hormones before orchiectomy in men with testicular cancer. *J Clin Oncol.* 1999;17(3):941-947. doi:10.1200/jco.1999. 17.3.941.

39. Xavier R, de Carvalho RC, Fraietta R. Semen quality from patients affected by seminomatous and non-seminomatous testicular tumor. *Int Braz J Urol.* 2021; 47(3):495-502. doi:10.1590/s1677-5538.Ibju.2021.99.01.

40. Dohle GR. Male infertility in cancer patients: review of the literature. *Int J Urol.* 2010;17(4):327-331. doi:10.1111/j.1442-2042.2010.02484.x.

41. Molokwu CN, Doull RI, Townell NH. A novel technique for repair of testicular rupture after blunt trauma. *Urology.* 2010;76(4):1002-1003. doi:10.1016/j.urology.2010.06.011.

42. Xu F, Ye L, Hu Y, et al. A novel protein biochip screening serum anti-sperm antibody expression and natural pregnancy rate in a follow-up study in Chinese infertility. *Biosci Rep.* 2020;40:1-10.

43. Cui D, Han G, Shang Y, et al. Antisperm antibodies in infertile men and their effect on semen parameters: a systematic review and meta-analysis. *Clin Chim Acta.* 2015;444:29-36. doi:10.1016/j.cca.2015.01.033.

44. Momen MN, Fahmy I, Amer M, Arafa M, Zohdy W, Naser TA. Semen parameters in men with spinal cord injury: changes and aetiology. *Asian J Androl.* 2007;9(5): 684-689. doi:10.1111/j.1745-7262.2007.00277.x.

45. Lauridsen LL, Arendt LH, Støvring H, Olsen J, Ramlau-Hansen CH. Is age at puberty associated with semen quality and reproductive hormones in young adult life? *Asian J Androl.* 2017;19(6):625-632. doi:10.4103/1008-682x.190328.

46. Goel P, Rawat JD, Wakhlu A, Kureel SN. Undescended testicle: An update on fertility in cryptorchid men. *Indian J Med Res.* 2015;141(2):163-171. doi:10.4103/0971-5916.155544.

47. Rodprasert W, Virtanen HE, Mäkelä JA, Toppari J. Hypogonadism and cryptorchidism. *Front Endocrinol (Lausanne).* 2019;10:906. doi:10.3389/fendo.2019.00906.

48. Skarin Nordenvall A, Chen Q, Norrby C, et al. Fertility in adult men born with hypospadias: A nationwide register-based cohort study on birthrates, the use of assisted reproductive technologies and infertility. *Andrology.* 2020;8(2):372-380. doi:10.1111/andr.12723.

49. Gersh I. Surgical procedures affecting male fertility; indications and contraindications. *Fertil Steril.* 1955;6(3):228-235. doi:10.1016/s0015-0282(16)31983-5.

50. Harlev A, Agarwal A, Gunes SO, Shetty A, du Plessis SS. Smoking and male infertility: an evidence-based review. *World J Mens Health.* 2015;33(3):143-160. doi:10.5534/wjmh.2015.33.3.143.

51. Guthauser B, Boitrelle F, Plat A, Thiercelin N, Vialard F. Chronic excessive alcohol consumption and male fertility: a case report on reversible azoospermia and a literature review. *Alcohol Alcohol.* 2014;49(1):42-44. doi:10.1093/alcalc/agt133.

52. Grover S, Mattoo SK, Pendharkar S, Kandappan V. Sexual dysfunction in patients with alcohol and opioid dependence. *Indian J Psychol Med.* 2014;36(4):355-365. doi:10.4103/0253-7176.140699.

53. Fronczak CM, Kim ED, Barqawi AB. The insults of illicit drug use on male fertility. *J Androl.* Jul-Aug 2012;33(4): 515-528. doi:10.2164/jandrol.110.011874.

54. Sharma A, Mollier J, Brocklesby RWK, Caves C, Jayasena CN, Minhas S. Endocrine-disrupting chemicals and male reproductive health. *Reprod Med Biol.* 2020;19(3):243-253. doi:10.1002/rmb2.12326.

55. Kenkel S, Rolf C, Nieschlag E. Occupational risks for male fertility: an analysis of patients attending a tertiary referral centre. *Int J Androl.* 2001;24(6):318-326. doi:10.1046/j.1365-2605.2001.00304.x.

56. Hamilton TR, Mendes CM, de Castro LS, et al. Evaluation of lasting effects of heat stress on sperm profile and oxidative status of ram semen and epididymal sperm. *Oxid Med Cell Longev.* 2016;2016:1687657. doi:10.1155/2016/1687657.

57. Baschat AA, Küpker W, al Hasani S, Diedrich K, Schwinger E. Results of cytogenetic analysis in men with severe subfertility prior to intracytoplasmic sperm injection. *Hum Reprod.* 1996;11(2):330-333. doi:10.1093/humrep/11.2.330.

58. Sokol RZ. Infertility in men with cystic fibrosis. *Curr Opin Pulm Med.* 2001;7(6):421-426. doi:10.1097/00063198-200111000-00011.

59. Inhorn MC, Kobeissi L, Nassar Z, Lakkis D, Fakih MH. Consanguinity and family clustering of male factor infertility in Lebanon. *Fertil Steril.* 2009;91(4):1104-1109. doi:10.1016/j.fertnstert.2008.01.008.

60. Lotti F, Maggi M. Sexual dysfunction and male infertility. *Nat Rev Urol.* 2018;15(5):287-307. doi:10.1038/nrurol.2018.20.

61. Agarwal A, Deepinder F, Cocuzza M, Short RA, Evenson DP. Effect of vaginal lubricants on sperm motility and chromatin integrity: a prospective comparative study. *Fertil Steril.* 2008;89(2):375-379. doi:10.1016/j.fertnstert.2007.02.050.

62. Wilcox AJ, Weinberg CR, Baird DD. Timing of sexual intercourse in relation to ovulation. Effects on the probability of conception, survival of the pregnancy, and sex of the baby. *N Engl J Med.* 1995;333(23):1517-1521. doi:10.1056/nejm199512073332301.

63. Leisegang K, Sengupta P, Agarwal A, Henkel R. Obesity and male infertility: Mechanisms and management. *Andrologia*. 2021;53(1):e13617. doi:10.1111/and.13617.

64. Kahn BE, Brannigan RE. Obesity and male infertility. *Curr Opin Urol*. 2017;27(5):441-445. doi:10.1097/mou.0000000000000417.

65. Chavarro JE, Toth TL, Wright DL, Meeker JD, Hauser R. Body mass index in relation to semen quality, sperm DNA integrity, and serum reproductive hormone levels among men attending an infertility clinic. *Fertil Steril*. 2010;93(7):2222-2231. doi:10.1016/j.fertnstert.2009.01.100.

66. Sermondade N, Faure C, Fezeu L, et al. BMI in relation to sperm count: an updated systematic review and collaborative meta-analysis. *Hum Reprod Update*. 2013;19(3):221-231. doi:10.1093/humupd/dms050.

67. Agarwal A, Majzoub A, Baskaran S, et al. Sperm DNA fragmentation: a new guideline for clinicians. *World J Mens Health*. 2020;38(4):412-471. doi:10.5534/wjmh.200128.

68. Panner Selvam MK, Sengupta P, Agarwal A. Sperm DNA fragmentation and male infertility. In: Arafa M, Elbardisi H, Majzoub A, Agarwal A, eds. *Genetics of Male Infertility: A Case-Based Guide for Clinicians*. Cham, Switzerland: Springer International Publishing; 2020:155-172.

69. Umul M, Köse SA, Bilen E, Altuncu AG, Oksay T, Güney M. Effect of increasing paternal body mass index on pregnancy and live birth rates in couples undergoing intracytoplasmic sperm injection. *Andrologia*. 2015;47(3):360-364. doi:10.1111/and.12272.

70. Schliep KC, Mumford SL, Ahrens KA, et al. Effect of male and female body mass index on pregnancy and live birth success after in vitro fertilization. *Fertil Steril*. 2015;103(2):388-395. doi:10.1016/j.fertnstert.2014.10.048.

71. Behre HM, Nashan D, Nieschlag E. Objective measurement of testicular volume by ultrasonography: evaluation of the technique and comparison with orchidometer estimates. *Int J Androl*. 1989;12(6):395-403. doi:10.1111/j.1365-2605.1989.tb01328.x.

72. Chapple CR, Steers WD, eds. *Practical Urology: Essential Principles and Practice*. London, UK: Springer-Verlag London Limited; 2011. doi:10.1007/978-1-84882-034-0_4.

73. Zini A, Buckspan M, Berardinucci D, Jarvi K. Loss of left testicular volume in men with clinical left varicocele: correlation with grade of varicocele. *Arch Androl*. 1998;41(1):37-41. doi:10.3109/01485019808988544.

74. Patel SR, Sigman M. Prevalence of testicular size discrepancy in infertile men with and without varicoceles. *Urology*. 2010;75(3):566-568. doi:10.1016/j.urology.2009.08.084.

75. Besiroglu H, Otunctemur A, Dursun M, Ozbek E. The prevalence and severity of varicocele in adult population over the age of forty years old: a cross-sectional study. *Aging Male*. 2019;22(3):207-213. doi:10.1080/13685538.2018.1465913.

76. McCullough R, Marshall FF, Berry SJ, Detweiler C. The influence of epididymal agenesis on the development and maturation of the testis: experimental model and clinical correlations. *Urol Res*. 1984;12(3):165-170. doi:10.1007/bf00255916.

77. Kolettis PN. Is physical examination useful in predicting epididymal obstruction? *Urology*. 2001;57(6):1138-1140. doi:10.1016/s0090-4295(01)00956-6.

78. Nickel JC. Chronic epididymitis: a practical approach to understanding and managing a difficult urologic enigma. *Rev Urol*. 2003;5(4):209-215.

79. de Souza DAS, Faucz FR, Pereira-Ferrari L, Sotomaior VS, Raskin S. Congenital bilateral absence of the vas deferens as an atypical form of cystic fibrosis: reproductive implications and genetic counseling. *Andrology*. 2018;6(1):127-135. doi:10.1111/andr.12450.

80. McCallum T, Milunsky J, Munarriz R, Carson R, Sadeghi-Nejad H, Oates R. Unilateral renal agenesis associated with congenital bilateral absence of the vas deferens: phenotypic findings and genetic considerations. *Hum Reprod*. 2001;16(2):282-288. doi:10.1093/humrep/16.2.282.

81. Yang DM, Yoon MH, Kim HS, et al. Comparison of tuberculous and pyogenic epididymal abscesses: clinical, gray-scale sonographic, and color Doppler sonographic features. *AJR Am J Roentgenol*. 2001;177(5):1131-1135. doi:10.2214/ajr.177.5.1771131.

82. Dubin L, Amelar RD. Varicocele size and results of varicocelectomy in selected subfertile men with varicocele. *Fertil Steril*. 1970;21(8):606-609. doi:10.1016/s0015-0282(16)37684-1.

83. Walsh TJ, Hotaling JM, Lue TF, Smith JF. How curved is too curved? The severity of penile deformity may predict sexual disability among men with Peyronie's disease. *Int J Impot Res*. 2013;25(3):109-112. doi:10.1038/ijir.2012.48.

84. Steggall MJ. Digital rectal examination. *Nurs Stand*. 2008;22(47):46-48. doi:10.7748/ns2008.07.22.47.46.c6633.

85. Villanueva Herrero JA, Abdussalam A, Kasi A. *Rectal Exam*. Treasure Island (FL): StatPearls Publishing; 2021.

86. Colbert GB, Venegas-Vera AV, Lerma EV. Utility of telemedicine in the COVID-19 era. *Rev Cardiovasc Med*. 2020;21(4):583-587. doi:10.31083/j.rcm.2020.04.188.

87. Gadzinski AJ, Ellimoottil C. Telehealth in urology after the COVID-19 pandemic. *Nat Rev Urol*. 2020;17(7):363-364. doi:10.1038/s41585-020-0336-6.

88. Novara G, Checcucci E, Crestani A, et al. Telehealth in urology: a systematic review of the literature. How much can telemedicine be useful during and after the COVID-19 pandemic? *Eur Urol*. 2020;78(6):786-811. doi:10.1016/j.eururo.2020.06.025.

89. Zhu A, Andino JJ, Chopra Z, Daignault-Newton S, Ellimoottil C, Dupree JMIV. Telehealth for male-infertility is feasible and saves patients' time and money. *Fertil Steril*. 2020;114(3):e60-e61. doi:10.1016/j.fertnstert.2020.08.187.

8

Basic Semen Analysis

Marion Bendayan and Florence Boitrelle

KEY POINTS

- Basic sperm tests are first-line tests for males who wish to conceive.
- The World Health Organization (WHO) manual is a very detailed technical guide that sets the standards for performing semen analysis.
- In the current edition of the WHO manual, the concept of standards and reference values has been abandoned.
- The 5th percentile values of each sperm parameter established in males according to their ability to conceive naturally are not enough to predict the heterosexual couple's fertility.
- These 5th percentile values should be used to refer the patient to a specialized andrology consultation. This specialized consultation will focus on reinterviewing the patient and examining him for potential causes of infertility.

INTRODUCTION

Infertility is defined as "the inability to achieve a spontaneous pregnancy within 12 months despite regular unprotected sexual intercourse" and estimated to affect between 40 million and 120 million couples worldwide,[1,2] i.e., approximately one in six couples of childbearing age. A male causal factor is found in approximately 50% of cases:[3,4] either alone (20% of cases) or as part of couples' infertility (30% of cases).[3,4] There are many causes of male infertility, but before diagnosing them, the clinician must be able to explore the male reproductive function in a "simple way." Thus the cornerstone of the evaluation of male infertility is the conventional semen analysis, which provides a baseline measure of the male reproductive system. It is usually the first test ordered for the male partner of a heterosexual couple, as it is noninvasive and relatively inexpensive. According to the latest recommendations for the management of infertile males and couples, basic sperm examinations are indeed the first analyses to prescribe for males who consult for infertility.[5] This examination is prescribed after questioning the male about his history, symptoms, and sexual and reproductive history, and preferably before the male's clinical examination.[5]

The evaluation of semen parameters is currently based on the standards defined in the laboratory manual for the examination and processing of human semen created by the World Health Organization (WHO).[5-8] From the first edition of the WHO laboratory manual, published in 1980, to the current 6th edition, significant progress has been made by incorporating recent developments in semen examination techniques and incorporating methods for quality control and quality assurance.[9,10] According to the 6th edition of the WHO manual, basic semen analysis should allow the diagnosis of male reproductive disorders, the identification of lines of investigation, the choice of appropriate initial and follow-up therapy, and the selection of appropriate assisted reproductive technology (ART) procedures, if needed.[8]

In this chapter, we detail different tests that are grouped in the WHO manual under the term "Basic semen examination," highlight the main changes made in the current edition of the WHO manual, and discuss the "concept of reference thresholds, standards" of these semen examinations.

BASIC SEMEN EXAMINATION— CHANGES IN THE WORLD HEALTH ORGANIZATION MANUAL, 6TH EDITION

The term "basic semen examination" covers several tests:

- Examination of macroscopic semen parameters (viscosity, macroscopic appearance, odor, ejaculate volume, pH)
- Quantitative and qualitative study of sperm motility and determination of the presence of agglutinates and aggregates
- Sperm vitality
- Sperm concentration and sperm count
- Quantitative and qualitative study of sperm morphology

In the 6th edition of the WHO manual, some adjustments have been made concerning the basic parameters of semen. These are detailed in subsequent paragraphs. The preanalytical steps for semen examination are detailed in the WHO manual and need to be followed. The period of sexual abstinence should be between 2 and 7 days, and the sperm collection should be performed in the laboratory in a suitable flared receptacle (Fig. 8.1) after clear explanation of the collection instructions.

Macroscopic Parameters

The volume of the ejaculate is measured by weighing the semen using a balance (see Fig. 8.1). pH is measured using strips (Fig. 8.2).

Assessment of semen odor has been added, and the manual states that "odors of urine or putrefaction may be of clinical interest." It should be noted that the assessment of semen odor is subjective, making standardization of this parameter very complicated. Furthermore, the addition of this parameter is against recommendations for the safety of laboratory personnel and personal protection against emerging viruses in the next decade, and from which respiratory transmission could not be excluded.[9]

Among the macroscopic parameters, one of the most important is the volume of semen. It should be noted that the WHO manual deletes all pathological terms related to low or high thresholds. For example, the term hypospermia, which represents the fact that the volume of ejaculate is below the 5th percentile values, has disappeared. It is important to keep in mind that in practice, clinicians will still use the 5th percentile values to adjust their work-up and order certain additional tests. Thus in case of hypospermia, the clinician will be able to look for dysfunction of the ejaculatory reflex (which may be responsible for partial retrograde ejaculation) and anatomical and/or functional abnormalities of the genital tract and glands. Among the latter, we find mainly mutations of the *CFTR* gene, which may lead to bilateral absence of the vas deferens, which will be the cause of hypospermia associated with azoospermia but also isolated

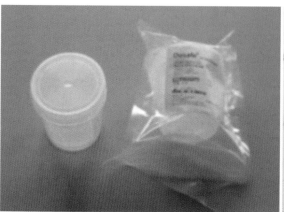
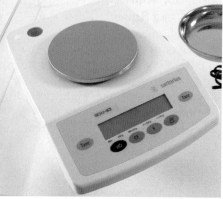

Fig. 8.1 Receptacle adapted for semen collection *(left)*, and scale adapted for semen weighing *(right)*.

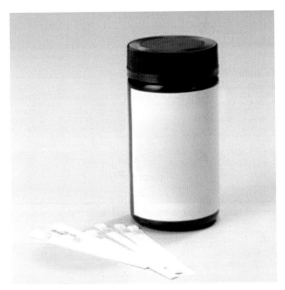

Fig. 8.2 pH measurement strips.

TABLE 8.1 Main Etiologies of Hypospermia

Mechanism	Etiologies
Ejaculatory reflex dysfunction responsible for partial retrograde ejaculation	• Neurological pathologies (multiple sclerosis, diabetic neuropathy, medullary trauma, etc.) • Surgical iatrogeny (lomboaortic curage, colorectal surgery, etc.) • Drug iatrogeny (neurotropics, psychotropics, etc.)
Anatomical and/or functional abnormalities of the genital tract and glands	• Endocrine pathologies (hypogonadotropic hypogonadism, hyperprolactinemia, etc.) • Bilateral or unilateral absence of the vas deferens, with or without seminal vesicle abnormalities (embryological development defect, *CFTR* gene mutation) • Obstructions of the ejaculatory ducts and other urogenital anatomical anomalies (cysts of the seminal vesicles, lithiasis of the ejaculatory ducts, etc.)

Based on Robin G, Marcelli F, Mitchell V, Marchetti C, Lemaitre L, Dewailly D, et al. Pourquoi et comment réaliser un bilan d'hypospermie? *Gynécologie Obstétrique Fertil.* 2008 Oct;36(10):1035–42 Copyright © 2008 Elsevier Masson SAS.

abnormalities of the seminal vesicles. The main etiologies of hypospermia are summarized in Table 8.1. The presence of hypospermia, even if isolated, should lead to a precise questioning of the patient (in particular to look for a problem of collection) and to complementary examinations if necessary. Particular attention should be paid to the presence of retrograde ejaculation. An endocrine work-up and an anatomical exploration of the genital and urinary tracts will be performed, and genetic analyses, in particular the search for a mutation of the *CFTR* gene, will be carried out in case of anatomical anomaly.[11]

Quantitative and Qualitative Study of Sperm Motility and Determination of the Presence of Agglutinates and Aggregates

Sperm motility is estimated with a phase contrast microscope. The 6th edition of the WHO manual has readopted the distinction of progressive motility into two categories (grades a and b). This distinction was made in the 4th edition (and valid until 2009) but was abandoned from 2010 to 2021.[12] Thus the categorization of sperm motility reverted to rapid progressive motility, slow progressive motility, nonprogressive motility, and immobility (grade a, b, c, or d, respectively). The distinction of rapid or slow progressive motility requires preincubation of clean microscope slides at 37°C. To justify this choice, the WHO manual cites older articles stating that rapid motility (grade a) is of clinical value.[13–21] However, the dissemination of this technique throughout the world could pose problems because it requires an adjustment of laboratory practices and the purchase of adapted and metrologically monitored heating plates. Moreover, because this distinction was dropped in the 5th edition of 2010, the distinction of progressive motility into two categories was not evaluated like the other parameters (by comparing data obtained from males whose time to pregnancy of a female partner is ≤12 months with those of males who remain childless). It is therefore surprising that this distinction of motility is added to the 6th edition without any recent studies (after 2010) demonstrating its utility in andrology or routine diagnosis.[9] It is important to correlate asthenozoospermia with necrozoospermia. The presence of a large proportion of live sperm (more than 25%–30%) but totally immotile spermatozoa may indicate structural defects in the flagellum.[22]

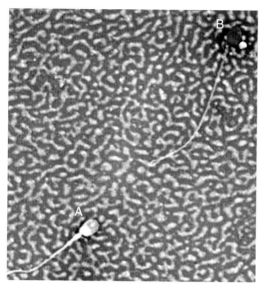

Fig. 8.3 Eosin-nigrosin staining of a live spermatozoon (white, on the left, *A*) and a dead spermatozoon (pink, on the right, *B*).

TABLE 8.2   Main Etiologies of Necrozoospermia
• Genital tract infections
• Testicular hyperthermia
• Varicocele
• Hyperthyroidism
• Spinal cord injury
• Polycystic kidney disease
• Antisperm antibodies
• Advanced male age
• Gonadotoxic substances
• Idiopathic

From Agarwal A, Sharma RK, Gupta S, et al. Sperm vitality and necrozoospermia: diagnosis, management, and results of a global survey of clinical practice. *World J Mens Health*. 2022;40(2):228.

Sperm Vitality

The study of sperm vitality can be done by different methods, including the eosin-nigrosin staining method. Eosin is a vital dye; a spermatozoon with a pinkish color is evaluated as dead (Fig. 8.3). Regarding the indications for sperm vitality assessment, the 6th edition corrected an inconsistency regarding sperm vitality assessment that existed in the previous 5th edition. In the 6th edition, sperm vitality assessment is recommended when total sperm motility is less than 40%.

The most common etiologies and risk factors for necrozoospermia are genital tract infections and testicular hyperthermia.[22] Other causes include varicocele, hyperthyroidism, spinal cord injury, polycystic kidney disease, and also the intake of gonadotoxic substances (tobacco, cannabis, etc.). The main causes of necrozoospermia are summarized in Table 8.2. In case of absolute necrozoospermia, it will be necessary to evaluate the sperm DNA fragmentation, which will allow to decide the best strategy for the management of the patient, that is practionner, to use ejaculated or testicular sperm for intracytoplasmic sperm injection.

Sperm Concentration, Sperm Count, and Round Cell Concentration

The evaluation of sperm concentration, sperm count, and round cell count is done with counting cells, such as the modified Neubauer cell. For the evaluation of the sperm count, the sperm dilutions have been simplified in the 6th edition, but 200 sperm must be counted per replicate. In the previous version of the manual, the observation of 0 to 4 sperm per field at 400× magnification could provide a sufficient indication for the evaluation of the concentration. According to the 5th edition of the WHO manual, sperm concentration could be reported as less than 2×10^6/mL.[12] In the 6th edition, the evaluation of low sperm concentrations ($<2 \times 10^6$/mL) must be assessed more precisely. Azoospermia is recorded when no sperm is found in the ejaculate after centrifugation. The etiologies of azoospermia are mainly endocrine diseases (hypogonadotropic hypogonadism such as Kallman syndrome), genetic abnormalities (karyotype abnormalities or microdeletions of the Y chromosome), or anatomical abnormalities (such as bilateral absence of the vas deferens). The management of azoospermia therefore should include a genetic and endocrine work-up as well as evaluation of the urogenital anatomy to exclude obstructive pathology.[4]

Quantitative and Qualitative Study of Sperm Morphology

The evaluation of sperm morphology using a systematic approach is described in the new 6th edition with multiple, higher-quality micrographs of sperm from untreated semen samples considered normal, borderline, or abnormal. They are accompanied by explanations of the classification of each evaluation, making it a useful guide. The evaluation of morphological abnormalities of the head, midpiece, and tail is described. The importance of recording the presence of large cytoplasmic droplets is emphasized.

The examination of sperm morphology is carried out on stained smear and must give the details of the anomalies, namely the anomalies of the head, the neck, the midpiece, the tail, and the excess residual cytoplasm. It is necessary to observe at least 200 sperm and to note also the presence of immature germ cells and nonsperm cells.

Evaluation of sperm morphology is clinically important in order to detect monomorphic abnormalities, that is, when the majority of the spermatozoa have a single abnormality. The main monomorphic anomalies are globozoospermia and macrozoospermia. Globozoospermia is characterized by an abnormality of the sperm head, which is round and without acrosome. The origin is usually genetic, and globozoospermic sperm are not able to fertilize the oocyte. In fact, the acrosome is essential to initiate the activation of the oocyte and the resumption of meiosis. Macrozoospermia is characterized by the presence of spermatozoa with a large head and often multiple flagella. In this case, there are often high levels of polyploidy and aneuploidy. The main cause is a mutation in the aurora kinase C gene, which is essential for meiosis.

Other abnormalities of sperm morphology include tail defects, which are often associated with asthenozoospermia and may be due to ciliary dyskinesia; residual cytoplasmic droplets, which reflect a defect in sperm maturation; and tapered sperm heads, which may be secondary to testicular hyperthermia related to a varicocele or obesity.

It is therefore important to take into account sperm morphology to guide the management of infertile patients.[23]

REFERENCE VALUES

In the 5th and 6th editions of the WHO manual of human semen analyses, 5th percentile values were measured in males for whom natural paternity was assessed in less than 12 months of regular unprotected intercourse. The reference thresholds for basic sperm parameters used in the 5th edition, and those described as "useful values" in the 6th edition, are compared in Table 8.3. The incorporation of additional regions and continents and the addition of more participants and

TABLE 8.3 WHO 2010 (5th ed.) and 2021 (6th ed.) Lower Fifth Percentile of Semen Parameters

	WHO 2010[a]	WHO 2021[a]
Semen volume (mL)	1.5 (1.4–1.7)	1.4 (1.3–1.5)
Total sperm number (10^6 per ejaculate)	39 (33–46)	39 (35–40)
Total motility (%)	40 (38–42)	42 (40–43)
Progressive motility (%)	32 (31–34)	30 (29–31)
Nonprogressive motility (%)	1	1 (1–1)
Immotile sperm (%)	22	20 (19–20)
Vitality (%)	58 (55–63)	54 (50–56)
Normal forms (%)	4 (3–4)	4 (3.9–4)

[a]95% confidence interval in parentheses.
WHO, World Health Organization.

samples in the final analysis give greater statistical power to the 5th percentile values recorded in the 6th edition, despite lack of significant difference from those reported in the 5th edition (see Table 8.1).

If the changes mentioned so far are slight adjustments, there is a more important change in this 6th edition: a paradigm shift. It should be noted that the 6th edition has taken the decision to remove the notion of "reference values," as well as "normality and abnormality." As previously mentioned, throughout the 280 pages of the 6th edition, the terms "hypospermia," "normozoospermia," "asthenozoospermia," "necrozoospermia," and "teratozoospermia" have been removed. These terms have been deliberately removed because the editors of the manual explain that reference thresholds alone are meaningless, and that multiple criteria must be applied to establish a diagnosis of male infertility. The latter statement is correct, but in actual practice, clinicians are likely to encounter some degree of confusion in the absence of reference values. To rely on other reference values, clinicians will need to search the literature for other sources. This can be time consuming and difficult. Therefore there remains a possibility that clinicians will continue to use the 5th percentile values, which were designed in the 5th edition to compare fertile and infertile males with the criterion of time to pregnancy of a female partner of less than or equal to 12 months.[9]

Clearly, these standards have little clinical value on their own, but they had the advantage of being able to direct the patient to specialized management. These 5th percentile values can therefore continue to be used, bearing in mind that they are one element among others in the evaluation of the infertile male.

Furthermore, it should also be kept in mind that these 5th percentile values are only of interest in the diagnosis of spontaneous fertility and infertility. They do not determine the type of management or treatment or the type of ART to be selected in infertile couples. The current WHO manual does not provide thresholds or reference ranges for sperm parameters to be used in conventional in vitro fertilization or intracytoplasmic sperm injection.

CONCLUSION

Basic semen analysis is the first-line examination for males who consult for fertility evaluation. Overall, the 5th edition of the WHO manual has made significant contributions to the practice of male infertility, from both a clinical and research perspective, and the incorporation of data from reference subsets is part of an ongoing attempt to define male fertility in numbers. The new 6th edition, published in July 2021, praises the importance of sperm analyses as a tool to (1) aid in fertility/infertility diagnosis, (2) assess male reproductive health and function to guide management, (3) guide the choice of ART procedure, (4) monitor response to treatment, and (5) measure the effectiveness of male contraception. A major deviation from the previous 5th version is the abandonment of reference values. In this 6th edition, it is clearly stated that the 5th percentile values are only one way to interpret the results of sperm analyses, and that the use of the 5th percentile alone is not sufficient to diagnose male infertility. The world of andrology and reproductive medicine is on the way to the 7th edition of the WHO manual, which should ideally combine standardization, technical quality, and clinical relevance of semen examinations to allow this examination to become a real diagnostic asset in the assessment of male infertility.

SUMMARY

For males seeking fertility assessment, a baseline semen analysis is the initial test. Overall, from both a clinical and research standpoint, the World Health Organization (WHO) manual's 5th edition has significantly advanced the field of male infertility, and the inclusion of data from reference subsets is a part of a continuing effort to quantify male fertility. The newly released 6th edition, which was released in July 2021, emphasizes the value of semen analysis as a tool to: (1) aid in the diagnosis of fertility/infertility; (2) assess male reproductive health and function to guide management; (3) guide the choice of assisted reproductive procedure; (4) monitor response to treatment; and (5) measure the effectiveness of male contraception. The removal of baseline values is a significant deviation from the 5th version. This 6th edition makes it very obvious that using the 5th percentile readings alone is insufficient for diagnosing male infertility. In this chapter, we describe the technical principles of basic semen analysis, outline the main etiologies associated with identified sperm abnormalities, and summarize what the physician can expect from basic semen analysis.

REFERENCES

1. Boivin J, Bunting L, Collins JA, Nygren KG. International estimates of infertility prevalence and treatment-seeking: potential need and demand for infertility medical care. *Hum Reprod.* 2007;22(6):1506-1512.
2. Datta J, Palmer MJ, Tanton C, et al. Prevalence of infertility and help seeking among 15 000 women and men. *Hum Reprod.* 2016;31(9):2108-2118.
3. Agarwal A, Mulgund A, Hamada A, Chyatte MR. A unique view on male infertility around the globe. *Reprod Biol Endocrinol.* 2015;13:37.
4. Agarwal A, Baskaran S, Parekh N, et al. Male infertility. *Lancet.* 2021;397(10271):319-333.
5. Schlegel PN, Sigman M, Collura B, et al. Diagnosis and treatment of infertility in men: AUA/ASRM guideline part I. *Fertil Steril.* 2021;115(1):54-61.
6. Barratt CLR, Björndahl L, De Jonge CJ, et al. The diagnosis of male infertility: an analysis of the evidence to support the development of global WHO guidance-challenges and future research opportunities. *Hum Reprod Update.* 2017;23(6):660-680.
7. Guzick DS, Overstreet JW, Factor-Litvak P, et al. Sperm morphology, motility, and concentration in fertile and infertile men. *N Engl J Med.* 2001;345(19):1388-1393.
8. World Health Organization. *WHO Laboratory Manual for the Examination and Processing of Human Semen.* 2021. Available at: https://apps.who.int/iris/handle/10665/343208.
9. Boitrelle F, Shah R, Saleh R, et al. The sixth edition of the WHO manual for human semen analysis: a critical review and SWOT analysis. *Life (Basel).* 2021;11(12):1368.

10. Wang C, Mbizvo M, Festin MP, Björndahl L, Toskin I, other Editorial Board Members of the WHO Laboratory Manual for the Examination and Processing of Human Semen. Evolution of the WHO "Semen" processing manual from the first (1980) to the sixth edition (2021). *Fertil Steril.* 2022;117(2):237-245.

11. Robin G, Marcelli F, Mitchell V, et al. Pourquoi et comment réaliser un bilan d'hypospermie? *Gynécologie Obstétrique Fertil.* 2008;36(10):1035-1042.

12. World Health Organization. *WHO Laboratory Manual for the Examination and Processing of Human Semen.* 5th ed. WHO; 2010:271.

13. Aitken RJ, Sutton M, Warner P, Richardson DW. Relationship between the movement characteristics of human spermatozoa and their ability to penetrate cervical mucus and zona-free hamster oocytes. *J Reprod Fertil.* 1985;73(2):441-449.

14. Barratt CL, McLeod ID, Dunphy BC, Cooke ID. Prognostic value of two putative sperm function tests: hypo-osmotic swelling and bovine sperm mucus penetration test (Penetrak). *Hum Reprod.* 1992;7(9):1240-1244.

15. Björndahl L. The usefulness and significance of assessing rapidly progressive spermatozoa. *Asian J Androl.* 2010;12(1):33-35.

16. Bollendorf A, Check JH, Lurie D. Evaluation of the effect of the absence of sperm with rapid and linear progressive motility on subsequent pregnancy rates following intra-uterine insemination or in vitro fertilization. *J Androl.* 1996;17(5):550-557.

17. Comhaire FH, Vermeulen L, Hinting A, Schoonjans F. Accuracy of sperm characteristics in predicting the in vitro fertilizing capacity of semen. *J In Vitro Fert Embryo Transf.* 1988;5(6):326-331.

18. Eliasson R. Semen analysis with regard to sperm number, sperm morphology and functional aspects. *Asian J Androl.* 2010;12(1):26-32.

19. Irvine DS, Aitken RJ. Predictive value of in-vitro sperm function tests in the context of an AID service. *Hum Reprod.* 1986;1(8):539-545.

20. Mortimer D, Pandya IJ, Sawers RS. Relationship between human sperm motility characteristics and sperm penetration into human cervical mucus in vitro. *J Reprod Fertil.* 1986;78(1):93-102.

21. Van den Bergh M, Emiliani S, Biramane J, Vannin AS, Englert Y. A first prospective study of the individual straight line velocity of the spermatozoon and its influences on the fertilization rate after intracytoplasmic sperm injection. *Hum Reprod.* 1998;13(11):3103-3107.

22. Agarwal A, Sharma RK, Gupta S, et al. Sperm vitality and necrozoospermia: diagnosis, management, and results of a global survey of clinical practice. *World J Mens Health.* 2022;40(2):228.

23. Agarwal A, Sharma R, Gupta S, et al. Sperm morphology assessment in the era of intracytoplasmic sperm injection: reliable results require focus on standardization, quality control, and training. *World J Mens Health.* 2022;40(3):347.

9

Sperm DNA Fragmentation Tests

Hussein Kandil and Ralf Reinhold Henkel

KEY POINTS

- Sperm genetic structure exhibits greater nuclear compaction compared to somatic cells, leading to significant chromatin condensation.
- Sperm DNA fragmentation comes in various forms, such as single or double-strand DNA fragmentation, and has diverse underlying causes contributing to its development.
- Sperm DNA fragmentation has been demonstrated to have an adverse effect on male fertility and reproductive outcomes.

- Various tools are widely being used to assess sperm DNA fragmentation, employing different methods and varying accuracy and clinical applications.
- Despite its clinical utility in managing male infertility, obstacles continue to impede the widespread adoption of sperm DNA fragmentation testing.
- Relevant case scenarios are being examined to illustrate how sperm DNA fragmentation is clinically applied in the context of managing male infertility.

INTRODUCTION

Although semen analysis (SA) was standardized by the World Health Organization (WHO) since its first publication of the "Laboratory Manual for the Examination and Processing of Human Semen" in 1980 until the most recent edition of the WHO manual in 2021,[1] conventional SA was repeatedly criticized because of its limited predictive value for the male reproductive potential.[2,3] Consequently, scientists and clinicians were looking for more advanced and more accurate diagnostic methods to predict male fertility potential and reproductive outcomes after natural and assisted reproductive techniques. Initially, various sperm function tests such as acrosome reaction[4] or sperm zona binding ability[5] were developed. However, these tests also have problems in terms of accuracy, repeatability, and reliability. On the other hand, one must accept that the fertilization process is a multifactorial process to which the individual sperm functions contribute in different proportions. Hence attention was drawn to sperm DNA integrity, as this is one of the last sperm

functions determining reproductive success. In addition, like sperm morphology, sperm DNA integrity is regarded as a more stable parameter with less biological variability and therefore is more reliable than sperm concentration or motility.[6] In the following years, several different tests to evaluate sperm DNA integrity were developed, based on different principles and methods. In this chapter, an overview of the most frequently used tests and their clinical relevance are discussed.

SPERM DNA STRUCTURE

The structural organization of the sperm DNA demonstrated by its complex condensation and compaction is considered a critical aspect to sperm development and maturity. This stems from the limited space within the sperm head to accommodate the genetic information, mandating a complex process of compaction to the sperm DNA, in a process that achieves a nuclear condensation that is six to seven times higher than in somatic cells.[7] The process of chromatin packaging and compaction takes place during spermatogenesis, starting in step 12 with the exchange of testicular histones by transition protein-1[8] and ending in the final replacement of the transition proteins by protamines in steps 14 to 16.[9] This process offers protection to the sperm DNA during the sperm transit.[10] The structural changes undergone by the developing sperm involve the replacement of histones by transition proteins and subsequently protamines (85%–90%), which harbor small cysteine residues capable of forming disulfide bridges between neighboring sulfhydryl groups, thereby offering potent chromatin stabilization. In addition, this process results in a neutralization of the negatively charged DNA by the arginine groups of the protamines, enabling the structural change of the sperm chromatin from supercoiled to linear arrays, thus a significantly higher compaction[11] and protection against damaging assaults.

Protamination takes place in the testis and continues in the epididymis during the sperm transition.[10] Zinc is believed to stabilize sperm DNA through its competent bonding with chromatin and, once eliminated following fertilization, it renders the DNA strands more dissociated, which happens upon the exposure to the seminal vesicle fluid, which dissociates zinc from chromatin.[12] Protamines appear in the nucleus at equal amounts in two forms, protamine-1 (P1) and protamine-2 (P2), and are rich in cysteine. The latter enables cross-linkage and ultimately chromatin condensation.[7] Interestingly, approximately 15% of the histones persist, even in the ejaculated mature sperm nuclei.[13] If the P1:P2 ratio is too high[14] or if the proportion of remaining histones is too high, this will render the sperm more prone to damage due to poor structural integrity.[15]

TYPES OF SPERM DNA FRAGMENTATION

DNA integrity is fundamental for male reproductive function. As mentioned earlier, several structural changes are necessary to convey the desired protection of the sperm genetic material, and any aberration involving these steps would render the sperm DNA susceptible for damage.[16] Sperm DNA damage can present either as single- or double-strand breaks, which are two different pathologic entities.[17] Double-strand breaks can occur secondary to failure in the repair system to mend aberrations occurring during remodeling and the absence or dysfunction of DNA repair mechanisms during meiosis,[18] whereas single-strand breaks are believed to result from oxidative damage.[19] Since single-strand breaks are

irreversible and have therefore a more serious impact on reproductive outcomes, double-strand damage can still be repaired by homologous recombination, nonhomologous end joining (NHEJ), and alternative NHEJ pathways.[20] Therefore double-strand breaks are associated with more serious consequences that can negatively affect pregnancy, where significant delays in embryo development and lower implantation rates were observed after intracytoplasmic sperm injection (ICSI).[21]

In cases where sperm are exposed to extensive oxidative stress (OS), sperm membranes will also be damaged by lipid peroxidation,[22] leading not only to a loss of sperm motility but also to DNA damage through direct oxidation, as well as indirect damage by genotoxic products deriving from lipid peroxidation. Consequently, these processes will negatively impact reproductive outcomes.[23] Both forms of damage are associated with reduced male fertility.[24] The presence of double-strand breaks can be associated with recurrent pregnancy loss, poor embryo development, and assisted reproductive technology (ART) failure.[21,25] Most DNA integrity tests cannot discern single- from double-strand breaks, except for the two-tailed comet assay. However, due to its complexity, variability of its results, and complexity of interpretation, it is considered of limited utility.[1,25]

DNA REPAIR

DNA integrity is crucial for normal male reproduction, and aberrations involving the sperm DNA are prone for transmission to the offspring.[26] Repair of DNA damage can take place during the initial phases of spermatogenesis, but it is absent following spermiogenesis when transcription and translation are terminated, offering the sperm no chance for repair during transport and storage, after which the only remaining possibility of repair would be the oocyte and early embryo.[19] However, in the zygote, DNA repair is needed to avoid transfer of damages to the germ line.[27] The oocyte is a vital source of repair to the sperm DNA, as demonstrated by the expression of DNA reparative genes, with evidence that this process tends to decline with advanced female age. In a study conducted in mice, the expression of 21 DNA repair genes was reduced in the older versus younger germinal vesicle oocytes ($p < 0.05$).[28] Sperm with fragmented DNA may undergo apoptosis if the oocyte reparative process fails to mend DNA breaks, resulting in pregnancy loss.[28] Sperm with damaged DNA can still fertilize oocytes, and the oocyte is still able to repair some DNA abnormalities when the degree of the damage is below 8%.[29] Otherwise, further development will either stop at the 4- to 8-cell stage when the paternal genome is switched on,[30] or this event will result in abnormal embryonic development and pregnancy loss.[28] Yet, checking for DNA damage and its effective repair is crucial and are done by the oocyte and the embryo. In this process, the triggering of checkpoints results in a delay of further development to allow for DNA repair or apoptosis.[31,32] However, it appears that the G1/S checkpoint is not activated in zygotes where the oocytes were inseminated with DNA-damaged sperm, resulting in no delay in the cell cycle earlier than the S-phase.[27,33]

CAUSES OF SPERM DNA FRAGMENTATION

During the different stages of spermatid maturity, DNA breaks are initiated by the enzyme topoisomerase II to relieve structural tension and allow for protamination, after which topoisomerase II is responsible for the relinking of the open nicks.[34,35] Failure of this repair can result in the ejaculation of sperm with fragmented DNA.[19,36] As mentioned earlier, the histone-to-protamine transition allows for chromatin compaction and established DNA integrity; hence, abnormalities in the P1:P2 ratio can be associated with SDF and subsequent poor fertilization and embryo development.[14,37] It has been shown that OS is correlated with increased levels of sperm with fragmented DNA and chromatin disruption, as reflected by the increased expression of 8-hydroxy-2′-deoxyguanosine ($p < 0.001$).[38] OS can be caused by an excessive production of reactive oxygen species from immature germ cells or leukocytes and is associated with reduced fertility due to its negative impact on the mature sperm DNA integrity.[26,39] It has been shown that sperm DNA is subject to deterioration in a timely fashion after ejaculation, with increased susceptibility of aberrations in sperm DNA.[19] Furthermore, cryopreservation has been associated with detrimental sperm structural and functional changes, reduced DNA quality, and altered sperm function.[40,41]

Clinical varicocele is the most common reversible cause of male infertility, affecting nearly 35% to 81% of patients presenting with primary and secondary infertility, respectively,[42] and a common cause of SDF, as shown in several studies with evidence of higher SDF among patients with varicocele compared to their healthy

counterparts.[43] The mechanism underlying varicocele-induced SDF resides in the increased level of OS, which is attributed to hyperthermia and abnormalities in testicular perfusion due to an increased venous pressure above the arteriolar pressure, with resultant accumulation of toxic byproducts.[44] Despite the solid knowledge regarding its contribution to male infertility, yet there remains a dispute concerning the role of varicocele repair in the management of male infertility. In a study by Esteves et al. evaluating SDF and sperm harboring degraded DNA in 593 semen tests from males presenting for fertility evaluation, it was found that in infertile patients with varicocele, the degradation index of the sperm DNA was two times higher compared with patients with other pathologies and fertile controls ($p < 0.0001$).[45] Studies have demonstrated the improvement in DNA integrity and reduction of OS following varicocele repair.[46] In a meta-analysis by Qiu et al. analyzing 11 studies, the sperm DNA fragmentation index decreased following varicocele repair by 5.79 (95% confidence interval [CI]: -7.39, -4.19), and when one study was removed due to its heterogeneity, the average decline was 6.14 (95% CI: -6.90, -5.37).[47] In another systematic review and metaanalysis by Lira Neto et al., which included 1070 infertile males from 19 studies, it was shown that varicocele repair was associated with significant improvement in sperm DNA integrity, with weighted mean differences of -7.23% (95% CI: -8.86, -5.59).[48] In a metaanalysis by Wang et al. it was shown that compared to fertile controls, the mean difference in SDF levels among varicocele patients was higher, reaching 9.84% (95% CI: 9.19, 10.49; $p < 0.00001$), and was significantly reduced to reach -3.37% (95% CI: -4.09, -2.65; $p < 0.00001$) following varicocele repair.[49] The decision to proceed with varicocele repair is sometimes challenging, especially when the outcome is unpredictable, a fact that calls for more advanced tests to support the clinical decision. Though most guidelines indicate varicocele repair only for clinical varicocele that is associated with abnormal semen parameters, a state of confusion exists when it comes to grade 2/3 varicocele and normal conventional semen parameters. In such case, there is evidence of the role of SDF to better identify patients with clinical varicocele who may need repair, even if conventional semen parameters are normal.[50,51]

Compared to fertile males, patients with genital tract infections (e.g., *Chlamydia trachomatis*) were shown to harbor higher levels of SDF.[52] Pagliuca et al. showed that males with evidence of genital infection were six times more prone to have sperm DNA abnormalities.[53] Age has also been shown to be associated with SDF.[54] In one study, lower SDF rates were observed in younger males (≤35 years), measuring 15.7%, compared to older males (36–39 years and ≥40 years), where SDF measured 18.2% (p = 0.034) and 18.3% (p = 0.022), respectively.[55] Another study has shown that the odds ratio of harboring elevated SDF was doubled in older males compared to their younger counterparts.[56] Furthermore, smoking and tobacco use have been linked to increased SDF due to elevated OS levels. Smoking is a common cause of altered sperm DNA, with evidence of a higher negative impact on chromatin integrity observed among smokers compared to nonsmokers (p < 0.001) and which is correlated with the intensity and duration of exposure.[57] Additionally, consuming alcoholic beverages, especially when consumed along with tobacco, is associated with increased SDF due to OS, reflected by the imbalance in the ratio observed between antioxidant activity and oxidative stressors.[58]

IMPACT OF SDF ON REPRODUCTIVE OUTCOMES

Natural Pregnancy

Several studies demonstrated the negative association between SDF and poor fertility, especially in heterosexual couples complaining of delayed or no pregnancy. A study by Evenson et al. and another by Spano et al. used the cells outside the main population (COMPαT) as a reflect to sperm with DNA integrity and have shown that a value above 30% is associated with poor fertility.[59] In their study, no natural pregnancy was achieved when COMPαT was greater than or equal to 30%.[59] In a metaanalysis analyzing three studies, Zini showed that the occurrence of a natural pregnancy is challenged among patients with elevated SDF, with an odds ratio of 7.01 (95% CI: 3.68, 13.36; p < 0.001).[60] Another metaanalysis by Tan et al. showed that in heterosexual couples experiencing idiopathic recurrent pregnancy loss, males had higher SDF levels when compared to fertile controls, with an average mean difference of 11.98 (95% CI: 6.64, 17.32; p < 0.001).[61] The probability of pregnancy was higher when SDF as measured by the sperm chromatin structure assay (SCSA) was less than 30% as compared to higher values.[59] Finally, a metaanalysis by McQueen et al. that included 13 studies demonstrated an elevated SDF in the cohort of 579 males of heterosexual couples suffering recurrent pregnancy loss when compared to 434 controls, with a mean difference of 11.91 (95%

CI: 4.97, 18.86).[62] Similar results were obtained by more recent metaanalyses for abortion (mean difference: 1.60; 95% CI: 1.04, 2.17)[63] and recurrent miscarriages (mean difference: 8.45; 95% CI: 1.48, 15.42).[64]

Assisted Reproductive Technology

Although intrauterine insemination (IUI) is less frequently used within the context of assisted reproduction,[65] many still adopt this method as the first line of management of some types of patients. Several studies have examined the impact of SDF on IUI outcome, but the results are less consistent. Bungum et al. noted that when measured with SCSA, an SDF of greater than 30% is associated with lower pregnancy rates following IUI.[66] Another study by Duran et al. has demonstrated that no pregnancy occurred when the SDF was greater than 12% using terminal deoxynucleotidyl transferase dUTP nick-end labeling (TUNEL) in males undergoing IUI.[67] Rilcheva et al. suggested a poor outcome following IUI when SCSA was greater than 27%.[68] On the other hand, Siddhartha et al., comparing the outcome of IUI and ICSI between patients with DNA fragmentation index (DFI)-positive and DFI-negative counterparts, showed no significant difference between both groups when IUI was performed (17.6% vs. 11.8%).[69] In a systematic review and metaanalysis of nine studies, a weak association was demonstrated between SDF and in vitro fertilization (IVF)-related pregnancy, with a combined odds ratio of 1.57 (95% CI: 1.18, 2.07; p < 0.05).[70] Another metaanalysis of 56 studies involving 8086 IVF/ICSI or mixed treatments reports a negative significant association of SDF and pregnancy, with a combined odds ratio of 1.68 (95% CI: 1.49, 1.89; p < 0.0001).[71] A similar result was also demonstrated by Zhao et al. in their metaanalysis of 16 studies reporting the negative association of high SDF on pregnancy rate in patients undergoing IVF, with an odds ratio of 0.66 (95% CI: 0.48, 0.90; p = 0.008).[72]

In a study on patients with elevated DFI undergoing ICSI cycles, the pregnancy rate was significantly lower (16.7%) compared to patients with low DFI (47.4%).[69] On the contrary, Host et al. found only a significant relationship between SDF and fertilization after IVF (p < 0.01) but not with ICSI (p > 0.05), thus attributing this to the possibility of selecting sperm with normal morphology for the ICSI procedure.[73]

Generally, in the context of ART failure, multiple variables including female age, type of SDF assay used, and the sperm source must be considered.[74] A systematic review and metaanalysis of studies examining the impact of DNA integrity on IVF/ICSI outcome showed that pregnancy loss was significantly more pronounced in the context of aberrant sperm DNA, with a combined odds ratio of 2.48 (95% CI: 1.52, 4.04; p < 0.0001).[70] Another systematic review and metaanalysis of 16 cohort studies that included treatments with IVF (n = 11) and ICSI (n = 14) was conducted to evaluate SDF impact on miscarriage. This study found a significant increase in the miscarriage rate in the high SDF group compared to their low SDF counterparts, with a risk ratio of 2.16 (95% CI: 1.54, 3.03; p < 0.001). The authors further suggest that pregnancy losses could be reduced if it were possible to select non–DNA-damaged sperm for injection purposes in a nondestructive manner, and specifically mention hyaluronan binding for the selection of morphologically normal sperm with reduced DNA damage and "physiological ICSI" as possible options.[75,76] However, more recent studies, including several Cochrane reviews, concluded that there is insufficient evidence from low-quality trials supporting the assumption that hyaluronan binding and physiological ICSI result in improved live birth rates. Yet, intracytoplasmic morphologically selected sperm injection may reduce the miscarriage rate.[77,78]

Assessment Tools for Sperm DNA Fragmentation

Conventional SA is not an ideal tool to discern fertile from infertile males due to its inability to assess the fertilizing capability of the sperm[79] and detect DNA damage.[80] Since SDF is a common cause of male infertility, it has recently gained recognition by the WHO as a tool of male fertility evaluation.[1] It has also been shown that SDF is more crucial when it comes to assessing the functional aspect of the sperm compared to conventional SA testing.[80] SDF testing may serve in patients at risk of harboring sperm DNA damage, especially in those with unexplained male infertility-whose semen parameters are within normal limits.[81] The currently available tests used for SDF evaluation are the TUNEL assay, SCSA, sperm chromatin dispersion (SCD) test, and the Comet assay. Although the TUNEL and SCSA assays are the most frequently used tests,[82] the other test systems are also regularly used for the clinical evaluation of SDF. However, direct comparisons of the different test systems reveal only moderate association as different aspects of DNA damage are assessed.[83] The variable degrees of standardization and complexity, as well as the predictive value of these tests, have been discussed in the literature.

TERMINAL DEOXYNUCLEOTIDYL TRANSFERASE dUTP NICK-END LABELING ASSAY

The TUNEL assay is one of the most commonly used SDF assays (30.6%).[82] This utilizes flow cytometry or fluorescence microscopy in the examination of positive sperm and is capable of detecting single- as well as double-stranded DNA breaks.[84] In a study of 261 infertile males compared against 95 controls using TUNEL assay, an SDF value of 16.8% had an estimated sensitivity and specificity of 32.6% and 91.6%, respectively, in differentiating infertile from control counterparts.[85] A systematic review and metaanalysis suggests that the TUNEL assay together with the comet assay has the highest predictive accuracy for pregnancy as compared with SCSA and SCD.[86] An earlier systematic review and metaanalysis the TUNEL found most predictive to miscarriage, with a risk ratio of 3.94 (95% CI: 2.45, 6.32, p < 0.00001).[75] Therefore the TUNEL assay is considered by many laboratories as the method of choice, as it can robustly test 10,000 cells.[87] On the other hand, it is criticized that the TUNEL assay is labor intensive.[88]

SPERM CHROMATIN STRUCTURE ASSAY

The SCSA is regarded the most standardized SDF test, as it has a strict, relatively easy protocol.[88] Like the TUNEL assay, this test uses flow cytometry to assess the integrity of sperm DNA. However, in contrast to the TUNEL assay, this assay involves an acid denaturation and subsequent fluorescent staining using acridine orange, a fluorescent dye that interacts electrostatically and intercalates with the DNA. It stains single-stranded (denatured) DNA red, while double-stranded (native) DNA is stained green.[89] The flow cytometer used for the SCSA enables the rapid assessment of 5000 to 10,000 cells.[90] An SCSA threshold of 25% can be associated with a range of concerns from delayed spontaneous pregnancy to failure of pregnancy or miscarriage, and if the threshold exceeds 25%, the couple could be counseled to undergo ICSI. Moreover, for males with SCSA greater than 50%, ICSI using intratesticular sperm is advised.[91]

SPERM CHROMATIN DISPERSION TEST

In contrast to the TUNEL and SCSA assays, the SCD is a slide-based, microscopic test that like the SCSA, assesses SDF using acid-induced denaturation. DNA damage is then identified by means of the specific halos around the sperm. The size of the halo indicates intact DNA that represents the dispersion of the DNA loop. In other words, failure of formation of such halos or the formation of only small halos is associated with SDF. Other than its accuracy and simplicity, this test is inexpensive and is reproducible.[92] Chohan et al. found that SDF results from normal and infertile males using SCSA, TUNEL, and SCD are significantly correlated (r > 0.866; p < 0.001).[93] On the other hand, a metaanalysis by Cissen et al. indicates poor predictive accuracy.[86]

COMET ASSAY (SINGLE-CELL GEL ELECTROPHORESIS)

The comet assay is also a slide-based test and therefore only a limited number of sperm can be evaluated. This assay can detect sperm single- and double-stranded DNA breaks at the single-cell level.[94] It was shown that the comet assay can predict the outcome of IVF treatment.[95] A threshold above 25% using the alkaline comet assay was associated with likelihood of infertility, with an odds ratio of 117.33 (95% CI: 12.72, 2731.84, RR: 8.75).[95] Ribas-Maynou et al. reported that the alkaline comet assay has the highest sensitivity compared to TUNEL, SCD, and SCSA.[96] In their metaanalysis, Cissen et al. report a fair predictive accuracy for pregnancy.[86] In addition, the 6th edition of the WHO manual suggests that the use of the comet assay may not be appropriate in clinical practice in some laboratories because of a high level of interlaboratory variations.[1]

CURRENT RECOMMENDATIONS OF SPERM DNA FRAGMENTATION TESTING BY PROFESSIONAL SOCIETIES

The European Association of Urology (EAU) addresses SDF in its guidelines, which strongly recommend sperm DNA testing for males of heterosexual couples with recurrent pregnancy loss, whether from natural or ART-related pregnancy and in the context of unexplained infertility.[97] Recently, the 6th edition of the WHO laboratory manual for the examination and processing of human semen was released, and SDF examination was listed with a detailed narrative of the different assays, yet no actual guidance regarding the clinical implication and indications, and stating that determining and validating the thresholds are tasks that the laboratories must perform.[1] Agarwal et al. have published several guideline reports highlighting the indication of SDF, according to which SDF testing is recommended in the context of unexplained male infertility, idiopathic male infertility, recurrent pregnancy loss, before starting or following failed IUI and IVF, recurrent ICSI failure, in patients with clinical varicocele and normal SA, and in patients with subclinical varicocele and borderline SA (recommendation grade C). Additionally, when managing high SDF, weight loss and dietary adjustments, in addition to oral antioxidants, could be used in reducing elevated SDF (recommendation grade C). Finally, in the context of oligozoospermia, recurrent failed IVF, and elevated SDF, testicular sperm may offer better outcome compared to ejaculated sperm (recommendation grade B–C).[50,74] Esteves et al. published another guideline report and stated that TUNEL, SCSA, SCD, and alkaline comet assay are reliable SDF tests (grade B) and used a threshold of 20% for TUNEL, SCSA, and SCD as a value to differentiate between fertile and infertile males (grade B).[98] In contrast, however, in their 2020 recommendations, the American Urology Association/American Society for Reproductive Medicine states that SDF is not recommended within the initial evaluation of infertile males, and that males of heterosexual couples suffering recurrent pregnancy loss should be offered a sperm DNA testing (moderate recommendation: grade C level of evidence).[99]

CHALLENGES OF SPERM DNA FRAGMENTATION TESTING IN CLINICAL PRACTICE

Despite the strong evidence over the utility of SDF in the qualitative evaluation of the male reproductive potential and evaluating the contribution of intact sperm DNA towards the time-to-pregnancy and proper embryo development, SDF has been marginally introduced in the daily management of the infertile male. Many concerns in such context still exist, including the variability of the available assays, less abundant availability, concerns regarding the standardization of the used tests, technical and interobserver variation, and financial concerns. In addition, there is no universal agreement on[100] which test should be used, as the WHO recommends the use of the TUNEL, SCD, comet, and acridine orange flow cytometry.[1]

CLINICAL SCENARIOS

CASE 1

A 38-year-old male patient presented complaining of secondary infertility with his 32-year-old healthy wife. He did not smoke or drink alcohol. He has worked in the petrochemical industry for more than 10 years. His first child was conceived naturally 7 years ago and over the past 3 years, the couple was unsuccessful in achieving pregnancy. His physical evaluation was unremarkable, with normal testes, vasa, and epididymises and no palpable varicocele. His initial laboratory evaluation revealed an SA with sperm concentration of 8 million/mL, 15% progressive motility, and 1% normal forms. Hormonal evaluation revealed normal total testosterone, luteinizing hormone (LH), follicle-stimulating hormone (FSH), estradiol, and prolactin. A TUNEL assay was done and resulted in 38% DFI. The patient was advised to minimize exposure to petrochemical fumes and to start a 3-month course of antioxidant therapy. Upon re-evaluation following the third month of treatment and cessation of hazardous exposure, his SA improved, with a sperm concentration of 17 million/mL, 27% progressive motility, and 4% normal forms. Six months later, the couple was able to conceive naturally.

CASE 2

A 45-year-old male patient presented complaining of a 4-years history of secondary infertility. The patient is a heavy smoker and obese, with a body mass index (BMI) of 39. His wife is 35 years old and was otherwise healthy. His clinical evaluation was consistent with increased truncal adiposity and normal genital examination. Laboratory evaluation was consistent with mildly elevated estradiol level and normal total testosterone, LH, and FSH. SA showed a sperm concentration of 10 million/mL, 12% progressive motility, and 1% normal forms. SDF testing was done using SCSA, which revealed a DFI of 45%. The patient was advised to lose weight and adopt a healthier lifestyle, maintaining

regular exercise and refraining from smoking. After 8 months, he returned for evaluation and, after losing significant weight, his BMI became 32 and he had quit smoking. His SA improved, with sperm concentration reaching 22 million/mL, 29% progressive motility, and 3% normal forms. Repeated SCSA testing showed a decline in DFI, reaching 24%. The couple was offered a trial of IUI, which successfully resulted in pregnancy.

CASE 3

A 28-year-old male patient presented complaining of primary infertility with his 25-year-old wife. His physical evaluation was consistent with left-sided epididymal tenderness. His sexual history revealed long-term urinary symptoms consistent with dysuria and occasional urethral discharge. SA revealed normal sperm count but low progressive motility (15%) and normal forms (2%). SCD was requested and revealed a DFI of 30%. Following a thorough investigation, both partners had positive genitourinary cultures for *Chlamydia trachomatis*, which was successfully treated with an antibiotic therapy, and repeated cultures confirmed resolution of infection. After 6 months, the patient persisted to showed Improvement in the preexisting urinary symptoms, and repeat SA was completely normal, with a DFI of 12% as revealed by SCD. The couple successfully achieved a natural pregnancy 3 months later.

CASE 4

A 35-year-old male patient presenting with a 2-year history of primary infertility and an associated sense of dull, aching scrotal discomfort for 1 year. His partner was 28 years old and was otherwise healthy. Physical evaluation was consistent with a left palpable grade 3 varicocele and moderately reduced left testicular size. Hormonal evaluation was unremarkable. SA revealed a concentration of 15 million/mL, progressive motility of 25%, and normal forms of 2%. A TUNEL assay was performed and revealed a DFI of 30%. The patient was advised to undergo left varicocele repair and was given a course of antioxidants for 3 months. Upon evaluation 6 months later, his SA showed a rise in sperm count, reaching 23 million/mL, progressive motility of 32%, and persistent normal forms at 2%. A repeat TUNEL was done and the result showed improvement in DFI, reaching 18%. The couple opted to try natural conception, which successfully happened 5 months later.

CASE 5

A 27-year-old male presented with his otherwise healthy 25-year-old female partner, complaining of primary infertility for 4 years. His history was remarkable for bilateral orchidopexy done at the age of 5 years for undescended testes, with a resultant decline in his sperm count. His laboratory evaluation revealed severe oligoasthenoteratozoospermia, with a sperm concentration of 1 million/mL, 5% progressive motility, and 1% normal forms. Endocrine evaluation was remarkable for a mildly elevated FSH level (12 mIU/mL). The couple had failed several ICSI treatments in the past. DFI measured by SCSA was 48%. The condition persisted despite a long-term course of antioxidants. Upon the current ICSI trial, the couple was advised to undergo an ICSI cycle using intratesticular sperm, which was retrieved using testicular aspiration. The fertilization was more successful than prior cycles, and pregnancy occurred following the second attempt of testicular sperm aspiration/ICSI.

SUMMARY

Scientific work to improve the predictive value of SA has been made during recent years, and more accurate, robust, and reliable tests than conventional SA have been developed, of which SDF appears to be the most important one. Despite the repeated evidence of its value in diagnosing male infertility factors,[24,50] the routine use of SDF as a test to make clinical recommendations remains controversial.[99] In contrast, the EAU clearly recommends that "SDF testing should be performed in the assessment of couples with RPL from natural conception and ARTs, or males with unexplained infertility."[97] Furthermore, the fact that the WHO recommends SDF testing in the chapter "Extended Examination" of the 2021 WHO manual[1] is a major step forward in the right direction. Although the existing evidence clearly indicates the value of SDF testing and each of the current SDF testing methods has its own advantages and limitations, these test systems need to be refined and standardized, and robust cut-off values to distinguish between fertile and infertile males need to be established, so that a clear methodological recommendation can be given.

REFERENCES

1. World Health Organization. *WHO Laboratory Manual for the Examination and Processing of Human Semen*. 6th ed. Geneva: World Health Organization; 2021.
2. Snow-Lisy D, Sabanegh E. What does the clinician need from an andrology laboratory? *Front Biosci (Elite Ed)*. 2013;5(1):289-304.
3. Barbăroşie C, Agarwal A, Henkel R. Diagnostic value of advanced semen analysis in evaluation of male infertility. *Andrologia*. 2021;53(2):e13625.
4. Henkel R, Müller C, Miska W, Gips H, Schill WB. Determination of the acrosome reaction in human spermatozoa is predictive of fertilization in vitro. *Hum Reprod*. 1993;8(12):2128-2132.
5. Burkman LJ, Coddington CC, Franken DR, Kruger TF, Rosenwaks Z, Hogen GD. The hemizona assay (HZA): development of a diagnostic test for the binding of human spermatozoa to the human hemizona pellucida to predict fertilization potential. *Fertil Steril*. 1988;49(4):688-697.
6. Zini A, Kamal K, Phang D, Willis J, Jarvi K. Biologic variability of sperm DNA denaturation in infertile men. *Urology*. 2001;58(2):258-261.
7. Champroux A, Torres-Carreira J, Gharagozloo P, Drevet JR, Kocer A. Mammalian sperm nuclear organization: resiliencies and vulnerabilities. *Basic Clin Androl*. 2016;26(1):17.
8. Heidaran MA, Showman RM, Kistler WS. A cytochemical study of the transcriptional and translational regulation of nuclear transition protein 1 (TP1), a major chromosomal protein of mammalian spermatids. *J Cell Biol*. 1988;106(5):1427-1433.
9. Yu YE, Zhang Y, Unni E, et al. Abnormal spermatogenesis and reduced fertility in transition nuclear protein 1-deficient mice. *Proc Natl Acad Sci U S A*. 2000;97(9):4683-4688.
10. Shamsi MB, Kumar R, Dada R. Evaluation of nuclear DNA damage in human spermatozoa in men opting for assisted reproduction. *Indian J Med Res*. 2008;127(2):115-123.
11. Ward WS, Coffey DS. DNA packaging and organization in mammalian spermatozoa: comparison with somatic cells. *Biol Reprod*. 1991;44(4):569-574.
12. Björndahl L, Kvist U. Human sperm chromatin stabilization: a proposed model including zinc bridges. *Mol Hum Reprod*. 2010;16(1):23-29.
13. Tanphaichitr N, Sobhon P, Taluppeth N, Chalermisarachai P. Basic nuclear proteins in testicular cells and ejaculated spermatozoa in man. *Exp Cell Res*. 1978;117(2):347-356.
14. Ni K, Spiess AN, Schuppe HC, Steger K. The impact of sperm protamine deficiency and sperm DNA damage on human male fertility: a systematic review and meta-analysis. *Andrology*. 2016;4(5):789-799.

15. Sati L, Ovari L, Bennett D, Simon SD, Demir R, Huszar G. Double probing of human spermatozoa for persistent histones, surplus cytoplasm, apoptosis and DNA fragmentation. *Reprod Biomed Online*. 2008;16(4):570-579.
16. Björndahl L, Kvist U. Structure of chromatin in spermatozoa. *Adv Exp Med Biol*. 2014;791:1-11.
17. García-Rodríguez A, Gosálvez J, Agarwal A, Roy R, Johnston S. DNA damage and repair in human reproductive cells. *Int J Mol Sci*. 2018;20(1):31.
18. Puzuka A, Alksere B, Gailite L, Erenpreiss J. Idiopathic infertility as a feature of genome instability. *Life*. 2021;11(7):628.
19. González-Marín C, Gosálvez J, Roy R. Types, causes, detection and repair of DNA fragmentation in animal and human sperm cells. *Int J Mol Sci*. 2012;13(11):14026-14052.
20. Kim JS, Krasieva TB, Kurumizaka H, Chen DJ, Taylor AMR, Yokomori K. Independent and sequential recruitment of NHEJ and HR factors to DNA damage sites in mammalian cells. *J Cell Biol*. 2005;170(3):341-347.
21. Casanovas A, Ribas-Maynou J, Lara-Cerrillo S, et al. Double-stranded sperm DNA damage is a cause of delay in embryo development and can impair implantation rates. *Fertil Steril*. 2019;111(4):699-707.e1.
22. John Aitken R, Clarkson JS, Fishel S. Generation of reactive oxygen species, lipid peroxidation, and human sperm function. *Biol Reprod*. 1989;41(1):183-197.
23. Zabludovsky N, Eltes F, Geva E, et al. Relationship between human sperm lipid peroxidation, comprehensive quality parameters and IVF outcome. *Andrologia*. 1999;31(2):91-98.
24. Agarwal A, Barbăroşie C, Ambar R, Finelli R. The impact of single- and double-strand DNA breaks in human spermatozoa on assisted reproduction. *Int J Mol Sci*. 2020;21(11):3882.
25. Ribas-Maynou J, Benet J. Single and double strand sperm DNA damage: different reproductive effects on male fertility. *Genes (Basel)*. 2019;10(2):105.
26. Aitken RJ, Baker MA, Sawyer D. Oxidative stress in the male germ line and its role in the aetiology of male infertility and genetic disease. *Reprod Biomed Online*. 2003;7(1):65-70.
27. Derijck A, van der Heijden G, Giele M, Philippens M, de Boer P. DNA double-strand break repair in parental chromatin of mouse zygotes, the first cell cycle as an origin of de novo mutation. *Hum Mol Genet*. 2008;17(13):1922-1937.
28. Horta F, Catt S, Ramachandran P, Vollenhoven B, Temple-Smith P. Female ageing affects the DNA repair capacity of oocytes in IVF using a controlled model of sperm DNA damage in mice. *Hum Reprod*. 2020;35(3):529-544.
29. Ahmadi A, Ng SC. Fertilizing ability of DNA-damaged spermatozoa. *J Exp Zool*. 1999;284(6):696-704.
30. Henkel R, Hajimohammad M, Stalf T, et al. Influence of deoxyribonucleic acid damage on fertilization and pregnancy. *Fertil Steril*. 2004;81(4):965-972.
31. Shiloh Y. ATM and related protein kinases: safeguarding genome integrity. *Nat Rev Cancer*. 2003;3(3):155-168.
32. Martin JH, Aitken RJ, Bromfield EG, Nixon B. DNA damage and repair in the female germline: contributions to ART. *Hum Reprod Update*. 2019;25(2):180-201.
33. Wang B, Li Z, Wang C, et al. Zygotic G2/M cell cycle arrest induced by ATM/Chk1 activation and DNA repair in mouse embryos fertilized with hydrogen peroxide-treated epididymal mouse sperm. *PLoS One*. 2013;8(9):e73987.
34. Cuvier O, Hirano T. A role of topoisomerase II in linking DNA replication to chromosome condensation. *J Cell Biol*. 2003;160(5):645-655.
35. Meyer-Ficca ML, Lonchar JD, Ihara M, Meistrich ML, Austin CA, Meyer RG. Poly(ADP-Ribose) polymerases PARP1 and PARP2 modulate topoisomerase II beta (TOP2B) function during chromatin condensation in mouse spermiogenesis. *Biol Reprod*. 2011;84(5):900-909.
36. Mengual L, Ballescá JL, Ascaso C, Oliva R. Marked differences in protamine content and P1/P2 ratios in sperm cells from Percoll fractions between patients and controls. *J Androl*. 2003;24(3):438-447.
37. Rogenhofer N, Dansranjavin T, Schorsch M, et al. The sperm protamine mRNA ratio as a clinical parameter to estimate the fertilizing potential of men taking part in an ART programme. *Hum Reprod*. 2013;28(4):969-978.
38. de Iuliis GN, Thomson LK, Mitchell LA, et al. DNA damage in human spermatozoa is highly correlated with the efficiency of chromatin remodeling and the formation of 8-hydroxy-2'-deoxyguanosine, a marker of oxidative stress. *Biol Reprod*. 2009;81(3):517-524.
39. Gil-Guzman E, Ollero M, Lopez MC, et al. Differential production of reactive oxygen species by subsets of human spermatozoa at different stages of maturation. *Hum Reprod*. 2001;16(9):1922-1930.
40. Alvarez JG, Storey BT. Evidence for increased lipid peroxidative damage and loss of superoxide dismutase activity as a mode of sublethal cryodamage to human sperm during cryopreservation. *J Androl*. 1992;13(3):232-241.
41. Gualtieri R, Kalthur G, Barbato V, di Nardo M, Adiga SK, Talevi R. Mitochondrial dysfunction and oxidative stress caused by cryopreservation in reproductive cells. *Antioxidants (Basel)*. 2021;10(3):337.

42. Gorelick JI, Goldstein M. Loss of fertility in men with varicocele. *Fertil Steril.* 1993;59(3):613-616.
43. Zini A, Dohle G. Are varicoceles associated with increased deoxyribonucleic acid fragmentation? *Fertil Steril.* 2011;96(6):1283-1287.
44. Cho CL, Esteves SC, Agarwal A. Novel insights into the pathophysiology of varicocele and its association with reactive oxygen species and sperm DNA fragmentation. *Asian J Androl.* 2016;18(2):186-193.
45. Esteves SC, Gosálvez J, López-Fernández C, et al. Diagnostic accuracy of sperm DNA degradation index (DDSi) as a potential noninvasive biomarker to identify men with varicocele-associated infertility. *Int Urol Nephrol.* 2015;47(9):1471-1477.
46. Tiseo B, Esteves S, Cocuzza M. Summary evidence on the effects of varicocele treatment to improve natural fertility in subfertile men. *Asian J Androl.* 2016;18(2):239.
47. Qiu D, Shi Q, Pan L. Efficacy of varicocelectomy for sperm DNA integrity improvement: a meta-analysis. *Andrologia.* 2021;53(1):e13885.
48. Lira Neto FT, Roque M, Esteves SC. Effect of varicocelectomy on sperm deoxyribonucleic acid fragmentation rates in infertile men with clinical varicocele: a systematic review and meta-analysis. *Fertil Steril.* 2021;116(3): 696-712.
49. Wang YJ, Zhang RQ, Lin YJ, Zhang RG, Zhang WL. Relationship between varicocele and sperm DNA damage and the effect of varicocele repair: a meta-analysis. *Reprod Biomed Online.* 2012;25(3):307-314.
50. Agarwal A, Majzoub A, Baskaran S, et al. Sperm DNA fragmentation: a new guideline for clinicians. *World J Mens Health.* 2020;38(4):412.
51. Kandil H, Shah R. Grades 2/3 varicocele and normal conventional semen analysis. In: Esteves S, Cho CL, Majzoub A, Agarwal A, eds. *Varicocele and Male Infertility.* Cham: Springer International Publishing; 2019:537-543.
52. Gallegos G, Ramos B, Santiso R, Goyanes V, Gosálvez J, Fernández JL. Sperm DNA fragmentation in infertile men with genitourinary infection by *Chlamydia trachomatis* and *Mycoplasma. Fertil Steril.* 2008;90(2):328-334.
53. Pagliuca C, Cariati F, Bagnulo F, et al. Microbiological evaluation and sperm DNA fragmentation in semen samples of patients undergoing fertility investigation. *Genes (Basel).* 2021;12(5):654.
54. Gonzalez DC, Ory J, Blachman-Braun R, Nackeeran S, Best JC, Ramasamy R. Advanced paternal age and sperm DNA fragmentation: a systematic review. *World J Mens Health.* 2022;40(1):104-115.
55. Vagnini L, Baruffi R, Mauri A, et al. The effects of male age on sperm DNA damage in an infertile population. *Reprod Biomed Online.* 2007;15(5):514-519.
56. Rosiak-Gill A, Gill K, Jakubik J, et al. Age-related changes in human sperm DNA integrity. *Aging.* 2019;11(15):5399-5411.
57. Mostafa RM, Nasrallah YS, Hassan MM, Farrag AF, Majzoub A, Agarwal A. The effect of cigarette smoking on human seminal parameters, sperm chromatin structure and condensation. *Andrologia.* 2018;50(3):1-8.
58. Aboulmaouahib S, Madkour A, Kaarouch I, et al. Impact of alcohol and cigarette smoking consumption in male fertility potential: Looks at lipid peroxidation, enzymatic antioxidant activities and sperm DNA damage. *Andrologia.* 2018;50(3):e12926.
59. Evenson DP, Jost LK, Marshall D, et al. Utility of the sperm chromatin structure assay as a diagnostic and prognostic tool in the human fertility clinic. *Hum Reprod.* 1999;14(4):1039-1049.
60. Zini A. Are sperm chromatin and DNA defects relevant in the clinic? *Syst Biol Reprod Med.* 2011;57(1-2):78-85.
61. Tan J, Taskin O, Albert A, Bedaiwy MA. Association between sperm DNA fragmentation and idiopathic recurrent pregnancy loss: a systematic review and meta-analysis. *Reprod Biomed Online.* 2019;38(6):951-960.
62. McQueen DB, Zhang J, Robins JC. Sperm DNA fragmentation and recurrent pregnancy loss: a systematic review and meta-analysis. *Fertil Steril.* 2019;112(1):54-60.e3.
63. Li J, Luo L, Diao J, et al. Male sperm quality and risk of recurrent spontaneous abortion in Chinese couples: A systematic review and meta-analysis. *Medicine.* 2021;100(10):e24828.
64. Dai Y, Liu J, Yuan E, Li Y, Shi Y, Zhang L. Relationship among traditional semen parameters, sperm DNA fragmentation, and unexplained recurrent miscarriage: a systematic review and meta-analysis. *Front Endocrinol (Lausanne).* 2021;12:802632.
65. Schorsch M, Gomez R, Hahn T, Hoelscher-Obermaier J, Seufert R, Skala C. Success rate of inseminations dependent on maternal age? An analysis of 4246 insemination cycles. *Geburtshilfe Frauenheilkd.* 2013;73(08):808-811.
66. Bungum M, Humaidan P, Axmon A, et al. Sperm DNA integrity assessment in prediction of assisted reproduction technology outcome. *Hum Reprod.* 2007;22(1): 174-179.
67. Duran EH, Morshedi M, Taylor S, Oehninger S. Sperm DNA quality predicts intrauterine insemination outcome: a prospective cohort study. *Hum Reprod.* 2002;17(12):3122-3128.
68. Rilcheva VS, Ayvazova NP, Ilieva LO, Ivanova SP, Konova EI. Sperm DNA integrity test and assisted reproductive technology (ART) outcome. *J Biomed Clin Res.* 2016;9(1):21-29.
69. Siddhartha N, Reddy N, Pandurangi M, Muthusamy T, Vembu R, Kasinathan K. The effect of sperm DNA

fragmentation index on the outcome of intrauterine insemination and intracytoplasmic sperm injection. *J Hum Reprod Sci.* 2019;12(3):189.

70. Zini A, Sigman M. Are tests of sperm DNA damage clinically useful? Pros and cons. *J Androl.* 2009;30(3):219-229.

71. Simon L, Zini A, Dyachenko A, Ciampi A, Carrell DT. A systematic review and meta-analysis to determine the effect of sperm DNA damage on IVF and ICSI outcome. *Asian J Androl.* 2017;19(1):80-90.

72. Zhao J, Zhang Q, Wang Y, Li Y. Whether sperm deoxyribonucleic acid fragmentation has an effect on pregnancy and miscarriage after in vitro fertilization/intracytoplasmic sperm injection: a systematic review and meta-analysis. *Fertil Steril.* 2014;102(4):998-1005.e8.

73. Høst E, Lindenberg S, Smidt-Jensen S. The role of DNA strand breaks in human spermatozoa used for IVF and ICSI. *Acta Obstet Gynecol Scand.* 2000;79(7):559-563.

74. Agarwal A, Majzoub A, Esteves SC, Ko E, Ramasamy R, Zini A. Clinical utility of sperm DNA fragmentation testing: practice recommendations based on clinical scenarios. *Transl Androl Urol.* 2016;5(6):935-950.

75. Robinson L, Gallos ID, Conner SJ, et al. The effect of sperm DNA fragmentation on miscarriage rates: a systematic review and meta-analysis. *Hum Reprod.* 2012;27(10):2908-2917.

76. Parmegiani L, Cognigni GE, Bernardi S, Troilo E, Ciampaglia W, Filicori M. "Physiologic ICSI": hyaluronic acid (HA) favors selection of spermatozoa without DNA fragmentation and with normal nucleus, resulting in improvement of embryo quality. *Fertil Steril.* 2010;93(2):598-604.

77. Gatimel N, Parinaud J, Leandri RD. Intracytoplasmic morphologically selected sperm injection (IMSI) does not improve outcome in patients with two successive IVF-ICSI failures. *J Assist Reprod Genet.* 2016;33(3):349-355.

78. Lepine S, McDowell S, Searle LM, Kroon B, Glujovsky D, Yazdani A. Advanced sperm selection techniques for assisted reproduction. *Cochrane Database Syst Rev.* 2019;7:CD010461.

79. Wang C, Swerdloff RS. Limitations of semen analysis as a test of male fertility and anticipated needs from newer tests. *Fertil Steril.* 2014;102(6):1502-1507.

80. Santi D, Spaggiari G, Simoni M. Sperm DNA fragmentation index as a promising predictive tool for male infertility diagnosis and treatment management - meta-analyses. *Reprod Biomed Online.* 2018;37(3):315-326.

81. El-Sakka AI. Routine assessment of sperm DNA fragmentation in clinical practice: commentary and perspective. *Transl Androl Urol.* 2017;6(S4):S640-S643.

82. Majzoub A, Agarwal A, Cho CL, Esteves SC. Sperm DNA fragmentation testing: a cross sectional survey on current

practices of fertility specialists. *Transl Androl Urol.* 2017;6(suppl 4):S710-S719.

83. Henkel R, Hoogendijk CF, Bouic PJD, Kruger TF. TUNEL assay and SCSA determine different aspects of sperm DNA damage. *Andrologia.* 2010;42(5):305-313.

84. Hassanen E, Elqusi K, Zaki H, Henkel R, Agarwal A. TUNEL assay: Establishing a sperm DNA fragmentation cut-off value for Egyptian infertile men. *Andrologia.* 2019;51(10):e13375.

85. Sharma R, Ahmad G, Esteves SC, Agarwal A. Terminal deoxynucleotidyl transferase dUTP nick end labeling (TUNEL) assay using bench top flow cytometer for evaluation of sperm DNA fragmentation in fertility laboratories: protocol, reference values, and quality control. *J Assist Reprod Genet.* 2016;33(2):291-300.

86. Cissen M, Wely M van, Scholten I, et al. Measuring sperm DNA fragmentation and clinical outcomes of medically assisted reproduction: a systematic review and meta-analysis. *PLoS One.* 2016;11(11):e0165125.

87. Sharma R, Iovine C, Agarwal A, Henkel R. TUNEL assay-standardized method for testing sperm DNA fragmentation. *Andrologia.* 2021;53(2):e13738.

88. Rex AS, Aagaard J, Fedder J. DNA fragmentation in spermatozoa: a historical review. *Andrology.* 2017;5(4):622-630.

89. Darzynkiewicz Z, Traganos F, Sharpless T, Friend C, Melamed MR. Nuclear chromatin changes during erythroid differentiation of friend virus induced leukemic cells. *Exp Cell Res.* 1976;99(2):301-309.

90. Bungum M, Bungum L, Giwercman A. Sperm chromatin structure assay (SCSA): a tool in diagnosis and treatment of infertility. *Asian J Androl.* 2011;13(1):69-75.

91. Evenson DP. Sperm chromatin structure assay (SCSA®). *Methods Mol Biol.* 2013;927:147-164.

92. Fernández JL, Muriel L, Rivero MT, Goyanes V, Vazquez R, Alvarez JG. The sperm chromatin dispersion test: a simple method for the determination of sperm DNA fragmentation. *J Androl.* 2003;24(1):59-66.

93. Chohan KR, Griffin JT, Lafromboise M, de Jonge CJ, Carrell DT. Comparison of chromatin assays for DNA fragmentation evaluation in human sperm. *J Androl.* 2006;27(1):53-59.

94. Enciso M, Sarasa J, Agarwal A, Fernández JL, Gosálvez J. A two-tailed Comet assay for assessing DNA damage in spermatozoa. *Reprod Biomed Online.* 2009;18(5):609-616.

95. Simon L, Lutton D, McManus J, Lewis SEM. Sperm DNA damage measured by the alkaline Comet assay as an independent predictor of male infertility and in vitro fertilization success. *Fertil Steril.* 2011;95(2):652-657.

96. Ribas-Maynou J, García-Peiró A, Fernández-Encinas A, et al. Comprehensive analysis of sperm DNA

fragmentation by five different assays: TUNEL assay, SCSA, SCD test and alkaline and neutral Comet assay. *Andrology*. 2013;1(5):715-722.

97. Tharakan T, Bettocchi C, Carvalho J, et al. European Association of Urology guidelines panel on male sexual and reproductive health: a clinical consultation guide on the indications for performing sperm DNA fragmentation testing in men with infertility and testicular sperm extraction in nonazoospermic men. *Eur Urol Focus*. 2022;8(1):339-350.

98. Esteves SC, Zini A, Coward RM, et al. Sperm DNA fragmentation testing: Summary evidence and clinical practice recommendations. *Andrologia*. 2021;53(2):e13874.

99. Schlegel PN, Sigman M, Collura B, et al. Diagnosis and treatment of infertility in men: AUA/ASRM guideline part I. *Fertil Steril*. 2021;115(1):54-61.

100. Tadros NN, Sabanegh Jr E. Commentary on clinical utility of sperm DNA fragmentation testing: Practice Recommendations of Sperm DNA Fragmentation Testing: Expert Commentaries by Invited Authors and Replies by Guest Editors Contributors from North America. *Transl Androl Urol*. 2017;6(suppl 4):S374-S376.

10

Genetic and Genomic Tests of Infertile Males

Paraskevi Vogiatzi, Ana Navarro-Gomezlechon, Evangelini Evgeni, and Nicolas Garrido Puchalt

KEY POINTS

- Male infertility is highly complex and genetically heterogeneous among individuals.
- Over 3000 genes are dynamically involved in the process of spermatogenesis and reproduction.
- The most frequent genetic aberrations retrieved in infertile males are sex chromosome aberrations, Y chromosome microdeletions, and mutations/polymorphisms in the *CFTR* gene.
- Genetic and genomic testing allow the diagnosis, facilitates assisted reproductive technology (ART) management, and prevents transmission of genetic defects to future generations.

- Genomics, epigenomics, and transcriptomics may enable targeted diagnostics in male infertility by the identification of genetic variants.
- Aberrant "omics" are associated with sperm quality, fertility dynamics, ART outcomes, and offspring health.
- Next-generation sequencing rapidly and accurately sequences large portions of the human genome and is a promising tool in male infertility.
- The difficulty surrounding genomic studies is the large number of genes that are analyzed to identify possible biomarkers and define future therapies.

INTRODUCTION

Male infertility may be the result of a wide array of genetic disorders, including chromosomal aberrations, monogenic disorders, and multifactorial genetic alterations such as epigenetic modifications, that affect fertility at pre- and post-testicular levels and specifically involve the hypothalamic pituitary axis, testicular function, spermatogenic defects, and specific expression/function of mapped genes and areas of critical importance outside the coding regions. Over 3000 genes are considered to be dynamically involved in the process of spermatogenesis and male reproductive pathway adequacy,[1] thus revealing a highly complex genetic interplay with increased heterogeneity in male infertility presentations among individuals. Currently, genetic abnormalities are defined in 13% to 30% of infertile males,[2] with severe presentations of infertility, oligozoospermia, or azoospermia validated in 20% to 30% of the cases, while 12% to 40% of infertile males lacking a definite diagnosis are suspected to have a background of genetic linkage.[3,4]

The most commonly used genetic tests include karyotyping to detect chromosomal abnormalities (such as Klinefelter syndrome [KS]), Y-chromosome microdeletion (YCM) screening, and cystic fibrosis transmembrane conductance regulator (*CFTR*) variant testing,[5–7] although frequently circumscribed to the most severe cases. However, in 30% to 40% of male infertility cases, the etiology remains unknown, characterized as "idiopathic." These cases may be associated with genetic abnormalities, although the genes involved, their individual influence, and perhaps the implicated effect in reproductive function remain undiscovered.[7–10] The clinical evaluation of male infertility does not systematically examine certain aspects of the reproductive system and sperm physiology related to fertility dynamics and genetic integrity; thus male infertility remains poorly understood at the molecular level.[5,11] These acknowledged scientific and diagnostic gaps motivate the need to identify novel biomarkers and develop new approaches in identifying the underlying cause of male infertility and to direct possible therapy and personalized treatment.[8]

To this end, spermatozoa are extremely specialized cells responsible for transmitting to progeny not only genetic material but also RNA, protein, and epigenetic information.[5,8,12] The complex process of spermatogenesis involves the coordination of numerous genes and during this process, spermatozoa exhibit huge variations in their genetic, cellular, and chromatin structures, resulting in optimal/suboptimal spermatozoa production.[8] Complete functionality of the sperm depends on its genome, epigenome, transcriptome, and proteome. In the attempt to identify underlying infertility causes, investigations were driven into the study of the genes involved in male infertility and the epigenetic modifications as well as the identification of other molecular biomarkers that may improve diagnostic capability.[8,9] Genetic and genomic testing in male infertility already serve to provide a more comprehensive understanding of the pathophysiology of male infertility,[13] determine heritable conditions that may be passed to offspring, contribute to a better diagnosis,[5,7,11,13] improve treatment options[5,7,13] and selection of sperm cells,[7] evaluate conditions that may impact the success of assisted reproductive technologies (ART) and the health of the affected individual, and ideally, direct research on potential therapeutics of the underlying genetic defects. In this chapter, an overview of the current clinical setting of genetic and genomic tests in male infertility is provided, along with essential information for healthcare professionals to utilize in routine practice in order to identify genetic and genomic abnormalities to improve medical management, as well as research landmarks to signify the direction of this medical field.

GENETIC TESTS

The most frequent genetic findings in male infertility include sex chromosome aberrations, Y-chromosome microdeletions, certain mutations, and genetic polymorphisms such as in the *CFTR* gene and their resulting anatomical deviations with congenital bilateral absence of the vas deferens (CBAVD). Genetic testing is considered and offered either in cases with strong indications of an involved genetic background (e.g., affected phenotype, clinical manifestations, family history) or in the incidence of unexplained infertility that surrounds 30% to 40% of total infertility cases,[14] where a more comprehensive and extensive diagnostic work-up may identify the underlying cause in four out of five infertile males.[15]

There are three main groups of genetic tests in male infertility currently applied in clinical diagnostic applications: cytogenetic tests (karyotyping) to detect chromosomal numerical and structural aberrations, polymerase chain reaction (PCR) technologies for Y-chromosome microdeletions, and gene sequencing technologies for genetic mutations.[4] Genetic testing allows the diagnosis of the infertility factor that in sequence facilitates management optimization through ART approaches. Importantly, by identifying the underlying genetic abnormality, prohibitory measures can be considered to avoid transmission to future generations that in some cases could mean severe health problems and a compromised quality of life for the affected individuals. In addition, several genetic mechanisms are shared and affect multiple physiological features and functions of the body. For example, inactivation of DNA repair genes such as the *EXO1* will not only produce spermatogenic defects but will also predispose an individual to tumor formation.[16] This is especially true for several other genetic defects; thus it has been established that infertility due to genetic factors may impose greater risk of mortality[17] and for other health problems such as malignancies[18] and autoimmune disorders[19] that appear to increase along with the severity of male infertility. Clinical evaluation, accurate diagnosis, and conclusive counseling enable targeted management and the protection of the male individual and the future generations from such possible health risks.

Chromosomal Abnormalities and Karyotype Analysis

Chromosomal aberrations comprise numerical abnormalities (loss or gain of chromosome/s) either in the autosomes or sex chromosomes, disrupting various aspects of health and reproductive potential, while structural abnormalities include duplications, deletions, insertions, or inversions in an area of a chromosome, or an exchange between parts of chromosomes, altering their location. Karyotype abnormalities may be presented in mosaic forms, meaning that the same individual may carry a mixture of normal and abnormal cell lines at various complementing percentages, as noted, for instance, in mosaic forms of KS (47,XXY/46,XY).

Karyotyping is a cytogenetic method that analyzes both the number and the gross structural characteristics of the chromosomes, allowing visualization of aneuploidies and other genetic changes such as chromosomal deletions, insertions, duplications, inversions, or translocations. This is succeeded by culturing lymphocytes from peripheral blood specimens and chemical arresting them in the metaphase of the mitotic cycle, while molecular staining techniques (e.g., Giemsa) are applied to reveal banding patterns of each chromosome (e.g., G-banding). Apart from its obvious clinical usefulness and compared with the currently available technologies, karyotyping possesses the lowest resolution, as it can identify DNA abnormalities greater than 5 megabase (Mb) in size.[16] Karyotype analysis is often proven imperative in male infertility investigation since it has been suggested from previous reports that around 14% of patients with nonobstructive azoospermia (NOA) have an abnormal karyotype, with a predominant 73% diagnosed with KS, 12% with other sex chromosome abnormalities, and 5% with autosomal translocations,[20] while approximately 5% of patients with oligozoospermia exhibit cytogenetic aberrations.[21]

Klinefelter Syndrome

KS (47,XXY) and its variants (e.g., 48,XXXY) or mosaic forms (47,XXY/46,XY) is identified in 1:600 males among the general population and is the most frequent chromosomal aneuploidy observed in azoospermic and severely oligozoospermic males.[22] Semen analysis in these individuals can be differential, as there are variant manifestations such as oligozoospermia, cryptozoospermia, and even the rare occurrence of natural pregnancies (mostly mosaic forms).[16] The clinical phenotype may also exhibit variant presentations but usually reflects hypogonadism and androgen deficiency, with possible gynecomastia and undervirilization, added to other general health problems such as metabolic syndrome, autoimmune diseases, and cognitive disturbances.[23] In the event of azoospermia, a systematic review and metaanalysis by Corona et al. (2017) revealed that the average successful testicular sperm extraction (TESE, microTESE) for KS cases with azoospermia is 50%, thus allowing a possibility for these patients to have a biological offspring through ART and intracytoplasmic sperm injection (ICSI).[24] In terms of offspring health, due to the increased incidence of sex chromosome and autosomal abnormalities, preimplantation genetic testing (PGT) or targeted prenatal screening should be considered to avoid transmission of defects to the progeny, even in cases where spermatogenic function is present, invariantly of the degree.[25,26]

46,XX Male, de la Chapelle Syndrome

The 46,XX testicular disorder of sex development is a rare genetic condition affecting 1:20,000 individuals,[27] characterized by a male gonad presence in an individual with a female genotype. Up to 90% of the cases have part of the Y chromosome and specifically, the sex-determining region Y (SRY) embodied in another chromosomal location, usually the p arm of the X chromosome.[27] In these individuals male genitalia are present even with prohibited appropriate function due to their female genetic constitution, missing the crucial azoospermia factors (AZFa, AZFb, AZFc) necessary for initiation of spermatogenesis.[28] Phenotype appears to share common characteristics with KS patients, although with shorter statures, while SRY-negative variants will mostly present with severe undervirilization defects.[29] Complete spermatogenic failure and NOA with Sertoli cell–only syndrome (SCOS) is established in these cases; therefore approaches such as TESE and assisted reproduction with their own gametes are not possible, and patients should be offered the option of gamete donation.

47,XYY, Jacobs Syndrome

47,XYY is a relatively frequent karyotype anomaly affecting 1:750 individuals due to parental nondisjunction at meiosis II, leading to the acquisition of an extra copy of chromosome Y in the genetic constituent of the offspring.[30] The affected males have frequently taller statures and may possibly present with learning and speech disabilities, while their fertility status can range from azoospermia and severe oligozoospermia to normozoospermia.[2] As with other male karyotype anomalies, these individuals exhibit an increased frequency of sperm aneuploidies[31] or chromosomal imbalances.[32] Complementary sperm fluorescence in situ hybridization (FISH) analysis may surface an increased risk of chromosomal aneuploidies and provide additional information for the genetic contribution to succeeding generations.[33] Thus in the event of infertility and/or increased rate of sperm aneuploidies, ART with/without PGT may be considered.

Mixed Gonadal Dysgenesis (45,X/46,XY Mosaicism)

45,X/46,XY is a rare event of mosaicism with a broad spectrum of phenotypes, including normal males with normal virilization, individuals with ambiguous genitalia, and females with Turner syndrome.[34] Normal male genitalia are determined in approximately 90% of these rarely described cases in the literature, with the remaining 10% presenting with either female or ambiguous reproductive physiology[4]. Mixed gonadal dysgenesis is defined in approximately 10% to 30% of the population carrying this mosaicism[35] and upon clinical assessment, an abnormal testis along with contralateral streak gonad is often present.[36] NOA is typically prevalent among populations with abnormal gonad formation, with one occurrence of successful TESE reported and a few scattered incidences of proven spermatogonia presence.[37]

Translocations

Chromosomal translocations have a pivotal role in male infertility, as these account for up to 13% of males with severely compromised semen parameters and exhibit a higher incidence of unbalanced spermatozoa capable of transmitting translocations, inversions, and other sex chromosome imbalances to their offspring.[28,38] Translocations can cause loss of essential genetic material at the involved breakpoints, meiotic disturbances during spermatogenesis leading to abnormal embryonic genetic content with gains or losses, with the risk of miscarriage and recurrent pregnancy loss being significantly increased in these cases.[39] The most common form found in infertile males is the Robertsonian translocation (ROB), which typically involves the fusion of the long arms of chromosomes 13, 14, 15, 21, and 22 and the genetic loss of the respective short arms. ROB carriers are phenotypically normal since the lost genetic material from the fusion of the involved short chromosome arms is considered inessential. Spermatogenic disturbances may, however, be present due to faulty segregation of the fused chromosomes,[1] with increased incidence in oligozoospermic (1.6%) and azoospermic males (0.09%), rates that are significantly higher by nine-fold compared with the general population.[40–42] Reciprocal translocations involve chromosomal content exchange between autosomes and autosomes/sex chromosomes, and their incidence rate is 0.7% in oligospermic and azoospermic males.[38,43] These carriers will often exhibit spermatogenic defects with

meiotic arrest due to disruption of the function of certain genes close to the breakpoints, while males with spermatogenesis are anticipated to have greater than 50% of sperm carrying chromosomal imbalances.[38,44] Recent genome sequencing of balanced translocations revealed that these complex rearrangements promoted gene disruptions/dysregulations and single-gene mutations in locations involved in male germ cell development, apoptosis, and spermatogenesis.[45] Key investigations may allow proper management of infertility, while the diagnosis and future reproductive plans should carefully consider potential transmission, as translocations can harbor significant health implications for the offspring such as trisomy 21 (Down syndrome), trisomy 13 (Patau syndrome), uniparental disomy, and Prader–Willi syndrome.[38] In vitro fertilization (IVF)/ICSI with PGT should be considered in this context.

Inversions

Inversions may either represent an incidental polymorphism without any clinical significance or may inflict a cascade of variable impacts on male fertility and reproductive outcomes. Reproductive spermatogenic impairment or poor semen analysis parameters, as well as normal reproductive parameters with an accompanying high risk of carrying genetically abnormal gametes that could result in either a spontaneous abortion or partial duplication/deletion in the embryonic genetic constitution, may be secondary to inversions. According to the literature, a pericentric inversion in chromosome 1 presents a risk of spermatogenic breakdown and azoospermia[46]; however, other data indicate that carriers of inversion may as well exhibit normal fertility and familial transmission,[47] and this depends on the specific breakpoints involved. Indeed, different clinical manifestations are found in inversion carriers of other chromosomes such as in chromosomes 6,[48] 9,[49] 10,[50] and 21,[51] where different types of infertility exist (recurrent miscarriages, azoospermia, oligoasthenozoospermia). Inversions may as well occur in the Y chromosome, promoting subsequent deletions in the AZFc region and causing spermatogenic failure.[52] Due to the heterogeneous infertility statuses and reproductive outcomes of such cases, careful assessment and consultation are required to ensure embryo health and a safe reproductive outcome, while sometimes ART with PGT is considered as the "golden" option to select an embryo with balanced chromosomal content and increased chances of a viable pregnancy, especially in cases with an inversed segment greater than 100 Mb.[53]

Y-Chromosome Microdeletion Screening

YCMs occurring in the AZF region of the Y chromosome constitute the second most common genetic cause of male infertility, with a frequency ranging from 3% to 55%.[54] Severe oligozoospermia and NOA are linked to the presence of YCMs in 6% to 8% and 3% to 15% of patients, respectively,[55] and YCM detection ranges widely among different countries (United States: 12%; Iran: 24.2%; Japan: 7%; Germany and Austria: 2%).[56] Current evidence supports the following classification of clinically relevant YCMs (Fig. 10.1): AZFa; AZFb (P5/proximal P1); AZFbc (P5/distal P1 or P4/distal P1); AZFc (b2/b4).

The most frequent deletion type is the AZFc (»80%), followed by AZFa (0.5%–4%), AZFb (1%–5%), and AZFbc (1%–3%), while extensively combined deletions such as AZFabc are most probably related to abnormal karyotypic findings such as 46,XX male or iso(Y).[57] AZFc microdeletions contribute to 5% to 10% of azoospermic and 2% to 5% of severe oligozoospermic cases[58] and are associated with major repercussions in spermatogenetic failure. Four main genes correspond to the AZFc region: Deleted in azoospermia (DAZ), chromodomin Y-linked 1 gene (CDY1), protein tyrosine phosphatase-non-receptor type 13–like on the Y chromosome 2 gene (PRY2), and basic protein on Y chromosome 2 gene (BPY2).[59] These AZFc-related gene families encode proteins with important regulatory functions in spermatogenesis, such as: transcriptional regulation and chromatin remodeling,[60] germ cell apoptosis,[61] protein ubiquitination,[62] and transport, storage, and translation activation of developmental regulatory transcripts.[63]

The particular type of deletions in the AZF region determines the extent of spermatogenic failure exhibited in the male patient. Males presenting with complete deletions of AZFa, AZFb, or any combination experience severely impaired spermatogenesis and are nearly always azoospermic, with no chance of sperm retrieval from the testis. The presence of deletions in AZFc often does not completely eliminate sperm production, providing the likelihood of successful sperm retrieval. Histologically, 46% of males with AZFc deletions demonstrate SCOS on biopsy, 38.2% exhibit maturation arrest, and 15.7% hypospermatogenesis. The possibility to retrieve sperm from patients with AZFc deletions using microTESE ranges from 13% to 100%, with a mean sperm retrieval rate of 47%.[64] AZFa deletions are mainly associated with SCOS,[65] while AZFb region deletions often result in meiotic arrest.[66] According to studies, among AZFa, AZFb, and AZFc loci, hypospermatogenesis is the most common for the AZFc microdeletion (16%), followed by AZFb (13%) and AZFa (2%). However, these figures should be interpreted cautiously due to the use of different techniques applied for the characterization of AZF deletions, which in some cases may reflect a combination of complete and partial deletions.

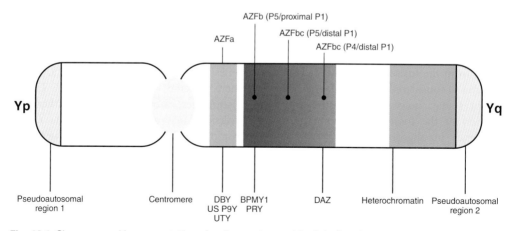

Fig. 10.1 Chromosome Y representation of variant regions, with clinically relevant microdeletions attributed to severe oligozoospermia and nonobstructive azoospermia.

Y-Chromosome Microdeletion Screening

The most widely adopted technique for the detection of YCMs is multiplex PCR amplification of genomic DNA, using the ZFX/ZFY as an internal PCR control. PCR amplification of selected regions of the Y chromosome is conducted using male-specific region of the Y chromosome–specific sequence-tagged site (STS) primers that amplify both anonymous sequences of the chromosome or genes.[67] Importantly, the panel of STS primers should derive from nonpolymorphic regions of the Y chromosome to specifically apply on clinically relevant microdeletion patterns. The set of PCR primers of choice for the diagnosis of YCMs includes: sY14 (SRY), ZFX/ZFY, sY84, sY86 (AZFa), sY127, sY134 (AZFb), and sY254 and sY255 (both in the *DAZ* gene) (AZFc),[68,69] covering over 95% of the deletions reported in the literature in the three AZF regions.[70]

The European Academy of Andrology (EAA) and the European Molecular Genetics Quality Network recommend YCM screening in the context of genetic routine testing for severe male infertility.[70] According to the Practice Committee of the American Society for Reproductive Medicine (ASRM), the prevalence of YCMs in the general population does not exceed 2%,[71] while the EAA estimates a much lower incidence of YCMs in unselected populations at a rate of 1 in 4000 (0.025%).[70] In brief, azoospermic or severely olizospermic males are indicated for YCM screening, while this approach should be also considered prior to TESE/ICSI, before varicocelectomy, and in nonidiopathic cases, according to the relevant medical indications. Screening is contraindicated in cases of diagnosed chromosomal abnormalities (except for the 46,XY/45,X karyotype), obstructive azoospermia (apart from cases with elevated FSH levels), or hypogonadotropic hypogonadism (HH).[72]

Patient Reproductive Potential

The efficiency of sperm retrieval may vary substantially between centers or among the experience and specialization of the involved healthcare professionals, although a higher chance of finding specific sites of sperm production may be expected when an extensive mapping and focused selection of tissue sampling is performed.[64] Although sperm retrieval can be achieved in AZFc male carriers, decreased fertilization, clinical pregnancy, and live birth rates are observed in ICSI in comparison with males producing chromosomally intact sperm. Testicular and ejaculated sperm of AZFc males provide comparable clinical outcomes[73] and levels of sperm DNA fragmentation, thus the use of ejaculated sperm is prioritized over testicular retrieval for ICSI.[72] In AZFc-deleted males undergoing assisted reproduction, the success rates may reach a fertilization rate of 59.8%, a clinical pregnancy rate of 28.6%, and a live birth rate of 23.4%. When successful, the YCM is inevitably transmitted to the male offspring at an equal or enlarged deletion size. A minimal or absent association of YCMs with abnormalities in the offspring or recurrent pregnancy loss has been reported so far, although the data remain limited.[74] The male progeny of AZFc ICSI fathers retain a high risk of spermatogenic and reproductive discrepancy, which is currently not fully elucidated.

Monogenic Diseases, Gene Mutations, Polymorphisms, and Copy Number Variations
Hypothalamic Disorders

Pretesticular causes of NOA involve either hypothalamic or pituitary disorders and encompass a wide spectrum of genotypes that characterize each. HH presents with a deficiency in gonadotrophin-releasing hormone (GnRH) or its receptor that disrupts the hormonal reproductive pathway, with a rare incidence of 1:8000 males.[75] HH can be either congenital or adult onset, may present with partial to complete anosmia (Kallmann syndrome) or with normal olfactory function, or can occur through obesity-associated syndromes such as Prader–Willi syndrome and Laurence–Moon–Biedl syndrome. The molecular basis of HH is as complex as the disorders involved in this state; for example, Kallmann syndrome has been partly genetically discovered with multiple modes of heredity (autosomal dominant, autosomal recessive, and X-linked) as also sporadic cases, with six frequent gene mutations (*KAL1* or *ANOS1*, *FGFR1*, *PROK2*, *PROKR2*, *CHD7*, *FGF8*) among 35 candidate genes covering only 35% of the total cases, and other genetic abnormalities being described, such as translocations (e.g., 10, 12) and copy number variations (CNVs) (e.g., in chromosomes 1, 2, 8, 14, and X).[4,76,77] While it is widely accepted that some abnormalities and particularly several genes are shared in both anosmic and normosmic HH, with the most common gene mutations being *KAL1*, *FGFR1*, and *GnRHR*, other possible genetic variations may occur, such as inversions and lack of genetic expression secondary to deletions of uniparental disomy, as occurs in Prader–Willi syndrome, and particularly in the q11 to q13 area of chromosome 15.[4] Due to high degree of variability surrounding HH occurrence, with a wide array of heredity modes, causative mutations, and sporadic chromosomal and structural genome deviations, genetic testing is often secondary to GnRH assessment and following exclusion of all secondary forms (e.g., pituitary disorders and tumors). For this case, a specific genetic panel is tested in a next-generation sequencing (NGS) platform that can provide a relevant diagnosis to approximately 40% of cases.[23]

Pituitary Disorders

Hypogonadism secondary to pituitary disorders may occur in males with either anterior pituitary hormone deficiency or a selective gonadotropin deficiency that both lead to a defective FSH and LH secretion, which is essential in reproductive function by promoting spermatogenesis and testosterone production. Several mutations have been described in males with pituitary disorders, and most involve genes coding for signaling molecules and transcription factors that interfere with early or late embryonic development of the pituitary gland,[4] such as *PROP1, PROKR2, FGFR1, FGFR8, FSHR, HESX1, LHX3, LHX4, SOX2,* and *WDR11* and mutation in the β subunit gene located in chromosome 11.[78] Genetic test panels are not readily available, as there are marked gaps in the genetic elucidation of such conditions, and the list of causative genes is rapidly increasing, especially in the past 5 years, due to the identification of variants.[78] NGS should allow an insight in some described mutations, and further data from inheritance patterns may assist in assessing the relevant risks for the offspring and the need for PGT.

Noonan Syndrome

Noonan syndrome is an autosomal dominant genetic disorder with an incidence between 1:1000 and 1:2500.[4] In this condition, germline mutations are detected across nearly 20 identified genes (including *PTPN11, SOS1, KRAS, NRAS, RAF1, BRAF, SHOC2, MEK1,* and *CBL*) that affect the signaling cascade of the RAS-GTPase and MAPK signaling transduction pathways.[79] The resulting clinical manifestations involve, among other general and anatomical health issues, unilateral and bilateral cryptorchidism occurring in up to 77% of the patients, and delayed or absent puberty secondary to testicular failure.[80,81] In these individuals, infertility

with oligospermia or azoospermia is secondary to cryptorchidism and testicular failure, while diagnosis of the syndrome usually precedes fertility assessments due to the severity of other general health concerns. As in all other autosomal dominant conditions, genetic counseling along with the option for screening of the embryos for such conditions should be routed for the affected individuals, while no rigid data support the option of testicular retrieval and its relevant success rates.

Cystic Fibrosis Transmembrane Conductance Regulator (CFTR) Gene Screening

Cystic fibrosis (CF) is an autosomal recessive disease with an incidence of 1:2500 that occurs following a mutation in the *CFTR* gene on chromosome 7q31.2.[82] Mutation in the *CFTR* gene results in CBAVD, with the hallmark of obstructive azoospermia in all CF patients, while carriers have also an increased risk for CBAVD varying according to ethnicity (1:25 in White populations).[28,83] Patients with CBAVD exhibit low semen volume that is devoid of spermatozoa and acidic pH following absence of the alkaline and fructose seminal vesicle fluidic contributions on the seminal fluid.

CFTR mutation has over 2000 variants described in the literature, with the most common occurrence being F508del and the 5T, 7T, and 9T variants.[23,84] *CFTR* genetic testing has been well established, with the screening of the most common mutations in the population and extended panels covering over 100 mutations and T polymorphisms. CF, or CBAVD in the absence of CF, mandates genetic testing of the male for diagnostic purposes and also the female partner to avoid transmission of the condition to the offspring through IVF/ICSI with PGT. TESE in these cases is anticipated to be successful since the condition does not interfere with testicular function and spermatogenesis.

X-Chromosome Genetic Factors

Male infertility is highly dependent on X-chromosome integrity as well as the function and expression of certain genes, with possible implications on the existence of variants and the involvement of other areas that are currently deemed important in male reproductive potential. These genetic factors comprise a modality of X-linked inherited diseases, mutations located in the X chromosome, CNVs, and polymorphisms. To this end, KS heterogenetic inheritance may commonly involve X-linked inheritance, while the *KAL-1* gene inherited in an X-linked recessive mode is responsible for congenital HH accounting for 30% to 60% of familial Kallmann syndrome cases and a further 10% to 15% of sporadic cases.[4,85,86] Normosmic HH diagnosed in infertile males has been previously been attributed to *DAX1* deletions and point mutations that cause X-linked congenital hypoplasia.[87] Mutations in the *USP26* and *SOX3* genes located in the q arm of the X chromosome have been linked with severe spermatogenic defects/hypogonadism and severe oligozoospermia/hypopituitarism, respectively, while *USP26* polymorphisms, even if they do not result in amino acid changes, are accountable for various aspects of infertility, with some haplotypes such as the TGGTC being overtransmitted in infertile males with astheno- and oligoasthenozoospermia.[88–90] Other mutations in X-linked genes previously implied include *TAF7L, DAZL, MTHFR, ER1, ER2* and *FSHR*,[4] while specifically *TEX11* mutations are a common cause of meiotic arrest and azoospermia in infertile males.[91] More recently a no-stop mutation in *MAGEB4* has been recognized as a possible cause of azoospermia and oligozoospermia.[92]

The androgen receptor (*AR*) gene located in the q arm of the X chromosome contains a critical region of CAG repeats in the exon 1, which once affected either by elongated or reduced presence of repeats, may lead to its inactivation.[1] This condition has been previously linked to the pathophysiology of KS and is correlated with the severity of the syndrome.[93] To date, only *AR* mutation screening has a clinical diagnostic significance indicated in males with hypoandrogenization and a high androgen sensitivity index, which is scarce, with only rare occurrences in the infertile population of up to 1.7%.[30,94] Obstructive infertility has been described in *ADGRG2* mutation carriers, with five pathogenic variants being reported and an accountable 11% to 15% of the CBAVD cases; thus testing for the specific mutations requires prior exclusion of *CFTR* gene, and testing should be performed to rule out X-linked transmission.[30,95] CNVs localized in the X chromosome have also been held accountable for male infertility, with currently three main types recognized in idiopathic infertility (CNVs 64-67-69).[96] Single nucleotide polymorphisms (SNPs) determined in the coding region of the *PGAM4* gene in the X chromosome of infertile patients imply possible connections to the reproductive phenotype due to its nature as a fundamental gene in male reproduction.[97]

Monogenic Defects and Gene Mutations

Genetic mutations can produce various phenotypes of male infertility, with over 3000 genes involved at various aspects of male reproductive dynamics and only an adversely small proportion being validated and utilized in clinical diagnosis[98] (Fig. 10.2). Nowadays, screening for mutations in candidate genes and monomorphic forms that affect sperm population, parameters, and function is largely dependent to NGS technology. NGS in idiopathic NOA cases revealed that more than 10% had monogenic and oligogenic mutations, as those in *SOHLH1* and *TEX1*, with an additional 20% found to have multiple molecular alterations.[99] NGS has been also proven useful in the elucidation of the cause of bilateral anorchia (vanishing testis syndrome). This rare congenital disease (1 in 20,000) presents with complete absence of the testis in phenotypically and genotypically normal individuals and may occur following a mutation in the steroidogenic factor-1 gene (*NR5A1*) on chromosome 9q33 that may result in midgestational testicular regression.[100]

Single-gene mutations have been detected and validated in various manifestations of male infertility, and these may involve sperm production sequences, such as SCOS or spermatocytic arrest, or interfere with sperm quality and functional characteristics such as reduced sperm count (*TEX11, TEX15, DDX3Y, NR5A1, HSF2, DMRT1*), compromised morphology and movement, and impaired sperm capacitation and fertilizing capacity (*CATSPER1, CATSPER2*)[98] (Fig. 10.2). In anatomical context, sperm head may appear round (globozoospermia), thus missing the acrosomal cap that enables the acrosome reaction and interaction with the oocyte; heads may appear elongated (macrozoospermia), possibly interfering with the normal fertilization process (polyploidy); may be absent (acephaly), precluding any reproductive potentiality; or may present with multiple morphological abnormalities of the flagella (MMAF), with absent, coiled, bent, irregular, or short tails, prohibiting normal movement.[23] On the functional aspect, both MMAF and primary ciliary dyskinesia (PCD) or Kartagener syndrome may promote compromised movement patterns to the extent that sperm–oocyte interaction is infrequent or impossible due to the inability of the spermatozoa to reach the ampulla region of the fallopian tube.[2] The indications for an underlying genetic cause for these patients mainly derive from specific observations during a conventional semen analysis,

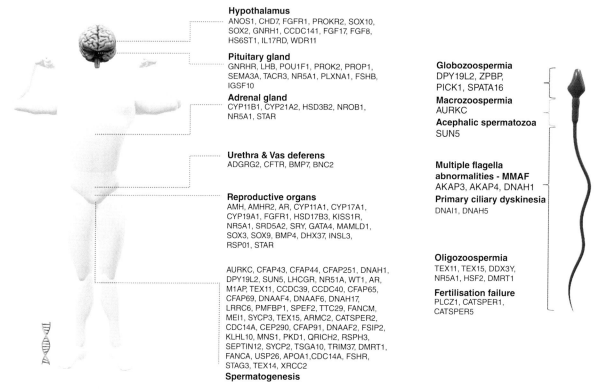

Hypothalamus
ANOS1, CHD7, FGFR1, PROKR2, SOX10, SOX2, GNRH1, CCDC141, FGF17, FGF8, HS6ST1, IL17RD, WDR11

Pituitary gland
GNRHR, LHB, POU1F1, PROK2, PROP1, SEMA3A, TACR3, NR5A1, PLXNA1, FSHB, IGSF10

Adrenal gland
CYP11B1, CYP21A2, HSD3B2, NROB1, NR5A1, STAR

Urethra & Vas deferens
ADGRG2, CFTR, BMP7, BNC2

Reproductive organs
AMH, AMHR2, AR, CYP11A1, CYP17A1, CYP19A1, FGFR1, HSD17B3, KISS1R, NR5A1, SRD5A2, SRY, GATA4, MAMLD1, SOX3, SOX9, BMP4, DHX37, INSL3, RSPO1, STAR

AURKC, CFAP43, CFAP44, CFAP251, DNAH1, DPY19L2, SUN5, LHCGR, NR51A, WT1, AR, M1AP, TEX11, CCDC39, CCDC40, CFAP65, CFAP69, DNAAF4, DNAAF6, DNAH17, LRRC6, PMFBP1, SPEF2, TTC29, FANCM, MEI1, SYCP3, TEX15, ARMC2, CATSPER2, CDC14A, CEP290, CFAP91, DNAAF2, FSIP2, KLHL10, MNS1, PKD1, QRICH2, RSPH3, SEPTIN12, SYCP2, TSGA10, TRIM37, DMRT1, FANCA, USP26, APOA1,CDC14A, FSHR, STAG3, TEX14, XRCC2

Spermatogenesis

Globozoospermia
DPY19L2, ZPBP, PICK1, SPATA16

Macrozoospermia
AURKC

Acephalic spermatozoa
SUN5

Multiple flagella abnormalities - MMAF
AKAP3, AKAP4, DNAH1

Primary ciliary dyskinesia
DNAI1, DNAH5

Oligozoospermia
TEX11, TEX15, DDX3Y, NR5A1, HSF2, DMRT1

Fertilisation failure
PLCZ1, CATSPER1, CATSPER5

Fig. 10.2 Schematic overview of genes involved in male infertility and spermatozoa quality and function deviations. (Figure partly adapted from Houston BJ, Riera-Escamilla A, Wyrwoll MJ, et al. A systematic review of the validated monogenic causes of human male infertility: 2020 update and a discussion of emerging gene-disease relationships. *Hum Reprod Update.* 2021;28(1):15-29; Spermatozoon three-dimensional model based on Philippe C. Spermatozoide humain. SketchFab website. https://sketchfab.com/3d-models/spermatozoide-humain-9cda311825bb43b4b5341dc900cd0441.)

and these should be indicative for further genetic assessment for clinically validated mutations. Management is based on the characteristics of the individual pathology, as ICSI allows sperm selection with morphological criteria and allows the recruitment of adjuvant tools to assess sperm vitality (other than motility) or to promote oocyte activation (calcium ionophore), while reproductive prognosis is variable and also dependent to the individual pathology, ranging from poor anticipated results (macrozoospermia, acephalic spermatozoa, PCD) to effective treatment through ICSI modalities (globozoospermia, MMAF, *CATSPER* mutations).

Genetic Polymorphisms

A genetic polymorphism involves one or more variants of a particular DNA sequence, with the most common occurrence being a variation of a single base pair, SNPs,

or longer stretches of DNA in other instances (length polymorphism). In a similar manner to CNVs, these are currently studied by genome sequencing and have been validated to be involved with diseases and various phenotypes, mainly as putative or predisposing factors. Several hundred polymorphisms have been identified in the literature to be linked with male infertility, although some of the presented forms have been proven as discordant between variable populations. Thus their validation has failed, or significantly more clinical data are required.[16,101] An early metaanalysis by Tüttelmann et al. (2007) identified significant associations between polymorphisms and male infertility for *AZF* gr/gr deletions and *MTHFR* C677T, but failed to demonstrate such effect for *POLG*, *DAZL*, *USP26*, and *FSHR*, while other candidate genes remained doubtful.[102] Current evidence supports an etiological relationship of polymorphisms of the *MTHFR* and *AR* genes and male infertility,[103,104] while *CFTR* polymorphisms have presented some rigid data in the past with the uncovering of *CFTR* polymorphism involvement in CBAVD through alterations in the intronic region of exon 8.[105] Such involvement has also been validated in more recent studies.[106] Newer studies also demonstrate a role of *TEX15, TNP2, CATSPER1, SPATA16,* and *MT-CYB* gene polymorphisms as factors involved in male infertility with severe oligozoospermia or idiopathic azoospermia, while contrastingly presenting an absence of a significant association with *USP26* and *TEX11* polymorphisms.[107,108]

Copy Number Variations

CNVs have been identified as a major cause of structural variation in the genome, with accumulating evidence of active involvement in population diversity and various health disorders. While it is a genomic structural deviation in nature, these alterations are typically too small (between 1000 bp and 5 Mb) to be identified through karyotypic analysis. Therefore molecular platforms with higher resolution were used to systematically identify CNVs, such as microarray comparative genomic hybridization (array CGH) or genotyping, which was rapidly substituted by the high-resolution data offered by NGS.[109] These are common features of the human genome and may include either duplications or deletions of a genomic segment or alternatively, a DNA sequence. Current data support their involvement in male fertility, either by introducing changes in genetic structure and function, or through gene mutation that consequently affects expression in testicular tissues.

Some studies have validated an involvement of CNVs on the sex chromosomes and autosomes in NOA[99] and SCOS, characterized by complete absence of germ cells in the seminiferous tubules of the testis.[110] Specifically, one study identified 73 CNVs in the X chromosome that are related to spermatogenesis, among which *CNV64, CNV67,* and *CNV69* were linked with idiopathic infertility in White populations.[96] Another study supported that CNVs, and especially duplications in the X chromosome, may contribute to the KS phenotype.[111] CNVs have also been identified within the AZF region of the Y chromosome, correlated with idiopathic male infertility.[112] In addition, CNVs are implicated in the pathogenesis of CBAVD through alterations of the *CFTR* gene.[113]

Genetic Testing Recommendations

Genetic testing in current clinical practice is overall recommended in populations with an increased probability of chromosomal and genetic abnormalities, in the presence of several indications (e.g., recurrent pregnancy loss, family history, phenotype), or as an extended evaluation of individuals with idiopathic infertility. Whenever there are no prior indications or suggestive family history, genetic testing is applied in cases with severe spermatogenic defects such as severe oligozoospermia or in azoospermia. According to the formal guidelines of the European Association of Urology (EAU), karyotype analysis is suggested in the event of azoospermia or oligozoospermia (<10 million sperm/mL), or in recurrent spontaneous miscarriages, a family history of malformations, and cognitive deficiencies.[114,115] The American Urological Association (AUA) and the ASRM, in their recent update on male fertility investigations, indicate that karyotyping should be performed in cases of azoospermia and oligozoospermia (<5 million/mL), along with other clinical indications of testicular failure, such as elevated FSH and atrophy, while additionally incorporating recurrent miscarriage with more than two events of spontaneous pregnancy loss.[116,117] The European Society of Human Reproduction and Embryology has additionally suggested the incorporation of the ART groups with more than three events of implantation failure as potential cases with marked chromosomal deficiencies.[118] Both AUA/ASRM and EAU guidelines recommend genetic analysis for YCMs in the presence of azoospermia or severe oligozoospermia, with a concentration less than 5 million/mL added to increased levels of serum FSH and indications of spermatogenic failure, such as testicular atrophy,[115–117] Furthermore, the EAU recommends *CFTR* mutation analysis in males with CBAVD.[115]

Genetic Counseling and Management

Genetic testing and counseling should always precede any medical management approach, following thorough discussion of the limitations and benefits of each procedure, along with the risks that accompany each genetic disorder. In medical practice, counseling provides and supports specialized information for patients/family and allows informed decisions on their life and family plans by assessing and weighting potential risks on individual and progeny health, as well as the course of personalized management. Genetic counseling should cover three main areas: (1) risk of genetic abnormality transmission to the offspring, the specific prospect of pregnancy progression, progeny overall health, and their reproductive potential; (2) management options of infertility (biopsy, ART with ICSI, PGT, gamete donation) and the respective transmission risks along with the anticipated success of such procedures; (3) further required testing, parallel risks on the male individual health (e.g., malignancies secondary to genetic abnormalities), and the chance of an affected relative according to the respective inheritance patterns (e.g., KS). On these grounds, each condition and their heritability roots should be adequately described and explained to the patient, and the heritability mode should be exhaustively explored according to current knowledge in order to reveal the potential risks to the pregnancy and the offspring as well as reveal the probability of an affected relative. Apart from specialized genetic counselors, the reproductive specialists themselves should acquire basic knowledge of the properties of common genetic disorders and their effect/risks on reproductive outcome[119] in order to promote genetic testing, avoid involuntary transmission of a defect to the embryo, and recognize instances that will benefit either from genetic testing and/or consultation.

Management of severe oligozoospermia and azoospermia usually resorts to ICSI in conjunction with TESE, microTESE, or other aspiration techniques, which have an overall high rate of successful sperm retrieval, reaching almost 60% through TESE.[120,121] Severe oligozoospermia and NOA may be effectively managed by personalized hormonal therapy using human chorionic gonadotropin followed by microTESE with ICSI, except for the cases of 46,XX male syndrome and AZFa or AZFb deletions. Although results remain inconsistent, it seems that testosterone levels may play a significant predictive role in the success of sperm retrieval rate, with a concentration of 250 ng/dL being a cut-off providing 22% higher sperm retrieval rate.[2] ART combined with PGT provides the benefit of advancing the time of diagnosis at the embryo stage,[14] avoiding the transmission of genetic disorders to the progeny, and enabling the selection of genetically normal embryos, thereby improving reproductive success outcomes in genetically infertile males.[2] Specialized forms of PGT attend different genetic deviations such as PGT for structural rearrangements addressed for chromosomal rearrangements such as translocations and inversions

and PGT for monogenic/single gene disorders (PGT-M) address the presence of monogenic disorders and other established mutations such as for CF, thalassemia, spinal muscular atrophy, hereditary hemoglobinopathies, and Huntington disease,[2] X-linked, Y-linked, and autosomal gene mutations can be detected by PGT-M, by a priori testing of the parents to signify the appropriate testing panels for the embryo, thus enabling preimplantation embryo diagnosis and preventing transmission by selective uterine transfer of embryos screened negative for the respective mutations.[2]

GENOMIC TESTS

Male fertility is a dynamic state dependent on many heterogeneous factors, such as the orchestrated function of probably thousands of genes, a balanced hormonal and physiological function, and environmental/lifestyle factors. Thus current knowledge often proves insufficient to reach its clinical diagnosis. This is clearly evident through the justification that even in our ever-expanding knowledge of the genetic contribution in male infertility, significant diagnostic gaps remain, with 30% to 40% infertile males being classified as idiopathic, even though there are indications of a genetic linkage to the condition.[122] To this end, the emergence of omic sciences is currently permitting novel insights into male infertility by identifying key molecules of the eminent biological processes, by discovering certain molecules that can act as future biomarkers or therapeutic targets, and by translating this information into clinical practice.[5,8,9,11]

Technological evolution has allowed significant developments in the omic sciences, altering the way genetic/genomic discovery occurs and, most importantly, how this is perceived in terms of biological impact to how these findings are translated in routine practice. Thus we live in an era where cornerstone technologies such as cytogenetic analysis, FISH, and CGH are quickly abandoned for more rigorous technologies such as NGS with whole-genome sequencing (WGS) and genome-wide association studies (GWAS) that in turn reveal novel areas of interest. NGS enables omics approaches by providing more powerful tools to study the genome, epigenome, and transcriptome, allowing the investigation of the underlying causes of male infertility. This rapidly acquired progression is evident by a snapshot of a timeline of such discoveries (Fig. 10.3).[7,8,13,98] Gene sequencing and NGS have allowed major insights into

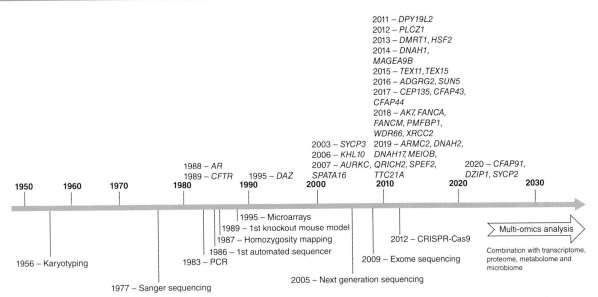

Fig. 10.3 Historical timeline of technological innovations and key genes identified in male infertility. (Adapted from Shiraishi K. Genome medicine in male infertility: from karyotyping to single-cell analysis. *J Obstet Gynaecol Res.* 2021;47(8):2586-2596; Xavier MJ, Salas-Huetos A, Oud MS, Aston KI, Veltman JA. Disease gene discovery in male infertility: past, present and future. *Hum Genet.* 2021;140(1):7-19.)

numerous mutations and genetic defects, as well as the eminent establishment of a diagnostics panel, with all the significant areas of interest that would allow rapid identification for presumably a good proportion of the idiopathic/undiagnosed cases. This can possibly include certain areas of emerging clinical significance that lie outside the coding regions, subtle genomic variations, and transcriptomic and epigenomic changes. WGS as an NGS application is an established technology constantly gaining ground in the etiopathogenesis of male infertility, since it allows concomitant sequencing of coding and intergenic regions and also smaller areas of interest in male infertility such as CNVs, SNPs, and chromosomal rearrangements that can inevitably surface hidden and very subtle genetic factors.

Genomics

The field of genomics studies the complete set of genes of an individual. In recent years, with the development of more powerful molecular techniques, there has been an increase in the identification of genes related to human male fertility.[5,98] Genomics can be helpful in discovering the molecular targets and the networks involved in the development of the male gamete and male infertility.[8] The genomic techniques available to

explore the genetic causes of male infertility include: arrays, CGH, and NGS (targeted sequencing, whole-exome sequencing [WES], and WGS).[8,9,98] These technologies have been proven promising for the identification of potential biomarkers and candidate genes in male infertility.[9] They enable the identification of the genes in infertile males, whose mutations or genetic variants could serve as diagnostic biomarkers of male infertility.[5]

In 2020, a study aimed to investigate the yield of a genomics first approach to male infertility on patients with severe oligospermia and NOA using exome sequencing in parallel with the standard practice of chromosomal analysis and controls. About 10.5% of patients had evidence of chromosomal aberrations, while 24.2% had a potential monogenic form of male infertility. They detected variants in genes with established links to male infertility (*CFAP44, NANOS1, SLC26A8, SYCP2, TEX11, TTC21A, USP9Y,* and *ZMYND15*), variants in established disease genes so far unrelated to male infertility (*HFM1, SGOL2, SPIDR, TDP1,* and *CEP250*), variants in previously reported candidate genes (*CCDC155, DNAH6, DZIP1, FAM47C, SPAG17,* and *TDRD6*), and 36 variants in 33 novel candidate genes (*TERB1, PIWIL2, ZSWIM7, AKAP9,*

ASZ1, CCDC146, CEP131, DAZL, DDX25, ELMO1, ESR2, HIPK4, HORMAD1, MAGEE2, MMRN1, ODF4, PGK2, ROS1, SPATA3, STRA8, TBCCD1, TTLL9, CST1, DMRTA2, DNAH7, MOSPD2, NLGN4Y, PPP1R36, RIOK2, SIRPG, STAG2, TCEANC, and *ZNF541*).[11]

In addition, several studies have emerged identifying genetically susceptible loci for NOA. A study in Han Chinese males consisting of three-stage GWAS of NOA individuals and controls identified significant associations between NOA risk and common variants near *PRMT6* (rs12097821 at 1p13.3), *PEX10* (rs2477686 at 1p36.32), and *SOX5* (rs10842262 at 12p12.1).[123] In 2014, a case-control study of these three SNPs and NOA against healthy controls in an independent Han Chinese population by direct DNA sequencing found that rs10842262 in the *SOX5* gene was significantly associated with NOA but did not support the association of rs12097821 and rs2477686 with NOA, therefore supporting the *SOX5* polymorphism as a risk factor for NOA in the Han Chinese population.[124] Another three-stage GWAS of the Han Chinese population (NOA and controls) consisting of a discovery stage and two confirmation stages identified variants at the human leukocyte antigen (*HLA*) regions that were independently associated with idiopathic NOA risk (*HLA-DRA*, rs3129878; C6orf10 and *BTNL2*, rs498422).[125]

Our group analyzed the effect in the Iberian population of six SNPs previously associated with NOA risk in Han Chinese and genotyped infertile males (NOA and severe oligospermia) and unaffected controls for variants *PRMT6*-rs12097821, *PEX10*-rs2477686, *CDC42BPA*-rs3000811, *IL17A*-rs13206743, *ABLIM1*-rs7099208, and *SOX5*-rs10842262, finding an association of *CDC42BPA*-rs3000811, *ABLIM1*-rs7099208 ,and *PEX10*-rs2477686 with different manifestations of severe spermatogenic failure in Iberians of European descent, likely by influencing gene expression and lincRNA deregulation.[126] A similar genetic association study involving similar patients and controls evaluated five SNPs (*USP8*-rs7174015, *DPF3*-rs10129954, *EPSTI1*-rs12870438, *PSAT1*-rs7867029, and *TUSC1*-rs10966811) previously associated with reduced fertility in Hutterites, finding that *EPSTI1*-rs12870438 and *PSAT1*-rs7867029 were associated with severe oligospermia, *USP8*-rs7174015 may contribute to the genetic susceptibility to NOA, and *TUSC1*-rs10966811 was associated with a higher predisposition to NOA hypospermatogenesis and with a higher probability of TESE success.[127]

High-throughput genome-wide sequencing was applied in a study to determine CNVs in patients with chromosomal abnormalities and patients with unexplained azoospermia, detecting 16 CNVs in 11 patients with chromosome abnormalities and 26 CNVs in 16 males with azoospermia. The involved genes included *EDDM3A, EDDM3B, HLA-DRB1, HLA-DQA1, POTE B, GOLGA8C, DNMT3L, ALF, NPHP1, NRG1, RID2, ADAMTS20, TWF1, COX10, MAK,* and *DNEL1.* They provided evidence that CNVs contribute to male infertility and presented a number of candidate genes as potential risk factors for spermatogenic failure.[6]

In 2018, a systematic review was published, including 23 studies in which NGS technologies were used to discover variants causing male infertility in humans, and altogether these studies showed variants in 28 genes causing male infertility. Regarding quantitative anomalies (azoospermia and oligospermia), 19 genes have been found to be implicated in causing quantitative defects in spermatogenesis by NGS: *ADGRG2, CFTR, DNAH6, DNMT3L, HLA-DQA1, HLA-DRB1, MAGEB4, MEIOB, NPAS2, SIRPA, SIRPG, SPINK2, SYCE1, SYCP3, TAF4B, TDRD9, TEX14, TEX15,* and *ZMYND15.* In terms of morphological anomalies (teratozoospermia, macrozoospermia, globozoospermia, and acephalic spermatozoa syndrome), causative variants have been detected in five genes: *BRDT, CEP135, DNAH1, NPHP4,* and *SUN5.* Investigation of motility anomalies (asthenozoospermia and flagellar abnormalities impairing movement) using NGS has identified five unique genes: *CFAP43, CFAP44, CFAP65, DNAH1,* and *SPAG17.* Moreover, while CBAVD is usually caused by *CFTR* mutations, a study has discovered mutations in *ADGRG2.* A *CFTR* mutation has also been discovered in a patient with unilateral absence of vas deferens.[7]

The investigation of the role of de novo mutations (DNMs) in the human genome on male infertility has also gained interest. In this regard, a trio-based WES study in 13 infertile males with idiopathic azoospermia and their parents was conducted, and the findings were further evaluated in independent males. Trio WES identified 11 DNMs in 10 genes, 5 of which were considered potential candidates for male infertility (*NEURL4, BRD2, SEMA5A, CD1D,* and *CD63*). It also identified rare, potentially pathogenic mutations in four genes previously implicated in male infertility (*FKBPL, UPF2, CLCA4,* and *NR0B1*).[128] A recent study analyzed trio-based WES data of 185 infertile males (unexplained azoospermia and oligozoospermia) and their unaffected parents, identifying 192 rare DNMs, including 145 protein-altering DNMs, 29 of which were likely causative for the infertility phenotype. They identified a number of promising candidate genes for male infertility, including the mRNA splicing gene *RBM5*.[10] Both studies support a potential role for DNMs in severe male infertility, propose new potential candidate genes for male infertility, and address the need for further investigation.

In 2021, a systematic review of evidence for monogenic causes of isolated or syndromic male infertility, as well as endocrine disorders or reproductive system abnormalities affecting the male sex organs, described an updated clinical validity assessment for 657 gene-disease relationships involving 596 genes and identified 104 genes linked to 120 male infertility or abnormal genitourinary development phenotypes with sufficient evidence for use in gene panels (Table 10.1).[98]

Precone et al. developed a NGS gene panel, including 65 additional prediagnostic genes that were used in 12 patients who were negative to a diagnostic genetic test for male infertility disorders consisting of 110 genes. Variants in prediagnostic genes were identified in 10 patients. Seventeen filtered variants were detected in 12 of the 65 genes analyzed: two pathogenic variants of *DNAH5* and *CFTR*; three uncertain significance variants of *DNAI1*, *DNAH11*, and *CCDC40*; three variants with high impact in *AMELY*, *CATSPER2*, and *ADCY10*; and variants of *DNAH10*, *GALNTL5*, *KLK4*, and *KLK14*. Almost half of the variants identified belonged to the cytoplasmic dynein genes. Genetic diagnosis testing and male infertility clinical management can be improved by developing NGS custom-made panel tests, including prediagnostic genes.[129]

Male infertility is a heterogeneous disorder, which complicates its diagnosis and management.[5] Although many research efforts have been done on male infertility

TABLE 10.1 List of Genes Linked to Male Infertility or Abnormal Genitourinary Development Phenotypes

	Disorder	Gene
Isolated infertility	Acephalic sperm	*PMFBP1, SUN5, TSGA10*
	Globozoospermia	*DPY19L2*
	Macrozoospermia	*AURKC*
	Multiple morphological abnormalities of the sperm flagella	*ARMC2, CFAP251, CFAP43, CFAP44, CFAP65, CFAP69, CFAP91, DNAH1, DNAH17, FSIP2, QRICH2, SEPTIN12, SPEF2, TTC29*
	Nonobstructive azoospermia or oligozoospermia	*AR, DMRT1, FANCM, KLHL10, MIAP, MEI1, STAG3, SYCP2, SYCP3, TEX11, TEX14, TEX15, USP26, XRCC2*
	Congenital bilateral absence of the vas deferens	*ADGRG2, CFTR*
	Fertilization failure	*PLCZ1*
Syndromic infertility	Primary ciliary dyskinesia	*CCDC39, CCDC40, DNAAF2, DNAAF4, DNAAF6, LRRC6, RSPH3, SPEF2*
	Other syndromes	*APOA1, CATSPER2, CDC14A, CEP290, FANCA, MNS1, NLRP3, PKD1, TRIM37*
Endocrine disorder/ reproductive system syndrome	Disorders of sexual development and hypogonadotropic hypogonadism	*CYP11B1, CYP17A1, CYP19A1, DHX37, GATA4, HSD17B3, MAMLD1, MYRF, NR5A1, SOX3, SOX9, SRD5A2, SRY, WT1, AMH, AMHR2, ANOS1, AR, BMP4, BMP7, BNC2, CCDC141, CHD7, CYP11A1, CYP19A1, CYP21A2, FGF17, FGF8, FGFR1, FSHB, FSHR, GNRH1, GNRHR, HS6ST1, HSD3B2, IGSF10, ILI7RD, INSL3, KISSR1R, LHB, LHCGR, NR0B1, PLXNA1, POU1F1, PROK2, PROKR2, PROP1, RSPO1, SEMA3A, SOX10, SOX2, STAR, TACR3, WDR11, WDR11*

Adapted from Houston BJ, Riera-Escamilla A, Wyrwoll MJ, et al. A systematic review of the validated monogenic causes of human male infertility: 2020 update and a discussion of emerging gene-disease relationships. *Hum Reprod Update.* 2021;28(1):15-29.

genetics, identification of new causative genes has remained challenging.[128] As we improve our understanding of the risk genes, we would be able to design a multigene panel testing for male infertility, enabling a more efficient and comprehensive clinical evaluation and management.[5,129] In recent years, the application of NGS technologies in male infertility research has allowed the identification of candidate genes and the validation of its relation with disease, which is essential for further translation of these findings to the clinical practice.[98]

Transcriptomics

The field of transcriptomics studies the total content of RNA within cells or tissues.[5] Spermatozoa contain RNA that is relevant to reproductive success and is transmitted to the offspring. Sperm RNA plays a key role in fertilization and early embryonic development, and these molecules could affect phenotypic characteristics of the embryo and offspring, hence the importance of their evaluation.[5,130–134] Although mature sperm are transcriptionally and translationally inert, several studies have revealed a diverse and complex population of RNA in sperm consisting of coding and noncoding RNAs. Spermatozoa retain, in a selective and specific manner, certain transcripts reflective of the anterior spermatogenic process and the subsequent fertilization and embryonic development.[135,136] Therefore RNA from sperm could be used as a potential infertility biomarker to explain the cases of idiopathic male infertility and to constitute a diagnostic test.[5,130,131,137] In this context, transcriptomic studies provide a better understanding of the sperm RNA content in fertile and infertile males.[5]

Advances in transcriptomic technologies have increased the knowledge of the role of sperm RNA. Several high-throughput technologies are available to explore the transcriptomic cause of male infertility, including microarrays and NGS (targeted sequencing, whole-transcriptome sequencing, mRNA sequencing, or miRNA sequencing), which have permitted the identification of some relevant transcripts involved in male infertility. Microarray technology has been used to study the transcriptomic profile of sperm as potential biomarkers of male infertility, obtaining promising results.[131] Different transcriptomes have been found in studies comparing fertile and infertile patients,[138,139] comparing infertile patients who achieved pregnancy with those who did not in intrauterine insemination

(IUI) or ICSI,[130,140] in patients with SCOS, obstructive azoospermia, NOA, or asthenozoospermia, and in patients with fertilization failures and idiopathic infertility.[5,130]

Ostermeier et al., using microarrays, defined sperm mRNA profiles of normal fertile males.[134] A later microarray study showed a set of RNAs that remained stable in sperm after various cycles of freezing/thawing, suggesting that they could be used as biomarkers for the prognostic evaluations of male factor infertility.[141] Another study comparing asthenozoospermic infertile patients with fertile controls detected differentially expressed genes between both groups, where the lower abundance found of the transcripts annexin A2 and bromodomain 2 could be associated with asthenozoospermia, potentially useful as a marker to evaluate the male fertility status.[137] Moreover, some transcripts have been suggested as potential biomarkers of different male infertility conditions, such as *PRM1/PRM2*, *SPZ-1*, *SPATA-4*, *MEA-1*, *CREM*, *NIPBL*, *PARK7*, *DDX3X*, *JMJD1A*, *PLCZ1*, *ACRV1*, *SPAM1*, *ODF1-4*, *CUL3*, *PRM1*, *HSPCD35*, *TPX-1*, and *TNFAIP3*.[5,133]

More recently, a microarray analysis including individuals with known fertility, idiopathic infertility (normozoospermic), and asthenozoospermia found several transcripts differentially expressed between the groups. Some were upregulated in the idiopathic group, including genes encoding ribosomal proteins (*RPS25*, *RPS11*, *RPS13*, *RPL30*, *RPL34*, *RPL27*, *RPS5*), *HINT1*, *HSP90AB1*, *SRSF9*, *EIF4G2*, and *ILF2*, but downregulated in the asthenozoospermic group compared to controls. They also found transcripts specific of the idiopathic group, upregulated: *CAPNS1*, *FAM153C*, *ARF1*, *CFL1*, *RPL19*, and *USP22*; or downregulated: *ZNF90*, *SMNDC1*, *c14orf126*, and *HNRNPK*. Other transcripts specific to the asthenozoospermic group, upregulated: *RPL24*, *HNRNPM*, *RPL4*, *PRPF8*, *HTN3*, *RPL11*, *RPL28*, *RPS16*, *SLC25A3*, *C2orf24*, *RHOA*, *GDI2*, *NONO*, and *PARK7*; or downregulated: *HNRNPC*, *SMARCAD1*, *RPS24*, *RPS24*, *RPS27A*, and *KIFAP3*.[136] However, microarrays have limited use in male infertility studies,[130,132] while RNA sequencing seems a more powerful tool to provide information of male infertility molecular mechanisms and biomarkers for diagnosing infertility.[132] Several studies have already used this technology to analyze the transcriptome of spermatic samples.[142,143]

Sendler et al. performed the first study using RNAseq to characterize the population of coding and noncoding transcripts in sperm of healthy donors, identifying known and novel sperm transcripts.[135] In 2015, a study using RNAseq to study sperm RNA from couples with idiopathic infertility identified sperm RNA elements that reflected fecundity status. They identified several required sperm RNA elements, the absence of which reduced the probabilities of achieving live birth in timed intercourse and IUI, while not being critical for IVF or ICSI. Moreover, approximately 30% of the heterosexual couples with idiopathic infertility had an incomplete set of the required sperm RNA elements, suggesting male factor infertility. They concluded that the analysis of sperm RNA elements has the potential to predict individual success rates of the different fertility treatments. Nevertheless, the identification of which sperm RNA elements are more useful is not yet established.[132] A recent study consisting of the expression analysis of miRNAs through RNAseq suggested that hsa-mir-191-5p could be used as a potential biomarker to detect high quality sperm to improve success rates in IVF.[144]

Although a lot of research efforts have been placed in sperm transcriptomics, retrieving valuable information suggestive of the potential role of sperm RNAs as male infertility biomarkers, further investigations are needed to better understand human spermatozoa RNA content, identify the most relevant transcripts, and unravel the underlying molecular mechanisms. The current and future advancements could be used to improve the evaluation and diagnosis of infertile males and the prediction of reproductive success.[5,136]

Epigenomics

Epigenetics is the study of the changes in gene regulation and function due to modifications in DNA and histone structure without altering the DNA sequence.[8] The mechanisms of epigenetic regulation include histone tail modifications, DNA methylation, chromatin remodeling, and small noncoding RNAs. Several studies have demonstrated an association of the epigenetic mechanisms with male infertility/subfertility condition.[8,9,145] Epigenomics is the study of the epigenetics of the whole genome, and it can be analyzed with array-based and NGS-based technologies.[8]

Spermatogenesis is regulated by epigenetic modifications and results in the formation of spermatozoa with a unique epigenome. Spermatozoa undergo several epigenetic changes to ensure that the DNA delivered to the future embryo is adequate. Chromatin compaction

by protamination (replacement of histones by protamines) is a form of epigenetic regulation because after DNA compaction, no more nuclear activity occurs in sperm. However, approximately 5% to 10% of the DNA remains bound to histones and is part of the epigenetic signature of sperm.[8,146] An appropriate paternal epigenome is essential for adequate sperm function and embryo development.[8,146] Additionally, epigenetic inheritance, in terms of paternal effect, consists of the possible modification of the epigenetics of the offspring by certain environmental exposure alterations that the father obtained prior to offspring conception, and this can justify epigenetic transmission to the offspring. Several studies have demonstrated that sperm epigenetic reprogramming can be altered by lifestyle, nutrition, physical activity, endocrine disruptors, stress, and environmental factors affecting male fertility, and this trait can be transmitted to offspring. Therefore paternal epigenome can impact sperm quality, early embryogenesis, and possibly even overall health of the progeny.[9,146] Several studies have demonstrated an association between epigenetic signatures and male infertility, with evidence suggesting that altered sperm epigenetics, mainly DNA methylation, can be associated with abnormal semen parameters, gene regulation in unexplained male infertility, pregnancy rate in ART, and male subfertility.[8,9,146,147]

Houshdaran et al. measured sperm DNA methylation, finding that DNA methylation at numerous sequences was increased in poor quality semen in terms of concentration, motility, and morphology. Improper erasure of DNA methylation during epigenetic reprogramming of the male germ line could be responsible for these epigenetic changes.[8,148] Moreover, a genome-wide sperm DNA methylation microarray study identified two genomic regions where significantly decreased methylation appeared to be associated with decreased pregnancy rates (*HSPA1L* and *HSPA1B*) and three genomic regions where significantly increased methylation appeared to be associated with pregnancy outcome (*USP6NL*, *SPON2*, and *PTPRN2*). These results suggest that alterations in DNA methylation at specific genomic loci appear to be associated with decreased fecundity.[9,145] More recently, a metaanalysis on sperm DNA methylation that included studies with males with oligozoospermia, oligoasthenoteratozoospermia, or idiopathic infertility and fertile controls found an association between male infertility and reduced sperm *H19* methylation and increased *MEST* and *SNRPN* methylation, and it did not find differences for *LINE-1* methylation levels.[9,146,147]

A pyrosequencing sperm DNA methylation study of *H19-ICR*, *KvDMR*, *SNRPN-ICR*, *IG-DMR*, and *MEG3-DMR*, including infertile males and fertile controls, found that infertile individuals have more spermatozoa with abnormal DNA methylation in regions regulated by genetic imprinting compared to controls, but these methylation anomalies did not influence ART outcomes.[149] In another array study, sperm DNA methylation was compared between infertile patients and fertile controls, identifying 696 differentially methylated CpGs (184 hypomethylated and 512 hypermethylated) associated with 501 genes (13 processes related to spermatogenesis) and 17 differentially methylated genes (some with functions related to spermatogenesis): *ATXN7L1*, *APCS*, *PATE4*, *PRDM1*, *ANK2*, *RPS6KA2*, *RHOBTB1*, *C6ORF118*, *ANKRD53*, *LOC100271702/ LINC00940*, *EIF2AK3*, *JAM3*, *NCAPD3*, *TEX261*, *CACNA2D4*, *FOXK1*, and *FOXK2*. Moreover, the study identified a significant association between *RPS6KA2* hypermethylation and advanced age, *APCS* hypermethylation and oligozoospermia, *JAM3/NCAPD3* hypermethylation and altered FISH pattern, and *ANK2* hypermethylation and lower pregnancy rate.[150]

A study by Camprubí et al., including infertile patients and fertile controls, found no differences in the distribution of the genotypes of *MTHFR* rs1801133 polymorphism and no associations between the genotypes and the characteristics of semen analysis or the presence of an abnormal sperm DNA hypomethylation pattern in paternally methylated *H19-ICR* or *IG-DMR*, suggesting that this polymorphism is not a risk factor for male infertility in the Spanish population. Moreover, they did not identify frameshift, nonsense, or missense mutations of the *CTCFL* gene, and *CTCFL* mutations were not associated with the pattern of sperm hypomethylation at paternally imprinting loci (*H19-ICR* and/ or *IG-DMR*).[151] In 2017, an array study trying to characterize the sperm methylome of fertile donors found that the sperm methylation profile is homogeneous and hypomethylated, and that hypomethylated gene promoters were related to spermatogenesis and embryogenesis processes. Sex chromosomes were the most hypomethylated, indicative of their essential role in spermatogenesis. Moreover, they found 94 genes resistant to demethylation, being strong candidates for transgenerational inheritance.[12] Interestingly, epigenetic alterations have been correlated with autism spectrum disorder. A recent sequencing genome-wide analysis for differential DNA methylation regions (low-density CpG regions) in sperm comparing fathers from autistic and nonautistic male children found 805 differential DNA methylation regions, of which in 303 have an increase and 502 have a decrease in DNA methylation in the autism group. These results show a highly significant set of 805 differential DNA methylated regions in sperm that can potentially act as a biomarker to identify offspring autism susceptibility transmitted from the father.[152]

Multiple studies have demonstrated an association between aberrant sperm epigenetics and sperm quality, ART outcomes, male subfertility, and more importantly, progeny health. These epigenetic marks might be considered as potential targets for diagnosis in male infertility cases, as well as improving clinical management and preventive and therapeutic options, along with assessing offspring health risks. Nevertheless, additional investigations are needed to elucidate the role and biological implication of epigenetic mechanisms in male subfertility.[9,145–148,152] Currently, there is a commercially available screening tool for sperm epigenetics called "Seed" that was developed by Episona Inc.[9]

Counseling and Management

The study of genomics, epigenomics and transcriptomics could be a potential area of targeted diagnostics in the setting of male infertility.[8,9] Advances in microarrays and NGS have provided more powerful tools to study the genome, epigenome, and transcriptome and have facilitated the identification of genetic variants that may play a role in male infertility.[13,98] These technologies have enormous clinical potential. The rapid introduction of NGS in the male infertility research field, together with the development of international sharing of data, expertise, and collaboration, are essential for the translation of these findings into the clinical practice.[13,98] There are several websites of data sharing initiatives (http://www.imigc.org and https://gemini.conradlab.org/) that are useful for data pooling, clinical assessment, and research purposes.[13] Some research laboratories study the genetics of male infertility with NGS methods; however, these techniques are not extensively used in clinical genetic diagnosis.[98] Genetic testing is not indicated for all infertile males; it is limited to the most common infertility manifestations, therefore depriving many patients of the benefits of a molecular diagnosis.[11,98] Healthcare professionals should always aim at providing a proper course of testing and management in infertile couples in order to protect the health and welfare of the patient and offspring and provide appropriate genetic counseling.[7,10]

CLINICAL/LABORATORY SCENARIOS

CASE 1

A patient presents for semen analysis with the following results: semen volume of 2.6 mL; sperm concentration of 65×10^6/mL; sperm motility of 0%; and vitality staining showing 45% viability. How will you manage this patient?

Solution
A genetic work-up focused on genes targeted for PCD is recommended, including *DNAI1* and *DNAH5* gene mutations, which account for up to 30% of all cases. A family history investigating provenance from consanguineous populations should be included. ICSI can be offered as a treatment modality, however, with low success rates. A higher risk for transmission of the entire spectrum of symptoms exists in case the female partner is also a carrier of a pathogenic mutation in the same gene. Testing of both partners prior to ICSI is advised, and PGD can be proposed if the mutation is commonly detected in the couple.

CASE 2

A patient presents for his initial semen analysis with the following results: semen volume of 2.5 mL with complete azoospermia. His body type exhibits high stature, long arms, and gynecomastia, and he reports the presence of mental retardation in his family history. How will you advise this patient?

Solution
A repetition of semen analysis within 1 to 3 months should be recommended to confirm the complete absence of spermatozoa in the ejaculate. A detailed andrological work-up including physical examination as well as hormonal evaluation to assess the levels of serum testosterone, FSH, and LH. A comprehensive medical examination to evaluate the possible presence of general health problems such as metabolic syndrome, autoimmune diseases, venous thromboembolism, and cognitive/psychiatric disturbances should be included.

Karyotypic analysis is strongly indicated to confirm or exclude the diagnosis of KS. If it is a validated case of KS, the patient should be further counseled for fertility preservation after microTESE as soon as possible to avoid time-dependent deterioration in germ cell quantity, given that a higher recovery rate is achieved under the age of 30 years. The average testicular sperm recovery rate is 50%, and spermatozoa can be used for the conception of a biological child through ART with ICSI. The need for PGT as a preventive option should be discussed with the patient in the context of possible risks to the offspring and the current literature evidence regarding the increased risk for autosomal chromosomal anomalies in children born from KS fathers which remains conflicting.

CASE 3

A heterosexual couple comes to a clinic and after semen analysis, no spermatozoa are found in the ejaculate of the male. Which genetic test would you advise to this couple?

Solution
In the case of obstructive azoospermia (mainly CBAVD), the first line recommended is *CFTR* testing and the second line is *ADGRG2* testing. Alternatively, for NOA cases, the recommendations for genetic testing point towards karyotyping and YCM as the first line and WES as a second line. In these NOA cases, genetic testing is very interesting because it can help elucidate the possibility of success of sperm retrieval after TESE. Additionally, genetic testing involving WES should go together with genetic counseling.

CASE 4

A patient comes to a clinic for a semen analysis, obtaining the following results: semen volume of 1.5 mL; sperm concentration of 40×10^6/mL; sperm motility of 50%; and normal morphology 0% with visible macrozoospermia. Which genetic test would you recommend to this patient?

Solution
Macrozoospermia is mainly due to *AURKC* mutations; therefore *AURKC* genetic screening is suggested as the first line, and WES is suggested as a second line. Moreover, genetic testing involving WES should go together with genetic counseling.

SUMMARY

The continuously emerging research and clinical evidence support a strong genetic basis in many types of male infertility. Healthcare professionals should conform to the established guidelines but should more-over possess a basic overview of potential genetic presentations in male infertility to enable the identification of individuals that require further testing, medically assisted reproductive management, and targeted counseling to protect their own and their progeny's health. Potential genetic contributions span from chromosomal abnormalities to gene mutations, transcriptional deviations, and epigenetic alterations, and current technological advancements permit clinical diagnosis on a significant proportion of males with genetic infertility. An equally significant proportion remains undiagnosed, either by missing the clinical indications or due to the lack of completeness of our current knowledge on genetic factors. Overall and at most instances, the genetically affected individuals have the option to father a biological child, and therefore this chance should be offered to them by granting targeted testing, accurate diagnosis, and reproductive management technologies.

A current soaring realization is that, despite recent advances, the genetic work-up of infertile males has remained relatively unchanged over the years. The scientific community has a long way to go to compile a final model of genetic infertility, but this process is accelerated by the means currently available. The modern sophisticated technologies have expanded over to sequencing and genetic expression of the whole genome, but these efforts require a copious engagement of multidisciplinary experts to combine and attribute the emerging data to specific conditions and disorders affecting male fertility. Specifically, the validation of the association between novel candidate genes and male infertility disease is essential for further diagnostic implementation of these approaches in male infertility. The guidelines implemented in clinical practice to explore genetic forms of infertility should evolve along with the emerging technologies and evidence and updated to best describe patients groups for which genetic testing is recommended, while encouraging the utilization of novel technologies. In the upcoming years, with the improvement in genetic testing and acquaintance of the realization of mechanisms that drive genomics, epigenomics, and transcriptomics in male infertility we should be able to improve prediction, prevention, management, counseling, diagnosis, and treatment, therefore advancing our ability to care for infertile couples.

FUNDING

Ana Navarro-Gomezlechon is granted by the Ministerio de Ciencia, Innovación y Universidades para la Formación de Profesorado Universitario (FPU19/06126), Spain.

REFERENCES

1. Neto FTL, Bach PV, Najari BB, Li PS, Goldstein M. Genetics of male infertility. *Curr Urol Rep.* 2016;17(10):70.
2. Lee SR, Lee TH, Song SH, et al. Update on genetic screening and treatment for infertile men with genetic disorders in the era of assisted reproductive technology. *Clin Exp Reprod Med.* 2021;48(4):283-294.
3. Dohle GR, Halley DJJ, Van Hemel JO, et al. Genetic risk factors in infertile men with severe oligozoospermia and azoospermia. *Hum Reprod.* 2002;17(1):13-16.
4. Hamada AJ, Esteves SC, Agarwal A. A comprehensive review of genetics and genetic testing in azoospermia. *Clinics (Sao Paulo).* 2013;68 Suppl 1(suppl 1):39-60.
5. Garrido N, Hervás I. Personalized medicine in infertile men. *Urol Clin North Am.* 2020;47(2):245-255.
6. Dong Y, Pan Y, Wang R, Zhang Z, Xi Q, Liu RZ. Copy number variations in spermatogenic failure patients with chromosomal abnormalities and unexplained azoospermia. *Genet Mol Res.* 2015;14(4):16041-16049.
7. Robay A, Abbasi S, Akil A, et al. A systematic review on the genetics of male infertility in the era of next-generation sequencing. *Arab J Urol.* 2018;16(1):53-64.
8. Sinha A, Singh V, Yadav S. Multi-omics and male infertility: Status, integration and future prospects. *Front Biosci - Sch.* 2017;9(3):375-394.
9. Krzastek SC, Smith RP, Kovac JR. Future diagnostics in male infertility: genomics, epigenetics, metabolomics and proteomics. *Transl Androl Urol.* 2020;9(7):S195-S205.
10. Oud MS, Smits RM, Smith HE, et al. A de novo paradigm for male infertility. *Nat Commun.* 2022;13(1):154.
11. Alhathal N, Maddirevula S, Coskun S, et al. A genomics approach to male infertility. *Genet Med.* 2020;22(12):1967-1975.
12. Camprubí C, Cigliano RA, Salas-Huetos A, Garrido N, Blanco J. What the human sperm methylome tells us. *Epigenomics.* 2017;9(10):1299-1315.

13. Shiraishi K. Genome medicine in male infertility: From karyotyping to single-cell analysis. *J Obstet Gynaecol Res.* 2021;47(8):2586-2596.

14. Cariati F, D'Argenio V, Tomaiuolo R. The evolving role of genetic tests in reproductive medicine. *J Transl Med.* 2019;17(1):267.

15. Ventimiglia E, Pozzi E, Capogrosso P, et al. Extensive assessment of underlying etiological factors in primary infertile men reduces the proportion of men with idiopathic infertility. *Front Endocrinol.* 2021;12:80125. Available at: https://www.frontiersin.org/article/10.3389/fendo.2021.801125.

16. Thirumavalavan N, Gabrielsen JS, Lamb DJ. Where are we going with gene screening for male infertility? *Fertil Steril.* 2019;111(5):842-850.

17. Del Giudice F, Kasman AM, Li S, et al. Increased mortality among men diagnosed with impaired fertility: analysis of US claims data. *Urology.* 2021;147:143-149.

18. Eisenberg ML, Li S, Brooks JD, Cullen MR, Baker LC. Increased risk of cancer in infertile men: analysis of U.S. claims data. *J Urol.* 2015;193(5):1596-1601.

19. Brubaker WD, Li S, Baker LC, Eisenberg ML. Increased risk of autoimmune disorders in infertile men: analysis of US claims data. *Andrology.* 2018;6(1):94-98.

20. Donker RB, Vloeberghs V, Groen H, Tournaye H, van Ravenswaaij-Arts CMA, Land JA. Chromosomal abnormalities in 1663 infertile men with azoospermia: the clinical consequences. *Hum Reprod.* 2017;32(12):2574-2580.

21. Yatsenko AN, Yatsenko SA, Weedin JW, et al. Comprehensive 5-year study of cytogenetic aberrations in 668 infertile men. *J Urol.* 2010;183(4):1636-1642.

22. Foresta C, Garolla A, Bartoloni L, Bettella A, Ferlin A. Genetic abnormalities among severely oligospermic men who are candidates for intracytoplasmic sperm injection. *J Clin Endocrinol Metab.* 2005;90(1):152-156.

23. Krausz C, Cioppi F, Riera-Escamilla A. Testing for genetic contributions to infertility: potential clinical impact. *Expert Rev Mol Diagn.* 2018;18(4):331-346.

24. Corona G, Pizzocaro A, Lanfranco F, et al. Sperm recovery and ICSI outcomes in Klinefelter syndrome: a systematic review and meta-analysis. *Hum Reprod Update.* 2017;23(3):265-275.

25. Levron J, Aviram-Goldring A, Madgar I, Raviv G, Barkai G, Dor J. Sperm chromosome analysis and outcome of IVF in patients with non-mosaic Klinefelter's syndrome. *Fertil Steril.* 2000;74(5):925-929.

26. Staessen C, Tournaye H, Van Assche E, et al. PGD in 47,XXY Klinefelter's syndrome patients. *Hum Reprod Update.* 2003;9(4):319-330.

27. Vorona E, Zitzmann M, Gromoll J, Schuring AN, Nieschlag E. Clinical, endocrinological, and epigenetic features of the 46,XX male syndrome, compared with 47,XXY Klinefelter patients. *J Clin Endocrinol Metab.* 2007;92(9):3458-3465.

28. Hotaling J, Carrell DT. Clinical genetic testing for male factor infertility: current applications and future directions. *Andrology.* 2014;2(3):339-350.

29. Abbas NE, Toublanc JE, Boucekkine C, et al. A possible common origin of "Y-negative" human XX males and XX true hermaphrodites. *Hum Genet.* 1990;84(4):356-360.

30. Krausz C, Riera-Escamilla A. Genetics of male infertility. *Nat Rev Urol.* 2018;15(6):369-384.

31. Egozcue S, Blanco J, Vendrell JM, et al. Human male infertility: chromosome anomalies, meiotic disorders, abnormal spermatozoa and recurrent abortion. *Hum Reprod Update.* 2000;6(1):93-105.

32. Gonzalez-Merino E, Hans C, Abramowicz M, Englert Y, Emiliani S. Aneuploidy study in sperm and preimplantation embryos from nonmosaic 47,XYY men. *Fertil Steril.* 2007;88(3):600-606.

33. Hwang K, Lipshultz LI, Lamb DJ. Use of diagnostic testing to detect infertility. *Curr Urol Rep.* 2011;12(1):68-76.

34. Martinerie L, Morel Y, Gay CL, et al. Impaired puberty, fertility, and final stature in 45,X/46,XY mixed gonadal dysgenetic patients raised as boys. *Eur J Endocrinol.* 2012;166(4):687-694.

35. Caglayan AO, Demiryilmaz F, Kendirci M, Ozyazgan I, Akalin H, Bittmann S. Mixed gonadal dysgenesis with 45,X/46,X,idic(Y)/46,XY,idic(Y) karyotype. *Genet Couns.* 2009;20(2):173-179.

36. Brosman SA. Mixed gonadal dysgenesis. *J Urol.* 1979;121(3):344-347.

37. Flannigan RK, Chow V, Ma S, Yuzpe A. 45,X/46,XY mixed gonadal dysgenesis: A case of successful sperm extraction. *J Can Urol Assoc.* 2014;8(1-2 FEB):45-47.

38. McLachlan RI, O'Bryan MK. Clinical Review#: State of the art for genetic testing of infertile men. *J Clin Endocrinol Metab.* 2010;95(3):1013-1024.

39. Suzumori N, Sugiura-Ogasawara M. Genetic factors as a cause of miscarriage. *Curr Med Chem.* 2010;17(29):3431-3437.

40. Johnson MD. Genetic risks of intracytoplasmic sperm injection in the treatment of male infertility: recommendations for genetic counseling and screening. *Fertil Steril.* 1998;70(3):397-411.

41. Meschede D, Lemcke B, Exeler JR, et al. Chromosome abnormalities in 447 couples undergoing intracytoplasmic sperm injection—prevalence, types, sex distribution and reproductive relevance. *Hum Reprod.* 1998;13(3):576-582.

42. De Braekeleer M, Dao TN. Cytogenetic studies in male infertility: a review. *Hum Reprod.* 1991;6(2):245-250.

43. Mau-Holzmann UA. Somatic chromosomal abnormalities in infertile men and women. *Cytogenet Genome Res.* 2005; 111(3-4):317-336.

44. Martin RH. Cytogenetic determinants of male fertility. *Hum Reprod Update.* 2008;14(4):379-390.

45. Kin Chau M, Li Y, Dai P, et al. Investigation of the genetic etiology in male infertility with apparently balanced chromosomal structural rearrangements by genome sequencing. *Asian J Androl.* 2022;24(3):248-254.

46. Balasar Ö, Zamani AG, Balasar M, Acar H. Male infertility associated with de novo pericentric inversion of chromosome 1. *Turkish J Urol.* 2017;43(4):560-562.

47. Li R, Fan H, Zhang Q, Yang X, Zhan P, Feng S. Pericentric inversion in chromosome 1 and male infertility. *Open Med (Warsaw, Poland).* 2020;15(1):343-348.

48. Fan H, Liu Z, Zhan P, Jia G. Pericentric inversion of chromosome 6 and male fertility problems. *Open Med.* 2022;17(1):191-196.

49. Xie X, Li F, Tan W, Tang J. Analysis of the clinical features of pericentric inversion of chromosome 9. *J Int Med Res.* 2020;48(9):300060520957820.

50. Zhang X, Shi Q, Liu Y, et al. Fertility problems in males carrying an inversion of chromosome 10. *Open Med (Warsaw, Poland).* 2021;16(1):316-321.

51. Beaumont M, Tucker EJ, Mary L, et al. Pseudodicentric chromosome originating from autosomes 9 and 21 in a male patient with oligozoospermia. *Cytogenet Genome Res.* 2019;159(4):201-207.

52. Hallast P, Kibena L, Punab M, et al. A common 1.6 mb Y-chromosomal inversion predisposes to subsequent deletions and severe spermatogenic failure in humans. *Elife.* 2021;10:e65420.

53. Anton E, Vidal F, Egozcue J, Blanco J. Genetic reproductive risk in inversion carriers. *Fertil Steril.* 2006;85(3):661-666.

54. Pan Y, Zhang HG, Xi QI, et al. Molecular microdeletion analysis of infertile men with karyotypic Y chromosome abnormalities. *J Int Med Res.* 2018;46(1):307-315.

55. Abur U, Gunes S, Ascı R, et al. Chromosomal and Y-chromosome microdeletion analysis in 1,300 infertile males and the fertility outcome of patients with AZFc microdeletions. *Andrologia.* 2019;51(11):e13402.

56. Kumar N, Singh AK. Trends of male factor infertility, an important cause of infertility: a review of literature. *J Hum Reprod Sci.* 2015;8(4):191-196.

57. Lange J, Skaletsky H, van Daalen SKM, et al. Isodicentric Y chromosomes and sex disorders as byproducts of homologous recombination that maintains palindromes. *Cell.* 2009;138(5):855-869.

58. Liu X, Qiao J, Li R, Yan L, Chen L. Y chromosome AZFc microdeletion may not affect the outcomes of ICSI for infertile males with fresh ejaculated sperm. *J Assist Reprod Genet.* 2013;30(6):813-819.

59. Navarro-Costa P, Gonçalves J, Plancha CE. The AZFc region of the Y chromosome: at the crossroads between genetic diversity and male infertility. *Hum Reprod Update.* 2010;16(5):525-542.

60. Caron C, Pivot-Pajot C, van Grunsven LA, et al. Cdyl: a new transcriptional co-repressor. *EMBO Rep.* 2003;4(9):877-882.

61. Stouffs K, Lissens W, Van Landuyt L, Tournaye H, Van Steirteghem A, Liebaers I. Characterization of the genomic organization, localization and expression of four PRY genes (PRY1, PRY2, PRY3 and PRY4). *Mol Hum Reprod.* 2001;7(7):603-610.

62. Wong EYM, Tse JYM, Yao KM, Lui VCH, Tam PC, Yeung WSB. Identification and characterization of human VCY2-interacting protein: VCY2IP-1, a microtubule-associated protein-like protein. *Biol Reprod.* 2004;70(3): 775-784.

63. Kee K, Angeles VT, Flores M, Nguyen HN, Reijo Pera RA. Human DAZL, DAZ and BOULE genes modulate primordial germ-cell and haploid gamete formation. *Nature.* 2009;462(7270):222-225.

64. Yuen W, Golin AP, Flannigan R, Schlegel PN. Histology and sperm retrieval among men with Y chromosome microdeletions. *Transl Androl Urol.* 2021;10(3): 1442-1456.

65. Kamp C, Huellen K, Fernandes S, et al. High deletion frequency of the complete AZFa sequence in men with Sertoli-cell-only syndrome. *Mol Hum Reprod.* 2001;7(10):987-994.

66. Soares AR, Costa P, Silva J, Sousa M, Barros A, Fernandes S. AZFb microdeletions and oligozoospermia—which mechanisms? *Fertil Steril.* 2012;97(4):858-863.

67. Skaletsky H, Kuroda-Kawaguchi T, Minx PJ, et al. The male-specific region of the human Y chromosome is a mosaic of discrete sequence classes. *Nature.* 2003;423(6942):825-837.

68. Liu X, Li Z, Su Z, et al. Novel Y-chromosomal microdeletions associated with non-obstructive azoospermia uncovered by high throughput sequencing of sequence-tagged sites (STSs). *Sci Rep.* 2016;6(1):21831.

69. Rabinowitz MJ, Huffman PJ, Haney NM, Kohn TP. Y-chromosome microdeletions: a review of prevalence, screening, and clinical considerations. *Appl Clin Genet.* 2021;14:51-59.

70. Krausz C, Hoefsloot L, Simoni M, Tüttelmann F. EAA/EMQN best practice guidelines for molecular diagnosis of Y-chromosomal microdeletions: state-of-the-art 2013. *Andrology.* 2014;2(1):5-19.

71. Practice Committee of the American Society for Reproductive Medicine. Diagnostic evaluation of the infertile male: a committee opinion. *Fertil Steril.* 2015;103(3): e18-e25.

72. Cioppi F, Rosta V, Krausz C. Genetics of azoospermia. *Int J Mol Sci*. 2021;22(6):3264.

73. Zhu YC, Wu TH, Li GG, et al. Decrease in fertilization and cleavage rates, but not in clinical outcomes for infertile men with AZF microdeletion of the Y chromosome. *Zygote*. 2015;23(5):771-777.

74. Krausz C, Cioppi F. Genetic factors of non-obstructive azoospermia: consequences on patients' and offspring health. *J Clin Med*. 2021;10(17):4009.

75. Boehm U, Bouloux PM, Dattani MT, et al. Expert consensus document: European Consensus Statement on congenital hypogonadotropic hypogonadism—pathogenesis, diagnosis and treatment. *Nat Rev Endocrinol*. 2015;11(9):547-564.

76. Bhagavath B, Podolsky RH, Ozata M, et al. Clinical and molecular characterization of a large sample of patients with hypogonadotropic hypogonadism. *Fertil Steril*. 2006;85(3):706-713.

77. Trarbach EB. Copy number variation associated with Kallmann syndrome: new genetics insights from genome-wide studies. *Asian J Androl*. 2011;13(2):203-204.

78. Gregory LC, Dattani MT. The molecular basis of congenital hypopituitarism and related disorders. *J Clin Endocrinol Metab*. 2020;105(6):dgz184.

79. Tartaglia M, Gelb BD, Zenker M. Noonan syndrome and clinically related disorders. *Best Pract Res Clin Endocrinol Metab*. 2011;25(1):161-179.

80. Sharland M, Burch M, McKenna WM, Paton MA. A clinical study of Noonan syndrome. *Arch Dis Child*. 1992;67(2):178-183.

81. Kelnar CJH. Noonan syndrome: the hypothalamo-adrenal and hypothalamo-gonadal axes. *Horm Res Paediatr*. 2009;72(suppl 2):24-30.

82. Rommens JM, Iannuzzi MC, Kerem B, et al. Identification of the cystic fibrosis gene: chromosome walking and jumping. *Science*. 1989;245(4922):1059-1065.

83. Samli H, Samli MM, Yilmaz E, Imirzalioglu N. Clinical, andrological and genetic characteristics of patients with congenital bilateral absence of vas deferens (CBAVD). *Arch Androl*. 2006;52(6):471-477.

84. Radpour R, Gourabi H, Dizaj AV, Holzgreve W, Zhong XY. Genetic investigations of CFTR mutations in congenital absence of vas deferens, uterus, and vagina as a cause of infertility. *J Androl*. 2008;29(5):506-513.

85. Albuisson J, Pêcheux C, Carel JC, et al. Kallmann syndrome: 14 novel mutations in KAL1 and FGFR1 (KAL2). *Hum Mutat*. 2005;25(1):98-99.

86. Georgopoulos NA, Pralong FP, Seidman CE, Seidman JG, Crowley WFJ, Vallejo M. Genetic heterogeneity evidenced by low incidence of KAL-1 gene mutations in sporadic cases of gonadotropin-releasing hormone deficiency. *J Clin Endocrinol Metab*. 1997;82(1):213-217.

87. Muscatelli F, Strom TM, Walker AP, et al. Mutations in the DAX-1 gene give rise to both X-linked adrenal hypoplasia congenita and hypogonadotropic hypogonadism. *Nature*. 1994;372(6507):672-676.

88. Shi Y, Wei L, Cui Y, et al. Association between ubiquitin-specific protease USP26 polymorphism and male infertility in Chinese men. *Clin Chim Acta*. 2011;412(7-8):545-549.

89. Solomon NM, Ross SA, Forrest SM, et al. Array comparative genomic hybridisation analysis of boys with X-linked hypopituitarism identifies a 3.9 Mb duplicated critical region at Xq27 containing SOX3. *J Med Genet*. 2007;44(4):e75.

90. Stouffs K, Lissens W, Tournaye H, Van Steirteghem A, Liebaers I. Possible role of USP26 in patients with severely impaired spermatogenesis. *Eur J Hum Genet*. 2005;13(3):336-340.

91. Yatsenko AN, Georgiadis AP, Röpke A, et al. X-linked TEX11 mutations, meiotic arrest, and azoospermia in infertile men. *N Engl J Med*. 2015;372(22):2097-2107.

92. Okutman O, Muller J, Skory V, et al. A no-stop mutation in MAGEB4 is a possible cause of rare X-linked azoospermia and oligozoospermia in a consanguineous Turkish family. *J Assist Reprod Genet*. 2017;34(5):683-694.

93. Zitzmann M, Depenbusch M, Gromoll J, Nieschlag E. X-chromosome inactivation patterns and androgen receptor functionality influence phenotype and social characteristics as well as pharmacogenetics of testosterone therapy in Klinefelter patients. *J Clin Endocrinol Metab*. 2004;89(12):6208-6217.

94. Ferlin A, Vinanzi C, Garolla A, et al. Male infertility and androgen receptor gene mutations: clinical features and identification of seven novel mutations. *Clin Endocrinol (Oxf)*. 2006;65(5):606-610.

95. Patat O, Pagin A, Siegfried A, et al. Truncating mutations in the adhesion G protein-coupled receptor G2 gene ADGRG2 cause an x-linked congenital bilateral absence of vas deferens. *Am J Hum Genet*. 2016;99(2):437-442.

96. Krausz C, Giachini C, Lo Giacco D, et al. High resolution X chromosome-specific array-CGH detects new CNVs in infertile males. *PLoS One*. 2012;7(10):e44887.

97. Okuda H, Tsujimura A, Irie S, et al. A single nucleotide polymorphism within the novel sex-linked testis-specific retrotransposed PGAM4 gene influences human male fertility. *PLoS One*. 2012;7(5):e35195.

98. Houston BJ, Riera-Escamilla A, Wyrwoll MJ, et al. A systematic review of the validated monogenic causes of human male infertility: 2020 update and a discussion of emerging gene-disease relationships. *Hum Reprod Update*. 2021;28(1):15-29.

99. Nakamura S, Miyado M, Saito K, et al. Next-generation sequencing for patients with non-obstructive azoospermia: implications for significant roles of monogenic/oligogenic mutations. *Andrology*. 2017;5(4):824-831.

100. Philibert P, Zenaty D, Lin L, et al. Mutational analysis of steroidogenic factor 1 (NR5a1) in 24 boys with bilateral anorchia: a French collaborative study. *Hum Reprod*. 2007;22(12):3255-3261.

101. Nuti F, Krausz C. Gene polymorphisms/mutations relevant to abnormal spermatogenesis. *Reprod Biomed Online*. 2008;16(4):504-513.

102. Tüttelmann F, Rajpert-De Meyts E, Nieschlag E, Simoni M. Gene polymorphisms and male infertility—a meta-analysis and literature review. *Reprod Biomed Online*. 2007;15(6):643-658.

103. Ghadirkhomi E, Angaji SA, Khosravi M, Mashayekhi MR. Association of novel single nucleotide polymorphisms of genes involved in cell functions with male infertility: a study of male cases in northwest Iran. *J Reprod Infertil*. 2021;22(4):258-266.

104. Metin Mahmutoglu A, Hurre Dirie S, Hekim N, Gunes S, Asci R, Henkel R. Polymorphisms of androgens-related genes and idiopathic male infertility in Turkish men. *Andrologia*. 2022;54(2):e14270.

105. Chillón M, Casals T, Mercier B, et al. Mutations in the cystic fibrosis gene in patients with congenital absence of the vas deferens. *N Engl J Med*. 1995;332(22):1475-1480.

106. Tan MQ, Huang WJ, Lan FH, Xu YJ, Zheng MY, Tang Y. Genetic mutation analysis of 22 patients with congenital absence of vas deferens: a single-center study†. *Biol Reprod*. 2022;106(1):108-117.

107. Ghadirkhomi E, Angaji SA, Khosravi M, Mashayekh MR. Correlation of novel single nucleotide polymorphisms of USP26, TEX15, and TNP2 genes with male infertility in north west of Iran. *Int J Fertil Steril*. 2022;16(1):10-16.

108. Behvarz M, Rahmani SA, Siasi Torbati E, Danaei Mehrabad S, Bikhof Torbati M. Association of CATSPER1, SPATA16 and TEX11 genes polymorphism with idiopathic azoospermia and oligospermia risk in Iranian population. *BMC Med Genomics*. 2022;15(1):47.

109. Pös O, Radvanszky J, Buglyó G, et al. DNA copy number variation: Main characteristics, evolutionary significance, and pathological aspects. *Biomed J*. 2021;44(5):548-559.

110. Sharma A, Jain M, Halder A, Kaushal S. Identification of genomic imbalances (CNVs as well as LOH) in sertoli cell only syndrome cases through cytoscan microarray. *Gene*. 2021;801:145851.

111. Rocca MS, Pecile V, Cleva L, et al. The Klinefelter syndrome is associated with high recurrence of copy number variations on the X chromosome with a potential role in the clinical phenotype. *Andrology*. 2016;4(2):328-334.

112. Zhou R, Cheng J, Ma D, et al. Identifying novel copy number variants in azoospermia factor regions and evaluating their effects on spermatogenic impairment. *Front Genet*. 2019;10:427.

113. Ma C, Wang R, Li T, Li H, Wang B. Analysis of CNVs of CFTR gene in Chinese Han population with CBAVD. *Mol Genet Genomic Med*. 2020;8(11):e1506.

114. *Sexual and Reproductive Health EAU Guidelines*. EAU website; 2021. Available at: https://uroweb.org/guideline/sexual-and-reproductive-health/#10.

115. Jungwirth A, Giwercman A, Tournaye H, et al. European Association of Urology guidelines on male infertility: the 2012 update. *Eur Urol*. 2012;62(2):324-332.

116. Schlegel PN, Sigman M, Collura B, et al. Diagnosis and treatment of infertility in men: AUA/ASRM guideline part II. *Fertil Steril*. 2021;115(1):62-69.

117. Schlegel PN, Sigman M, Collura B, et al. Diagnosis and treatment of infertility in men: AUA/ASRM guideline part I. *Fertil Steril*. 2021;115(1):54-61.

118. Cimadomo D, Craciunas L, Vermeulen N, Vomstein K, Toth B. Definition, diagnostic and therapeutic options in recurrent implantation failure: an international survey of clinicians and embryologists. *Hum Reprod*. 2021;36(2):305-317.

119. Katagiri Y, Tamaki Y. Genetic counseling prior to assisted reproductive technology. *Reprod Med Biol*. 2021;20(2):133-143.

120. Schlegel PN, Li PS. Microdissection TESE: sperm retrieval in non-obstructive azoospermia. *Hum Reprod Update*. 1998;4(4):439.

121. Schiff JD, Palermo GD, Veeck LL, Goldstein M, Rosenwaks Z, Schlegel PN. Success of testicular sperm extraction [corrected] and intracytoplasmic sperm injection in men with Klinefelter syndrome. *J Clin Endocrinol Metab*. 2005;90(11):6263-6267.

122. Oud MS, Volozonoka L, Smits RM, Vissers LELM, Ramos L, Veltman JA. A systematic review and standardized clinical validity assessment of male infertility genes. *Hum Reprod*. 2019;34(5):932-941.

123. Hu Z, Xia Y, Guo X, et al. A genome-wide association study in Chinese men identifies three risk loci for non-obstructive azoospermia. *Nat Genet*. 2012;44(2):183-186.

124. Zou S, Li Z, Wang Y, et al. Association study between polymorphisms of PRMT6, PEX10, SOX5, and nonob-

structure azoospermia in the Han Chinese population. *Biol Reprod.* 2014;90(5):1-4.

125. Zhao H, Xu J, Zhang H, et al. A genome-wide association study reveals that variants within the HLA region are associated with risk for nonobstructive azoospermia. *Am J Hum Genet.* 2012;90(5):900-906.

126. Cerván-Martín M, Bossini-Castillo L, Rivera-Egea R, et al. Effect and in silico characterization of genetic variants associated with severe spermatogenic disorders in a large Iberian cohort. *Andrology.* 2021;9(4): 1151-1165.

127. Cerván-Martín M, Bossini-Castillo L, Rivera-Egea R, et al. Evaluation of male fertility-associated loci in a european population of patients with severe spermatogenic impairment. *J Pers Med.* 2021;11(1):1-19.

128. Hodžić A, Maver A, Plaseska-Karanfilska D, et al. De novo mutations in idiopathic male infertility—A pilot study. *Andrology.* 2021;9(1):212-220.

129. Precone V, Cannarella R, Paolacci S, et al. Male infertility diagnosis: improvement of genetic analysis performance by the introduction of pre-diagnostic genes in a next-generation sequencing custom-made panel. *Front Endocrinol (Lausanne).* 2021;11:605237.

130. Garrido N, García-Herrero S, Meseguer M. Assessment of sperm using mRNA microarray technology. *Fertil Steril.* 2013;99(4):1008-1022.

131. Garrido N, Remohi J, Martínez-Conejero JA, García-Herrero S, Pellicer A, Meseguer M. Contribution of sperm molecular features to embryo quality and assisted reproduction success. *Reprod Biomed Online.* 2008;17(6): 855-865.

132. Jodar M, Sendler E, Moskovtsev SI, et al. Absence of sperm RNA elements correlates with idiopathic male infertlity. *Sci Transl Med.* 2015;7(295):295re6.

133. Hamatani T. Human spermatozoal RNAs. *Fertil Steril.* 2012;97(2):275-281.

134. Ostermeier GC, Dix DJ, Miller D, Khatri P, Krawetz SA. Spermatozoal RNA profiles of normal fertile men. *Lancet.* 2002;360(9335):772-777.

135. Sendler E, Johnson GD, Mao S, et al. Stability, delivery and functions of human sperm RNAs at fertilization. *Nucleic Acids Res.* 2013;41(7):4104-4117.

136. Bansal SK, Gupta N, Sankhwar SN, Rajender S. Differential genes expression between fertile and infertile spermatozoa revealed by transcriptome analysis. *PLoS One.* 2015;10(5):1-21.

137. Jodar M, Kalko S, Castillo J, Ballescà JL, Oliva R. Differential RNAs in the sperm cells of asthenozoospermic patients. *Hum Reprod.* 2012;27(5):1431-1438.

138. Garrido N, Martínez-Conejero JA, Jauregui J, et al. Microarray analysis in sperm from fertile and infertile men without basic sperm analysis abnormalities reveals a significantly different transcriptome. *Fertil Steril.* 2009;91(suppl 4.):1307-1310.

139. García-Herrero S, Garrido N, Martínez-Conejero JA, Remohí J, Pellicer A, Meseguer M. Ontological evaluation of transcriptional differences between sperm of infertile males and fertile donors using microarray analysis. *J Assist Reprod Genet.* 2010;27(2-3):111-120.

140. García-Herrero S, Meseguer M, Martínez-Conejero JA, Remohí J, Pellicer A, Garrido N. The transcriptome of spermatozoa used in homologous intrauterine insemination varies considerably between samples that achieve pregnancy and those that do not. *Fertil Steril.* 2010; 94(4):1360-1373.

141. Ostermeier GC, Goodrich RJ, Diamond MP, Dix DJ, Krawetz SA. Toward using stable spermatozoal RNAs for prognostic assessment of male factor fertility. *Fertil Steril.* 2005;83(6):1687-1694.

142. Corral-Vazquez C, Blanco J, Aiese Cigliano R, et al. The RNA content of human sperm reflects prior events in spermatogenesis and potential post-fertilization effects. *Mol Hum Reprod.* 2021;27(6):1-15.

143. Schuster A, Tang C, Xie Y, Ortogero N, Yuan S, Yan W. SpermBase: A database for sperm-borne RNA contents. *Biol Reprod.* 2016;95(5):99-99.

144. Xu H, Wang X, Wang Z, et al. MicroRNA expression profile analysis in sperm reveals hsa-mir-191 as an auspicious omen of in vitro fertilization. *BMC Genomics.* 2020;21(1):1-9.

145. Jenkins TG, Aston KI, Meyer TD, et al. Decreased fecundity and sperm DNA methylation patterns. *Fertil Steril.* 2016;105(1):51-57.e3.

146. Ibrahim Y, Hotaling J. Sperm epigenetics and its impact on male fertility, pregnancy loss, and somatic health of future offsprings. *Semin Reprod Med.* 2018;36(3-4): 233-239.

147. Santi D, De Vincentis S, Magnani E, Spaggiari G. Impairment of sperm DNA methylation in male infertility: a meta-analytic study. *Andrology.* 2017;5(4): 695-703.

148. Houshdaran S, Cortessis VK, Siegmund K, Yang A, Laird PW, Sokol RZ. Widespread epigenetic abnormalities suggest a broad DNA methylation erasure defect in abnormal human sperm. *PLoS One.* 2007;2(12):e1289.

149. Camprubí C, Pladevall M, Grossmann M, Garrido N, Pons MC, Blanco J. Semen samples showing an increased rate of spermatozoa with imprinting errors

have a negligible effect in the outcome of assisted reproduction techniques. *Epigenetics.* 2012;7(10): 1115-1124.

150. Camprubí C, Salas-Huetos A, Aiese-Cigliano R, et al. Spermatozoa from infertile patients exhibit differences of DNA methylation associated with spermatogenesis-related processes: an array-based analysis. *Reprod Biomed Online.* 2016;33(6):709-719.

151. Camprubí C, Pladevall M, Grossmann M, Garrido N, Pons MC, Blanco J. Lack of association of MTHFR rs1801133 polymorphism and CTCFL mutations with sperm methylation errors in infertile patients. *J Assist Reprod Genet.* 2013;30(9):1125-1131.

152. Garrido N, Cruz F, Egea RR, et al. Sperm DNA methylation epimutation biomarker for paternal offspring autism susceptibility. *Clin Epigenetics.* 2021;13(1):6.

11

Computer-Assisted Semen Analysis

Hanae Pons-Rejraji, Marion Bendayan, and Florence Boitrelle

KEY POINTS

- There are several computed-assisted semen analysis (CASA) systems, with two different technologies (phase-contrast microscopy or electrooptics).
- CASA systems have the advantage of saving technical time and improving the standardization of analyses.
- CASA systems allow a fine analysis of flagellar movement.

- Sperm analysis with CASA systems is limited to normal or subnormal quality sperm.
- CASA systems are less reliable for patients with severe oligospermia.
- CASA analysis of sperm morphology has not yet been proven to be reliable.

INTRODUCTION

Infertility affects approximately 8% to 12% of couples, and in 50% of cases infertility in heterosexual couples is at least partially of male origin.[1,2] Standard semen analysis is the first-line examination to explore heterosexual couple infertility.[3] World Health Organization (WHO) laboratory manuals for the examination and processing of human semen analysis[4] defined technical procedures and reference thresholds in order to measure semen parameters, most notably sperm concentration, motility, vitality, and morphology.[4,5] In addition, to allow a rapid and noninvasive diagnosis of male sub/infertility, sperm analysis is useful to guide assisted reproductive technique (ART) management.[5,6] Standard semen analysis is carried out mainly manually, and consequently, the results suffer from a strong intra- and interlaboratory variability.[7,8] The last two versions of the WHO manual[4,5] have emphasized the need to standardize semen analyses and make them more objective. However, in the current edition of the WHO laboratory manual for the examination and processing of human semen, computer-aided semen analysis

(CASA) systems are placed in the chapter "advanced semen examinations," which corresponds to analyses not used routinely but which can be used in research.[5] In this chapter, CASA systems will be detailed, benefits and drawbacks of CASA systems will be described, and their interest in the diagnosis of male infertility and in the framework of ART will be assessed. Emerging technologies using smartphones will also be mentioned.

DESCRIPTION OF DIFFERENT TYPES OF COMPUTED-ASSISTED SEMEN ANALYSIS SYSTEMS

Systems Using Phase-Contrast Microscopy

The first automated system for sperm parameters analysis, the CASA system, appeared in the 1980s with the development of computers and imaging techniques.[9,10] This system consists of acquiring successive images of a sperm sample placed in a count cell using a phase-contrast microscope equipped with a camera connected to a computer. Using algorithms, the software calculates sperm concentration by identifying them by their size and luminosity. Sperm motility and velocity were assessed by following their movement. The trajectory of each spermatozoon is reconstructed, with its head as referent point. Quickly, the systems evolved to allow reliable measurement of sperm concentration and sperm velocity by distinguishing them from debris and round cells. Numerous CASA systems are commercialized and offer a broad range of analyses, whether semi- or fully automated.[11,12] The most widespread come from Hamilton Thorne Research (Fig. 11.1, Hamilton-Thorn Sperm Analyzers IVOS and CEROS, Beverly, MA, USA) and Microptic Automatic Systems SL (see Fig. 11.1, Sperm Class Analyzer SCA Scope and Evolution, Microptic Automatic Systems SL, Barcelona, Spain). These systems are updated regularly and their analysis software is constantly evolving. Current versions assess sperm vitality, morphology, and sperm DNA fragmentation using different magnifications and staining. Some CASA systems could even use fluorescence microscopy. CASA systems with fluorescent staining can distinguish sperm cells from nonsperm particles, as well as living from dead spermatozoa. CASA systems can also be equipped with an automatized and/or temperature-controlled objective stage. The IVOS and SCA Scope systems perform automatic analysis with the set-up of the correct calibration, optics, and focus.

Systems Using Electrooptics

More recently, a second system has been developed, the Sperm Quality Analyzer V (Fig. 11.2, SQA-V Vison and Gold, Medical Electronic Systems Ltd., Caesarea, Israel). It does not correspond to the strict definition of a CASA system, given that it combines technology in electrooptics, computer algorithms, and video microscopy spectrophotometry. The system assesses

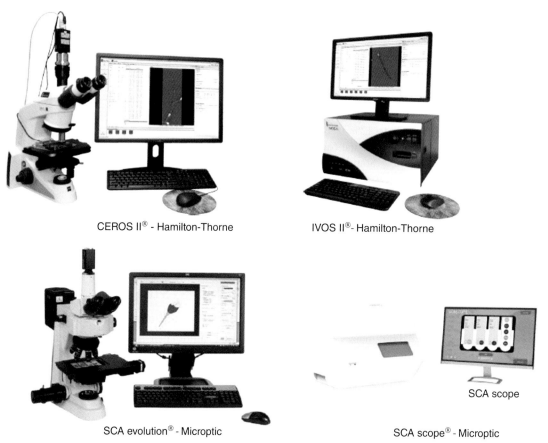

CEROS II® - Hamilton-Thorne

IVOS II®- Hamilton-Thorne

SCA evolution® - Microptic

SCA scope

SCA scope® - Microptic

Fig. 11.1 Computer-Assisted Sperm Analysis (CASA) Systems Using Phase-Contrast Microscopy.

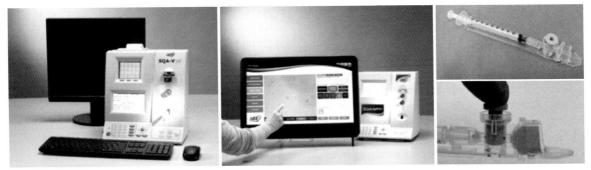

SQA-V® vision and gold - Medical electronic systems Ltd   Capillary and cuvette

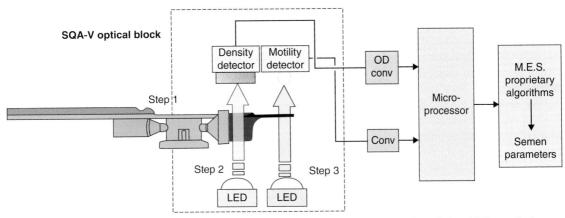

Fig. 11.2 Sperm Analysis Systems Using Electrooptics. *LED*, Light-emitting diode; *MES*, medical electronic systems; *OD*, optical density.

sperm concentration and sperm motility in a unique measurement of a sperm sample placed in a specific capillary containing two sections: a "thin capillary" and a "cuvette" (see Fig. 11.2). Motile sperm concentration (MSC) and progressive motile sperm concentration (PMSC) are measured using microscopy spectrophotometric in the thin capillary section. Sperm cell movement causes light disturbances as they move through a light beam. The light disturbances are converted into electronic signals that are analyzed by microprocessor software based on an algorithm and translated into motility parameters. Sperm concentration is assessed using electrooptic technology in the cuvette. An optical density (OD) detector measures the amount of light (with a specific wavelength) absorbed by spermatozoa and converts it to OD (see Fig. 11.2). The OD reading is translated into sperm concentration by a microprocessor based on algorithms. Total and progressive motility are calculated using the measured issue from both capillary sections. The percentage of typical morphology spermatozoa is calculated using a specific algorithm. The two latest versions, the SQA-V Gold and the SQA-Vision, distinguish sperm total and progressive motility and are discriminating as to the presence of debris and round cells.[13-19] The main advantage of this equipment is to permit a unique, simple, and quick analysis but only at ambient temperature and with low possibility of adjustments.

SEMEN EXAMINATIONS USING COMPUTER-ASSISTED SEMEN ANALYSIS

Computer-Assisted Semen Analysis Systems User Guide

Nature and Quality of Semen

All the systems proposed adapted programs regarding the nature and quality of semen. Most of the CASA systems proposed different options to analyze sperm concentration and motility, depending on if it is native semen, washed, selected spermatozoa (by density gradient or swim-up), or freeze-thawed spermatozoa. Some systems offer "postvasectomy" and "azoospermia" testing protocols. Semen volume, pH, viscosity, appearance, presence of debris or round cells, and presence of polymorphonuclear neutrophils (PMNs) must be previously and, usually manually, measured. A few systems, such as SCA, propose an integrated protocol to assay PMN concentration. These parameters must be assessed initially and some of these results will condition the CASA use (or manual measurement) and, secondly, the program choice. For example, a volume higher than 0.5 mL is required to measure sperm motility and sperm concentration with SQAV. For a low volume (<0.5 mL), the system proposes to dilute the sample or to use the thin section requiring 20 μL and calculate only MSC and PMSC. For almost all CASA systems, a volume of 2 to 20 μL is necessary to measure sperm concentration and sperm motility, depending on counting slides or hemocytometer. The other parameters (vitality and morphology) required equivalent sperm and preparation than manual measured (usually a 50-μL per slide smear). The most important preanalytical parameter is the presence of cell debris and round cells, notably PMNs. It must be measured beforehand because this variable will intervene in the program choice of most of system or even make it impossible to use the CASA.

Dilution and Pretreatment

WHO laboratory manuals recommend that sperm concentration measured with the CASA systems should be from 2×10^6 to 50×10^6 spermatozoa/mL.[4,5] The protocols of concentration by centrifugation and dilution are described in detail in the WHO manual. For dilution, it is recommended to centrifuge the sperm sample and diluted it with its own seminal plasma. Some suppliers propose their own dilution media and range dilution. For example, using SQA-V, it is recommended to dilute the semen sample volume by volume (1:1) if the concentration is higher than 50×10^6 spermatozoa/mL. Microptic recommends to use SCA for sperm concentrations between 5×10^6 to 95×10^6 spermatozoa/mL and, if the concentration is above, to dilute 1:20. Most CASA systems have difficulty analyzing samples with a concentration lower than 2 to 5×10^6 spermatozoa/mL regarding supplier's description. Numerous studies

reports that accuracy decreases in the case of oligozoospermia (sperm concentration lower than 15×10^6 spermatozoa/mL).[11,20,21] For the centrifuged semen sample, it should be marked in the detection report. In these conditions, motility analysis must be assessed separately from concentration measurement.

For accurate motility analyses, it is essential to ensure that there are not too many sperm on screen (high sperm concentration), and it is recommended to work within the concentration range from 2×10^6 to 20 to 50×10^6 spermatozoa/mL, depending on the CASA system. Many studies have reported that high sperm concentrations distort the results of sperm count, motility, and kinetic parameters.[5]

Staining protocols, notably for vitality and morphology analysis, are required to follow supplier recommendations and to be specifically adapted to and validated for the CASA systems. The different CASA suppliers propose commercial kits validated for their systems, but usually they can also analyze spermatozoa labeled with Papanicolaou or Shorr staining.

Sources of Errors

Many factors affect the performance of CASA systems.[11,22,23] First, it is necessary to rigorously homogenize semen sample, notably when the measuring volume is small. High-viscosity sperm is also difficult to analyze by CASA and requires mechanical or/and enzymatic pretreatment. For the SQA-V, it needs ensuring that no air bubbles are aspirated into the capillary, which could distort the wavelength measures. For the other CASA systems, the depth (10, 20, or 30 μm) and the type (Makler, Leja, and MicroCell) of sperm counting chamber influence sperm concentration and motility results and should be standardized for accurate analysis.[5,22,24,25] The WHO manual recommends scoring 2 counting chambers with a depth of 20 μm. At least 5 different fields or 200 spermatozoa should be assessed per chamber. The frame rate has also direct effect on sperm motions parameters: while 60 Hz is sufficient for the analysis of sperm concentration, motility, and general dynamics, the analysis of sperm capacitation requires 80 to 100 Hz.[26]

In the 6th edition, the WHO manual recommends analyzing motility at 37°C because sperm motion is very sensitive to temperature. The temperature of 37°C is notably required to measure sperm motion and to discriminate spermatozoa with rapid (≥ 25 μm/s) and slow (5 to <25 μm/s) progressive motility. Most CASA systems, except SQA-V, can be equipped with a temperature-controlled object stage to maintain the sample at a stable temperature.

Finally, the use of suitable quality controls, such as bead solutions with standardized concentrations and video recordings, are essential to ensure the performance and accuracy of CASA systems. Regular maintenance according to the supplier's cleaning protocols is essential, and for most systems, cleaning and self-calibration must be performed daily. Finally, considering the preparation of the sample, the choice of adapted protocol and settings, and the verification of the absence of measurement bias, it is required that the operators are properly trained to the CASA systems but also to manual analysis of standard sperm parameters. It is indeed not uncommon for the manual method to be required to assess sperm concentration and sperm motility (values below or above the acceptability thresholds of the devices). It is therefore essential to have a trained operator to take a step back from the given analyses and, to date, it is not possible to carry out CASA analysis without human intervention.

Decision Trees

To summarize, decision trees can be drawn for each system. For the SQA-V system (Fig. 11.3A), a minimal volume of 0.5 mL is required to measure sperm concentration and motility. If it is below 0.5 mL, two options are possible: to dilute by 2 to obtain of volume of 0.5 mL or to measure only PMSC and MSC with the low-volume procedure (20 μL). Both measures are useful for ART but not sufficient for a diagnostic report. If these two options do not meet the need, we must switch to manual methods. The manual method is also required if the sperm appearance is altered too much (cell debris, round cells, PMNs, red blood cells), if the viscosity is too high, if the sperm cell concentration is higher than 50 M/mL before or after dilution, or if the sperm cell concentration is lower than 2×10^6/mL. Vitality requires manual measurement using SQA-V or an external microscope. SQA-V can give a percentage of spermatozoa with typical morphology higher than 2% without quantifying specific abnormalities. This parameter may be overestimated by SQA-V and only weakly correlated with the manual method.[11] In conclusion, although limited, the SQA-V is useful as a screening tool for distinguishing between samples with normal versus abnormal concentration, motility, and morphology.

For CASA systems (Fig. 11.3B), notably Hamilton and Microptic systems, the minimal volume required is lower than what is used for manual measurement. Using commercial chambers, the volume can be lower than 10 μL for concentration and motility measurement.

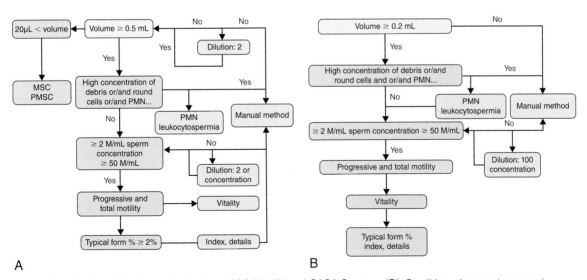

A   B

Fig. 11.3 Decision Trees for the Use of SQA-V (A) and CASA Systems (B). Conditions that require manual analysis to complement the automated analysis are presented in green. *MSC,* Motile sperm concentration, *PMN,* polymorphonuclear neutrophil; *PMSC,* progressive motile sperm concentration.

High viscosity and "dirty" sperm can be difficult to analyze, but recent versions of the different systems propose an adapted protocol to discriminate spermatozoa from other cells and debris, notably by using fluorescent labeling. Concentration of spermatozoa must be between 2 and 50 $\times$ 10^6/mL for optimal measurement. Sperm concentration can be remeasured after adapted dilution or concentration by indicating it in the system because they can distort motility and morphology analysis. Using supplementary modules, sperm vitality and PMN concentration can be measured as well as the details of abnormality, notably of the head and flagellum midpiece and principal piece.

Comparison of Automated and Manual Analysis Methods
Sperm Concentration and Total Sperm Count
The majority of studies concerning the measurement of sperm concentration and total motile sperm count show a good correlation between manual and

automated methods (Table 11.1). The study by Lammers et al. published in 2014 compares the analysis of 250 semen samples using manual and automated methods with two systems: SQA-V Gold and CASA-CEROS.[21] They show no significant difference in sperm concentration for either system, except for patients with severe oligospermia. Vernon et al.'s study published in 2014 also showed no significant difference in sperm concentration measurement between the manual and automated method with the SCA version 5.1.[27] However, the samples were not semen samples but Accu-Beads. Dearing et al. published a study, also in 2014, comparing sperm concentration measurement with SCA (version 4.0) and manual methods.[20] They showed a high correlation between the two methods ($r^2 = 0.95$, $p < 0.0001$). Engel et al.'s 2018 study of 100 semen samples showed no significant difference between manual and SQA-Vision sperm count measurement, even for oligozoospermic patients (concentration $<15 \times$ 10^6/mL).[28] However, this study reported three cryptozoospermic

TABLE 11.1 Studies Comparing Manual and Automated Methods for Sperm Parameter Assessment

Study	Comparison	Concentration	Motility	Morphology
Lammers et al., 2014	SQA-V vs. CASA CEROS vs. manual method	No difference between the three methods	No difference between the three methods	Significant difference with manual methods
Engels et al., 2018	SQA-V vs. manual method	No difference except for very low-concentration sperm (cryptozoospermia)	No difference for total motility but significant difference for progressive motility	Significant difference
Shubert et al., 2018	SCA 5.4. vs. manual method	No difference	No difference	No difference (measured with David modified classification)
Talarczyk-Desole et al., 2017	SCA 5.4 vs. manual method	Significant difference	Significant difference for progressive motility; no difference for non-progressive motility	Significant difference
Vernon et al., 2014	SCA 5.1 vs. manual method	Not different (measured with Accu-Beads)	Not achieved	Not achieved
Singh et al., 2011	SQA-V vs. manual method	Not achieved	Not achieved	High correlation for screening test
Dearing et al., 2014	SCA 4.0 vs. manual method	High correlation between the two methods	Not achieved	Not achieved
Dearing et al., 2019	SCA 4.1 vs. manual method	Not achieved	Significant difference	Not achieved

patients using the manual method who were classified as azoospermic with SQA analysis. Schubert et al.'s study published in 2019 analyzed 150 samples in manual and automated methods (by SCA) and showed no significant difference in sperm concentration measurement, even for low-concentration samples (<1 M/mL).[29] This study also analyzed the repeatability and showed that the coefficients of variation were lower with the automated method. On the contrary, the study by Talarczyk-Desole et al. in 2017 shows a significant difference for sperm concentration between the manual analysis performed on 184 semen samples using the manual method and the automated method by the SCA.[30] Overall, automated sperm concentration analysis appears to be a good alternative to the manual reference method for normozoospermic patients. This method seems less reliable when the sperm concentration is low.[31] Larger-scale studies are needed to conclude. It is probably for this reason that these CASA tests have been described as research tests, under development, by the WHO laboratory manual.

Sperm Motility

Many studies have compared manual and automated methods for sperm motility analysis (Table 11.1). The study by Lammers et al. published in 2014 compared the measurement of total motility in 250 semen samples by manual or automated methods with SQA-V Gold and CEROS and showed no significant difference in this parameter for either method.[21] In 2021, they presented similar resulting comparing manual or automated methods with SQA-V Gold and SCA.[32] Engel et al.'s 2018 study showed no significant difference in the measurement of total motility between manual and automated methods using SQA-Vision (n = 77).[28] However, the same study showed a more significant difference in progressive motility. Talarczyk-Desole et al.'s 2017 study, conducted on 184 semen samples, also showed a significant difference on progressive motility performed by manual or automated SQA method but did not show a significant difference regarding nonprogressive motility.[30] In 2019, Dearing et al.'s team analyzed the motility of more than 4400 semen samples using the SCA (version 4.1.)[33] They also showed a significant difference between the two manual and automated methods in the measurement of this parameter. In contrast, Schubert et al. compared the measurement of progressive motility on 30 samples using manual and automated (SCA) methods and showed no significant difference.[29] Hence automated motility analysis seems to be a good alternative to the manual method. In addition, automated analysis makes it easier to differentiate between rapid progressive sperm and slow progressive sperm, as recommended in the 6th edition of the WHO laboratory manual for the examination and processing of human semen.[5]

Velocity parameters. Automated analysis provides new parameters, called velocity parameters, which provide additional information to the analysis of sperm motility. The measured values are shown in Fig. 11.4 and described in the WHO laboratory manual[5] as:
- VCL, velocity along the curvilinear path (μm/s)
- VSL, velocity along the straight-line path (μm/s)
- VAP, velocity along the average path (μm/s)
- ALH, the amplitude of the lateral displacement of the head (μm)
- MAD, mean angular displacement (degrees)

Other commonly used measures are derived from the calculation of these five variables:
1. LIN, linearity
2. WOB, wobble
3. STR, straightness
4. BCF, beat-cross frequency (Hz)
5. D, fractal dimension

The measurement of these parameters is not possible by manual methods and allows the assessment of sperm hyperactivation, which is a biological process that will induce a behavioral change in the flagellar waveform. So, with these data, the measurement of sperm trajectory can be analyzed by CASA. However, a study published in 1992 shows that the depth of the chamber used (10, 20, or 200 μm) can significantly affect the results, especially in the analysis of rapid sperm movements (hyperactive sperm).[34] Zhu et al. in 1994 also showed an impact on the percentage of hyperactivation, mean VCL, mean VSL, ALH, and percentage LIN, depending on the image frequency used.[35] Kraemer et al.'s 1998 study showed variations in these analyses depending on different factors (temperature, chamber depth, gray level, image frequency, and maximum burst speed) and recommended that a set of conditions be respected for a reliable analysis.[36] Mortimer in 2015 confirmed these variations in results, depending on the depth of the chamber used.[37] Another study, also published in 1992, showed on the analysis of 30 semen samples that the kinematic variables (VSL, VCL, LIN,

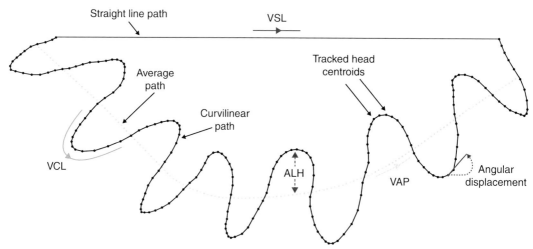

Fig. 11.4 Standard terminology for variables measured by CASA computer-assisted semen analysis systems according to the WHO. *ALH,* Amplitude of the lateral displacement of the head; *VAP,* velocity along the average path; *VCL,* velocity along the curvilinear path; *VSL,* velocity along the straight-line path. (From *WHO Laboratory Manual for the Examination and Processing of Human Semen.* 6th ed. World Health Organization 2021. https://www.who.int/publications-detail-redirect/9789240030787.)

and ALH) can vary significantly from one machine to another.[38] The automated analysis thus provides additional information that is not obtained by the manual method. It should be noted, however, that for these parameters, the WHO manual does not define reference values, which makes their interpretation difficult.

Sperm Morphology

The CASA system for the analysis of sperm morphology is also called computer-aided sperm morphology analysis. The analysis of sperm morphology by manual methods requires considerable expertise and time. Studies have focused on the analysis of sperm morphology by automated systems and the reliability of the results obtained (see Table 11.1). CASA systems have the advantage of allowing analysis of large numbers of sperm as well as greater reproducibility and accuracy.[39,40] However, the results can be distorted by the presence of debris or staining problems, especially when the count is low. Menkveld et al. in 1997 compared different stains and showed a difference in the analysis of morphology by automated methods.[41] The study conducted by Singh et al. in 2011 compared the analysis of sperm morphology on 201 semen samples from infertile males by the manual method with Papanicolaou staining and by the automated method

with the SQA-V.[19] The automated method showed a sensitivity of 85.5% and a specificity of 87.3% in detecting teratozoospermia (defined by the authors as a percentage of normal forms less than 30%, applying the WHO criteria). The authors concluded that the correlation is significant for a screening test, but the manual method remains the gold standard for sperm morphology analysis. In 2014, Lammers et al.'s study on 250 semen samples showed a significant difference between morphology measurements performed by manual or automated methods, regardless of the automaton (SQA-V Gold or CEROS).[21] In 2018, Engel et al.'s study showed significant discordance in sperm morphology measured by manual or automated methods with SQA-V (n = 74).[28] Similarly, Talarczyk-Desole et al.'s 2017 study showed a significant difference for sperm morphology between manual analysis performed on 184 semen samples using the manual and automated methods with the SCA.[30] Schubert et al.'s study published in 2019 compared morphology analysis with the modified David classification by manual and automated methods (by SCA version 5.4.0.0) on 90 samples.[29] They showed acceptable agreement between the two techniques. It should be noted that the technique for measuring sperm morphology differs for the SQA system compared to other CASA systems: the result is an estimate of the morphology thanks to an algorithm taking into account the motility results and the kinetic parameters. This system does not allow for double reading or correction by the operator. Automated analysis of sperm morphology does not seem to be reliable enough at the moment and therefore cannot be recommended as routine.

RECOMMENDATIONS, ADVANTAGES, AND DISADVANTAGES OF COMPUTER-ASSISTED SEMEN ANALYSIS SYSTEMS

International Recommendations

The good practice guide defined by the European Society for Human Reproduction and Embryology in 1998 considers that CASA systems have limited use.[42] However, technology advances of the different CASA systems had allowed improving their performances. In the 5th edition of the WHO manual,[4] CASA systems are described in advanced semen analysis. They should permit to increase objectivity and standardization of semen analysis, notably for motility and morphology. CASA systems are described in the new 6th edition of the WHO manual in the section of "advanced semen examinations."[5] The manual indicates that they are useful for the kinematic analysis of spermatozoa, but warns that percentage motility can be unreliable in the presence of cell debris. It indicates that CASA system must maintain the sample at a stable 37°C and could analyze motility of sperm samples with a concentration of between 2 and 50×10^6 spermatozoa/mL without dilution. Automated morphology analysis should permit greater objectivity, precision, and reproducibility than manual measurement. However, numerous endogenous (concentration of spermatozoa, agglutinates, cell debris, and round cells) and exogenous (sample preparation and staining, focus, illumination) factors can bias the automated measures. Despite the emerging results of comparative studies (see Table 11.1), the WHO manual states that there is still not enough evidence to allow the wide use of CASA in clinical practice. Therefore, although limited for some, CASA systems are useful as screening tools for distinguishing between samples with normal versus abnormal parameters.

Advantages

It has been suggested that CASA systems can be a valid alternative for sperm concentration and motility measurements in diagnostic practice.[21] The analysis of sperm parameters is performed on a larger number of cells, which in theory improves the accuracy of the results obtained.[39,40] In addition, automated analysis limits inter- and intraoperator variability. Since human eyes are attracted by movement, CASA systems provide objective analysis of sperm movement, if spermatozoa and cell debris concentrations are not too high. Moreover, CASA systems assess velocity parameters and can distinguish clearly between different types of motility. The discrimination of rapid, progressively motile (grade a) from slow, progressively motile (grade b) could be clinically relevant, since the number of rapid progressively motile (grade a) spermatozoa pre- and postselection are correlated with sperm cervical mucus penetration, fertilization, and pregnancy rate.[12,43-48] In addition, the analysis of sperm movement provides additional information compared to the manual method. Thus CASA allows for the detection of sperm hyperactivation abnormalities by measuring trajectory, head movements, and flagellum movements, and by analysis via algorithms.[49-51] This makes it possible to determine the ability of the sperm to pass through the cervical mucus and fertilize the oocyte. The analysis of these parameters thus allows the diagnosis of infertility associated with flagellar abnormalities and in particular, slippery spermatozoa, as shown in the study by Feneux et al. published in 1985.[52] In this study, automated analysis of four semen samples from patients with unexplained infertility revealed a form of flagellar dyskinesia not identifiable by manual methods. The sperm had a higher beat frequency and a lower beat efficiency.

Furthermore, if a CASA system is well mastered, in addition to a gain in reproducibility, it has been demonstrated as a tool than can help in saving time, reducing operator failure, and certainly providing a better analysis yield. However, the WHO does not provide reference values, and the interpretation of the results obtained can be complex. During an ART attempt, the advantage of automated analysis is that it saves a considerable amount of time and makes it possible to obtain sperm concentration and sperm motility values that allow intrauterine insemination (IUI), conventional in vitro fertilization (IVF), or intracytoplasmic sperm injection (ICSI) techniques to be performed. This allows standardization of values within a laboratory and is sufficient for sperm evaluation before insemination or fertilization. Sperm motion parameters using the CASA system were correlated with successful IVF rate.[46-48] Hirano et al. showed in 2001,[46] using a Hamilton Thorne CASA, significant correlations between fertilization rates obtained by conventional IVF and CASA velocity parameters such as ALH, VCL, VSL, and rapid progressive motility before and after swim-up. Shibahara et al. in 2004[47] showed on 682 cycles of IUI that typical sperm morphology, rapid progressive motility, VCL value, VSL value, and VAP value are correlated with pregnancy outcome. Thus CASA systems could allow a better analysis of sperm mobility and a better choice of ART technique (conventional IVF or ICSI). Studies are needed to confirm the interest of the automated method and to allow the integration of CASA analysis in the "extended semen examinations" section of the next edition of the WHO manual.

Disadvantages

The first drawback is that CASA systems and dedicated consumables and reagents are expensive.[53-56] The second is that manual intervention is necessary to control and to complete CASA results, such as determination of PMN concentration, sperm vitality, and morphology (see Fig. 11.3). Most CASA systems do measure those parameters currently. Few, such as CEROS and SCA, can perform them with additional module that increase their cost. Moreover, numerous endogenous factors can bias sperm parameters measured by CASA systems (appearance, viscosity, cell debris, agglutinates, high or low sperm concentration) and limit their use to normal or subnormal quality semen so as not to waste too much time analyzing. Numerous studies showed that CASA systems are not optimal for patients with severe oligozoospermia.[28,57] In addition, the analysis of sperm morphology seems to be limited in routine use. The performance differs from one CASA system to another, and many studies show a significant difference in results compared to the manual method.[28,30,57] Parameter settings, protocol choices, and quality control require trained operators. Thus the manual method is until today the gold standard for the analysis of sperm parameters, as confirmed by the 6th edition of the WHO laboratory manual for the examination and processing of human semen.[5]

PERSPECTIVES AND EMERGING TECHNOLOGIES

Sperm DNA Fragmentation and Acrosome Reaction Tests using Computer-Assisted Semen Analysis Systems

The most recent CASA systems offer analyses of parameters that are not in standard use. Notably, some automated systems now offer sperm DNA fragmentation analysis in complements of morphology and PMN analysis (Fig. 11.5). For example, the SCA uses the sperm chromatin dispersion (SCD) method. The SCA will then automatically capture and analyze over 500 sperm per sample. It will then classify the sperm as fragmented or unfragmented, based on halo size. Only one study, published in 2016 by Sadeghi et al., compared two commercial sperm DNA fragmentation measurement kits based on the SCD technique using the ISAS v1 automaton.[58] They show on seven semen samples a significant difference between the two kits. However, there are no studies comparing conventional and automated methods for this analysis. The measurement of sperm DNA fragmentation by automated methods has therefore not yet been proven to be effective and cannot be recommended for routine use.

The SCA-Evolution system can measure acrosome quality using agglutinin labeled with fluorescein isothiocyanate. *Arachis hypogea* (peanut) agglutinin binds the outer acrosomal membrane of spermatozoa (Fig. 11.5D). Sperm cells with their acrosomal membranes showed marked fluorescence on the acrosomal region, while those that had lost their acrosomal membrane were either devoid of fluorescence or showed a fluorescent mark along the equatorial segment.[5] To date, automated or manual analysis of the acrosomic reaction has not shown any particular clinical interest. For this reason, the WHO manual has classified these tests as "advanced semen examinations." Larger-scale studies are needed to conclude whether they are of clinical interest.

Emerging Technologies

New systems are able to follow and to analyze individually spermatozoa tracks and at much higher sperm concentration than usual CASA systems,[59] notably by following flagella waveforms.[59-62] Using new software tools[61] or new plug-ins[62] for CASA systems,

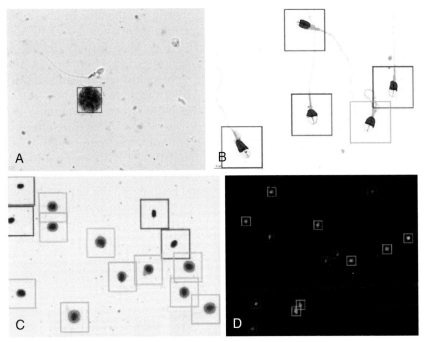

Fig. 11.5 Polynuclear/leukocytospermia (A), sperm morphology (B), sperm DNA fragmentation (C), and acrosome integrity (D) analysis using SCA Evolution.

they can visualize the head and/or flagellum of progressive cells in high-viscosity[61] or microfluidic[62] environments. Moreover, artificial intelligence (AI) methods are especially objective and suited for videos, images, text, or tabular treatments.[63,64] In recent years, algorithms have been developed that automatically learn from data without being explicitly programmed. They correspond to machine learning (ML), a subfield within AI.

Few AI systems have been also developed to detect and classify sperm motility,[64,65] kinetic motion,[49,66] and sperm DNA integrity.[67] Hicks et al. in 2019[64] compared their AI prediction of sperm motility classification against manual methods with good results. Agarwal et al.[68,69] showed high correlation between their new AI system using optical microscopic technology (Lens-Hooke® X1 PRO device) compared with IVOS CASA and manual methods regarding sperm concentration, total motility, and progressive motility. More recent studies have been performed to improve morphology assessments.[63] ML shows promise in improving notably ICSI by guiding the clinicians to objectively select sperm.[63,70] Some AI have been developed to analyze

whole spermatozoa morphology,[65,71] and others concentrate on head predicting.[60,65,72-74] Recent models for morphological assessment based on images of unstained spermatozoa are under development to improve ICSI techniques by classifying images in real time[75,76] but are not yet complete. For recognizing and interpreting images of spermatozoa at the pixel level, segmentation is the common approach.[71] Recent studies showed high classification accuracy for morphological classification,[65] and most of them have both trained and validated the models on freely available datasets/dictionaries.[74,77] These studies show how AI can be useful to classify and select spermatozoa. However, prospective multicenter studies with different cohorts and randomized controlled trials comparing these manual methods and/or CASA systems are needed to evaluate the real benefits and the routine application of these systems in clinical practice.

Numerous kits and applications, notably using smartphones equipped with high-quality digital cameras, are expanding because they are less expensive than a clinical analysis and can be done at home.[53-56,78] Besides, standard semen analysis in clinic can be laborious, and even stressful and embarrassing, which may stop patients who suffer infertility from seeking diagnostic services. Moreover, the user friendliness and cost effectiveness of home semen analysis kits increase accessibility for patients. They combine innovative technology and chromatographic immunoassays, colorimetric reactions, microfluidics, and smartphone-based microscopy.[53-56,78]

The SpermCheck Fertility test (Princeton BioMeditech Corp., Monmouth Junction, NJ, USA, Fig. 11.6) is a rapid qualitative test to detect the presence of sperm in human semen.[54] It combines solid-phase chromatographic immunoassay technology and comprises an immunochromatographic strip in a single cassette. One test strip is calibrated to give a positive result if the sperm concentration is 2×10^7 sperm/mL or greater. The Trak Male Fertility Testing System (Sandstone Diagnostics, Inc., Livermore CA, USA, see Fig. 11.6) is a more sophisticated microfluidic device that combines a colorimetric reaction with centrifugation and resistive pulse device to determine sperm cell count. It delivers results within three categories: low ($<15 \times 10^6$ sperm/mL), moderate ($15–55 \times 10^6$ sperm/mL), and optimal ($>55 \times 10^6$ sperm/mL).[53] SwimCount Sperm Quality®Test (MotilityCount ApS, Valby, Denmark) and Fertility-SCORE kits can determine the concentration of live sperm or motile sperm within a range when the sperm concentration exceeds a certain threshold.

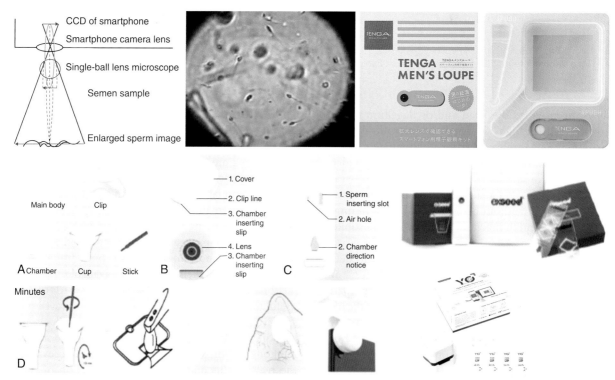

Fig. 11.6 Sperm Analysis Systems Using Smartphones. (From Kobori Y, Pfanner P, Prins GS, Niederberger C. Novel device for male infertility screening with single-ball lens microscope and smartphone. *Fertil Steril.* 2016;106(3):574-578; Onofre J, Geenen L, Cox A, et al. Simplified sperm testing devices: a possible tool to overcome lack of accessibility and inconsistency in male factor infertility diagnosis. An opportunity for low- and middle- income countries. *Facts Views Vis Obgyn.* 13(1):79-93; and Park MJ, Lim MY, Park HJ, Park NC. Accuracy comparison study of new smartphone-based semen analyzer versus laboratory sperm quality analyzer. *Investig Clin Urol.* 2021;62(6):672-680.)

They function by using an antibody reaction for colorimetric signals. SwimCount Sperm Quality Test presents the advantage to discriminate normal motile spermatozoa with low sperm DNA fragmentation using a microfluidic chamber. The males's Loupe (Tenga Health Care, Torrance, CA, USA, see Fig. 11.6), SEEM (Recruit Lifestyle Co., Ltd., Tokyo, Japan, see Fig. 11.6), O'VIEW-M PRO (Intin, Daegu, Korea, see Fig. 11.6), and ExSeed (Medical Electronics Systems, Los Angeles, CA, USA, see Fig. 11.6) are kits that use smartphones. These systems contain a lens microscope, which is inserted into a support and needs to be paired with smartphone camera for measuring sperm concentration, motility, and number of motile sperm. YO Home Sperm Test (Medical Electronics Systems, Los Angeles, CA, USA, see Fig. 11.6) uses a miniature microscope, smartphone camera, and light source to analyze sperm motility but displays only a qualitative result. Studies demonstrated that results from these different devices showed a strong correlation with CASA or manual method results[55,79-82] (see Fig. 11.6). Another example of smartphone use is Bemaner (Shenzhen Createcare Technology Co). Bemaner results showed good correlation for total and MSC ($r = 0.65$, $p < 0.001$; $r = 0.84$, $p < 0.001$, respectively) and percentage of motility ($r = 0.90$, $p < 0.001$) in comparison with manual values obtained by well-trained andrologists.[83] Most of these devices are approved by the US Food and Drug Administration and/or have European conformity (CE) marking. New approaches to home semen testing are being developed using lensless on-chip microscopy, paper-based diagnosis, or digital holography.[54] However, these devices still cannot compete with the performance of a traditional CASA system and the need for a full semen analysis performed in clinic, but they can be considered as a first screening step before consulting for infertility.

SUMMARY

Computer-assisted semen analysis (CASA) systems are equipment that use different methodologies. When a laboratory wishes to acquire these systems, it is important to know how they perform. CASA has been "relegated" to the "advanced semen examinations" section in the latest version of the World Health Organization (WHO) lab manual because there is a lack of literature to demonstrate its full utility in routine infertility diagnosis. However, some systems perform very well in assessing sperm motility and sperm count. In the context of assisted reproductive techniques (ARTs), these systems save time and can provide a standardized assessment of the characteristics of semen prepared for ART. CASA systems are evolving steadily, artificial (AI) systems are being developed, and smartphone-based sperm analysis systems are now available for home analysis. It is clear that andrology and ART are rapidly changing fields, whereas AI and automation are only just beginning. But in a few years' time, there is no doubt that these CASA systems should improve further and enable what the WHO manual has been calling for since 2010: greater reproducibility and standardization.

REFERENCES

1. Agarwal A, Baskaran S, Parekh N, et al. Male infertility. *Lancet*. 2021;397(10271):319-333. doi:10.1016/S0140-6736(20)32667-2.
2. Vander Borght M, Wyns C. Fertility and infertility: Definition and epidemiology. *Clin Biochem*. 2018;62:2-10. doi:10.1016/j.clinbiochem.2018.03.012.
3. Schlegel PN, Sigman M, Collura B, et al. Diagnosis and treatment of infertility in men: AUA/ASRM guideline part II. *Fertil Steril*. 2021;115(1):62-69. doi:10.1016/j.fertnstert.2020.11.016.
4. World Health Organization *WHO Laboratory Manual for the Examination and Processing of Human Semen*. 5th ed. Geneva: World Health Organization; 2010.
5. *WHO Laboratory Manual for the Examination and Processing of Human Semen*. 6th ed. World Health Organization; 2021. Available at: https://www.who.int/publications-detail-redirect/9789240030787.
6. Tomlinson MJ. Uncertainty of measurement and clinical value of semen analysis: has standardisation through professional guidelines helped or hindered progress? *Andrology*. 2016;4(5):763-770. doi:10.1111/andr.12209.
7. Keel BA, Quinn P, Schmidt CF, Serafy NT, Serafy NT, Schalue TK. Results of the American Association of Bioanalysts national proficiency testing programme in andrology. *Hum Reprod*. 2000;15(3):680-686. doi:10.1093/humrep/15.3.680.
8. Auger J, Eustache F, Ducot B, et al. Intra- and inter-individual variability in human sperm concentration, motility and vitality assessment during a workshop involving ten laboratories. *Hum Reprod*. 2000;15(11):2360-2368. doi:10.1093/humrep/15.11.2360.
9. David G, Serres C, Jouannet P. Kinematics of human spermatozoa. *Gamete Res*. 1981;4(2):83-95. doi:10.1002/mrd.1120040202.

10. Katz D, Dott H. Methods of measuring swimming speed of spermatozoa. *J Reprod Fertil.* 1975;45:263-272. doi:10.1530/jrf.0.0450263.

11. Finelli R, Leisegang K, Tumallapalli S, Henkel R, Agarwal A. The validity and reliability of computer-aided semen analyzers in performing semen analysis: a systematic review. *Transl Androl Urol.* 2021;10(7):3069-3079. doi:10.21037/tau-21-276.

12. Mortimer ST, van der Horst G, Mortimer D. The future of computer-aided sperm analysis. *Asian J Androl.* 2015;17(4):545-553. doi:10.4103/1008-682X.154312.

13. Bartoov B, Ben-Barak J, Mayevsky A, Sneider M, Yogev L, Lightman A. Sperm motility index: a new parameter for human sperm evaluation. *Fertil Steril.* 1991;56(1):108-112. doi:10.1016/s0015-0282(16)54427-6.

14. Mahmoud AM, Gordts S, Vereecken A, et al. Performance of the sperm quality analyser in predicting the outcome of assisted reproduction. *Int J Androl.* 1998;21(1):41-46. doi:10.1046/j.1365-2605.1998.00090.x.

15. Martínez C, Mar C, Azcárate M, Pascual P, Aritzeta JM, López-Urrutia A. Sperm motility index: a quick screening parameter from sperm quality analyser-IIB to rule out oligo- and asthenozoospermia in male fertility study. *Hum Reprod.* 2000;15(8):1727-1733. doi:10.1093/humrep/15.8.1727.

16. Shibahara H, Suzuki T, Obara H, et al. Accuracy of the normal sperm morphology value by Sperm Quality Analyzer IIC: comparison with the strict criteria. *Int J Androl.* 2002;25(1):45-48. doi:10.1046/j.1365-2605.2002.00322.x.

17. Fuse H, Akashi T, Nozaki T, Nishio R, Mizuno I. Assessment of sperm quality analyzer II B: comparison with manual semen analysis and CASA. *Arch Androl.* 2005;51(1):65-67. doi:10.1080/014850190513012.

18. Akashi T, Mizuno I, Okumura A, Fuse H. Usefulness of sperm quality analyzer-V (SQA-V) for the assessment of sperm quality in infertile men. *Arch Androl.* 2005;51(6):437-442. doi:10.1080/014850190959081.

19. Singh S, Sharma S, Jain M, Chauhan R. Importance of papanicolaou staining for sperm morphologic analysis: comparison with an automated sperm quality analyzer. *Am J Clin Pathol.* 2011;136(2):247-251. doi:10.1309/AJCPCLCSPP24QPHR.

20. Dearing CG, Kilburn S, Lindsay KS. Validation of the sperm class analyser CASA system for sperm counting in a busy diagnostic semen analysis laboratory. *Hum Fertil (Camb).* 2014;17(1):37-44. doi:10.3109/14647273.2013.865843.

21. Lammers J, Splingart C, Barrière P, Jean M, Fréour T. Double-blind prospective study comparing two automated sperm analyzers versus manual semen assessment. *J Assist Reprod Genet.* 2014;31(1):35-43. doi:10.1007/s10815-013-0139-2.

22. Lu JC, Huang YF, Lü NQ. Computer-aided sperm analysis: past, present and future. *Andrologia.* 2014; 46(4):329-338. doi:10.1111/and.12093.

23. Yeste M, Bonet S, Rodríguez-Gil JE, Rivera Del Álamo MM. Evaluation of sperm motility with CASA-Mot: which factors may influence our measurements? *Reprod Fertil Dev.* 2018;30(6):789-798. doi:10.1071/RD17475.

24. Dardmeh F, Heidari M, Alipour H. Comparison of commercially available chamber slides for computer-aided analysis of human sperm. *Syst Biol Reprod Med.* 2021;67(2):168-175. doi:10.1080/19396368.2020.1850907.

25. Mortimer ST. CASA—practical aspects. *J Androl.* 2000;21(4):515-524. doi:10.1002/j.1939-4640.2000.tb02116.x.

26. Bompart D, García-Molina A, Valverde A, et al. CASA-Mot technology: how results are affected by the frame rate and counting chamber. *Reprod Fertil Dev.* 2018;30(6):810-819. doi:10.1071/RD17551.

27. Vernon DD, Johnson JE, Houwing AM, Higdon HL, Boone WR. Accu-Beads as a quality control measure for manual and automated methods of measuring sperm concentration—an observational study. *J Assist Reprod Genet.* 2014;31(1):25-33. doi:10.1007/s10815-013-0107-x.

28. Engel KM, Grunewald S, Schiller J, Paasch U. Automated semen analysis by SQA Vision® versus the manual approach-A prospective double-blind study. *Andrologia.* 2019;51(1):e13149. doi:10.1111/and.13149.

29. Schubert B, Badiou M, Force A. Computer-aided sperm analysis, the new key player in routine sperm assessment. *Andrologia.* 2019;51(10):e13417. doi:10.1111/and.13417.

30. Talarczyk-Desole J, Berger A, Taszarek-Hauke G, Hauke J, Pawelczyk L, Jedrzejczak P. Manual vs. computer-assisted sperm analysis: can CASA replace manual assessment of human semen in clinical practice? *Ginekol Pol.* 2017;88(2):56-60. doi:10.5603/GP.a2017.0012.

31. Yis OM. Comparison of fully automatic analyzer and manual measurement methods in sperm analysis and clinical affect. *Exp Biomed Res.* 2020;3(4):224-230. doi:10.30714/j-ebr.2020463605.

32. Lammers J, Chtourou S, Reignier A, Loubersac S, Barrière P, Fréour T. Comparison of two automated sperm analyzers using 2 different detection methods versus manual semen assessment. *J Gynecol Obstet Hum Reprod.* 2021;50(8):102084. doi:10.1016/j.jogoh.2021.102084.

33. Dearing C, Jayasena C, Lindsay K. Can the Sperm Class Analyser (SCA) CASA-Mot system for human sperm motility analysis reduce imprecision and operator subjectivity and improve semen analysis? *Hum Fertil (Camb).* 2021;24(3):208-218. doi:10.1080/14647273.2019.1610581.

34. Lannou DL, Griveau JF, Pichon JPL, Quero JC. Effects of chamber depth on the motion pattern of human spermatozoa in semen or in capacitating medium. *Hum Reprod.* 1992;7(10):1417-1421. doi:10.1093/oxfordjournals.humrep.a137585.

35. Zhu JJ, Pacey AA, Barratt CLR, Cooke ID. Computer-assisted measurement of hyperactivation in human

spermatozoa: differences between European and American versions of the Hamilton-Thorn motility analyser. *Hum Reprod*. 1994;9(3):456-462. doi:10.1093/oxfordjournals.humrep.a138527.

36. Kraemer M, Fillion C, Martin-Pont B, Auger J. Factors influencing human sperm kinematic measurements by the Celltrak computer-assisted sperm analysis system. *Hum Reprod*. 1998;13(3):611-619. doi:10.1093/humrep/13.3.611.

37. Mortimer D, Mortimer S, van der Horst G. The future of computer-aided sperm analysis. *Asian J Androl*. 2015;17(4):545. doi:10.4103/1008-682X.154312.

38. Davis RO, Katz DF. Standardization and comparability of CASA instruments. *J Androl*. 1992;13(1):81-86.

39. Garrett C, Baker HW. A new fully automated system for the morphometric analysis of human sperm heads. *Fertil Steril*. 1995;63(6):1306-1317.

40. Menkveld R, Stander FSH, Kotze TJ, Kruger TF, van Zyl JA. The evaluation of morphological characteristics of human spermatozoa according to stricter criteria. *Hum Reprod*. 1990;5(5):586-592. doi:10.1093/oxfordjournals.humrep.a137150.

41. Menkveld R, Lacquet FA, Kruger TF, Lombard CJ, Sanchez Sarmiento CA, de Villiers A. Effects of different staining and washing procedures on the results of human sperm morphology evaluation by manual and computerised methods. *Andrologia*. 1997;29(1):1-7. doi:10.1111/j.1439-0272.1997.tb03141.x.

42. Guidelines on the application of CASA technology in the analysis of spermatozoa. ESHRE Andrology Special Interest Group. European Society for Human Reproduction and Embryology. *Hum Reprod*. 1998;13(1):142-145.

43. Barratt CLR, Björndahl L, Menkveld R, Mortimer D. ESHRE special interest group for andrology basic semen analysis course: a continued focus on accuracy, quality, efficiency and clinical relevance. *Hum Reprod*. 2011;26(12):3207-3212. doi:10.1093/humrep/der312.

44. Larsen L, Scheike T, Jensen TK, et al. Computer-assisted semen analysis parameters as predictors for fertility of men from the general population. The Danish First Pregnancy Planner Study Team. *Hum Reprod*. 2000;15(7):1562-1567. doi:10.1093/humrep/15.7.1562.

45. Mortimer D, Pandya IJ, Sawers RS. Relationship between human sperm motility characteristics and sperm penetration into human cervical mucus in vitro. *J Reprod Fertil*. 1986;78(1):93-102. doi:10.1530/jrf.0.0780093.

46. Hirano Y, Shibahara H, Obara H, et al. Relationships between sperm motility characteristics assessed by the computer-aided sperm analysis (CASA) and fertilization rates in vitro. *J Assist Reprod Genet*. 2001;18(4):213-218. doi:10.1023/a:1009420432234.

47. Shibahara H, Obara H, Ayustawati null, et al. Prediction of pregnancy by intrauterine insemination using CASA estimates and strict criteria in patients with male factor infertility. *Int J Androl*. 2004;27(2):63-68. doi:10.1111/j.0105-6263.2004.00437.x.

48. Sivanarayana T, Krishna ChR, Prakash GJ, et al. CASA derived human sperm abnormalities: correlation with chromatin packing and DNA fragmentation. *J Assist Reprod Genet*. 2012;29(12):1327-1334. doi:10.1007/s10815-012-9885-9.

49. Goodson SG, White S, Stevans AM, et al. CASAnova: a multiclass support vector machine model for the classification of human sperm motility patterns. *Biology of Reproduction*. 2017;97(5):698-708. doi:10.1093/biolre/iox120.

50. Mortimer D, Mortimer ST. Computer-Aided Sperm Analysis (CASA) of sperm motility and hyperactivation. *Methods Mol Biol*. 2013;927:77-87. doi: 10.1007/978-1-62703-038-0_8.

51. Ooi EH, Smith DJ, Gadêlha H, Gaffney EA, Kirkman-Brown J. The mechanics of hyperactivation in adhered human sperm. *R Soc Open Sci*. 2014;1(2):140230. doi:10.1098/rsos.140230.

52. Feneux D, Serres C, Jouannet P. Sliding spermatozoa: a dyskinesia responsible for human infertility? *Fertil Steril*. 1985;44(4):508-511.

53. Gonzalez D, Narasimman M, Best JC, Ory J, Ramasamy R. Clinical update on home testing for male fertility. *World J Mens Health*. 2021;39(4):615-625. doi:10.5534/wjmh.200130.

54. Kobori Y. Home testing for male factor infertility: a review of current options. *Fertil Steril*. 2019;111(5):864-870. doi:10.1016/j.fertnstert.2019.01.032.

55. Park MJ, Lim MY, Park HJ, Park NC. Accuracy comparison study of new smartphone-based semen analyzer versus laboratory sperm quality analyzer. *Investig Clin Urol*. 2021;62(6):672-680. doi:10.4111/icu.20210266.

56. Onofre J, Geenen L, Cox A, et al. Simplified sperm testing devices: a possible tool to overcome lack of accessibility and inconsistency in male factor infertility diagnosis. An opportunity for low- and middle- income countries. *Facts Views Vis Obgyn*. 13(1):79-93. doi:10.52054/FVVO.13.1.011.

57. Lammers J, Splingart C, Barrière P, Jean M, Fréour T. Double-blind prospective study comparing two automated sperm analyzers versus manual semen assessment. *J Assist Reprod Genet*. 2014;31(1):35-43. doi:10.1007/s10815-013-0139-2.

58. Sadeghi S, Garca-Molina A, Celma F, Valverde A, Fereidounfar S, Soler C. Morphometric comparison by the ISAS® CASA-DNA system of two techniques for the evaluation of DNA fragmentation in human spermatozoa. *Asian J Androl*. 2016;18(6):835-839. doi:10.4103/1008-682X.186875.

59. Urbano LF, Masson P, VerMilyea M, Kam M. Automatic tracking and motility analysis of human sperm in time-

lapse images. *IEEE Trans Med Imaging.* 2017;36(3): 792-801. doi:10.1109/TMI.2016.2630720.

60. Wei SY, Chao HH, Huang HP, Hsu CF, Li SH, Hsu L. A collective tracking method for preliminary sperm analysis. *Biomed Eng Online.* 2019;18(1):112. doi:10.1186/s12938-019-0732-4.

61. Gallagher MT, Cupples G, Ooi EH, Kirkman-Brown JC, Smith DJ. Rapid sperm capture: high-throughput flagellar waveform analysis. *Hum Reprod.* 2019;34(7): 1173-1185. doi:10.1093/humrep/dez056.

62. Elsayed M, El-Sherry TM, Abdelgawad M. Development of computer-assisted sperm analysis plugin for analyzing sperm motion in microfluidic environments using Image-J. *Theriogenology.* 2015;84(8):1367-1377. doi:10.1016/j.theriogenology.2015.07.021.

63. Riegler MA, Stensen MH, Witczak O, et al. Artificial intelligence in the fertility clinic: status, pitfalls and possibilities. *Hum Reprod.* 2021;36(9):2429-2442. doi:10.1093/humrep/deab168.

64. Hicks SA, Andersen JM, Witczak O, et al. Machine learning-based analysis of sperm videos and participant data for male fertility prediction. *Sci Rep.* 2019;9(1): 16770. doi:10.1038/s41598-019-53217-y.

65. Ilhan HO, Sigirci IO, Serbes G, Aydin N. A fully automated hybrid human sperm detection and classification system based on mobile-net and the performance comparison with conventional methods. *Med Biol Eng Comput.* 2020;58(5):1047-1068. doi:10.1007/s11517-019-02101-y.

66. Valiuškaitė V, Raudonis V, Maskeliūnas R, Damaševičius R, Krilavičius T. Deep learning based evaluation of spermatozoid motility for artificial insemination. *Sensors (Basel).* 2020;21(1):72. doi:10.3390/s21010072.

67. McCallum C, Riordon J, Wang Y, et al. Deep learning-based selection of human sperm with high DNA integrity. *Commun Biol.* 2019;2(1):1-10. doi:10.1038/s42003-019-0491-6.

68. Agarwal A, Panner Selvam MK, Ambar RF. Validation of LensHooke® X1 PRO and computer-assisted semen analyzer compared with laboratory-based manual semen analysis. *World J Mens Health.* 2021;39(3):496-505. doi:10.5534/wjmh.200185.

69. Agarwal A, Henkel R, Huang CC, Lee MS. Automation of human semen analysis using a novel artificial intelligence optical microscopic technology. *Andrologia.* 2019;51(11):e13440. doi:10.1111/and.13440.

70. You JB, McCallum C, Wang Y, Riordon J, Nosrati R, Sinton D. Machine learning for sperm selection. *Nat Rev Urol.* 2021;18(7):387-403. doi:10.1038/s41585-021-00465-1.

71. Movahed RA, Mohammadi E, Orooji M. Automatic segmentation of sperm's parts in microscopic images of human semen smears using concatenated learning approaches. *Comput Biol Med.* 2019;109:242-253. doi:10.1016/j.compbiomed.2019.04.032.

72. Ilhan HO, Serbes G. Sperm morphology analysis by using the fusion of two-stage fine-tuned deep networks. *Biomedical Signal Processing and Control.* 2022;71:103246. doi:10.1016/j.bspc.2021.103246.

73. Chandra S, Gourisaria MK, GM H, et al. Prolificacy assessment of spermatozoan via state-of-the-art deep learning frameworks. *IEEE Access.* 2022;10:13715-13727. doi:10.1109/access.2022.3146334.

74. Chang V, Garcia A, Hitschfeld N, Härtel S. Gold-standard for computer-assisted morphological sperm analysis. *Comput Biol Med.* 2017;83:143-150. doi:10.1016/j.compbiomed.2017.03.004.

75. Javadi S, Mirroshandel SA. A novel deep learning method for automatic assessment of human sperm images. *Comput Biol Med.* 2019;109:182-194. doi:10.1016/j.compbiomed.2019.04.030.

76. Abbasi A, Miahi E, Mirroshandel SA. Effect of deep transfer and multi-task learning on sperm abnormality detection. *Comput Biol Med.* 2021;128:104121. doi:10.1016/j.compbiomed.2020.104121.

77. Shaker F, Monadjemi SA, Alirezaie J, Naghsh-Nilchi AR. A dictionary learning approach for human sperm heads classification. *Comput Biol Med.* 2017;91:181-190. doi:10.1016/j.compbiomed.2017.10.009.

78. Yu S, Rubin M, Geevarughese S, Pino JS, Rodriguez HF, Asghar W. Emerging technologies for home-based semen analysis. *Andrology.* 2018;6(1):10-19. doi:10.1111/andr.12441.

79. Kobori Y, Pfanner P, Prins GS, Niederberger C. Novel device for male infertility screening with single-ball lens microscope and smartphone. *Fertil Steril.* 2016;106(3): 574-578. doi:10.1016/j.fertnstert.2016.05.027.

80. Cheon WH, Park HJ, Park MJ, et al. Validation of a smartphone-based, computer-assisted sperm analysis system compared with laboratory-based manual microscopic semen analysis and computer-assisted semen analysis. *Investig Clin Urol.* 2019;60(5):380-387. doi:10.4111/icu.2019.60.5.380.

81. Agarwal A, Panner Selvam MK, Sharma R, et al. Home sperm testing device versus laboratory sperm quality analyzer: comparison of motile sperm concentration. *Fertil Steril.* 2018;110(7):1277-1284. doi:10.1016/j.fertnstert.2018.08.049.

82. Yoon YE, Kim TY, Shin TE, et al. Validation of SwimCount™, a novel home-based device that detects progressively motile spermatozoa: correlation with World Health Organization 5th semen analysis. *World J Mens Health.* 2020;38(2): 191-197. doi:10.5534/wjmh.180095.

83. Tsai VF, Zhuang B, Pong YH, Hsieh JT, Chang HC. Web- and artificial intelligence–based image recognition for sperm motility analysis: verification study. *JMIR Med Inform.* 2020;8(11):e20031. doi:10.2196/20031.

12

Seminal Oxidative Stress and Reactive Oxygen Species Testing

Faith Tebatso Moichela, Ralf Reinhold Henkel, and Kristian Leisegang

KEY POINTS

- Reactive oxygen species (ROS) are essential for sperm physiological function and overall reproductive function in males.
- Oxidative stress (OS) due to excessive ROS or inefficient availability of antioxidants impairs male fertility.
- The role of OS in physiology and pathology warrants robust testing, with high sensitivity and specificity for research and clinical practice.

- Indirect and direct tests enable quantitative measurement of seminal ROS/antioxidants, but their clinical application is inherently limited by some disadvantages in terms of costs, time, ease of use, and standardization.
- Evidence suggests that a combination of tests may provide a comprehensive overview on levels of seminal ROS.

INTRODUCTION

It is widely understood that cyanobacteria paved the way for the multicellular life through the production of oxygen as a byproduct of cellular metabolism, and contributed to the Great Oxidation Event.[1,2] The increased oxygen concentration in the earth's atmosphere nearly 2.3 billion years ago necessitated an evolutionary adaptation of early life to toxic oxygen, necessitating the transformation of Archean life forms into more complex eukaryotes.[3] Consequently, there was a rapid diversification of multicellular life, supported by increased energy production through the emergence of aerobic respiration and mitochondria,[1,4,5] which, according to the endosymbiont hypothesis, developed from cyanobacteria that were ingested by archaea. Mitochondria reside in the cytoplasm of eukaryotic cells, where they mediate numerous physiological and pathophysiological functions, including the production of adenosine triphosphate (ATP), alongside reactive oxygen species (ROS) as a by-product. Furthermore, mitochondria contribute to cell proliferation, calcium metabolism,

lipid signaling, immune regulation, steroidogenesis, membrane biogenesis, autophagy, and apoptosis.[6]

A stable atom or molecule in a neutral state contains a complementary set of valence electrons in its outer orbit and is relatively inert.[7] Radicals are molecules with a single, unpaired electron in their outer orbit. Atmospheric oxygen is a diatomic diradical and remains in this state, as its electrons are in a parallel spin, until it and/or its derivatives are reduced to chemically unstable free radicals with an unpaired electron in their orbit.[8] Although not all ROS are technically reactive free radicals, their successive reduction produces highly reactive by-products; hence these reactive oxygen molecules are collectively referred to as "ROS."[7,8] In an attempt to reach an electrochemically inert state, the unstable electrons in their outer orbit will drive oxidative reactions in a cell.[9,10]

During mitochondrial oxidative phosphorylation (OxPHOS), ATP is produced via the electron transport chain (ETC) through a series of five transmembrane protein complexes of the respiratory chain.[6,10] Notably, complexes I, III, and IV use nicotinamide adenine dinucleotide as a substrate.[6,10,11] The utilization of oxygen in this way results in an inevitable leakage of electrons from the respiratory chain complexes I and III.[6,10] Superoxide ($O_2\cdot^-$) is the principal ROS produced through the mitochondrial OxPHOS in most mammalian cells, and it serves as the precursor of other endogenous ROS. Subsequently, $O_2\cdot^-$ is rapidly transformed into hydrogen peroxide (H_2O_2) through enzymatic or spontaneous dismutation.[7] Superoxide also reacts with H_2O_2 to form hydroxyl ($OH\cdot^-$) molecules in the presence of copper and iron,[7,12] with nitric oxide to form peroxynitrite ($ONOO^-$), and with chloride to form hypochlorite (ClO^-).[7,8] Other radicals formed in subsequent reductions or oxidations are singlet oxygen,($^1O_2$), hydroxyl ($OH\cdot$), peroxyl ($ROO\cdot$), and alkyl ($RO\cdot$) radicals.[7,8,13]

Physiologically, at low concentrations, ROS mediate numerous intracellular pathways, acting as phosphorylating/dephosphorylating switches in redox biology.[7,10] ROS act as modulators of cell division, caspases, kinases, phosphatase switches, and modifiers of synaptic plasticity of ion channels and receptors.[10] Furthermore, ROS regulate key genomic elements of signal transduction, such as transcription factors, and modify promoter proteins, in addition to playing a direct role in apoptosis, autophagy, immunity signaling, aging, and cell differentiation.[10,14,15]

In male reproduction, physiological levels of ROS serve as intracellular and extracellular messengers for essential processes such as spermatogenesis, epididymal sperm maturation, capacitation, acrosome reaction, hyperactivated motility, sperm–oocyte binding, fertilization, and pre- and postembryonic events.[7,11,16] Extrinsic and intrinsic factors play a role in the production of excess ROS, which culminates in seminal oxidative stress (OS), which causes sperm lipid peroxidation (LPO), sperm DNA damage, apoptosis, and eventually male infertility.[11,13,17] Excess ROS in the seminal fluid emanates from the spermatozoa and the leukocytes.[7,18,19]

Increasing ROS levels in the evolution of eukaryotes and multicellular organisms necessitated counteracting protective or regulatory systems that are commensurate with ROS production rates for optimum functionality. Antioxidants are substances produced endogenously or synthetically that decrease, confine, scavenge, delay, or completely inhibit cell damage arising from oxidizing agents, thereby maintaining redox balance in biological systems.[20,21] Endogenous antioxidants, such as catalase, glutathione, and superoxide dismutase (SOD), evolved

to neutralize excessive ROS in biological systems.[20,22,23] Exogenous antioxidants include vitamins, minerals, polyphenols, and amino acid analogs such as carnitines, cysteines, and glutamine[18,24,25] and have proven beneficial in neutralizing harmful ROS in OS.[25-27] Notwithstanding, excessive or dysregulated antioxidant supplementation can induce reductive stress, which is as detrimental to male reproductive processes as its redox counterpart, OS.[28,29] Therefore both extremes of the redox balance warrant-specific, reproducible, cost-effective, time-conserving tests that can reliably and rapidly detect seminal OS in males with unexplained or idiopathic infertility[18,30] and thereby provide indications of male fertility potential.

A number of different tests are available for direct and indirect ROS detection, such as chemiluminescence, fluorescence, DNA fragmentation assays, total antioxidant capacity (TAC), and oxidation-reduction potential (ORP).[18,31] This chapter aims to discuss the sources of ROS in the seminal milieu, their physiological role, OS, and their clinical assessment in the male fertility work-up.

SOURCES OF REACTIVE OXYGEN SPECIES IN THE MALE REPRODUCTIVE TRACT

Endogenous Reactive Oxygen Species
Defective and Immature Spermatozoa

During the last stage of spermiogenesis, spermatogonia extrude excess residual cytoplasm that is then phagocytosed by Sertoli cells before the sperm are released into the lumen to be transported into the epididymis for maturation.[32] In the event that spermatogenesis is disturbed or prematurely arrested, the midpiece of released spermatids will remain disproportionately unshed, which is strongly associated with male infertility.[33] Furthermore, immotile and defective spermatozoa also produce high levels of ROS.[11] The surplus intercellular space harbored by the residual cytoplasm is endowed with an armory of metabolic enzymes such as glucose-6-phosphate dehydrogenase, lactic acid dehydrogenase, and creatinine kinase.[33] The former dehydrogenases act putatively to increase the availability of nicotinamide adenine dinucleotide phosphate (NADPH) through the hexose monophosphate shunt, which exacerbates NADPH oxidase–based ROS production at the sperm membrane level.[9,17] While some authors have argued a protective value of the cytoplasmic droplets in containing free-radical antioxidant enzymes such as glutathione in other mammalian species,[11] in the human, their role in seminal oxidative physiology is unanimously recognized as defective when the cytoplasmic droplets are larger than one-third of the sperm head.[33]

Leukocytes

Leukocytes play a crucial role in immunosurveillance and inflammatory responses; however, their known role in the seminal plasma remains largely associated with testicular dysfunction and male infertility.[34-36] Testicular leukocytes originate from accessory gland secretions, with significant polymorphonuclear neutrophils (PMNs) deriving from the rete testis or the epididymis. PMNs and macrophages make up the bulk of the ROS-producing leukocytes in the testis, ranging between 50% and 60% and 30% and 20%, respectively.[36-48]

In the presence of genitourinary infections, leukocytes can produce 1000 times more ROS than sperm. In addition, leukocytes can cause a secondary immune response characterized by the release of proinflammatory cytokines.[13] Increased concentrations of leukocytes are closely associated with excessive seminal ROS, leading to impaired sperm motility, morphology, and viability.[34,35] However, some studies could not find any correlational or causative relationship between increased seminal leukocytes and biomarkers of seminal oxidative damage or even suggest that leukocytes may have beneficial roles.[39-42]

Exogenous Reactive Oxygen Species
Environmental Toxins, Pollution, Heat, and Radiation

Exposure to environmental and industrial pollutants, such as phthalates, pesticides, glycol ethers, dioxinlike compounds, perflourinated compounds, bisphenol A, polychlorinated biphenyls, plasticizers, and dioxins, has received increased attention due to their ubiquitous application in the manufacturing sector.[43,44] The increased release of these compounds into the environment has led to increased exposure of people to these substances, with increased serum levels of these toxins in human populations. In particular, the testes exhibit a unique susceptibility to the damaging effects of pollutants and toxins, especially those with endocrine-disrupting properties.[45-47] Among other mechanisms, these chemicals compromise the integrity of the blood–testis barrier,

which precipitates disruption in spermatogenesis, spermiogenesis, and sperm DNA integrity. Additionally, they may alter the lipid profile, increase lipid oxidation, and in turn, negatively affect the steroidogenic apparatus, sperm motility, capacitation, and acrosome reaction.[43,48] Accumulation, degradation, and metabolism of such compounds and/or their intermediates are also widely documented to negatively affect the hypothalamic-pituitary-testicular axis, thereby altering the hormonal balance.[49]

Genital heat stress is induced when the testicular temperature rises 2°C to 5°C above the baseline temperature and reportedly suppresses spermatogenesis, with a resultant decrease in semen quality.[50] Males may also be exposed to elevated temperatures through their workplace, such as foundry, glass, steel industries, bakeries, kitchens, and mines.[51,52] Testicular hyperthermia is further caused by sedentary occupations and lifestyles (sauna therapy, obesity, long-distance driving, cycling), clothing (tight underwear), and seasonal ambient temperatures.[51-53] Pathological conditions such as cryptorchidism and varicocele increase OS and sperm DNA fragmentation, partly through genital heat stress.[50] Ionizing/non-ionizing radiation increases scrotal temperature through interfering with surface conductive thermoregulation, which is vulnerable to electromagnetic waves.[13,50] Hyperthermic testicular OS is propagated through sperm mitochondrial degeneration, impaired ATP synthesis, antioxidant depletion, and alteration of the functional proteins, resulting in a culmination of pathological crosstalk that is mediated by OS and followed by defective sperm motility, acrosome reaction, increased apoptosis, and infertility.[54,55] Additionally, exposure of the genitourinary tract to high concentrations of heavy metals such as lead, arsenic, cadmium, mercury, selenium, copper, zinc, and manganese has been implicated in suboptimal semen quality and dysregulated antioxidant function, given their dualistic functions as adjuvants of enzymatic antioxidant enzymes and prooxidant systems.[46,51,55]

Individual Lifestyle Factors

Personal lifestyle factors such as smoking, alcohol consumption, use of recreational drugs, poor dietary habits, sleep deprivation, and work-related and non–work-related sedentary tendencies contribute to physical and psychological burden, especially in modern-day lifestyle.[13,46] These stressors may singly or synergistically promote accumulation of chemicals, toxins, metabolic intermediates, and by-products, which may shift the redox balance in favor of oxidants.[46,56] An increase in the oxidative status increases proneness to inflammation, type 2 diabetes mellitus, hypertension, hyperinsulinemia, obesity, and cardiovascular, autoimmune, and neurodegenerative diseases and infertility (see reviews[56,57]).

Evidence suggests a multidirectional, complex interplay of pathogenic mechanisms involving OS and other systemic derangements relating to male fertility.[46,58] For instance, chronic inflammation in metabolic derangement manifestations has been associated with the mitochondrial dysfunction, increased DNA damage, altered expression of antioxidant genes, hypogonadotropic hypogonadism, defective steroidogenesis, impaired semen parameters, and reduced fertility, as well as increased heritable epigenetic modifications in males.[13,46,58] Global increments in the prevalence of noncommunicable diseases unsurprisingly appear to increase in tandem with male infertility.[59,60] While numerous hypotheses have been proposed in linking the pathophysiologic factors involved in the eventual reproductive dysfunction, it is clear that OS and impaired inflammatory responses are the central molecular mediators of this progressive derangement, especially in the testes, and warrant further inquiry.[61]

ANTIOXIDANT REGULATION OF REACTIVE OXYGEN SPECIES IN THE MALE REPRODUCTIVE TRACT

Endogenous Antioxidants in the Male Reproductive Tract

Antioxidants neutralize deleterious effects of oxidation chain reactions by removing reactive intermediates through electron donation.[12] When the oxidizing potential of radicals is interrupted or delayed, the cascade of redox reactions and their potential toxicity is confined, reduced, or completely inhibited.[12,22] This coordinated regulation of redox homeostasis is achieved through interrelated endogenous and exogenous antioxidative free-radical scavenging systems, with the latter class supplied through diet.[22] Mammalian cells, including spermatozoa, have evolved to endogenously synthesize enzymatic antioxidants such as catalase (CAT),

SODs/superoxide reductases, glutathione peroxidases (GPx), and peroxiredoxins, and nonenzymatic antioxidants such as glutaredoxins or thioredoxins that are intracellularly synthesized in the diminutive cytoplasm of the spermatozoa and have also been characterized in the seminal fluid, suggesting vesicular or prostatic origin.[62,63]

Interestingly, proteomics revealed that polymorphisms of a number of genes such as NRF2, GST, GPx, SOD, or CAT have been linked to male infertility.[64] The activities between seminal enzymatic antioxidants SOD, CAT, and GPx, as well as their relationship with malondialdehyde (MDA), revealed that antioxidants confer protection to spermatozoa against peroxidative attacks inflicted by MDA.[63] These classes of antioxidant systems are found in either the cytosolic or extracellular spaces of the spermatozoa. Their catalytic efficiency is dependent on micronutrient cofactors such as zinc, selenium, copper, iron, and manganese.[12,65]

Additionally, bilirubin, ubiquitin, glucose-6-phosphate dehydrogenase, uric and lipoic acid, and melatonin offer antioxidant capacities that mediate mitochondrial function and ATP synthesis, thereby regulating sperm motility, ROS production, capacitation, hyperactivation, and acrosome reaction.[20,22,58,66] In fact, the antioxidative capacities of urate, thiol, albumin, and ferritin were found to be significantly reduced in infertile males compared to their fertile counterparts. The reduction was reportedly accompanied by increased sperm peroxidative damage confirmed by the levels of MDA and a reduction in total and progressive motility.[67] Melatonin, other than regulating circadian rhythms, exhibits antioxidant properties and is recommended for reducing age-related OS. In the testis, melatonin offers antioxidative properties through increased expression of antioxidant genes and suppression of leukocytospermia.[66] Metal-chelating, -sequestering, and -storing glycoproteins such as ferritin, lactoferrin, transferrin, ceruloplasmin, albumin, haptoglobin, and hemopexin exist in the sperm microenvironment and attenuate redox chain reactions in the testicular tissue, particularly at the sperm plasma membrane.[20,22,63] Albumin self-oxidizes, thereby sparing the adjacent sperm from ROS attack.[17] Plasmalogen and prostasomes have demonstrated free-radical quenching properties in various biological systems, including the seminal fluid.[22] Despite the assortment of endogenous defense mechanisms in the testis, sperm remain vulnerable to OS; hence dietary supplementation with antioxidants is proposed.[64]

Exogenous Antioxidants

Endogenous radical-quenching systems are complemented by non-enzymatic dietary or exogenously sourced antioxidants such as vitamins (ascorbates, tocopherols, retinols, carotenoids), lycopenes, polyphenols, and phenolic acids that can be derived from diet or herbal medicines.[20,58,68] Additional exogenous antioxidants involved in the neutralization of excess ROS in the reproductive tract are L-carnitine, lutein, L-acetyl carnitine, N-acetyl-cysteine, coenzyme Q10 (ubiquinol), selenium, taurine/hypotaurine, inositol, zinc, folate, zeaxanthin, and pentoxifylline.[25,26,69] These antioxidants are able to quench ROS, suppress pathways precipitating production of $O_2\bullet^-$ or its peroxidative sister radical hydrogen peroxide, and act as adjuvants or cofactors in the enzymatic or other formulations of antioxidants.[19,63,70] On the other hand, misuse or high intake of antioxidants will impair fundamental reproductive functions in which moderate ROS play a signaling role. Notwithstanding, excessive seminal ROS require neutralization that is not sufficiently fulfilled by the endogenous seminal antioxidants; hence it is reasonable to introduce exogenous supplementation.

Overdosage of Antioxidants and Reductive Stress

Gutteridge and Halliwell alluded to the "antioxidant paradox," which highlighted the dangers of overutilization or supplementation of dietary antioxidants with little or no quantifiable preventative or therapeutic effect.[71,72] While the mediatory role of OS in male infertility is comprehensively documented, there remain gaps in the understanding of the effects of reductive stress on male reproduction, as excess antioxidants may impair sperm functions as well.[29] Antioxidant therapy is recommended for infertile males when OS is identified as a cause of male infertility but can cause harm if the redox balance is pushed into a reductive stress situation by a high or inappropriate mixture of antioxidants.

Vitamin C, vitamin E, N-acetyl L-cysteine, carnitine, and coenzyme 10 (CoQ10), as well as selenium, zinc, and folic acid are commonly prescribed to infertile males.[25,29] Data reveal cases where such therapy could improve and restore seminal parameters, reverse damage, and confer protection against OS damage in infertile males.[24,28,26] However, it should be noted that other randomized clinical trials, including Cochrane studies, were unable to corroborate the acclaimed benefits of antioxidant supplementation in infertile males; instead, they reported an increase in levels of sperm DNA fragmentation and chromatin decondensation and no consistent data on improvement of live birth rates in infertility treatment–seeking couples.[25,73,74] Agarwal and collaborators have shed light on the discrepancies associated with arbitrary supplementation of antioxidants.[24] Among other concerns, lack of standardized dosages, small sample sizes, bias, poor methodologies, inconsistent reporting on clinical outcomes, and use of various combinations were found to add to the controversy and skepticism of antioxidant therapy for improvement of male semen parameters.[25,27,29,73,74]

PHYSIOLOGICAL ROLE OF REACTIVE OXYGEN SPECIES IN MALE REPRODUCTION AND FERTILITY

Despite their potential as damaging intermediates of aerobic respiration, ROS are critical to male reproductive physiology.[7] Key transcriptional and translational pathways in sperm functional signaling require a balanced redox state comprising a specific type and limited amount of ROS.[8,75] For instance, small quantities of seminal ROS promote oxidation and extrusion of cholesterol within the membrane and increase its fluidity during initiation of capacitation.[17,76,77] Additionally, ROS levels orchestrate the activation of Src kinases, accompanied by inhibition of the tyrosine/serine/threonine phosphatase; both occurrences induce a consequent increase in cyclic adenosine monophosphate (cAMP) pathways by Ca^{2+} or bicarbonate, which are essential in cytoplasmic alkanization.[9,77] Furthermore, ROS regulates downstream activation of protein kinase A (PKA), which is crucial for efficient sperm capacitation and acrosome reaction pathways, including the mitogen-activated protein kinase (MAPK) and extracellular-regulated kinase (ERK), as well phosphoinositide-3 kinase (PI3K)/Akt, and lastly, tyrosine phosphorylation of target proteins. ROS mediates spermatogenesis, sperm chromatin compaction, epididymal sperm maturation, chemotaxis, sperm–oocyte fusion, and maintains optimal viability post ejaculation.[7,78]

PATHOLOGICAL EFFECTS OF OXIDATIVE STRESS IN MALE REPRODUCTION

Lipid Peroxidation

Sperm membranes constitute a rich diversity of polyunsaturated fatty acids (PUFAs).[79] PUFAs are essential for membrane fluidity and flexibility, which augment capacitation, hyperactivation, and acrosome reaction.[80] At the same time, this unique composition renders this diminutive cell especially vulnerable to oxidative and peroxidative insults.[81] The susceptibility to peroxidative damages is due to their inherent excess ROS-generating tendencies, coupled with the limited cytoplasmic volume, which translates to reduced antioxidant availability and inability to repair or correct peroxidative damage themselves.[13,82,83] The presence of double bonds causes a weak methyl-carbon-hydrogen bond, which consequently makes the unattached hydrogen vulnerable to free radical attack in the sperm plasma membranes.[69,84]

In a self-perpetuating autocatalytic manner, ROS attacks of PUFA precipitate peroxyl (ROO•) and alkyl (RO•) radicals.[83] These radicals propagate cyclical generation of peroxides and further unstable radicals, especially in the presence of metals such as copper and iron in adjacent membranes unless counteracted by endogenous antioxidants.[69,82,83] Besides peroxides, further lipid breakdown by the abovementioned radicals produces highly reactive aldehydes, hydroxynonenal or alkenals (4-HNE and 2-propenal), isoprostanes, and ultimately a stable product, MDA. The former products have demonstrated pronounced genotoxic and mutagenic properties in sperm.[69,85] The unattenuated propagation of LPO propels a pathological chain reaction of damaging ROS and end products and ultimately precipitates mitochondrial dysfunction, poor motility, oxidation of ETC proteins and chromatin, and DNA damage in the sperm.[16,69,83]

Chromatin and DNA Damage

Although the human sperm nuclear DNA is highly compacted in protamines, it remains accessible to harmful effects of OS.[9,17] Spermatozoal DNA damage occurs through the following mechanisms: abortive apoptosis, defective compaction or incomplete protamination during spermiogenesis, the activity of endonucleases, unfavorable epididymal microenvironment, and lastly,

oxidative assaults through OS.[17,40] OS can directly oxidize guanosine components, yielding adducts such as 8-hydroxy-2-deoxyguanosine (8-OHdG), 1,N^6-etheno-2′-deoxyadenosine (ϵdA) ϵAdo, and 1,N^6-etheno-2′-deoxyguanosine (ϵdG), with the former resulting from a hydroxyl attack on the base and often assayed as a biomarker of oxidative DNA damage.[69] Thus higher sperm DNA fragmentation indices consistently correlate with poor motility, viability, mitochondrial membrane potential, capacitation, and acrosome reaction.[39,40,86] Additionally, sperm DNA damage exhibits strong negative correlations with reproductive outcomes such as fertilization, implantation, embryogenesis, pregnancy, and live birth.

Spermatozoa with oxidatively damaged DNA can successfully fertilize the ovum, although the embryos may not develop beyond blastocyst or early fetal state when the paternal genome is switched on.[17,87] In the event that damaged sperm DNA is extensive or evaded oocyte repair mechanisms and successfully fertilized an ovum, as may be the case in intracytoplasmic sperm injection (ICSI), the outcomes can be profoundly dire for the resulting offspring, especially when genetic defects involve Y-chromosome modifications.[17,87] Although poorly documented, childhood morbidities, reduced life span, and susceptibility to cancers are some of the repercussions for the offspring produced from DNA-damaged sperm.[17]

Apoptosis

Apoptosis balances the number of germ cells with the Sertoli cells' "nursing" capacities in ontogenic testes, while ensuring phagocytic clearance of excess or deformed sperm cells during spermatogenesis in adult testes.[40,69] When the homeostatic pathways are disrupted by stress, such as excess ROS, the cells are programmed by default to enter an intrinsic programmed death in a controlled manner.[40] The process is characterized by an assemblage of apoptotic genes such Fas, BAX, BAK1, BcL-x, phosphatidylserine, NOXA, and some caspases.[40,69] Following activation of other apoptogenic factors from the mitochondria, cytochrome c is released and triggers the effector caspases 3 and 9, which promote spermatozoal demise.[13,69] The expression of the aforementioned markers is pronounced in infertile semen samples in comparison to fertile ones.[69]

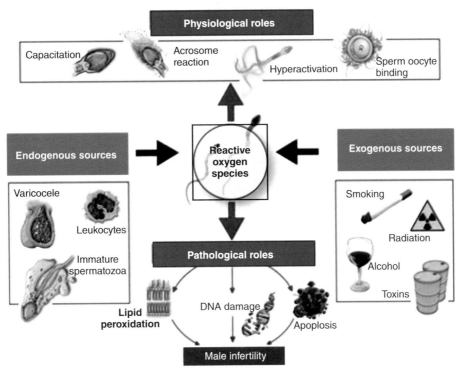

Sources of ROS in male infertility.

SEMINAL BIOMARKERS OF REACTIVE OXYGEN SPECIES AND OXIDATIVE STRESS

To date, various tests to determine ROS and seminal OS have been developed and marketed for their effectiveness in detecting, localizing, and quantifying OS in the seminal plasma and the spermatozoa themselves. Direct assays assess the level of ROS produced proportional to available oxidants or ROS producers, while indirect methods quantify the amount of ROS resulting secondary to ROS-induced damage to plasma membrane (lipids), DNA, and proteins and the antioxidant efficiency in neutralizing oxidants.[18]

Direct Methods
Chemiluminescence

Chemiluminescence is predominantly used for direct ROS quantification in clinical and research andrological laboratories. Perhaps its extensive application is due the high specificity and sensitivity.[18,88] The assay uses a luminometer (single/double or multiple) and luminescent probes to measure the intensity of light produced during a chemical reaction.[88] The most commonly used luminescent probes are luminol and lucigenin, which react with intracellular and extracellular ROS intermediates, and their excitation is quantified and expressed as relative light units (RLU), photons per minute, or millivolts per second (mV/s).[18,89]

The principle of the assay is oxidation or reduction of redox- or non–redox-sensitive probes producing light.[18] The intensity of the light in both probes depends on the concentration of endoperoxide or dioxetane, which is further metabolized to an excited product.[89] Lucigenin reacts specifically with extracellular $O_2^{\bullet-}$,[88] while luminol is preferred to its counterpart partly due to its diffusive characteristics, which allow indiscriminate detection of various ROS including $O_2^{\bullet-}$, H_2O_2, and $OH^{\bullet-}$.[18,77] The assay also has relatively well established ranges for distinguishing fertile and infertile males.[77] The set-up for luminol-based chemiluminescence includes a blank, a negative control, the test sample, and the positive control.[77] The inability to differentiate the sources of ROS in heterogeneous fluids such as semen and the costs associated with the luminometry apparatus limit its clinical use.[18,77] Furthermore, luminol chemiluminescence is produced by various chemical reactions in the sperm microenvironment, the probe is prone to oxidation at increased temperatures, and luminol requires large volumes of semen to reliably quantify levels of ROS (outlined in Table 12.1).[51,85]

Lastly, chemiluminescence is affected by other interfering factors such as prolonged incubation time, seminal pH, viscosity, and PMN contamination; hence these factors should be considered during interpretation of results. Nevertheless, chemiluminescence is touted as the accurate technique for ROS quantification in both diagnostic and research laboratories.

Intracellular Reactive Oxygen Species

Flow cytometry. Flow cytometry is a sophisticated technology that rapidly quantifies chemophysical properties of a single cell or subpopulations through multiparametric analysis.[90] The technique uses laser beams as sources of visible light that analyze intracellular and cellular expressions of molecules in individual cells or populations as they pass through a rapidly flowing fluid where the signals are transduced by either photodiode or photomultiplier tubes.[90,91] Cells can simultaneously be characterized for different features based on the type of probes used and their fluorescent intensities.[91] In both instances, light and fluorescent signals are converted into electrical signals analyzed by a cytometer and computationally normalized to a standard format (.fcs).[90]

The technology is suitable for heterogeneous mixtures such as semen, as it permits characterization of various populations of sperm suspensions (dead, live, DNA-damaged, apoptotic immature, round cells, PMNs, oxidatively or peroxidatively stressed cells). The system is also specialized to quantify the expression of seminal and spermatozoal biomarkers produced by these cells based on their light-scattering or fluorescent tendencies.[10,82,83,91] For ROS determination, sperm subpopulations are "gated" or sorted based on their $O_2^{\bullet-}$-producing capacities, in which 10,000 sperm-specific or non–sperm-specific events are captured by means of either fluorescence or light scattering (see configurations for excitation and emission wavelengths and filters in previous publications[82,83]).

Interestingly, flow cytometry can be combined with fluorescence where fluorochromes are localized by either confocal or scanning microscope.[82,83,92] For sperm

mitochondrial $O_2^{\bullet-}$ detection, fluorescent probes that measure mitochondrial ROS and the vitality of live ROS-producing sperm are utilized to yield high-throughput, accurate, reproducible analysis of ROS produced intracellularly.[82,83] The only limitations to the application of cytometry are costs required for the set-up, maintenance and the technical expertise (see Table 12.1).[91]

Fluorescence Microscopy

Fluorescence is a phenomenon that describes the two-phase process where light is absorbed at a shorter wavelength by a chemical fluorophore that is subsequently excited to emit light at a longer wavelength.[93] The spectral change in fluorescence enables visualization and localization of proteins, chromosomes, DNA, RNA, ROS, and other markers.[30]

For seminal and spermatozoal ROS, detection is achievable with fluorescent and labeling agents such dihydroethidium, hexyl triphenylphosphonium, monobromobimane (mbbr), and SYTOX Green for quantification of sperm mitochondrial ROS.[89,94] Another fluorophore for detection of ROS production in defective spermatozoa is nonfluorescent 2,7-dichlorofluorescein diacetate (DCFH2-DA). The probe is stable and cell impermeable; however, it deesterifies to a fluorescent 2,7-dichlorofluorescein in the presence of H_2O_2 and forms of ROS such as ONOO−, ClO−, and OH•.[40] Dihydrorhodamine, dihydroxyphonoxazine, etc. are also nonfluorescent dyes that produce highly fluorescent products when reacted with H_2O_2, in some instances ONOO−, cytochrome C, and ascorbates.[94,95]

Hydrocyanines such as hydro-Cy3, hydro-Cy5, and hydro-Cy7 have gained considerable relevance in in vivo and in vitro imaging of ROS intermediates. Although these fluorogenic sensors detect $O_2^{\bullet-}$ and OH• at very low concentrations, their weak fluorescence, autooxidation, and low solubility limit their clinical application.[96] The hydroxyl radical (OH•) in seminal preparations can be indirectly detected by non-fluorescent probes such as 1,3-chlorohexanedione, sodium terephthalate, coumarin/coumarin intermediates, etc., where hydroxylation of the probes produce fluorescent compounds that emit signals.[95] Additionally, dipyridamole and diphenyl-1-pyrenylphosphine are antioxidant-assessing fluorescent probes. They indirectly measure ROO•, OH•, and $O_2^{\bullet-}$ accumulation in biological samples, which is inversely proportional to the radical scavenging activity of antioxidants.[95]

TABLE 12.1 The Strengths and Limitations of Direct Tests for Quantification of Seminal Levels of Oxidative Stress

Direct Tests	Strengths	Limitations
Chemiluminescence	• High specificity and sensitivity	• Inability to distinguish between ROS sources, • Requires a large semen sample (800 µL) • High costs for luminometry apparatus • Prone to interferences with pH, temperature • Long incubation time • Sensitivity may be altered by the presence of reducing agents • Not suitable for analyzing azoospermic and hyperviscous samples
Intracellular measurement by fluorescence and cytometry	• Analyzes predefined subpopulations of sperm at high speed • Portable machinery • Quantifies multiple sperm parameters simultaneously • The techniques can be applied singly or in conjunction	• Requires expensive machinery and maintenance • Usage requires prior training/expertise
Nitroblue tetrazolium	• Easy to use, cost effective, and highly sensitive to ROS produced by various source in heterogeneous semen populations • Detects ROS at low concentrations of leukocytes (0.5×10^6 cells/mL)	• The presence and levels of oxidoreductases limit specificity for ROS • Interpretation of results is subjective to the observer
Cytochrome c reduction	• Low sensitivity but detects high production of extracellular ROS from neutrophils; has low specificity	• Electrons can be donated by other molecules or oxidases, which limits specificity for superoxide or NADPH activity; low levels of intracellular ROS are undetectable
Electron spin resonance	• Highly sensitive to various types of oxidative intermediates at low concentrations • Spin adducts from cyclic hydroxylamine have long half-lives • Highly specific to compounds with unpaired electrons • Detects high levels of ROS	• Metals, temperatures (requires ultracold temperatures), reducing agents, chemical and magnetic fields may affect spin adduct formation, spontaneous oxidation of spin-reagents • Hydroxylamine derivatives are always one nitrous compound (indistinguishable oxidants)
Oxidation-reduction potential	• Fast, easy to use, reliable, highly sensitive and specific system • The procedure is user friendly and requires no technical experience • Requires low volumes of semen (30 µL) • It functions as an advanced and independent indicator of reductants and oxidants in the semen sample • It has established cut-off values for both infertile and fertile males	• The running and maintenance costs of the entire system can be prohibitive • The technique is not suitable for viscous and azoospermic samples • There may be overlaps in cut-off values; interpretation should be supplemented by results from other tests (preferably direct)

NADPH, Nicotinamide adenine dinucleotide phosphate; *ROS*, reactive oxygen species.

Fluorescein and its derivatives, such as fluorescein isothiocyanate, are commonly conjugated into biological molecules, and fluorescein is oxidized by most free radicals.[89,94,95] Acridine orange (AO) is a fluorescent dye used for the evaluation of DNA damage that may indirectly measure ROS.[18,89,94] These dyes are often used to directly or indirectly assess both intracellular and extracellular ROS levels and can be used in conjunction with counterstains/DNA interchelators such as propidium iodide (PI), Hoechst stain, ethidium bromide (EtBr), *etc.* for indication of viability of the sperm producing ROS.[94] Alternatively, acetylated non-fluorescent membrane dyes such as SYBR-14 and SYTO-1 exhibit intense fluorescence when they incorporate sperm into intact plasma membrane; that way, ROS-producing sperm can be separated as live, apoptotic, or dead.[94] Fluorescence offers a promising approach for quantitative and qualitative visualization of ROS generation and resultant sperm damage; however, its application is still limited by labor-intensive assays, costly reagents, detection hardware, and lack of standardization for assisted reproduction.[30,82,94]

Nitroblue Tetrazolium Test

The nitroblue tetrazolium (NBT) test is often preferred for its affordability and its user-friendly properties. The principle of the assay is based on the ability of cytoplasmic molecules to reduce NBT (2,2'-bis[4-nitrophenyl]-5,5'-diphenyl-3,3'-[3,3'-dimethoxy-4,4'-diphenylene] ditetrazolium chloride) to purple-blue, water-insoluble precipitates of formazan, which are assessed with a microscope or spectrophotometer.[18,31,89] Typically, NADPH facilitates formation of superoxide through the oxidase system in the sperm and leukocytes.

The diformazan crystals can be released into extracellular environments by solubilizing agents such as dimethyl sulphoxide (DMSO) and measured spectrophotometrically at an absorbance range of 530 to 630 nm.[97] ROS production is expressed as μg formazan/10^7 sperm.[97] The percentage of NBT-positive cells is strongly negatively associated with sperm motility, concentration, and DNA integrity. It also shows a positive relationship with abnormal sperm, apoptosis, and excessive ROS production. Although widely applied due to its high sensitivity, the NBT test remains largely unused in clinical andrology. The reservations often cited in literature include observer subjectivity, the ability of any reductase enzyme in the seminal plasma to reduce NBT (creating false-positives), and the lack of clearly established cut-off values for male infertility from large cohorts (see Table 12.1).[77]

Cytochrome c Reduction

Cytochrome c is a small, water-soluble pro-apoptotic mitochondrial protein interspersed between the compartments of the inner and outer membranes of various proteins complexes of the ETC.[10] Apart from signaling early apoptotic status in a cell, the protein facilitates electron transfer between protein complexes III and IV of the ETC. Its role in the cellular respiratory events has been well established.[9]

In this technique, a ferricytochrome c reagent is loaded to sperm suspensions, where its iron-heme center is reduced to ferrocytochrome c through the NADPH-dependent reductase.[30,31] The colorimetric changes are followed using a spectrophotometer configured at a wavelength of 550 nm.[30,31] A buffer, a positive control (NADPH reductase), SOD enzyme, and oxidase inhibitor solution are required.[30,31] The rate at which SOD is able to inhibit ferricycytochrome reduction provides an estimate of the amount of superoxide that is extracellularly present and is expressed as the NADPH-cytochrome c reductase units.[31]

The clinical usage of this assay is still sparse, which may be partly due to its inability to detect intracellular ROS in sperm suspensions due to ferricytochrome c not penetrating membranes.[18,30] The test is only sensitive to substantial amounts of superoxide with high reductase activity. Any reductase in the sperm immediate environment can reduce ferricytochrome c and will provide an artifactual signal whose change in absorbance is not specific to $O_2^{\bullet-}$ (see Table 12.1).[30,31]

Electron Spin Resonance

This technique takes advantage of ROS's diminutive size, ubiquitous nature, and short half-life (nanoseconds to seconds) in biological systems.[30] Electron spin resonance (ESR) characterizes electrons by their kinetic behavior and spin energy (shift in absorption spectra) when a magnetic field is applied.[9] For ROS and nitrogen species to be identified, the ESR technique requires an ESR magnetic spectroscope and spin-trapping compounds and/or probes.[98] Spin traps bind covalently to ROS, while spin probes get oxidized to form unreactive intermediates.[30] The spin-trapping resonance commonly uses nitrous compounds: nitroso- and nitrone-based 5,5-dimethyl-1-pyrroline-*N*-oxide.[30,98] Essentially, the spin-trap reagent binds to a free radical molecule to form a spin-trap adduct that possesses a characteristic long life that can be quantified spectroscopically in terms of g-value, hyperfine coupling constant, and concentration.[98]

On the other hand, spin probes require the transfer of one electron to form a stable nitroxide that is detectable by ESR.[30] Various cyclic hydroxylamine probes (reviewed elsewhere[30]) form stable paramagnetic derivatives.[30,98] The ESR techniques offer objective means of detecting and determining ROS levels due to their ability to differentiate various types of ROS. Their limited application is due to their proneness to chemical and magnetic interferences. Buffers and metal chelators are required for efficient spin adduct formation, and the presence of antioxidants or any free radical–scavenging agent will inhibit any nitroxide or spin adduct formation (see Table 12.1).[30,98] While this method is widely employed for seminal plasma compositions and proteomic analyses, it is not employed in the clinical andrological setting for quantification of site-specific seminal ROS.

Oxidation Reduction Potential

ORP is a novel approach in the quantification of seminal OS.[18,26,77] ORP assesses the balance between oxidants and reductants as a function of the propensity of electrons to be transferred from one electrochemical entity to the next, thus measuring both sides of the redox balance. In this context, the ORP expresses real-time potential of electron movement from reductants to oxidants using galvanostatic circuitry (MiOYXSYS), and the calculated voltage difference is measured in mV.[18,31,69] The MiOYXSYS comprises an electrometer (analyzer) and a sensor that compares the voltage between the standard electrode and that of the semen sample. The results need to be normalized to the seminal sperm concentration and are expressed as mV/sperm concentration/mL (mV/10^6 cells/mL).[18] The measurement takes about 4 minutes and is thus much quicker than all other methods.

In its latest laboratory manual, the World Health Organization (WHO) lists this technique in Chapter 4, "Advanced Examinations."[77] The MiOYXSYS is comparatively easy to operate, requires little or no prior expertise, and rapidly provides the redox status in a relatively small semen sample (30 μL), and the results are reproducible in similar study designs.[18,77] However, its diagnostic and/or prognostic indications should be interpreted cautiously, as there seems to be no consensus yet on definitive threshold values.[77] For instance, in 2016, the normalized cut-off value for normal semen quality was set at 1.36 mV/10^6 sperm/mL, while cut-off value for identifying infertile from fertile males was set at 1.42 mV/10^6 sperm/mL. However, similar multicenter comparative studies reported the cut-off value to differentiate normal and abnormal semen quality to be 1.34 mV/10^6 sperm/mL, with 1.42 mV/10^6 sperm/mL distinguishing infertile males from fertile males.[18,31] In addition, these cut-off values were not established by using reproductive outcome parameters such as fertilization, pregnancy, or live birth as classification variables but distinguished between sperm donor and patient attending an andrology clinic.

The first study that used reproductive outcomes (fertilization, blastocyst development, implantation, pregnancy, and live birth) to calculate a cut-off value reported a value of 0.51 mV/10^6 sperm/mL after ICSI (Henkel et al., 2022),[99] a value that is even lower than the one published by Gill and coworkers for proven fertile males of 0.81 mV/10^6 sperm/mL.[100] Despite its robustness, the measurement of ORP is not recommended in cases of viscous and severe oligozoospermic or azoospermic samples.[18] Therefore ORP can be used in conjunction with other techniques to provide a complete redox picture in both fertile and infertile males.

Indirect Methods
Lipid Peroxidation

Determination of malondialdehyde. MDA is a potently reactive aldehyde produced as an end product of LPO.[16,82] The principle of the thiobabituric acid (TBA)-reactive substances (TBARS) is based on the reaction of MDA with two molecules of the TBA, forming an MDA:TBARS adduct whose red color is assessed by means of colorimetry or fluorometry.[9,69] Low levels of MDA are detectable by means of high-performance liquid chromatography (HPLC) or spectrofluorometry due to their sensitivity and specificity.[9,63] Although the TBA method is one of the oldest methods to evaluate membrane LPO and the resultant peroxidative damage, its inferences regarding OS-induced infertility require careful considerations. First of all, MDA is not the only by-product of sperm LPO, neither is it the only peroxidative aldehyde with which TBARS reacts. Lastly, not all LPO reactions end up with MDA produced as the end product (Table 12.2).[101] The assay furthermore requires appropriate controls, and HPLC is a sophisticated quantification system not readily available in every clinical and research setting.

***C11-BODIPY*[581/591]**. The C11-BODIPY[581/591]assay is seldom utilized for the quantification of human sperm LPO. However, it has been applied to bull, boar, stallion, rat, and equine spermatozoa.[82,83] Although quantification of "classic" LPO by-products paint a clear picture of the extent to which sperm plasma membrane unsaturated fatty acid had been oxidized, it falls short in indicating the subcellular resolution the membrane undergoes throughout the LPO.[63,92] Also, the levels of these by-products do not provide any information regarding which cytoskeletal elements of a single sperm cell are the preferred target for ROS attack (head, midpiece, or flagellum), nor do they indicate sperm subpopulations with increased sensitivity to LPO (see Table 12.2).[82,83,92]

For these reasons, alternative fluorescent fatty acid probes were developed. The fluorescent lipophilic analog 4,4-difluoro-5-(4-phenyl-1,3-butadienyl)-4-bora-3a,4a-diaza-s-indacene-3-undecanoic acid (C11-BODIPY[581/591]) offers unique properties for monitoring LPO, as it readily incorporates into the plasma membrane, eliminating artifacts with uptake and absorption of the probe by other organelle debris in the sperm microenvironment.[92] The dye is preferred for penetration-visualization studies due to its hydrophobic, photostable, readily adjustable photochemical behavior, as well as its sharp excitation/emission spectra.[102] Upon incorporating in the cell, C11-BODIPY[581/591] intercalates with intact membranes, producing an intense red fluorescence. As it undergoes further oxidation by any of the ROS or peroxynitrites, there is a spectral emission shift to an orange and intense green fluorescence to indicate advanced LPO.[82,92]

The probe can be visualized by epifluorescence and confocal microscopy, and the extent of LPO as measured by fluorescence intensity can be quantified by flow cytometry or a fluorescence multiplate reader.[82,92] It is apparent that this ratiometric fluorescent sensor provides a thorough quantification of LPO in the spermatozoa; however, a limitation to its widespread use remains the enormous expense, such as that of the confocal microscope and flow cytometry equipment.[82,83,92,103] Also, a mass spectrometric study found the assay to overestimate the extent of oxidative lipid damage, with accompanied underdetection of the reducing effect of α-tocopherol, as well as the probe

TABLE 12.2 **The Strengths and Limitations of Indirect Tests Used for Quantification of Levels of Seminal Oxidative Stress**

Indirect Tests	Strengths	Limitations
Lipid Peroxidation		
Malondialdehyde	• Rapid and easy to use without expertise • Fluorometric analysis may be relatively affordable	• The assay requires proper controls for reliability • Not all LPO reactions end up with MDA as the by-product • TBARS are not specific to MDA (react with other LPO adducts) • For low LPO detection, HPLC is a high-cost/high-maintenance detection system
C11-BODIPY[581/591]	• High specificity and sensitivity for localization and visualization of LPO • Provides site-specific visualization of sperm LPO • Provides information on the sperm cytoskeletal elements prone to ROS attack • The probe is resistant to environmental changes in the sperm milieu	• The assay is prone to exaggeration of the extent of single cell oxidative damage • The probe reportedly exhibits reductive potential, which interferes with true depiction of LPO in sperm cells (under detection of true antioxidant effect of reducing agents) • High costs required flow cytometric apparatus

HPLC, High-performance liquid chromatography; *LPO,* lipid peroxidation; *MDA,* malondialdehyde; *ROS,* reactive oxygen species; *TBARS,* thiobabituric acid–reactive substances.

exerting an antioxidative capacity of its own (summarized in Table 12.2).[104]

Myeloperoxidase

The latest WHO manual recommends orthotoluidine and the peroxidase-positive tests (granulocytes) for evaluation of leukocytospermia and recognizes the condition when white blood cells (WBCs) exceed the threshold of $1 \times 10^6/mL$ in semen samples.[41,105] The myeloperoxidase (Endtz) is an alternative to the abovementioned tests for assessing the presence of male genital tract infection, which has associations with seminal OS and male infertility.[38,41,106] This assay takes advantage of the ability of peroxidase-containing granulocytes to oxidize benzidine to an insoluble blue/brown compound that can be easily assessed by means of brightfield microscopy. This way, immature germ cells and other cellular debris are distinguished from the WBCs responsible for seminal ROS overproduction.[19,35] Despite its simplicity, the assay should be used in concert with other ROS-detecting techniques, as it is unable to give an account of the amount of ROS produced by the spermatozoa themselves; also, it is unable to detect peroxidase-devoid granulocytes (see Table 12.2).[69]

Sperm DNA Fragmentation

Terminal deoxynucleotidyl transferase–mediated deoxyuridine triphosphate nick ending labeling assay. Terminal deoxynucleotidyl transferase (TdT)-mediated deoxyuridine triphosphate (dUTP) nick ending labeling (TUNEL) has emerged as gold standard in predicting the fertilizing capacity in infertile males.[39] The assay works on the principle that fragmented DNA will have 3′-OH exposed terminals that can be fluorescently monitored through an enzymatic incorporation of dUTP.[18,40] The enzyme TdT transfers fluoresceinated dUTP to terminal 3'-OH of single- and double-strand breaks, and the labeled nucleotides can be quantified and followed by means of flow cytometry or fluorescence. Various commercial kits are available for assessing these breaks in DNA.[39] The assay is robust, requires low sample numbers, and can be performed with or without expensive equipment. Despite its high sensitivity, this assay remains to be standardized in both research and validated clinical studies (see Table 12.2).[31]

Sperm chromatin structure assay. The sperm chromatin structure assay (SCSA) assay is based on the susceptibility of DNA or chromatin structural integrity to acid or heat denaturation.[31] Briefly, the assay assesses the percentage of sperm with single- and/or double-strand DNA fragmentation by a metachromatic shift in fluorescence. This SCSA assay uses a cell-permeable fluorescent dye that transverses the sperm plasma membrane easily, Acridine orange (AO) to assess the sperm chromatin integrity. The monomeric binding of the fluorophore (AO) to native double-stranded DNA tends to produce an intense green fluorescence, while the polymeric intercalation with single-stranded DNA gives off a red fluorescence.[31,94] The summative reaction of AO and sperm DNA strands can be analyzed by means of cytometry or epifluorescence and expressed as DNA fragmentation index or high DNA stainability.[31,94] The assay requires a flow cytometer, and the user needs to be trained (see Table 12.2). Further, the assay requires that temperature and other laboratory conditions be maintained optimally, as slight changes in either produce significant changes in the results. On the other hand, the test is standardized and has a protocol in place. It is only proprietary without commercial kits. Just as with many of these assays, the SCSA yields variable observer differences either in the same laboratory or between laboratories.[18,31]

Sperm chromatin dispersion test. The sperm chromatin dispersion test, just like the SCSA, indirectly evaluates the susceptibility of deproteinized chromatin to acid denaturation. For this assay, sperm suspensions are dispersed in a low-melting agarose matrix after being lysed in an acid solution. Subsequently, the cells are stained with the 4′,6-diamidino-2-phenylindole (DAPI) or the stain provided in the kit. Intact DNA forms loops, resulting in characteristic halos, whereas damaged DNA does not form these loops.[31] The lack of halos or the formation of very small halos is indicative of DNA-damaged spermatozoa. The halo is visualized and determined using a bright-field or fluorescent microscope. This test is preferred for its rapid, simple, hassle-free application, with reproducible results that can be corroborated and correlated to those obtained from the SCSA (see Table 12.2). Despite not requiring fluorescence or light color intensity, being highly standardized, simple, fast and easy to use, there is not sufficient clinical reporting on the utility of this assay.[31]

Comet assay. The Comet assay is seldom performed in diagnostic laboratories, perhaps due to lack of standardized protocols. Referred to as single-cell gel electrophoresis, this assay separates DNA-fragmented sperm cells based on the exposed charges following exposure of loose DNA supercoils.[94] There are two different types of comet assays; namely the neutral comet, which detects double-stranded DNA breaks, and the alkaline comet which detects both double- and single-stranded DNA breaks. Cells are applied to a thin layer of agarose gel. When an electric field is applied, cleaved fragments of DNA migrate out of the sperm nucleus towards the positively charged pole of the anode.[31] The comet tail is monitored microscopically after staining with EtBR or DAPI.[94] The shape and length of a comet tail around the sperm head circumference correspond with the severity of sperm DNA damage in males with variable semen quality.[31] The assay is not immune to subjectivity and it is likely irreproducible. Although the technique is highly sensitive to variable levels of sperm DNA damage, it is arduous to perform and remains unstandardized. Another impediment to its clinical uptake is the strict requirement for a fresh semen sample, as well as interobserver variability, compounded by the need for the observer to be experienced (see Table 12.2).[31]

Total Antioxidant Capacity

The assay measures the total reductive capacities conferred by both enzymatic and non-enzymatic antioxidants, including macromolecules.[69] The assay is based on the combinational capacity of all antioxidants in the seminal plasma to reduce the 2,20-azino-di-[3-ethylbenzthiazolinesulfonate] (ABTS) to an ABTS·+ radical cation following exposure of a neat semen sample to H_2O_2. The proton-donating potential of all present antioxidants should inhibit the absorption of the ABTS radical at a maximum wavelength of 734 nm (750 nm in seminal plasma) compared to that of Trolox (vitamin E analog) used as the standard.[22,18] The combined reductive power of antioxidant in the system is measured colorimetrically, with a reference limit for normal or efficient seminal antioxidants set at 1950 micromoles of Trolox.[18] This implies that semen samples with a lower ROS-TAC score indicate a disequilibrium in favor of oxidants and also denotes reduced antioxidants ability to scavenge or suppress seminal OS.[22,18,26]

SUMMARY

Despite the important role of ROS in sperm to trigger essential physiological functions, if produced in excess, they cause a pathological state of OS when not acted upon by antioxidants. OS has been established as an independent etiological factor in male infertility.

Therefore time- and cost-effective, robust, and highly standardized methods for measuring OS are crucial in the management of male infertility. Despite numerous WHO-recommended techniques, their application presents pros and cons that require careful consideration, especially when results obtained from these tests influence the management of infertile heterosexual couples. Lastly, more studies are warranted for refinement of the current methods and the introduction of novel OS quantification techniques for improved diagnosis and evidence-based infertility therapies.

Oxygen is the main substrate of OxPHOS in the ETC in mammalian mitochondria. Its consumption during ATP production results in the generation of ROS as by-products of aerobic respiration in mitochondria. In the male reproductive tract, including the seminal milieu, low levels of ROS play an essential regulatory role as primary or secondary messengers of redox-dependent physiological processes such as capacitation, acrosome reaction, and fertilization. Optimal ROS levels are regulated by antioxidants synthesized endogenously and those sourced exogenously. When the level of seminal ROS exceeds the reducing capacities of antioxidant systems, the resultant redox disequilibrium precipitates OS, while excess antioxidants results in reductive stress, with implied consequences on reproductive function and fertility. Seminal OS in the testis plays an independent and assistive etiological role through induction of sperm LPO, DNA fragmentation, and apoptosis, among other mechanisms. Pathophysiological pathways can be initiated or enhanced by intrinsic and extrinsic factors, which complicate the diagnosis of male infertility. Testing and quantification of seminal ROS are therefore crucial in delineating the extent of OS in infertile males, especially in cases of idiopathic or unexplained infertility. Direct and indirect methods of assessing seminal ROS are discussed in this chapter.

REFERENCES

1. Sessions AL, Doughty DM, Welander PV, Summons RE, Newman DK. The continuing puzzle of the great oxidation event. *Curr Biol.* 2009;19(14):R567-R574.
2. Luo G, Ono S, Beukes N, Wang D, Xie S, Summons R. Rapid oxygenation of Earth's atmosphere 2.33 billion years ago. *Sci Adv.* 2016;2:e1600134.
3. Crowe SA, Døssing LN, Beukes NJ, et al. Atmospheric oxygenation three billion years ago. *Nature.* 2013;501 (7468):535-538.

4. Hammarlund EU. Harnessing hypoxia as an evolutionary driver of complex multicellularity. *Interface Focus.* 2020;10(4):20190101.

5. Picard M, Taivassalo T, Gouspillou G, Hepple RT. Mitochondria: isolation, structure and function. *J Physiol.* 2011;589(18):4413-4421.

6. Amaral A, Lourenço B, Marques M, Ramalho-Santos J. Mitochondria functionality and sperm quality. *Reprod Camb Engl.* 2013;146(5):R163-R174.

7. Du Plessis SS, Agarwal A, Halabi J, Tvrda E. Contemporary evidence on the physiological role of reactive oxygen species in human sperm function. *J Assist Reprod Genet.* 2015;32(4):509-520.

8. Ford WCL. Regulation of sperm function by reactive oxygen species. *Hum Reprod Update.* 2004;10(5):387-399.

9. Wagner H, Cheng JW, Ko EY. Role of reactive oxygen species in male infertility: an updated review of literature. *Arab J Urol.* 2017;16(1):35-43.

10. Zhao RZ, Jiang S, Zhang L, Yu ZB. Mitochondrial electron transport chain, ROS generation and uncoupling (Review). *Int J Mol Med.* 2019;44(1):3-15.

11. Pintus E, Ros-Santaella JL. Impact of oxidative stress on male reproduction in domestic and wild animals. *Antioxid Basel Switz.* 2021;10(7):1154.

12. Aprioku JS. Pharmacology of free radicals and the impact of reactive oxygen species on the testis. *J Reprod Infertil.* 2013;14(4):158-172.

13. Agarwal A, Leisegang K, Sengupta P. Chapter 2 - Oxidative stress in pathologies of male reproductive disorders. In: Preedy VR, editor. *Pathology.* Academic Press; 2020:15-27. Available at: https://www.sciencedirect.com/science/article/pii/B9780128159729000020.

14. Finelli R, Leisegang K, Kandil H, Agarwal A. Oxidative stress: a comprehensive review of biochemical, molecular, and genetic aspects in the pathogenesis and management of varicocele. *World J Mens Health.* 2022;40(1):87-103.

15. Sena LA, Chandel NS. Physiological roles of mitochondrial reactive oxygen species. *Mol Cell.* 2012;48(2):158-167.

16. Aitken RJ, Drevet JR, Moazamian A, Gharagozloo P. Male infertility and oxidative stress: a focus on the underlying mechanisms. *Antioxidants.* 2022;11(2):306.

17. Tremellen K. Oxidative stress and male infertility—a clinical perspective. *Hum Reprod Update.* 2008;14(3):243-258.

18. Agarwal A, Qiu E, Sharma R. Laboratory assessment of oxidative stress in semen. *Arab J Urol.* 2017;16(1):77-86.

19. Sabeti P, Pourmasumi S, Rahiminia T, Akyash F, Talebi AR. Etiologies of sperm oxidative stress. *Int J Reprod Biomed.* 2016;14(4):231-240.

20. Yadav A, Kumari R, Yadav A, Mishra JP, Srivastava S, Prabha S. Antioxidants and its functions in human body - A Review. *Res Environ Life Sci.* 2016;9:1328-1331.

21. Oroian M, Escriche I. Antioxidants: Characterization, natural sources, extraction and analysis. *Food Res Int Ott Ont.* 2015;74:10-36.

22. Flieger J, Flieger W, Baj J, Maciejewski R. Antioxidants: classification, natural sources, activity/capacity measurements, and usefulness for the synthesis of nanoparticles. *Mater Basel Switz.* 2021;14(15):4135.

23. Sheng Y, Abreu IA, Cabelli DE, et al. Superoxide dismutases and superoxide reductases. *Chem Rev.* 2014;114(7):3854-3918.

24. Agarwal A, Sekhon LH. The role of antioxidant therapy in the treatment of male infertility. *Hum Fertil.* 2010;13(4):217-225.

25. Henkel R, Sandhu IS, Agarwal A. The excessive use of antioxidant therapy: a possible cause of male infertility? *Andrologia.* 2019;51(1):e13162.

26. Agarwal A, Panner Selvam MK, Samanta L, et al. Effect of antioxidant supplementation on the sperm proteome of idiopathic infertile men. *Antioxidants.* 2019;8(10):488.

27. Agarwal A, Majzoub A. Role of antioxidants in assisted reproductive techniques. *World J Mens Health.* 2017;35(2):77-93.

28. Arafa M, Agarwal A, Majzoub A, et al. Efficacy of antioxidant supplementation on conventional and advanced sperm function tests in patients with idiopathic male infertility. *Antioxidants.* 2020;9:219.

29. Agarwal A, Nallella KP, Allamaneni SS, Said TM. Role of antioxidants in treatment of male infertility: an overview of the literature. *Reprod Biomed Online.* 2004;8(6):616-627.

30. Dikalov SI, Harrison DG. Methods for detection of mitochondrial and cellular reactive oxygen species. *Antioxid Redox Signal.* 2014;20(2):372-382.

31. Robert KA, Sharma R, Henkel R, Agarwal A. An update on the techniques used to measure oxidative stress in seminal plasma. *Andrologia.* 2021;53(2):e13726.

32. O'Donnell L. Mechanisms of spermiogenesis and spermiation and how they are disturbed. *Spermatogenesis.* 2014;4(2):e979623.

33. Rengan AK, Agarwal A, van der Linde M, du Plessis SS. An investigation of excess residual cytoplasm in human spermatozoa and its distinction from the cytoplasmic droplet. *Reprod Biol Endocrinol.* 2012;10(1):92.

34. Aziz N, Saleh RA, Sharma RK, et al. Novel association between sperm reactive oxygen species production, sperm morphological defects, and the sperm deformity index. *Fertil Steril.* 2004;81(2):349-354.

35. Thomas J, Fishel SB, Hall JA, Green S, Newton TA, Thornton SJ. Increased polymorphonuclear granulocytes in seminal plasma in relation to sperm morphology. *Hum Reprod.* 1997;12(11):2418-2421.

36. Khodamoradi K, Kuchakulla M, Narasimman M, et al. Laboratory and clinical management of leukocytospermia and hematospermia: a review. *Ther Adv Reprod Health.* 2020;14:2633494120922511.

37. Wolff H. The biologic significance of white blood cells in semen. *Fertil Steril.* 1995;63(6):1143-1157.

38. Henkel R, Offor U, Fisher D. The role of infections and leukocytes in male infertility. *Andrologia.* 2021;53(1):e13743. Available at: https://onlinelibrary. wiley.com/doi/10.1111/and.13743.

39. Lobascio AM, De Felici M, Anibaldi M, Greco P, Minasi MG, Greco E. Involvement of seminal leukocytes, reactive oxygen species, and sperm mitochondrial membrane potential in the DNA damage of the human spermatozoa. *Andrology.* 2015;3(2):265-270.

40. Mupfiga C, Fisher D, Kruger T, Henkel R. The relationship between seminal leukocytes, oxidative status in the ejaculate, and apoptotic markers in human spermatozoa. *Syst Biol Reprod Med.* 2013;59(6):304-311.

41. Tomlinson MJ, Barratt CL, Cooke ID. Prospective study of leukocytes and leukocyte subpopulations in semen suggests they are not a cause of male infertility. *Fertil Steril.* 1993;60(6):1069-1075.

42. Cavagna M, Oliveira JBA, Petersen CG, et al. The influence of leukocytospermia on the outcomes of assisted reproductive technology. *Reprod Biol Endocrinol RBE.* 2012;10:44.

43. Iwamoto T, Nozawa S, Yoshiike M. Semen quality of Asian men. *Reprod Med Biol.* 2007;6(4):185-193.

44. Turner TT, Lysiak JJ. Oxidative stress: a common factor in testicular dysfunction. *J Androl.* 2008;29(5):488-498.

45. Pant N, Kumar G, Upadhyay AD, Patel DK, Gupta YK, Chaturvedi PK. Reproductive toxicity of lead, cadmium, and phthalate exposure in men. *Environ Sci Pollut Res Int.* 2014;21(18):11066-11074.

46. Leisegang K, Dutta S. Do lifestyle practices impede male fertility? *Andrologia.* 2021;53(1):e13595. Available at: https://onlinelibrary.wiley.com/doi/10.1111/and.13595.

47. Ji H, Miao M, Liang H, et al. Exposure of environmental Bisphenol A in relation to routine sperm parameters and sperm movement characteristics among fertile men. *Sci Rep.* 2018;8(1):17548.

48. Dcunha R, Hussein RS, Ananda H, et al. Current insights and latest updates in sperm motility and associated applications in assisted reproduction. *Reprod Sci.* 2022;29(1):7-25.

49. Schuppe HC, Wieneke P, Donat S, Fritsche E, Köhn FM, Abel J. Xenobiotic metabolism, genetic polymorphisms and male infertility. *Andrologia.* 2000; 32(4-5):255-262.

50. Durairajanayagam D, Sharma RK, du Plessis SS, Agarwal A. Testicular heat stress and sperm quality. In: du Plessis SS, Agarwal A, Sabanegh ES, eds. *Male Infertility.* New York, NY: Springer New York; 2014: 105-125. Available at: http://link.springer. com/10.1007/978-1-4939-1040-3_8.

51. Kumar N, Singh AK. Impact of environmental factors on human semen quality and male fertility: a narrative review. *Environ Sci Eur.* 2022;34(1):6.

52. Thonneau P, Bujan L, Multigner L, Mieusset R. Occupational heat exposure and male fertility: a review. *Hum Reprod Oxf Engl.* 1998;13(8):2122-2125.

53. Durairajanayagam D, Sharma RK, du Plessis SF, Agarwal A. *2014 - Testicular Heat Stress and Sperm Quality.* [cited 2022 Apr 20]. Available at: https://www.clevelandclinic. org/reproductiveresearchcenter/docs/publications/93_ Durairajanayagam_et_al_Heat_Stress.pdf.

54. Cho CL, Esteves SC, Agarwal A. Novel insights into the pathophysiology of varicocele and its association with reactive oxygen species and sperm DNA fragmentation. *Asian J Androl.* 2016;18(2):186-193.

55. Blay RM, Pinamang AD, Sagoe AE, Owusu EDA, Koney NKK, Arko-Boham B. Influence of lifestyle and environmental factors on semen quality in Ghanaian men. *Int J Reprod Med.* 2020;2020:e6908458.

56. Yadav UCS, Rani V, Deep G, Singh RK, Palle K. Oxidative stress in metabolic disorders: pathogenesis, prevention, and therapeutics. *Oxid Med Cell Longev.* 2016;2016:e9137629.

57. Roberts CK, Hevener AL, Barnard RJ. Metabolic syndrome and insulin resistance: underlying causes and modification by exercise training. *Compr Physiol.* 2013;3(1):1-58.

58. Leisegang K, Roychoudhury S, Slama P, Finelli R. The mechanisms and management of age-related oxidative stress in male hypogonadism associated with non-communicable chronic disease. *Antioxidants.* 2021;10(11):1834.

59. Corona G, Mannucci E, Forti G, Maggi M. Hypogonadism, ED, metabolic syndrome and obesity: a pathological link supporting cardiovascular diseases. *Int J Androl.* 2009;32(6):587-598.

60. Dutta S, Biswas A, Sengupta P. Obesity, endocrine disruption and male infertility. *Asian Pac J Reprod.* 2019;8(5):195.

61. Monserrat-Mesquida M, Quetglas-Llabrés M, Capó X, et al. Metabolic syndrome is associated with oxidative stress and proinflammatory state. *Antioxidants.* 2020;9(3):236. Available at: https://www.ncbi.nlm.nih. gov/pmc/articles/PMC7139344/.

62. Geva E, Lessing JB, Lerner-Geva L, Amit A. Free radicals, antioxidants and human spermatozoa: clinical implications. *Hum Reprod Oxf Engl.* 1998;13(6): 1422-1424.

63. Tavilani H, Goodarzi M, Vaisi-Raygani A, Salimi S, Hassanzadeh T. Activity of antioxidant enzymes in seminal plasma and their relationship with lipid peroxidation of spermatozoa. *Int Braz J Urol.* 2008;34:485-491.

64. Dutta S, Sengupta P, Roychoudhury S, Chakravarthi S, Wang CW, Slama P. Antioxidant paradox in male infertility: 'a blind eye' on inflammation. *Antioxidants.* 2022; 11(1):167.

65. Zelko IN, Mariani TJ, Folz RJ. Superoxide dismutase multigene family: a comparison of the CuZn-SOD (SOD1), Mn-SOD (SOD2), and EC-SOD (SOD3) gene structures, evolution, and expression. *Free Radic Biol Med.* 2002;33(3):337-349.

66. Rossi SP, Windschuettl S, Matzkin ME, et al. Melatonin in testes of infertile men: evidence for anti-proliferative and anti-oxidant effects on local macrophage and mast cell populations. *Andrology.* 2014;2(3):436-449.

67. Palani AF. Effect of serum antioxidant levels on sperm function in infertile male. *Middle East Fertil Soc J.* 2018;23(1):19-22.

68. Gupta NP, Kumar R. Lycopene therapy in idiopathic male infertility—a preliminary report. *Int Urol Nephrol.* 2002;34(3):369-372.

69. Agarwal A, Virk G, Ong C, du Plessis SS. Effect of oxidative stress on male reproduction. *World J Mens Health.* 2014;32(1):1-17.

70. Mínguez-Alarcón L, Mendiola J, López-Espín JJ, et al. Dietary intake of antioxidant nutrients is associated with semen quality in young university students. *Hum Reprod.* 2012;27(9):2807-2814.

71. Halliwell B. The antioxidant paradox: less paradoxical now? *Br J Clin Pharmacol.* 2013;75(3):637-644.

72. Gutteridge JM, Halliwell B. Reoxygenation injury and antioxidant protection: a tale of two paradoxes. *Arch Biochem Biophys.* 1990;283(2):223-226.

73. Showell MG, Mackenzie-Proctor R, Brown J, Yazdani A, Stankiewicz MT, Hart RJ. Antioxidants for male subfertility. *Cochrane Database Syst Rev.* 2014;(12):CD007411. Available at: https://www.cochranelibrary.com/cdsr/doi/10.1002/14651858.CD007411.pub3/full.

74. Smits RM, Mackenzie-Proctor R, Yazdani A, Stankiewicz MT, Jordan V, Showell MG. Antioxidants for male subfertility. *Cochrane Database Syst Rev.* 2019;3: CD007411.

75. Sanocka D, Kurpisz M. Reactive oxygen species and sperm cells. *Reprod Biol Endocrinol.* 2004;2(1):12.

76. Ullah Khan A, Wilson T. Reactive oxygen species as cellular messengers. *Chem Biol.* 1995;2(7):437-445.

77. Castleton PE, Deluao JC, Sharkey DJ, McPherson NO. Measuring reactive oxygen species in semen for male preconception care: a scientist perspective. *Antioxidants.* 2022;11(2):264.

78. Mannucci A, Argento FR, Fini E, et al. The impact of oxidative stress in male infertility. *Front Mol Biosci.* 2022;8:799294.

79. Mandal R, Badyakar D, Chakrabarty J. Role of membrane lipid fatty acids in sperm cryopreservation. *Adv Androl.* 2014;2014:e190542.

80. Lenzi A, Picardo M, Gandini L, Dondero F. Lipids of the sperm plasma membrane: from polyunsaturated fatty acids considered as markers of sperm function to possible scavenger therapy. *Hum Reprod Update.* 1996;2(3): 246-256.

81. Thuwanut P, Axnér E, Johanisson A, Chatdarong K. Detection of lipid peroxidation reaction in frozen-thawed epididymal cat spermatozoa using BODIPY(581/591) C11. *Reprod Domest Anim Zuchthyg.* 2009;44(suppl 2): 373-376.

82. Koppers AJ, De Iuliis GN, Finnie JM, McLaughlin EA, Aitken RJ. Significance of mitochondrial reactive oxygen species in the generation of oxidative stress in spermatozoa. *J Clin Endocrinol Metab.* 2008;93(8):3199-3207.

83. Aitken RJ, Wingate JK, De Iuliis GN, McLaughlin EA. Analysis of lipid peroxidation in human spermatozoa using BODIPY C11. *Mol Hum Reprod.* 2007;13(4):203-211.

84. De Lamirande E, Gagnon C. Reactive oxygen species and human spermatozoa. *J Androl.* 1992;13(5):368-378.

85. Aitken RJ. Molecular mechanisms regulating human sperm function. *Mol Hum Reprod.* 1997;3(3):169-173.

86. Ozmen B, Caglar G, Köster F, Schopper B, Diedrich K, Al-Hasani S. Relationship between sperm DNA damage, induced acrosome reaction and viability in ICSI patients. *Reprod Biomed Online.* 2007;15:208-214.

87. Henkel R, Hajimohammad M, Stalf T, et al. Influence of deoxyribonucleic acid damage on fertilization and pregnancy. *Fertil Steril.* 2004;81(4):965-972.

88. Agarwal A, Allamaneni SS, Said TM. Chemiluminescence technique for measuring reactive oxygen species. *Reprod Biomed Online.* 2004;9(4):466-468.

89. Gosalvez J, Tvrda E, Agarwal A. Free radical and superoxide reactivity detection in semen quality assessment: past, present, and future. *J Assist Reprod Genet.* 2017;34(6):697-707.

90. McKinnon KM. Flow cytometry: an overview. *Curr Protoc Immunol.* 2018;120:5.1.1-5.1.11.

91. Verschoor CP, Lelic A, Bramson JL, Bowdish DME. An introduction to automated flow cytometry gating tools and their implementation. *Front Immunol.* 2015;6:380. Available at: https://www.frontiersin.org/article/10.3389/fimmu.2015.00380.

92. Brouwers JF, Silva PFN, Gadella BM. New assays for detection and localization of endogenous lipid peroxidation products in living boar sperm after BTS dilution or after freeze–thawing. *Theriogenology.* 2005;63(2):458-469.

93. Marshall J, Johnsen S. Fluorescence as a means of colour signal enhancement. *Philos Trans R Soc B Biol Sci.* 2017;372(1724):20160335.

94. Farah OI, Cuiling L, Jiaojiao W, Huiping Z. Use of fluorescent dyes for readily recognizing sperm damage. *J Reprod Infertil.* 2013;14(3):120-125.

95. Gomes A, Fernandes E, Lima JLFC. Fluorescence probes used for detection of reactive oxygen species. *J Biochem Biophys Methods.* 2005;65(2):45-80.

96. Espinoza EM, Røise JJ, Li IC, Das R, Murthy N. Advances in imaging reactive oxygen species. *J Nucl Med.* 2021;62(4):457-461.

97. Tunc O, Thompson J, Tremellen K. Development of the NBT assay as a marker of sperm oxidative stress. *Int J Androl.* 2010;33(1):13-21.

98. Kohno M. Applications of electron spin resonance spectrometry for reactive oxygen species and reactive nitrogen species research. *J Clin Biochem Nutr.* 2010;47(1):1-11.

99. Henkel R, Morris A, Vogiatzi P, et al. Predictive value of seminal oxidation-reduction potential analysis for reproductive outcomes of ICSI. *Reprod Biomed Online.* 2022;45(5):1007-1020.

100. Gill K, Kups M, Harasny P, et al. The negative impact of varicocele on basic semen parameters, sperm nuclear DNA dispersion and oxidation-reduction potential in semen. *Int J Environ Res Public Health.* 2021;18(11):5977.

101. Dorsey BM, Jones MA. Chapter 2 - Healthy components of coffee processing by-products. In: Galanakis CM, ed. *Handbook of Coffee Processing By-Products.* Cambridge, Massachusetts: Academic Press; 2017:27-62.

102. Porubský M, Gurská S, Stanková J, Hajdúch M, Džubák P, Hlaváč J. Amino-BODIPY as the ratiometric fluorescent sensor for monitoring drug release or "power supply" selector for molecular electronics. *RSC Adv.* 2019;9(43):25075-25083.

103. BALL Dr BA, Anthony V. Detection of lipid peroxidation in equine spermatozoa based upon the lipophilic fluorescent dye C11-BODIPY581/591. *J Androl.* 2002;23(2):259-269.

104. MacDonald ML, Murray IVJ, Axelsen PH. Mass spectrometric analysis demonstrates that BODIPY 581/591 C11 overestimates and inhibits oxidative lipid damage. *Free Radic Biol Med.* 2007;42(9):1392-1397.

105. Henkel RR. Leukocytes and oxidative stress: dilemma for sperm function and male fertility. *Asian J Androl.* 2011;13(1):43-52.

106. Lackner JE, Märk I, Sator K, Huber J, Sator M. Effect of leukocytospermia on fertilization and pregnancy rates of artificial reproductive technologies. *Fertil Steril.* 2008;90(3):869-871.

13

Assessment of Reproductive Hormones in Infertile Males

Gianmaria Salvio, Francesca Firmani, and Giancarlo Balercia

KEY POINTS

- Male hormones drive fetal gonadal development by a complex two-way mechanism that requires the anatomical and functional integrity of the hypothalamic-pituitary-gonadal axis.
- Alterations in fetal gonadal development (due to intrinsic and extrinsic factors) are accompanied by testicular disorders in adulthood, including infertility, hypogonadism, and testicular cancer.
- Several factors (both congenital and acquired) can alter the function of the hypothalamic-pituitary-gonadal axis and determine infertility. The study of sex hormones and their main regulators helps to distinguish the causes of testicular and pretesticular infertility.
- A correct diagnostic evaluation guides the subsequent therapeutic orientation and provides useful information on the reproductive prognosis of patients with male infertility.

INTRODUCTION

Reproductive hormones play a key role in determining and maintaining male fertility that spans from fetal development to adulthood. The aim of this chapter is therefore to explore the function of sex hormones and their complex interrelationships and guide the clinician interested in reproductive medicine in the management of the most common fertility issues.

- **Fetal development of the testes**

  The human testis arises from an intermediate mesoderm region shared with the primordial adrenal gland, the "adrenogonadal primordium," from which the primordial adrenal gland and the bipotential gonad differentiate around 28 days post conception. This common origin explains some shared features of adrenal glands and gonads, such as the ability to synthesize steroids,[1] as well as the development of ectopic lesions of adrenal origin in the gonads, the so-called "testicular adrenal rest tumors" observed in congenital adrenal hyperplasia resulting from 21-hydroxylase enzyme deficiency.[2] The presence of the Y chromosome in the developing embryo, around 41 days post conception, leads to transient expression of the sex-determining region Y (*SRY*) gene, which in turn directs the bipotential gonad toward testicular development. Subsequently, at 7 to 8 weeks post conception, anti-Müllerian hormone (AMH) secreted by Sertoli cells causes the regression of Müllerian structures (uterus and upper vagina), whereas testosterone (especially in its active form, dihydrotestosterone [DHT]) synthetized by Leydig cells stimulates the development of Wolffian structures and external genitalia (Fig. 13.1).[1] During its development, the testicle undergoes a two-step process of descent into the scrotum, with a first intraabdominal phase and a second inguinoscrotal phase, dependent, respectively, on insulin-like peptide 3 (INSL3) and testosterone, both of which are produced by Leydig cells.[3] Improper development of the testis at this level could lead to impaired proliferation/differentiation of the embryonic germ cells that may be associated with oligozoospermia and/or testicular cancer during adulthood.[4] This is the case of fetal exposure to environmental factors called "endocrine disruptors," such as phthalates and bisphenol A, that are linked to testicular dysgenesis syndrome (TDS), a condition associated with deficiency of fetal androgen production, of which components are undescended testis (or cryptorchidism), hypospadias, poor semen quality, and testicular germ cell tumor.[4,5] In addition, incomplete sexual development (with micropenis at birth) and cryptorchidism could also be the consequence of congenital hypogonadotrophic hypogonadism (CHH): during early fetal life, the initial masculinization of external genitalia is supported by placental human chorionic gonadotropin (hCG), which stimulates Leydig cells to produce testosterone, but subsequent luteinizing hormone (LH) production by the fetal pituitary is needed to complete growth of the penis and testicular descent.[3] Cryptorchidism is therefore an important sign to investigate because it may represent an early manifestation of reduced production of fetal androgens, as these determine the structural changes of the gubernaculum testis that conducts the testicle in the scrotal site,[6] and it is frequently associated with oligo- and azoospermia and with testicular tumor during adult life.[7]

- **Male hormones and sperm production**

  In the adult male, sex hormone secretion and spermatogenesis are regulated by the hypothalamic-pituitary-gonadal (HPG) axis (Fig. 13.2).[8] At the upper level of the HPG axis, the hypothalamus produces a decapeptide named gonadotrophin-releasing hormone (GnRH) that reaches the pituitary through the hypophysial portal circulation in a pulsatile manner.[9] The size and frequency of pulsatile GnRH secretion stimulates the release of LH or follicle-stimulating hormone (FSH) by the pituitary, which in turn regulate testicular androgen production and spermatogenesis: LH binds to its receptors on Leydig cells, activating gonadal steroid hormone production, whereas FSH acts on Sertoli cells to create a microenvironment supportive for spermatogenesis. FSH, LH, and steroids, in turn, act at the hypothalamic and pituitary level through a negative feedback mechanism.[8]

- **Gonadotrophin-releasing hormone**

  GnRH is a 10-amino acid peptide (pGlu-His-Trp-Ser-Tyr-Gly-Leu-Arg-Pro-GlyNH2) encoded by the genes *GnRH1* and *GnRH2*, which are located on chromosome 8p11.2-p21 and 20p13, respectively, and is produced by hypothalamic neurosecretory cells (GnRH neurons).[9] The pulsatile pattern of GnRH release seems to be regulated by the neuropeptide kisspeptin produced by non-GnRH neurons in the medial basal hypothalamus region, which exerts its function inducing the transcription of *GnRH1* and GnRH receptor genes, but its exact mechanism has not been fully elucidated.[8] In this purpose, testosterone inhibits GnRH release by the hypothalamus, but GnRH neurons do not express androgen receptor (AR). Since the expression of estrogen receptor has been described in kisspeptin neurons, on which estradiol exerts an inhibitory effect, a similar mechanism has been hypothesized for testosterone, either mediated by testosterone itself or through its conversion to estradiol.[9]

  During fetal life, GnRH neurons originate outside the central nervous system, in the olfactory placode, and migrate to reach their definitive location in the hypothalamus under the guidance of several molecular regulators, including anosmin (see later). Any failure involving GnRH development or migration results in CHH and impairs complete sexual maturation.[9]

GONADOTROPINS

The binding between GnRH and GnRH receptor, a member of the rhodopsin-like G protein–coupled receptor (GPCR) superfamily, stimulates the hypophyseal release of gonadotropins, including LH and FSH. They are glycoprotein hormones composed of a common α-subunit and a specific β-subunit (FSHβ and LHβ).[9] The α-subunit is also shared with placental hCG and pituitary thyroid-stimulating hormone (TSH).[8] LH receptor (LHR) is a member of GPCR family located on the surface of Leydig cells that binds both LH and hCG with high affinity. The binding with LH stimulates androgen production, including androstenedione, DHT,

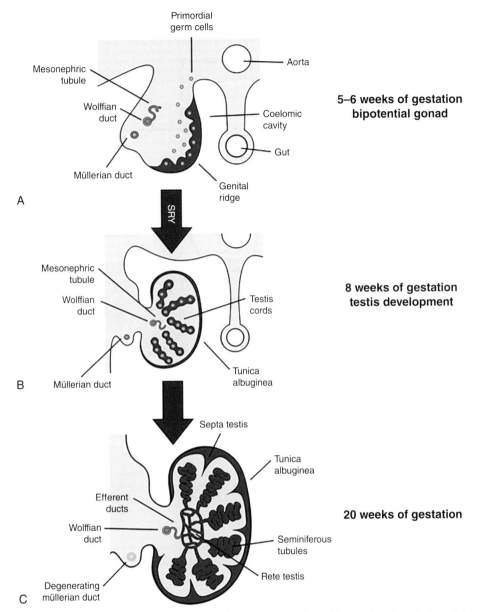

Fig. 13.1 Fetal Development of the Testes. (A) The gonadal development begins with the migration of primordial germ cells from the wall of the yolk sac to the genital ridge by approximately 5 weeks of gestation. By the 6th week of gestation, primordial germ cells have completely invaded the genital ridge and divide to reach about 3000 cells, with activation of gametogenic genes and inactivation of pluripotency genes. The genital ridge originates from the intermediate mesoderm that resides in the coelomic cavity, beside the dorsal mesentery, and it is constituted by proliferating coelomic epithelial cells. Another fundamental structure is the Wolffian (or mesonephric) duct, which contributes to the formation of the epididymis, seminal vesicles, and vas deferens. The Müllerian (or paramesonephric) duct runs in parallel to the Wolffian duct and undergoes degeneration following male sex determination. (B) The presence of the Y chromosome leads to the expression of the sex-determining region of the Y chromosome (SRY). The latter encodes for a transcription factor that activates the testis-specific enhancer of the autosomal gene *SOX9* (SRY-box transcription factor 9), which is essential for the initiation of Sertoli cell differentiation from supporting cell precursors. At 7–8 weeks of gestation, Sertoli cells secrete anti-Müllerian hormone, which prevents the development of Müllerian structures (uterus and upper vagina), whereas the testosterone synthetized by Leydig cells stimulates the development of Wolffian structures and external genitalia. The genital ridge gives rise the capsule, connective tissue, stroma, and septa of the testis, whereas the coelomic epithelium covering the genital ridge gives the testis cords. (C) The testis cords become seminiferous tubules: their straight ends become the rete testis, which joins the mesonephric tubules (efferent ducts).

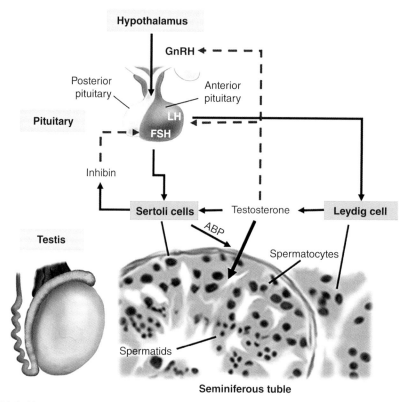

Fig. 13.2 Male Hormones and Testicular Function. The hypothalamus produces the gonadotrophin-releasing hormone *(GnRH)* that reaches the pituitary through the hypophyseal portal circulation in a pulsatile manner, stimulating luteinizing hormone *(LH)* and follicle-stimulating hormone *(FSH)* release. LH binds to its receptors on Leydig cells, activating gonadal steroid hormone production (mainly testosterone), whereas FSH acts on Sertoli cells to secrete paracrine/autocrine factors that support germ cells, growth and development, including androgen-binding protein *(ABP)*, which increases intratesticular testosterone concentration. In addition, Sertoli cells release inhibin B, which downregulates the production of FSH. FSH, LH, and steroids, in turn, act at the hypothalamic and pituitary level through a negative feedback mechanism.

and testosterone.[8,9] Similar to LHR, FSH receptor (FSHR) is a member of GPCR family, but it is localized on Sertoli cells and it has affinity for FSH only. The binding with FSH stimulates Sertoli cells to secrete paracrine/autocrine factors that support germ cell growth and development, including androgen-binding protein, which increases intratesticular testosterone concentration.[8] In recent years, the binding affinity between FSH and FSHR, influenced by genetic factors, such as variants in the gene encoding the FSH subunit B (*FSHB*) and FSHR polymorphisms, has gained increasing interest in the study of infertility, but data are still inconclusive (see later).[10] Moreover, despite animal models showing that adult mice lacking FSHR have a reduced number of Sertoli cells but are still fertile, males lacking FSH are almost invariably infertile.[8]

In addition to GnRH, several regulators expressed at all levels of the HPG axis modulate gonadotropin secretion, including activin, inhibin, and follistatin. Activin and inhibin are both gonadal glycoprotein hormones belonging to the transforming growth factor-β (TGF-β) superfamily. Inhibins are disulfide-linked dimers consisting of an α-subunit (common) and a β-subunit (βA or βB), with two possible isoforms, inhibin A (A-βA) and inhibin B (A- βB), the latter representing the major human form. Activins are dimers of two β-subunits, giving rise to three activin isoforms, A (βA-βA), B (βA-βB), and C (βB-βB).[9] Both activins and inhibins exert numerous autocrine and paracrine modulatory effects on germ cells and Sertoli cells, but the best-known mechanism is that of regulating pituitary release of FSH. Indeed, activin A stimulates the release of FSH from the pituitary, whereas inhibin B suppresses its secretion.[11] In turn, FSH increases inhibin B expression in testes, so that serum inhibin B levels are inversely correlated with serum FSH levels and positively correlated with Sertoli cell number.[9] Follistatin, in addition, is a monomeric polypeptide expressed in gonadal tissue and in pituitary gonadotrophs that binds to activin A and B, decreasing their bioactivity and indirectly suppressing FSH release.[11]

Finally, very recent evidence has shown a possible role of AMH in the hormonal regulation of the HPG axis. AMH, which has already been mentioned for its role in the virilization of the external genitalia during fetal life,[1] is a homodimeric glycoprotein belonging to the TGF-β superfamily (similar to activins and inhibins) mainly secreted by the Sertoli cells into the seminiferous tubules, whose role is the maturation and maintenance of germ cells. Recently, the discovery of AMH expression in GnRH neurons led to the evidence of a novel role for AMH in the regulation of HPG axis: AMH, indeed, acts on the hypothalamus, increasing the activity of GnRH neurons, which modulate LH secretion, and on pituitary-enhancing FSH synthesis.[12]

TESTOSTERONE AND TESTICULAR ANDROGENS

One of the fundamental actions of the testis is the production of steroid hormones, mainly represented by testosterone, secreted by Leydig cells. During fetal life, testosterone allows male gonadal differentiation and growth, while during adult life, it is necessary for the maintenance of sexual function and spermatogenesis.[13] All steroid-producing organs (mainly represented by adrenal glands and gonads) synthetize steroid hormones from cholesterol through a cascade of enzymes encoded by common genes. The specificity of hormones produced by the gonads (male or female) and adrenals depends on the local expression of some genes rather than others, which influences their secretion profile.[14] In the testis, binding between LH and LHR leads to the upregulation of genes related to steroidogenesis,[13] of which the first step is represented by the transport of cholesterol to the inner mitochondrial membrane by the steroidogenic

acute regulatory protein (Fig. 13.3). In the mitochondria, cholesterol is converted to pregnenolone by the side chain cleavage system (comprising the enzymes CYP11A1, ferrodoxin, and ferrodoxin-reductase). Pregnenolone is then converted to 17α-hydroxypregnenolone and dehydroepiandrosterone (DHEA) through the delta 5 pathway by CYP17A1, which owns 17 α-hydroxylase and 17,20 lyase activity supported, respectively, by P450 oxidoreductase (POR) alone and by POR and cytochrome b5. DHEA is then converted to androstenedione (by 3β-hydroxysteroid dehydrogenase type II) or androstenediol (by 17β-hydroxysteroid dehydrogenase 3), and both are then turned over to testosterone. Testosterone, in turn, may be converted to DHT, whose affinity for AR is about 10 times higher than that of testosterone. Its conversion is catalyzed by 5α reductase type II, which is expressed in genital skin and the prostate.[14] AR is localized in the cytoplasm of target cells and, after binding with testosterone or DHT, undergoes a conformational change, dissociating from heat shock proteins and translocating into the nucleus, where it binds to specific sequences of DNA (known as hormone response elements) to up- or downregulate specific gene transcription. Interestingly,

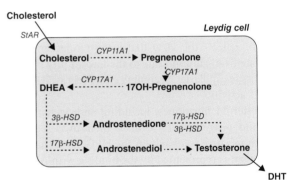

Fig. 13.3 Testicular Steroidogenesis Starts from the Transport of Cholesterol to the Inner Mitochondrial Membrane by the Steroidogenic Acute Regulatory Protein *(StAR)*. In the mitochondria, CYP11A1 converts cholesterol to pregnenolone, which in turn is converted to 17α-hydroxypregnenolone *(17OH-pregnenolone)* and dehydroepiandrosterone *(DHEA)* by CYP17A1. DHEA is then converted to androstenedione by 3β-hydroxysteroid dehydrogenase *(3β-HSD)* type II or androstenediol by 17β-hydroxysteroid dehydrogenase 3 *(17β-HSD)*. Finally, androstenedione and androstenediol are converted to testosterone by 17β-HSD or 3β-HSD, respectively. Once in the bloodstream, testosterone may be converted to dihydrotestosterone *(DHT)*, which has a 10-fold higher affinity for androgen receptor than testosterone does.

genetic variants of AR could be implicated in determining AR transcriptional activity, with subsequent sensitivity to androgen action. In detail, the AR gene is composed of eight exons and is located on the X chromosome (q11-q12). Exon 1 contains a polymorphic sequence of CAG repeats (usually ranging from 10 to 35 repeats) that encodes polyglutamine stretches of the AR transactivation domain, and recent findings have suggested that transcriptional activity of AR could be negatively correlated with CAG number.[15] In addition, 5α-reductase type II polymorphisms have been also described, with a potential impact of androgen effects due to the altered activation of testosterone.[16] Notably, circulating testosterone, usually referred as "total testosterone," is the sum of the concentrations of protein-bound and unbound testosterone. The major sex steroid hormones, indeed, bind to sex hormone–binding globulin (SHBG) and to human albumin, both secreted by the liver. SHBG binds testosterone with high affinity, whereas albumin has lower binding capacity, but its high concentration allows it to heavily influence total testosterone levels. The term "free testosterone" (FT) refers therefore to the unbound fraction of circulating testosterone, which represents only 1% to 4% of circulating testosterone and directly binds to its receptors on target tissues, whereas the sum of unbound and albumin-bound testosterone represents "bioavailable testosterone." The latter term reflects the view that testosterone can easily dissociate from albumin due to the low-affinity binding in the tissue capillaries, becoming effectively available for biologic activity.[17]

Sex steroid hormones, including androgens, estrogens, and progesterone, regulate their own secretion through negative feedback on the HPG axis. The main mechanism is represented by the binding with ARs and estrogen receptors in the hypothalamus, leading to inhibition of GnRH release by GnRH neurons, which in turn decreases gonadotropin production but a direct effect on the pituitary, and in particular, on the release of LH, has also been observed.[8]

THE HUMAN SPERMATOGENESIS

The fundamental element of male gametogenesis is represented by the seminiferous tubules. Each seminiferous tubule consists of a basement membrane, Sertoli cells, and germ cells at varying stages of maturation, measuring 70 to 80 cm when stretched, for a total length of 250 m of seminiferous tubules per testis. The peritubular tissue, on the other hand, is composed of myoid cells, responsible for the propulsion of the testicular fluid, which also support the function of Sertoli cells. Finally, Leydig cells are localized between vessels and seminiferous tubules and produce testosterone upon LH stimulation, which is released into the systemic circulation or stored in the intratesticular compartment, reaching, in the latter, concentrations 100 times higher than in serum.[18] Testosterone is also secreted by Sertoli cells in response to FSH and exerts paracrine effects to support spermatogenesis.[19]

So far, 13 types of germ cells have been identified. They are distributed within the seminiferous tubules in a highly organized manner: less mature cells occupy the basal layer, progressing to the adluminal compartment as maturation occurs. During fetal life, the primordial germ cells originating from extraembryonic tissue around the yolk sac migrate to the gonadal ridge and, between 3 and 5 weeks of development, differentiate into gonocytes (see Fig. 13.1).[18] This process is supported by testosterone secreted by Leydig cells under the stimulus of both placental hCG and fetal LH, as mentioned earlier.[3] Environmental factors and genetic defects occurring at this point and leading to disturbance in germ cell maturation have been invoked as causative elements of TDS, associated with risk of infertility and malignancy in adults.[20] After this, gonocytes remain mitotically inactive until birth.[18] Around 1 week of age, FSH and LH start to increase, peaking between 1 and 3 months and decreasing to prepubertal levels by 6 to 9 months of age. This phase of temporary HPG axis activation is called "minipuberty" and leads to an increase in testicular size and in the number of germ cells, Leydig cells, and Sertoli cells.[3] Notably, during this period, Sertoli cells do not express AR and spermatogenesis is not initiated, but gonocytes differentiate into spermatogonia. Then they stay quiescent until the age of 5 to 7 years, when they increase in number by mitosis and begin the differentiation progress at puberty.[3,18] Spermatogonia are diploid germ cells located in the basal compartment of the seminiferous tubules. They have the dual ability to undergo mitosis and self-renew, maintaining a stable pool of germ cells, or to undergo meiosis and differentiate to spermatozoa. According to their content of heterochromatin, spermatogonia are divided in three subtypes: A dark, A pale, and B. A dark and A pale spermatogonia are supposed to be, respectively, quiescent and active stem germ cells, the latter being able to self-renew or undergo further differentiation. B spermatogonia derive from A pale germ cells and undergo one mitotic division before initiating meiosis.[18] The inability of spermatogonia to differentiate or replicate can give rise to various pictures of impaired spermatogenesis, including hypospermatogenesis and maturational arrest, culminating in Sertoli cell–only syndrome.[21] B spermatogonia, after mitosis, become primary spermatocytes and cross the blood–testis barrier to reach the adluminal compartment of the seminiferous tubules. Here, primary spermatocytes are subclassified according to the stages of prophase 1: preleptotene, eptotene, zygotene, and pachytene. After the first meiosis, two secondary spermatocytes with a haploid number of chromosomes and 2n DNA content are formed and undergo second meiosis to form a total of four round spermatids with a haploid number of chromosome and n DNA content.[18] The final phase of spermatogenesis, called spermiogenesis, leads to the formation of the mature spermatozoon and is highly testosterone dependent.[19] During this stage, a series of cytoplasmatic and nuclear changes occur: (1) the acrosome is formed from the Golgi apparatus, (2) the nucleus become more condensed and moves to an eccentric position, (3) the tail originates from the centriole, (4) mitochondria increase in number and form the midpiece around the tail basis, and (5) excess cytoplasm is removed as residual body, phagocytized by Sertoli cells. When spermiogenesis is complete, spermatids are released in the lumen of the seminiferous tubule. This process is called spermiation, and it is dependent on both FSH and testosterone.[18]

- **Hormonal causes of male infertility**
  - **Epidemiology**

    Couple infertility, defined as the inability to achieve pregnancy after 1 year of regular unprotected intercourse, is a condition affecting more than 186 million people worldwide (corresponding to the 8%–12% of reproductive-aged couples). A male factor, alone or combined with a female factor, is involved in 50% of cases.[22] In about 90% of cases, poor sperm quality or a low sperm count can be identified, and genetic, hormonal, and anatomical causes of male infertility have been described.[23] Among these, endocrinopathies play a major role, since the testis performs the dual function of gametogenesis and testosterone production,

and these two activities appear to be closely related. In addition, chronic systemic diseases, including human immunodeficiency virus-1 infection, heart failure, chronic obstructive pulmonary disease, impaired renal function, and bowel inflammatory diseases, are able to suppress the HPG axis, inducing a state of functional hypogonadism.[24] For this reason, sperm quality and reproductive function are considered markers of general health,[25] and a hormonal cause of infertility should always be suspected.

- **Classification**

  Among the many classifications of the hormonal causes of infertility, it is particularly useful to refer to the HPG axis, distinguishing between pretesticular causes, which involve the hypothalamus and pituitary gland, and testicular causes, which directly involve the different cell populations constituting the male gonad. A further useful subclassification divides the causes of male infertility into congenital and acquired (Table 13.1). However, it should be kept in mind that this classification, although didactically useful, may be limited in clinical practice by the fact that sometimes more than one factor may be present at the same time.

PRETESTICULAR CAUSES: THE HYPOTHALAMUS-PITUITARY-GONADAL AXIS

- **Puberty and regulation of gonadotropin-releasing hormone secretion**

  The first marker of the onset of puberty is testicular growth above 4 mL, reflecting the increase in seminiferous tubule diameter mainly due to the proliferation of Sertoli cells and A spermatogonia promoted by FSH. Proceeding through puberty, further testicular growth is due to an increase in meiotic and haploid germ cells (spermatocytes and spermatids), mainly due to the effects of LH and testosterone.[26] As mentioned above, the release of gonadotropins is regulated by hypothalamic GnRH neurons, which are quiescent until the onset of puberty, when GnRH starts to be secreted into the hypophysial portal system in a pulsatile manner (about one pulse every 60–90 minutes) (Fig. 13.4). The organization of the pulsatile release of GnRH is under the control of a hypothalamic neuronal network named the "GnRH pulse generator," whose activity is modulated by stimulatory and inhibitory signals. Among these, the most important endogenous regulator of the GnRH pulse generation is the kisspeptin-neurokinin-dynorphin (KNDy) system, as demonstrated by the observation of delayed puberty or hypogonadism in males with loss-of-function mutations in genes encoding for kisspeptin and its receptor (KISS1R, also known as GPR54).[27]

Kisspeptin is a 54–amino acid polypeptide acting as a GnRH secretagogue released from the arcuate nucleus of the hypothalamus together with neurokinin B and dynorphin, the last two acting as a stimulator and an inhibitor, respectively, of kisspeptin release.[28] The onset of puberty is thought to be triggered by the release of a molecular "brake" on the KNDy-GnRH system, represented by makorin-3 (MKRN3).[27] Although its exact mechanism of action is not understood, the expression of MKRN3 abruptly decreases before the onset of puberty, and loss-of-function mutation in its gene causes precocious puberty.[28]

- **Causes of hypothalamic-pituitary-gonadal axis disruption (hypogonadotropic hypogonadism)**

  Alterations in the normal functioning of the GnRH pulse generator or pituitary abnormalities may alter gonadotropin release, leading to a condition of hypogonadotropic hypogonadism. The causes of hypogonadotropic hypogonadism are multiple and can be distinguished into congenital or acquired, accompanied by distinct clinical pictures. In the congenital forms (CHH, see previous sections), indeed, the lack of activation of the HPG axis during fetal life and in early postnatal life can be evident at birth with micropenis and cryptorchidism and, later in life, with absent or minimal virilization, eunuchoid proportions, low libido, erectile dysfunction, and absence of puberty.[29] Conversely, congenital postpubertal and acquired hypogonadotropic hypogonadism present with normal stature, normal size of penis and prostate, and testes of normal or slightly low volume, with the main complaints being by infertility, diminished libido, and erectile dysfunction.[30]

- Several causes of acquired hypogonadism exist. Depending on whether the HPG axis is anatomically intact or not, hypogonadotropic hypogonadism can be distinguished into functional or organic.[31] Among organic causes, pituitary/hypothalamic tumors represent a particularly insidious threat to male fertility. An incidental pituitary adenoma (or "incidentaloma") may be found in up to 10% of unselected subjects undergoing brain magnetic resonance imaging (MRI) scans, and in about 60% of cases, it may be associated with hormone hypersecretion, including prolactin (PRL) (32%–66%), growth hormone (GH)

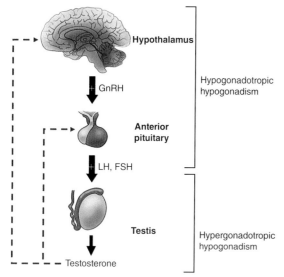

Fig. 13.4 The Hypothalamic-Pituitary-Gonadal Axis. Gonadotrophin-releasing hormone *(GnRH)* is released by the hypothalamus under the control of a hypothalamic neuronal network named the GnRH pulse generator and activity is modulated by stimulatory and inhibitory signals, mainly represented by the kisspeptin-neurokinin-dynorphin system. GnRH is secreted into the hypophyseal portal system and induces the synthesis and release of luteinizing hormone *(LH)* and follicle-stimulating hormone *(FSH)*. LH acts on testicular Leydig cells, stimulating testosterone production, which in turn regulates the release of GnRH and gonadotropin through negative feedback. A blockage at the level of the pituitary gland or higher prevents the release of gonadotropins, resulting in reduced testosterone production, a condition called hypogonadotropic hypogonadism. On the other hand, primary testicular insufficiency is accompanied by reduced testosterone production, resulting in reduced feedback on pituitary and hypothalamus and consequently, increased gonadotropin release. This condition is called hypergonadotropic hypogonadism.

(8%–16%), and adrenocorticotropic hormone (ACTH) (2%–6%). Rarely, pituitary tumor can also secrete TSH or gonadotropins, but these account for less than 1% of cases. Large tumors arising from the pituitary may also lead to hypogonadism due to their compressive effect on gonadotroph cells, but hypogonadism could also represent an indirect consequence of tumor treatments (e.g., transsphenoidal surgery and pituitary radiotherapy) as well. In addition, functional hypogonadotropic hypogonadism may also occur when hormone hypersecretion is present. Indeed, hyperprolactinemia and excess of GH (acromegaly) or ACTH (Cushing disease) are all associated with functional HPG impairment through the disruption of GnRH pulsatility, leading to hypogonadism. Moreover, the regulation of PRL release by the lactotroph cells is mainly due to the inhibitory effect of hypothalamic dopaminergic neurons, the axons of which are localized in the pituitary stalk. Hence hyperprolactinemia could result not only from PRL-hypersecreting tumors (prolactinomas) but also from any sellar lesion causing stalk deviation/interruption or drugs with inhibitory effects on the dopaminergic system (e.g., antidepressants and antipsychotics).[32]

- On the other hand, most CHH cases are due to genetic defects, and hypogonadism could be the only abnormality or be part of a complex syndrome (e.g., CHARGE syndrome and septooptic dysplasia).[29] According to the presence of an intact sense of smell or not, isolated CHH can be subdivided in normosmic (or idiopathic) CHH and anosmic CHH. The latter is also known as Kallmann syndrome, and it is due to mutations (mainly represented by nucleotide insertions or deletions resulting in frame shift mutations or a premature stop codon) of the *KAL1* (or *ANOS1*) gene, encoding anosmin, a protein involved in GnRH and olfactory neuron migration. *KAL1* gene mutations are involved in the recessive X-linked form of Kallmann syndrome, but several other gene defects (and different ways of inheritance) have been described.[30]

- **Treatment and reproductive outcomes**
The approach to hypogonadotropic hypogonadism is similar for congenital or acquired forms and depends on goals, such as development/maintenance of male sexual characteristics or induction of male fertility. Indeed, induction of virilization can be easily reached with testosterone (as transdermal testosterone or injectable esters such as enanthate, cypionate, or undecanoate), but full testicular growth and development of seminiferous tubules require gonadotropin replacement which can be achieved with GnRH or exogenous gonadotropins. In order to simulate physiologic pulsatile release, GnRH needs to be administered through a subcutaneous pump, whereas gonadotropins can be administered by less frequent subcutaneous injections (two to three times weekly) and are more commonly chosen. A typical regimen of puberty induction begins with hCG alone, with the addition of FSH if no sperm can be found in the ejaculate after 3 to 6 months. The prognosis, in terms of fertility, is good for patients with hypogonadotropic hypogonadism, but negative predictive factors are represented by previous history of cryptorchidism, prepubertal testicular volume of less than 4 mL, and low serum levels of inhibin B. In males with severely impaired sperm quality, gonadotropin replacement therapy combined with assisted reproductive technology (ART) could be considered.[33]

TESTICULAR CAUSES: PRIMARY TESTICULAR FAILURE

- **Causes of testicular failure (hypergonadotropic hypogonadism)**
In cases of male infertility due to testicular failure, the impairment of spermatogenesis and the decrease in serum testosterone determine a physiologic response of the HPG axis, leading to an increase in gonadotropin levels (hypergonadotropic hypogonadism).[34] Similarly to hypogonadotropic hypogonadism, clinical manifestations of hypergonadotropic (or primary) hypogonadism largely depend on the age of onset of androgen deficiency.[35] Notably, primary hypogonadism is only rarely functional and/or the consequence of endocrinopathies, with the sole exception of transient hypogonadism observed during ketoconazole therapy for Cushing syndrome.[36] Nonhormonal causes of primary hypogonadism are listed in Table 13.1.

TABLE 13.1	**Causes of Male Infertility**	
	Pretesticular Causes	**Testicular Causes**
Congenital	Kallmann syndrome	Klinefelter syndrome
	Idiopathic CHH	Myotonic dystrophy
		Cryptorchidism, anorchia
Acquired	Pituitary adenomas	Traumatic lesions
	Infiltrative disease of the pituitary	Orchidectomy
	Stalk deviation/section	Infections
	Hyperprolactinemia	Radiotherapy
	Hypothalamic tumors	Drugs (ketoconazole, chemotherapy)
	Hemochromatosis	
	Drugs (glucocorticoids, androgens, progestins, estrogens, GnRH agonists)	
	Opioids	
	Alcohol and marijuana abuse	
	Severe obesity	
	Chronic illness	

CHH, Congenital hypogonadotropic hypogonadism; *GnRH,* gonadotrophin-releasing hormone.

Most hypergonadotropic hypogonadism cases are related to the presence of an extra X chromosome, resulting in a 47,XXY karyotype, a condition known as Klinefelter syndrome. The genetic background of Klinefelter syndrome is represented by sex chromosome nondisjunction during maternal or paternal meiosis (nearly 50% each). In 10% to 20% of cases, a mosaicism (mainly 46,XY/47,XXY) is present. The prevalence of Klinefelter syndrome reaches up to 4% in infertile males, with an estimated overall frequency of 1:500 to 1:1000 males. In Klinefelter syndrome, the typical signs of hypogonadism are also associated with psychosocial problems, mainly represented by language and speech disabilities that worsen if more than one supernumerary X chromosome is present.[37] The genetic alteration leads to progressive testicular damage that first involves germ cells, degeneration of which begins in utero and progresses during infancy and adolescence, leading to extensive fibrosis and hyalinization of the seminiferous tubules, whereas the involvement of Leydig cells may occur later in life. As a result, the early manifestation of Klinefelter syndrome could be azoospermia alone, and the diagnosis could be delayed. Indeed, only 10% of patients with Klinefelter syndrome are diagnosed before puberty.[38]

As mentioned, other genetic and hormonal factors may be involved during fetal development of the male gonad, leading to infertility in adulthood. On this purpose, endocrine disruptors (environmental pollutants with hormonal action found in pesticides and plastic products) can interfere with gubernaculum testis development mediated by INSL3 and leucine-rich, repeat-containing G protein–coupled receptor 8 during testicular descent, leading to cryptorchidism.[39] Regarding additional genetic causes, Sertoli cells function seems to be influenced by the number of CAG repeats of AR,[40] whereas the effect of *FSHR* gene variants has been hypothesized but not clearly established.[41]

• **Treatment and reproductive outcomes**

Distinct from hypogonadotropic hypogonadism, hormonal replacement therapy can be initiated with the sole aim to induce and maintain male sexual characteristics because medical treatment is not likely to restore fertility in subjects with primary testicular failure.[42] For these patients, as well as for any patients with nonobstructive azoospermia due to testicular failure, ART with conventional or micro-testicular sperm extraction (TESE or m-TESE) and subsequent intracytoplasmic sperm injection (ICSI) could be offered.[43] Thanks to these techniques, the prognosis of these patients, in terms of reproductive capacity, has improved greatly in recent years, with average sperm retrieval rates reaching 50%.[44]

LABORATORY ASSESSMENT

The flowchart of the proposed diagnostic work-up is presented in Fig. 13.5. The initial minimum hormonal evaluation should include FSH, LH, and total testosterone. Evaluation of testosterone may be influenced by circadian variation and food intake, so the blood sample should be collected in the morning after an overnight fast.[45] The gold standard method for testosterone measurement is considered mass spectrometry (MS), but even though the introduction of gas chromatography (GC) and liquid

chromatography (LC) in association with MS (GC-MS and liquid chromatography tandem mass spectrometry, LC-MS/MS) made the analysis of steroids with these techniques simpler and quicker,[46] their complexity and high costs still limit their routine use, so most of the current commercial methods are immunoassays (IAs).[45] All IAs, including enzyme-linked immunosorbent assay (ELISA), chemiluminescence IA (CLIA), and radioimmunoassay (RIA), are based on binding between a first antibody and the analyte of interest (a hormone). In the case of ELISA, the substrate of a specific enzymatic reaction is used to determine the amount of the analyte in the sample. In CLIA, the binding with the analyte is highlighted with a chemiluminescent agent (e.g., luminol or isoluminol), where "chemiluminescence" is defined as the production

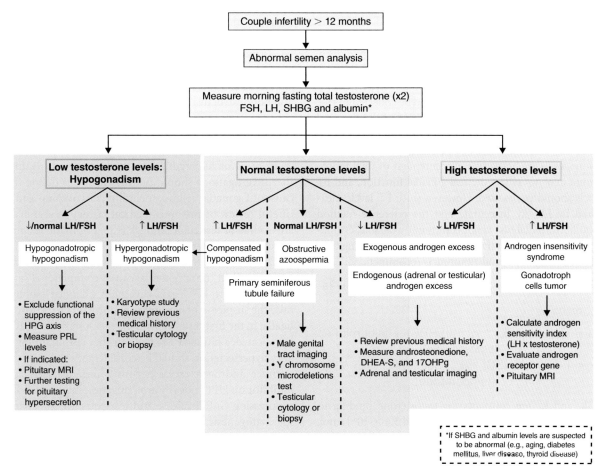

Fig. 13.5 Diagnostic Flowchart of Male Infertility. *17OHPg*, 17-Hydroxyprogesterone; *DHEA-S*, dehydroepiandrosterone sulfate; *FSH*, follicle-stimulating hormone; *HPG*, hypothalamic-pituitary-gonadal; *LH*, luteinizing hormone; *MRI*, magnetic resonance imaging; *PRL*, prolactin; *SHBG*, sex hormone–binding globulin.

of electromagnetic radiation from a chemical reaction yielding an electronically excited intermediate or end product after the addition of H_2O_2. Finally, in RIA, the analyte and a radiolabeled antigen are mixed with an antibody to which they bind competitively; then the analyte concentration is estimated by measuring the radioactivity of the sample after separating the bound from the free fractions (the lower the radioactivity, the higher the concentration of the analyte in the sample—unless it is an immunometric assay, where the antibodies are labeled instead).[47] The main limitation of all IAs is crossreactivity, which is particularly relevant for steroid hormones. In addition, in most laboratories, the total steroid hormone concentration, including the free hormone plus the hormone bound to binding proteins, is measured.[48] This is the case of total testosterone levels, for which concentrations greater than 12 nmol/L (350 ng/dL), including both FT and testosterone bound to albumin and SHBG, are considered normal.[45] Since SHBG levels could be lowered by obesity, diabetes, insulin resistance, hypothyroidism, and acromegaly and, on the other hand, increased by aging, chronic infections, liver disease, and hyperthyroidism,[17] a careful medical history should be collected to rule out these possible conditions that could make the total testosterone dosage unreliable. Indeed, when levels of albumin or SHBG are suspected to be abnormal or testosterone levels are borderline, measurement of total testosterone may not reflect the real gonadal function, and FT levels should be assessed. However, since FT levels measured by IAs are inaccurate and the reference method (equilibrium dialysis) is not commonly available, estimation of FT levels with the Vermeulen equation, using total testosterone, SHBG, and albumin, is recommended:[49]

$$FT \text{ (mol/L)} = (-b + \sqrt{(b^2 + 4 * [\text{testosterone}])})/2a$$

where:

$$a = k_{at} + k_t + (k_{at} * k_t) * ([\text{SHBG}] + [\text{albumin}] - [\text{testosterone}])$$
$$b = 1 + k_t * [\text{SHBG}] + k_{at} * [\text{albumin}] - (k_{at} + k_t) * [\text{testosterone}]$$

k_t and k_{at} are constants for testosterone binding to SHBG and albumin: 10×10^8 L/mol and 3.6×10^4 L/mol, respectively. FT levels less than 64 pg/mL (220 pmol/L) are considered diagnostic for hypogonadism.[42]

Alternatively, salivary testosterone measurement could be a good alternative as a direct measure of FT,

since saliva contains only the non–SHBG-bound fraction of testosterone, but technical issues regarding sample collection still limit its routine use.[50]

If testosterone concentrations in serum are low, a second measurement should be performed and, if total (or free) testosterone levels are confirmed to be reduced, a diagnosis of hypogonadism is confirmed.[42] At this point, gonadotropin levels could help in the localization of the cause of hypogonadism.

Low or normal FSH/LH values, measured by IAs, suggest secondary (or hypogonadotropic) hypogonadism,[42] whereas LH levels over 9.4 IU/L[51] and raised FSH levels (>7.6 IU/L)[52] in the context of hypogonadism are suggestive of primary gonadal failure. However, since FSH secretion is also downregulated by inhibin B produced by Sertoli cells, patients with infertility due to isolated spermatogenic failure may present with normal LH/testosterone and with high FSH levels being the only endocrine abnormality.[21] On the other hand, FSH levels could be normal in up to 40% of patients with impaired spermatogenesis.[52] In such cases, further examinations should be conducted to distinguish between obstructive and nonobstructive causes of infertility, especially if azoospermia is present, including imaging investigations (e.g., transrectal prostate ultrasound) and testicular tissue sampling (by fine-needle aspiration or biopsy).

In cases of hypergonadotropic hypogonadism, further investigations should be carried out to define the causes of gonadal failure, including karyotyping and a careful review of previous medical history in search of any source of testicular damage (e.g., traumatic lesions, infections, or drugs).[52]

On the other hand, the presence of hypogonadotropic hypogonadism (once potential causes of functional suppression of the HPG axis have been excluded) should raise the suspicion of a pituitary abnormality to be investigated in the first instance with the measurement of PRL. If indicated, a pituitary MRI and further testing for pituitary hypersecretion should be considered.[42]

Since androgen excess acts as a negative feedback inhibitor on HPG axis (by aromatization into estradiol), suppressing GnRH release and consequently impairing spermatogenesis, the presence of normal (or even high) testosterone levels in conjunction with low gonadotropins and impaired spermatogenesis may suggest exogenous androgen introduction (e.g., anabolic androgenic steroids abuse) or abnormal androgen synthesis. The latter could be related to adrenal diseases, including congenital adrenal hyperplasia and functional tumors, testicular tumors, or androgen insensitivity disorders.[53] In such cases, measurement of adrenal androgens, including androstenedione, DHEA sulfate, and 17-hydroxyprogesterone may be helpful in guiding the diagnosis.[54]

As well as androgen excess, high levels of estrogens may lead to direct GnRH suppression as observed in obese males due to aromatization of testosterone into estradiol by adipose tissue.[53] When a similar situation is suspected, serum estradiol levels could be measured, but it should be kept in mind that normal levels of estrogens in males are not well established and the current literature provides conflicting results.[55]

Finally, further investigation may be needed during initial evaluation of CHH diagnosed in children and adolescents, including GnRH and hCG stimulation tests and measurement of inhibin B, AMH, and INSL3,[33] but their use does not fall strictly within the framework of male infertility and is beyond the scope of the present chapter.

Clinical significance, biological aspects, and reference limits of the main hormones evaluated in the diagnostic work-up of the infertile male are shown in Table 13.2.

CLINICAL CASE SCENARIOS

In agreement with what has been discussed so far, the following scenarios illustrate some cases that may occur during the diagnostic work-up of male infertility.

CASE 1

A 26-year-old patient provided a semen sample for the laboratory showing normal volume (2.3 mL) and pH (7.8) but no sperm in the ejaculate (even after centrifugation). The patient was in good health. On physical examination, small and firm testes, tall stature with long extremities, and poor representation of secondary sexual characteristics were noted. Initial laboratory assessment showed: total testosterone = 254 ng/dL ($\downarrow$, reference range [RR] 270–1100), SHBG = 65.1 nmol/L ($\uparrow$, RR 18.3–54.8), LH = 23.6 IU/L ($\uparrow$, RR 1.3–9.0), FSH = 28.4 IU/L ($\uparrow$, RR 1.4–16.0).

How should the data be interpreted?
Solution: Levels of total testosterone between 230 and 350 ng/dL are considered borderline. In such

cases, once low or borderline levels of testosterone are confirmed by a second sampling, the estimation of FT using SHBG and albumin may be helpful. According to the Vermeulen equation, the patient shows low FT levels (31 pg/mL), confirming the diagnosis of hypogonadism. The increase in FSH and LH levels indicates a physiological response of the HPG axis to reduced testosterone levels, suggesting that the cause of hypogonadism may be related to primitive gonadal failure. A karyotype study was performed from peripheral lymphocytes, showing the presence of an extra X chromosome (47,XXY). The diagnosis, therefore, was hypergonadotropic hypogonadism resulting from Klinefelter syndrome.
Solution: Regarding the reproductive aspect, ART (TESE-ICSI) could be proposed to the patient. Subsequently, testosterone replacement therapy will help to correct the hypogonadism.

CASE 2

A 31-year-old patient provided a semen sample for the laboratory showing normal volume (2.2 mL) and pH (7.9) but no sperm in the ejaculate (even after centrifugation). Moreover, for several months, the patient had been complaining of decreased libido and moderate erectile dysfunction, whereas in the past, he had had no problems related to sexual health. On physical examination, nothing significant had emerged. Initial laboratory assessment showed: total testosterone = 184 ng/dL ($\downarrow$, RR 270–1100), SHBG = 54.3 nmol/L (normal, RR 18.3–54.8), LH = 1.2 IU/L ($\downarrow$, RR 1.3–9.0), FSH = 1.6 IU/L (low-normal, RR 1.4–16.0).

How should the data be interpreted?
The patient presents with symptoms and examination consistent with hypogonadotropic hypogonadism. Normal pubertal development suggests that this condition is an acquired issue. PRL measurement shows values of 986 ng/mL (normal 2–18 ng/mL). An MRI of the pituitary gland was then requested, which revealed the presence of a sellar mass of approximately 20 mm, compatible with prolactinoma.
Solution: Since the first-line treatment of PRL-hypersecreting adenomas is medical, cabergoline (a dopamine agonist) therapy may be proposed in this case, with the goal of restoring normal HPG axis function and testicular sperm production.

TABLE 13.2	**Male Hormones Involved in the Initial Assessment of Male Infertility**					
				REPRODUCTIVE CONSEQUENCES— INTERPRETATION		
Hormone	**Source**	**Target**	**Normal Values**	↑		↓
Testosterone	Testicular Leydig cells (+++) and Sertoli cells (+). Adrenal glands (++)	Germ cells	Total testoster- one: 240–950 ng/dL[a] 8.3–33.0 nmol/L[a] FT: >64 pg/mL[b] >220 pmol/L[b]	GnRH suppression and impaired spermatogenesis. Exclude androgen- secreting tumors or exogenous androgen abuse.		Impaired spermato- genesis. Hypogo- nadism warranting further investigation.
LH	Pituitary go- nadotroph cells	Leydig cells	1.8–13.4 IU/L[c]	In association with low testosterone levels indicates hy- pergonadotropic hy- pogonadism. Re- search potential causes of testicular disease.		In association with low testosterone levels indicates hy- pogonadotropic hy- pogonadism. Search for organic or func- tional causes of hypogonadotropic hypogonadism.
FSH	Pituitary gonado- troph cells	Sertoli cells	1.5–12.4 IU/L[a]	Sign of Sertoli cell in- jury and seminifer- ous tubule damage. Research potential causes of testicular disease.		In association with low LH and testosterone levels indicates hypogo- nadotropic hypogo- nadism. Search for organic or functional causes of hypogo- nadotropic hypogo- nadism.
SHBG	Liver	Circulating testoster- one	11.5–66.3 nmol/L[d]	Reduced testoster- one bioavailability and falsely normal or increased total testosterone levels. Causes: aging, chronic infections, liver disease, and hyperthyroidism.		Falsely low testoster- one levels. Causes: obesity, diabetes and insulin resis- tance, hypothyroid- ism, and acromegaly.

[a]Lindsay TJ, Vitrikas KR. Evaluation and treatment of infertility. *Am Fam Physician.* 2015;91(5):308-314.
[b]Bhasin S, Brito JP, Cunningham GR, et al. Testosterone therapy in males with hypogonadism: an Endocrine Society Clinical Practice Guideline. *J Clin Endocrinol Metab.* 2018;103(5):1715-1744.
[c]Grimstad F, Le M, Zganjar A, et al. Re: an evaluation of reported follicle-stimulating hormone, luteinizing hormone, estradiol, and prolactin reference ranges in the United States. *J Urol.* 2019;201(5):844-845.
[d]Yu S, Qiu L, Liu M, et al. Establishing reference intervals for sex hormones and SHBG in apparently healthy Chinese adult males based on a multicenter study. *Clin Chem Lab Med.* 2018;56(7):1152-1160.
FSH, Follicle-stimulating hormone; *FT,* free testosterone; *GnRH,* gonadotrophin-releasing hormone; *LH,* luteinizing hormone; *SHBG,* sex hormone–binding globulin.

CASE 3

A 38-year-old patient provided a semen sample for the laboratory showing normal volume (2.4 mL) and pH (7.8) but decreased sperm concentration (8 million/mL), decreased sperm motility (progressive 7% and total 26%), and decreased normal sperm morphology (3%). On physical examination, nothing significant had emerged. There had been no drug use in the previous 6 months and there was nothing relevant in the patient's medical history. Initial laboratory assessment showed: total testosterone = 566 ng/dL (normal, RR 270–1100), SHBG = 44.3 nmol/L (normal, RR 18.3–54.8), LH = 4.2 IU/L (normal, RR 1.3–9.0), FSH = 3.6 IU/L (normal, RR 1.4–16.0).

How should the data be interpreted?

The patient presents oligoasthenoteratozoospermia (OAT) with eugonadism (normal testosterone and gonadotropin levels). In the absence of elements that could justify these seminal abnormalities (e.g., drugs, varicocele, infections, etc.), the diagnosis is "idiopathic OAT."

Solution: The treatment of idiopathic OAT depends on several factors, both patient- and partner-related. Based on the impairment of semen quality and the presence of any ovarian, uterine, or tubal problems in a female partne as well as the age of the latter, medical therapy (e.g., treatment with antioxidants or exogenous gonadotropins) or ART may be proposed.

SUMMARY

Fetal gonad development is regulated by sex hormones in a complex two-way mechanism, which requires anatomical and functional integrity of the HPG axis. LH and FSH are the key hormones produced by the pituitary gland upon stimulation of hypothalamic GnRH and act at the testicular level by promoting sex steroid production and spermatogenesis. Testosterone is fundamental for the maintenance of sexual and reproductive function, so it represents the starting point in hormonal investigations of the infertile male. In case of reduced testosterone levels, the measurement of gonadotropins allows to divide the causes of hypogonadism into pretesticular (hypogonadotropic hypogonadism) and testicular (hypergonadotropic hypogonadism), which present different therapeutic options. Pretesticular causes may be reversible and have a better prognosis. Testicular causes, on the other hand, more frequently require ART and have a lower percentage of reproductive chances. However, it should be kept in mind that normal testosterone and gonadotropin levels can be associated with both obstructive and nonobstructive problems, which sometimes require the integration of further investigations.

In conclusion, the measurement of reproductive hormones represents a fundamental part of the diagnostic work-up of the infertile male, and the knowledge of the regulation of the HPG axis represents a fundamental requirement for gynecologists, andrologists, and reproductive scientists dealing with male infertility.

REFERENCES

1. del Valle I, Buonocore F, Duncan AJ, et al. A genomic atlas of human adrenal and gonad development. *Wellcome Open Res.* 2017;2:1-42. doi:10.12688/wellcomeopenres.11253.1.
2. Engels M, Span PN, Van Herwaarden AE, Sweep FCGJ, Stikkelbroeck NMML, Claahsen-Van Der Grinten HL. Testicular adrenal rest tumors: current insights on prevalence, characteristics, origin, and treatment. *Endocr Rev.* 2019;40(4):973-987. doi:10.1210/er.2018-00258.
3. Kuiri-Hänninen T, Sankilampi U, Dunkel L. Activation of the hypothalamic-pituitary-gonadal axis in infancy: Minipuberty. *Horm Res Paediatr.* 2014;82(2):73-80. doi:10.1159/000362414.
4. Rouiller-Fabre V, Habert R, Livera G. Effects of endocrine disruptors on the human fetal testis. *Ann Endocrinol (Paris).* 2014;75(2):54-57. doi:10.1016/j.ando.2014.03.010.
5. Selvi I, Ozturk E, Yikilmaz TN, Sarikaya S, Basar H. Effects of testicular dysgenesis syndrome components on testicular germ cell tumor prognosis and oncological outcomes. *Int Braz J Urol.* 2020;46(5):725-740. doi:10.1590/S1677-5538.IBJU.2019.0387.
6. Favorito LA, Costa SF, Julio-Junior HR, Sampaio FJB. The importance of the gubernaculum in testicular migration during the human fetal period. *Int Braz J Urol.* 2014;40(6):722-729. doi:10.1590/S1677-5538. IBJU.2014.06.02.
7. Hagiuda J, Nakagawa K, Oya M. Frequent azoospermia in patients with testicular germ cell cancer and a history of cryptorchidism: a report of nine cases and review of the literature. *Syst Biol Reprod Med.* 2021;67(3):189-192. doi:10.1080/19396368.2020.1867666.
8. Jin JM, Yang WX. Molecular regulation of hypothalamus-pituitary-gonads axis in males. *Gene.* 2014;551(1):15-25. doi:10.1016/j.gene.2014.08.048.

9. Kaprara A, Huhtaniemi IT. The hypothalamus-pituitary-gonad axis: tales of mice and men. *Metabolism.* 2018;86:3-17. doi:10.1016/j.metabol.2017.11.018.

10. Santi D, Potì F, Simoni M, Casarini L. Pharmacogenetics of G-protein-coupled receptors variants: FSH receptor and infertility treatment. *Best Pract Res Clin Endocrinol Metab.* 2018;32(2):189-200. doi:10.1016/j.beem.2018.01.001.

11. Wijayarathna R, de Kretser DM. Activins in reproductive biology and beyond. *Hum Reprod Update.* 2016;22(3):342-357. doi:10.1093/humupd/dmv058.

12. Silva MSB, Giacobini P. New insights into anti-Müllerian hormone role in the hypothalamic–pituitary–gonadal axis and neuroendocrine development. *Cell Mol Life Sci.* 2021;78(1):1-16. doi:10.1007/s00018-020-03576-x.

13. Barbagallo F, Condorelli RA, Mongioì LM, et al. Effects of bisphenols on testicular steroidogenesis. *Front Endocrinol (Lausanne).* 2020;11:373. doi:10.3389/fendo.2020.00373.

14. Flück CE, Pandey AV. Steroidogenesis of the testis - new genes and pathways. *Ann Endocrinol (Paris).* 2014;75(2):40-47. doi:10.1016/j.ando.2014.03.002.

15. Tirabassi G, Cignarelli A, Perrini S, et al. Influence of CAG repeat polymorphism on the targets of testosterone action. *Int J Endocrinol.* 2015;2015:298107. doi:10.1155/2015/298107.

16. Yeap BB, Knuiman MW, Handelsman DJ, et al. A 5α-reductase (SRD5A2) polymorphism is associated with serum testosterone and sex hormone–binding globulin in men, while aromatase (CYP19A1) polymorphisms are associated with oestradiol and luteinizing hormone reciprocally. *Clin Endocrinol (Oxf).* 2019;90(2):301-311. doi:10.1111/cen.13885.

17. Goldman AL, Bhasin S, Wu FCW, Krishna M, Matsumoto AM, Jasuja R. A reappraisal of testosterone's binding in circulation: physiological and clinical implications. *Endocr Rev.* 2017;38(4):302-324. doi:10.1210/ER.2017-00025.

18. Neto FTL, Bach PV, Najari BB, Li PS, Goldstein M. Spermatogenesis in humans and its affecting factors. *Semin Cell Dev Biol.* 2016;59:10-26. doi:10.1016/j.semcdb.2016.04.009.

19. Shiraishi K, Matsuyama H. Gonadotoropin actions on spermatogenesis and hormonal therapies for spermatogenic disorders. *Endocr J.* 2017;64(2):123-131. doi:10.1507/endocrj.EJ17-0001.

20. Jørgensen A, Lindhardt Johansen M, Juul A, Skakkebaek NE, Main KM, Rajpert-De Meyts E. Pathogenesis of germ cell neoplasia in testicular dysgenesis and disorders of sex development. *Semin Cell Dev Biol.* 2015;45:124-137. doi:10.1016/j.semcdb.2015.09.013.

21. Gashti NG, Ali M, Gilani S, Abbasi M. Sertoli cell-only syndrome: etiology and clinical management. *J Assist Reprod Genet.* 2021;38(3):559-572.

22. Vander Borght M, Wyns C. Fertility and infertility: definition and epidemiology. *Clin Biochem.* 2018;62:2-10. doi:10.1016/j.clinbiochem.2018.03.012.

23. Leaver RB. Male infertility: an overview of causes and treatment options. *Br J Nurs.* 2016;25(18):S35-S40. doi:10.12968/bjon.2016.25.18.S35.

24. Corona G, Goulis DG, Huhtaniemi I, et al. European Academy of Andrology (EAA) guidelines on investigation, treatment and monitoring of functional hypogonadism in males: endorsing organization: European Society of Endocrinology. *Andrology.* 2020;8(5):970-987. doi:10.1111/andr.12770.

25. Ferlin A, Garolla A, Ghezzi M, et al. Sperm count and hypogonadism as markers of general male health. *Eur Urol Focus.* 2021;7(1):205-213. doi:10.1016/j.euf.2019.08.001.

26. Koskenniemi JJ, Virtanen HE, Toppari J. Testicular growth and development in puberty. *Curr Opin Endocrinol Diabetes Obes.* 2017;24(3):215-224. doi:10.1097/MED.0000000000000339.

27. Livadas S, Chrousos GP. Molecular and environmental mechanisms regulating puberty initiation: an integrated approach. *Front Endocrinol (Lausanne).* 2019;10:828. doi:10.3389/fendo.2019.00828.

28. Spaziani M, Tarantino C, Tahani N, et al. Hypothalamo-pituitary axis and puberty. *Mol Cell Endocrinol.* 2021;520:111094. doi:10.1016/j.mce.2020.111094.

29. Young J, Xu C, Papadakis GE, et al. Clinical management of congenital hypogonadotropic hypogonadism. *Endocr Rev.* 2019;40(2):669-710. doi:10.1210/er.2018-00116.

30. Fraietta R, Zylberstejn DS, Esteves SC. Hypogonadotropic hypogonadism revisited. *Clinics.* 2013;68(suppl 1):81-88. doi:10.6061/clinics/2013(Sup01)09.

31. Grossmann M, Matsumoto AM. A perspective on middle-aged and older men with functional hypogonadism: focus on holistic management. *J Clin Endocrinol Metab.* 2017;102(3):1067-1075. doi:10.1210/jc.2016-3580.

32. Salvio G, Martino M, Giancola G, Arnaldi G, Balercia G. Hypothalamic–pituitary diseases and erectile dysfunction. *J Clin Med.* 2021;10(12):2551. doi:10.3390/jcm10122551.

33. Boehm U, Bouloux PM, Dattani MT, et al. Expert consensus document: European Consensus Statement on congenital hypogonadotropic hypogonadism-pathogenesis, diagnosis and treatment. *Nat Rev Endocrinol.* 2015;11(9):547-564. doi:10.1038/nrendo.2015.112.

34. Basaria S. Male hypogonadism. *Lancet.* 2014;383(9924):1250-1263. doi:10.1016/S0140-6736(13)61126-5.

35. Ross A, Bhasin S. Hypogonadism: its prevalence and diagnosis. *Urol Clin North Am.* 2016;43(2):163-176. doi:10.1016/j.ucl.2016.01.002.

36. Pivonello R, De Leo M, Cozzolino A, Colao A. The treatment of Cushing's disease. *Endocr Rev.* 2015;36(4):385-486. doi:10.1210/er.2013-1048.

37. Bonomi M, Rochira V, Pasquali D, et al. Klinefelter syndrome (KS): genetics, clinical phenotype and hypogonadism. *J Endocrinol Invest.* 2017;40(2):123-134. doi:10.1007/s40618-016-0541-6.

38. Aksglaede L, Juul A. Testicular function and fertility in men with Klinefelter syndrome: a review. *Eur J Endocrinol.* 2013;168(4):67-76. doi:10.1530/EJE-12-0934.

39. Duan S, Jiang X, Zhang X, et al. Diethylstilbestrol regulates the expression of LGR8 in mouse gubernaculum testis cells. *Med Sci Monit.* 2016;22:415-420. doi:10.12659/MSM.895089.

40. Giagulli VA, Carbone MD, De Pergola G, et al. Could androgen receptor gene CAG tract polymorphism affect spermatogenesis in men with idiopathic infertility? *J Assist Reprod Genet.* 2014;31(6):689-697. doi:10.1007/s10815-014-0221-4.

41. Cannarella R, Musso N, Condorelli RA, et al. Combined effects of the FSHR 2039 A/G and FSHR-29 G/A polymorphisms on male reproductive parameters. *World J Mens Health.* 2020;38(3):516-525. doi:10.5534/WJMH.200070.

42. Bhasin S, Brito JP, Cunningham GR, et al. Testosterone therapy in men with hypogonadism: an Endocrine Society Clinical Practice Guideline. *J Clin Endocrinol Metab.* 2018;103(5):1715-1744. doi:10.1210/jc.2018-00229.

43. Cioppi F, Rosta V, Krausz C. Genetics of azoospermia. *Int J Mol Sci.* 2021;22(6):3264. doi:10.3390/ijms22063264.

44. Corona G, Pizzocaro A, Lanfranco F, et al. Sperm recovery and ICSI outcomes in Klinefelter syndrome: a systematic review and meta-analysis. *Hum Reprod Update.* 2017;23(3):265-275. doi:10.1093/humupd/dmx008.

45. Kanakis GA, Tsametis CP, Goulis DG. Measuring testosterone in women and men. *Maturitas.* 2019;125:41-44. doi:10.1016/j.maturitas.2019.04.203.

46. Keevil BG. LC–MS/MS analysis of steroids in the clinical laboratory. *Clin Biochem.* 2016;49(13-14):989-997. doi:10.1016/j.clinbiochem.2016.04.009.

47. Shen Y, Prinyawiwatkul W, Xu Z. Insulin: a review of analytical methods. *Analyst.* 2019;144(14):4139-4148. doi:10.1039/c9an00112c.

48. Hillebrand JJ, Wickenhagen WV, Heijboer AC. Improving science by overcoming laboratory pitfalls with hormone measurements. *J Clin Endocrinol Metab.* 2021;106(4):1504-1512. doi:10.1210/clinem/dgaa923.

49. Agretti P, Pelosini C, Bianchi L, et al. Importance of total and measured free testosterone in diagnosis of male hypogonadism: immunoassay versus mass spectrometry in a population of healthy young/middle-aged blood donors. *J Endocrinol Invest.* 2021;44(2):321-326. doi:10.1007/s40618-020-01304-7.

50. Keevil BG, Adaway J. Assessment of free testosterone concentration. *J Steroid Biochem Mol Biol.* 2019;190:207-211. doi:10.1016/j.jsbmb.2019.04.008.

51. Tajar A, Forti G, O'Neill TW, et al. Characteristics of secondary, primary, and compensated hypogonadism in aging men: evidence from the European male ageing study. *J Clin Endocrinol Metab.* 2010;95(4):1810-1818. doi:10.1210/jc.2009-1796.

52. Thurston L, Abbara A, Dhillo WS. Investigation and management of subfertility. *J Clin Pathol.* 2019;72(9):579-587. doi:10.1136/jclinpath-2018-205579.

53. Sengupta P, Dutta S, Karkada IR, Chinni SV. Endocrinopathies and male infertility. *Life.* 2022;12(1):1-23. doi:10.3390/life12010010.

54. Speiser PW, Arlt W, Auchus RJ, et al. Congenital adrenal hyperplasia due to steroid 21-hydroxylase deficiency: an Endocrine Society clinical practice guideline. *J Clin Endocrinol Metab.* 2018;103:4043-4088. doi:10.1210/jc.2018-01865.

55. Smy L, Straseski JA. Measuring estrogens in women, men, and children: recent advances 2012–2017. *Clin Biochem.* 2018;62:11-23. doi:10.1016/j.clinbiochem.2018.05.014.

14

Imaging in Male Factor Infertility

Parviz K. Kavoussi

KEY POINTS

- Although the physical examination is most critical in assessing male fertility, imaging modalities have gained utility as adjuncts in the evaluation of male reproductive anatomy.
- Routine scrotal ultrasound should not be performed in the initial evaluation of the infertile male; specific case scenarios may indicate the need for scrotal sonography as an adjunct diagnostic modality.
- Scrotal Doppler ultrasound revealing multiple spermatic veins measuring greater than 2.5 to 3 mm correlate with the presence of a clinically significant varicocele.

- The vasogram is primarily a historic test of interest more so than a clinically useful test, except for in rare circumstances.
- Transrectal ultrasound is not recommended as part of the initial evaluation of the infertile male but should be considered when the semen analysis is suspicious for ejaculatory duct obstruction indicated by acidic pH, azoospermia, semen volume of less than 1.5 mL, normal serum testosterone levels, and palpable vas deferens.

INTRODUCTION

An understanding of male reproductive anatomy and imaging modalities is crucial for diagnosis and guidance of treatment options for the infertile male. Although the physical examination is the most critical anatomic evaluation of the infertile male, imaging may be used as an adjunct in specific circumstances. A fundamental understanding of gross anatomy is necessary to interpret imaging of the male reproductive anatomy. This chapter provides a basic gross anatomic description of the male reproductive system as a framework for imaging to follow.

MALE REPRODUCTIVE GROSS ANATOMY

Testis

The testicles are paired organs located in the scrotum for endocrine and reproductive function. In 85% of males the right testicle is lower than the left one. Normal

testicular dimensions include a length of 4 to 5 cm, a width of 3 cm, and a depth of 2.5 cm. The normal testicular volume ranges between 15 and 25 mL (Fig. 14.1).[1,2] The appendix testis is a small, sessile or pedunculated structure located at the upper pole of the testis. The testis is enveloped by tough capsule, which is comprised of the visceral tunical vaginalis (Figs. 14.2 and 14.3), the tunica albuginea, and the tunica vasculosa, from external to internal, prior to reaching the parenchyma of the testis (Fig. 14.4). Smooth muscle cells traverse the collagenous tissue of the tunica albuginea.[3] The mediastinum testis is formed by an invagination of the tunica albuginea into the testis and is where vessels and ducts traverse the testicular capsule.

Epididymis

The epididymis is a comma-shaped tubule attached to the posterolateral aspect of the testis. The epididymis is encapsulated in the tunica vaginalis sheath and tightly

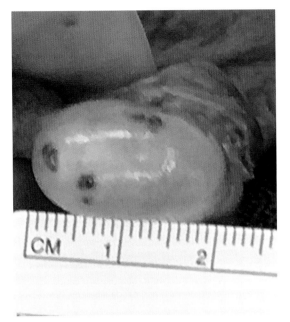

Fig. 14.1 The gross appearance of an atrophic testis.

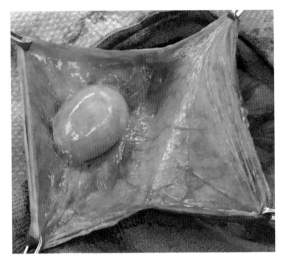

Fig. 14.3 The inner layer of the tunica vaginalis exposed during a hydrocelectomy revealing the white tunica albuginea covering the testis.

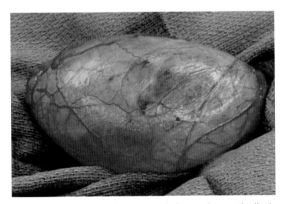

Fig. 14.2 The gross appearance of the tunica vaginalis in a male with a hydrocele.

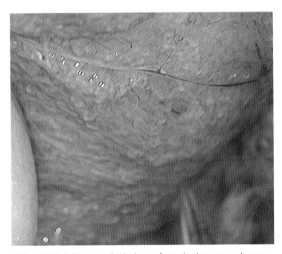

Fig. 14.4 Microsurgical view of testicular parenchyma.

coiled and would measure 3 to 4 m in length if it were stretched out.[4,5] Histologically characteristic areas are formed by septal extensions of the tunica vaginalis sheath into interductal spaces.[6] The three anatomic areas of the epididymis are the caput (head), the corpus (body), and the tail (cauda) (Fig. 14.5). The caput of the epididymis is comprised of eight to 12 ductuli efferentes. Multiple efferent ducts connect the caput of the epididymis to the testis. The tubule of the epididymis becomes continuous with the vas deferens at the most distal portion of the cauda of the epididymis. This duct is irregularly shaped and relatively large adjacent to the testis and becomes more concentric and narrower near the ductus epididymis junction (Fig. 14.6). The diameter of the duct is unchanged throughout the length of the corpus epididymis. The duct diameter enlarges and becomes irregularly shaped in the cauda epididymis and then progresses to form the vas deferens distally. The appendix of the epididymis is a sessile or pedunculated cystic body on the upper pole of the caput of the epididymis.

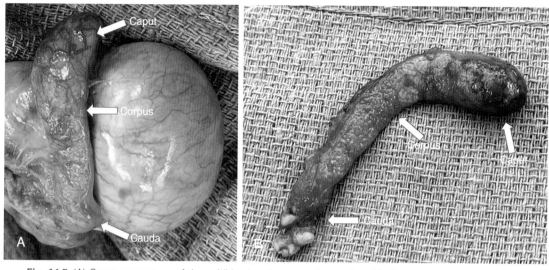

Fig. 14.5 (A) Gross appearance of the epididymis adjacent to the testis, with the caput, corpus, and cauda labeled. (B) Entirety of the epididymis after surgical excision, with the caput, corpus, and cauda labeled.

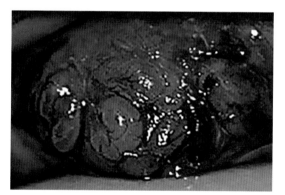

Fig. 14.6 Microsurgical appearance of the epididymal duct after being stained with methylene blue.

Vas Deferens

The vas deferens extends as a tubular structure formed from the distal end of the cauda epididymis. The vas deferens embryologic origin is from the mesonephric (Wolffian) duct. The convoluted vas deferens is the tortuous 2- to 3-cm segment leaving the epididymis, after which it becomes the straight vas deferens. The vas deferens measures 30 to 35 cm in length from its origin following the cauda epididymis to its termination at the ejaculatory duct. The vas deferens travels behind the spermatic cord vessels posteriorly (Fig. 14.7), travels through the inguinal canal, and enters the pelvis lateral to the epigastric vessels. The vas deferens separates from

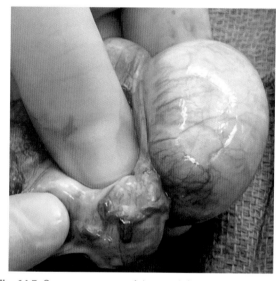

Fig. 14.7 Gross appearance of the vas deferens traveling in the posterior spermatic cord between the gloved fingers.

the testicular vessels after passing through the inguinal canal upon entering the pelvis (Fig. 14.8). After traveling medial to the pelvic sidewall, the vas deferens ultimately reaches the posterior base of the prostate gland. The vas deferens is divided into five anatomic segments. The first segment is the epididymal segment within the tunica vaginalis and is without a sheath. The second segment is within the scrotum, and the third is within

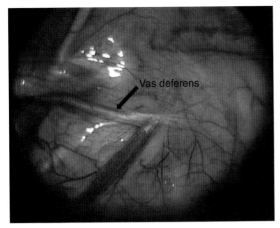

Fig. 14.8 Laparoscopic appearance of the pelvic vas deferens.

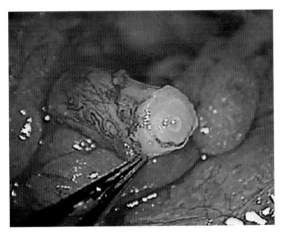

Fig. 14.9 Microsurgical appearance of transected straight portion of the vas deferens, demonstrating the microscopic lumen.

the inguinal canal. The fourth segment is the retroperitoneal segment, and the fifth is ampulla of the vas deferens.[7] Depending on the segment of the vas deferens, the lumen ranges between 0.2 and 0.7 mm in diameter. The outer diameter of the vas deferens tube ranges between 1.5 and 2.7 mm (Fig. 14.9).[8]

Seminal Vesicles and Ejaculatory Ducts

Posterior to the prostate and the bladder are a pair of visceral organs known as the seminal vesicles, which are lateral outpouchings of the vasa deferentia. Each seminal vesicle measures 5 to 7 cm in length and 1.5 cm in width, when not obstructed, and has the capacity to hold 3 to 4 mL of volume. This highly coiled single tube

forms several outpouchings that would measure 15 cm in length if stretched out. The junction of the vas deferens and the seminal vesicle creates the ejaculatory duct. The combination of the smooth muscle sheaths from the seminal vesicle and the vas deferens join at the prostatic base. The excretory duct of the seminal vesicle joins the duct of the ampullary vas deferens as it enters the prostate. The paired ejaculatory ducts empty through the verumontanum into the prostatic urethra. The ejaculatory duct is subdivided into three distinct anatomic regions. The regions include the extraprostatic (proximal), the intraprostatic (mid), and the distal region joining the lateral aspect of the verumontanum emptying into the prostatic urethra.[9]

Prostate Gland

The normal prostate is an ovoid gland weighing 18 to 20 g and measuring 3 cm in length, 4 cm in width, and 2 cm in depth and is positioned directly inferior to the bladder, with the prostatic urethra traveling through the prostate gland. The base of the prostate is located at the bladder-prostate junction, and the narrowed most inferior portion of the prostate is termed the apex, which is continuous with the striated urethral sphincter. An 0.5-mm thick prostatic capsule comprised of collagen and elastin envelopes the gland. There is no a true capsule at the apex of the prostate where prostate glands blend into the urethral sphincter's striated muscle, and there is no true capsule at the base separating the prostate from the bladder.[10] The prostate capsule is continuous with the endopelvic fascia on the anterior and anterolateral aspects of the prostate. The prostate has a point of fixation at the pubic bone anteriorly by the puboprostatic ligaments near the apex of the prostate. The levator ani's pubococcygeal portion hugs the lateral aspects of the prostate and is related to the overlying endopelvic fascia.

The prostate is divided into distinct anatomic zones, which are readily identified by endorectal ultrasonography. The smallest zone, making up 5% to 10% of the glandular tissue of the prostate, is the transition zone. The ducts of the transition zone start at the angle dividing the preprostatic and prostatic urethra, and they travel beneath the preprostatic sphincter to course along its lateral and posterior sides. The ducts of the central zone are positioned circumferentially, surrounding the openings of the ejaculatory ducts. The central zone of the prostate comprises 25% of the glandular tissue of the prostate. Seventy percent of the glandular tissue of the prostate is made up of the peripheral zone, the largest zone, making up the posterior and lateral aspects of the prostate.

BASIC PRINCIPLES OF ULTRASONOGRAPHY

The interaction of sound waves with tissues and anatomic structures results in ultrasound images. Waves of ultrasound are produced through the application of short bursts of alternating electrical current to a series of crystals contained within the transducer. A mechanical wave that is transmitted through a coupling medium to the skin and then into the tissue is created by alternating expansion and contraction of the crystals via the piezoelectric effect. Longitudinal waves are produced with particle motion in the same direction as the wave propagation. Areas of rarefaction and compression of tissue in the travel direction of the ultrasound wave are produced by this motion. Some of the wave is reflected towards the transducer, which receives the returning sound wave and reconverts the mechanical energy to electrical energy. The interaction of mechanical ultrasound waves with tissues and materials within in the body produces the sonographic image. Real-time images can be obtained as ultrasound waves are transmitted and received at frequent time intervals.[11] The principles of Doppler ultrasound are based on the concept that the frequency of the echo reflected from a moving target will be different than the incident frequency. The ultrasound transducer emits ultrasound waves that travel towards the blood vessel, and backscatter is produced by the moving blood cells to the receiving transducer of a slightly different frequency. The Doppler signal power is in accordance with the acoustical size and properties of the volume of blood flow through the beam.[12]

BASIC PRINCIPLES OF COMPUTED TOMOGRAPHY

Computed tomography (CT) imaging is produced by the attenuation of X-ray photons as they pass through the body. Three-dimensional (3D) images of internal structures are produced by recoding the passage of X-rays through different tissues within the body. Cross-sectional images are reconstructed by a computer based

on measurement of X-ray transmission through thin slices of the body.[13] Generation of a collimated X-ray beam on one side of the patient and the amount of transmitted radiation is measured by a detector opposite to the X-ray beam. Systematic repetition of these images with a series of exposures from different projections is made as the X-ray beams rotate around the patient. The recording of passage of different energy waves through various internal structures results in the production of a 3D image of internal structures of the body. Computerized algorithms reconstruct the data collected by the detectors in a viewable tomographic image.

BASIC PRINCIPLES OF MAGNETIC RESONANCE IMAGING

Magnetic resonance imaging (MRI) is performed by placing the patient on a gantry that passes through the bore of a magnet. A magnetic field of such strength causes the free water protons in the body to orient along the z-axis of the magnetic field, which is the "head-to-toe" axis through the bore of the magnet. A coil, radiofrequency antenna, is positioned over the area of interest for imaging. Radiofrequency pulses emitted from the coil transmit through the body, and when these pulses stop, energy is released from the protons, which is detected and processed to produce the image. Each type of tissue in the body absorbs and releases this energy based on tissue characteristics.[14]

TESTIS IMAGING

Doppler Ultrasonography

The primary imaging modality for assessing the testes and intrascrotal content is ultrasonography. Although per the American Urological Association/American Society for Reproductive Medicine guideline for diagnosis and treatment of infertility in males, routine scrotal ultrasound should not be performed in the initial evaluation of the infertile male, specific case scenarios may use scrotal sonography as an adjunct diagnostic modality.[15] Scrotal ultrasonography is performed with high-frequency linear array transducers (7.5–10 MHz) and real-time grayscale techniques, as well as power and color flow Doppler. Scrotal ultrasound is performed with the patient in the supine position with the transducer positioned on the scrotal skin after a coupling gel is applied. The scrotal wall without pathology is hypoechoic and measures 3 to 4 mm in thickness. A small amount of physiologic fluid between the parietal and visceral layers of the tunica vaginalis commonly appears as an anechoic area between the echogenic scrotal wall and the testicle. An echogenic band parallel to the epididymis may be visualized in the posterior testis and represents the mediastinum testis, which may vary in length and thickness depending on the individual.[16] Sonographically, the normal testis exhibits a uniform, fine, medium-level echo pattern, and measures approximately 5 cm × 3 cm × 2 cm.[17] Testicular vasculature can be imaged by color Doppler (Fig. 14.10).[18] The lower vascular resistance of the testis is demonstrated by low impedance patterns with high levels of diastolic flow waveforms from intratesticular arteries and testicular capsular arteries. Low-impedance waveforms from testicular, deferential, and cremasteric arteries are sonographically visible as supratesticular arteries.[19] Although diagnosis of a varicocele is primarily a finding on physical examination, ultrasonography may be useful when the examiner is uncertain whether a varicocele is present on an inconclusive physical examination.[20] Although there are no definitive evidence-based criteria, there is general agreement that multiple spermatic veins measuring greater than 2.5 to 3 mm correlate with the presence of a clinically significant varicocele (Fig. 14.11).[21]

Magnetic Resonance Imaging

Although ultrasonography is the primary modality of imaging the testis, MRI may be used as a secondary imaging modality when necessary. MRI can clearly depict the normal structures of the scrotum. The tunica

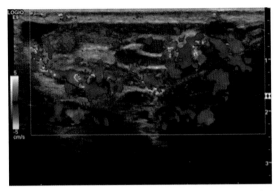

Fig. 14.11 Scrotal color duplex Doppler ultrasound of the dilated veins of a varicocele adjacent to the testis.

albuginea can be clearly differentiated from the parenchyma of the testis and the epididymis. Potential advantages of testicular MRI include delineation of normal and pathological structures greater than 1 mm and the ability to image bilateral hemiscrota and the inguinal region in a single imaging plane.[22] In males with a nonpalpable testis and an unclear history, magnetic resonance angiography has been utilized to identify inguinal testicular nubbin tissue.[23]

EPIDIDYMIS IMAGING

Ultrasonography

The normal epididymis appears either hyperechoic or isoechoic in comparison with the testis in posterolateral position to the testis.[18] The caput epididymis is typically isoechoic, the corpus epididymis is hypoechoic, and the vas deferens is anechoic in comparison with the testis.[24] Sonographically, the normal caput epididymis measures between 10 and 12 mm, and the normal corpus epididymis measures between 2 and 5 mm.[25] The appendix epididymis can be visualized by ultrasound as an isoechoic structure coming off of the caput epididymis.[26] In the nonpathological state, pulsed Doppler and color Doppler detect vascular flow in all areas of the epididymis, with a mean resistive index of 0.55.[27]

Magnetic Resonance Imaging

As with the testis, ultrasonography is the primary imaging modality of the epididymis; however, MRI may be used an adjunct form of epididymal imaging. High-resolution MRI demonstrates clear delineation of the epididymis by differences in signal intensity.[28]

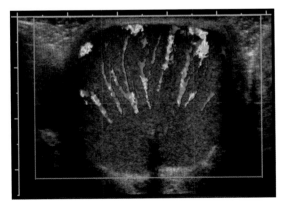

Fig. 14.10 Testicular color Doppler image demonstrating testicular vasculature originating from the mediastinum testis.

VAS DEFERENS IMAGING

Vasogram

The vasogram is primarily a historic test of interest, more so than a clinically useful test, except for in rare circumstances. A vasogram is performed through invasive measures by cannulating the lumen of the vas deferens, injecting contrast, and obtaining plain films or using fluoroscopy. Although it was previously considered to be the radiographic imaging of choice for assessment of the prostate, ejaculatory ducts, and seminal vesicles in the infertile male, it has largely been replaced by transrectal ultrasonography (TRUS). Currently, the vasogram is only used during reconstructive surgery, as it is invasive and may result in scar formation in the vasal lumen and, ultimately, obstruction.[29]

SEMINAL VESICLE AND EJACULATORY DUCT IMAGING

Transrectal Ultrasonography

TRUS is not recommended as part of the initial evaluation of the infertile male but should be considered when the semen analysis is suspicious for ejaculatory duct obstruction indicated by acidic pH, azoospermia, semen volume of less than 1.5 mL, normal serum testosterone levels, and palpable vas deferens.[15] As the seminal vesicles are anatomically positioned posteriorly at the base of the prostate, they can be imaged by TRUS. The normal seminal vesicles are hypoechoic in comparison to the prostate, paired, crescent-shaped, and symmetrical by ultrasonography. The measurements of the normal seminal vesicle are 2 cm in width and 4.5 to 5.5 cm in length. In the transverse plane, they are oriented horizontally. The seminal vesicles and the base of the prostate are separated sonographically by hypoechoic fatty tissue. TRUS may occasionally visualize the ejaculatory ducts as hypoechoic structures entering the prostate posteriorly. Ejaculatory duct obstruction is demonstrated by TRUS measurement of the seminal vesicle diameter in the anteroposterior plane of greater than 1.5 cm, with or without a midline prostatic cyst.[30,31]

Computed Tomography

The preferred imaging modality of the seminal vesicles and ejaculatory ducts is via TRUS; however, CT and MRI may be utilized as adjunct imaging modalities. Seminal vesicles can be imaged by CT and measure 3 cm in length and 1.5 cm in width in the nonpathologic state. The seminal vesicles do not demonstrate significant change in structure with age except for diminishing width of the seminal vesicles. Small punctate densities along the lateral aspects of the seminal vesicle represent the pudendal venous plexus by CT.[32]

Magnetic Resonance Imaging

MRI T1 imaging of the normal seminal vesicles demonstrates signal intensity similar to that of muscle or the bladder, and the seminal vesicles demonstrate signal intensity that is higher than the surrounding fat on T2 imaging.[33–35]

SUMMARY

Male infertility is on the rise worldwide. As with all fields in medicine, the appropriate diagnosis guides the appropriate treatment. For the infertile male, an anatomic evaluation is paramount. Although the physical examination is the most critical assessment, imaging modalities have gained utility as adjuncts in the evaluation of male reproductive anatomy. A fundamental understanding of gross male reproductive anatomy and the imaging modalities that may support the anatomical assessment are necessary to care for the infertile male.

REFERENCES

1. Prader A. Testicular size: assessment and clinical importance. *Triangle.* 1966;7(6):240-243.
2. Tishler PV. Diameter of testicles. *N Engl J Med.* 1971; 285(26):1489.
3. Langford GA, Heller CG. Fine structure of muscle cells of the human testicular capsule: basis of testicular contractions. *Science.* 1973;179(4073):573-575.
4. Turner TT. On the epididymis and its function. *Invest Urol.* 1979;16(5):311-321.
5. Von L, Neuhaeuser G. [Morphometric Analysis of the Human Epididymis]. *Z Anat Entwicklungsgesch.* 1964; 124:126-152.
6. Kormano M, Reijonen K. Microvascular structure of the human epididymis. *Am J Anat.* 1976;145(1):23-27.
7. Lich R Jr, Howerton LW, Amin M. Anatomy and surgical approach to the urogenital tract in the male. In: Harrison JH, Gittes RF, Perlmutter AD, et al., eds., *Campbell's Urology,* vol 1. 4th ed. Philadelphia: W.B. Saunders Co; 1978:3.
8. Middleton WD, Dahiya N, Naughton CK, Teefey SA, Siegel CA. High-resolution sonography of the normal extrapelvic vas deferens. *J Ultrasound Med.* 2009;28(7):839-846.

9. Nguyen HT, Etzell J, Turek PJ. Normal human ejaculatory duct anatomy: a study of cadaveric and surgical specimens. *J Urol.* 1996;155(5):1639-1642.

10. Epstein J. *The Prostate and Seminal Vesicles.* New York: Raven; 1989.

11. Gilbert BR. *Urinary Tract Imaging, Basic Principles of Urologic Ultrasonography.* Phildelphia, PA: Elsevier; 2021.

12. Atkinson P, Wells PN. Pulse-Doppler ultrasound and its clinical application. *Yale J Biol Med.* 1977;50(4):367-373.

13. WB. *Basic Principles.* Baltimore, MD: Williams and Brant Wilkins; 1999.

14. Bishoff JT, Rastinehad AR. *Urinary Tract Imaging, Basic Principles of CT, MRI, and Plain Film Imaging.* Philadelphia, PA: Elsevier; 2021.

15. Schlegel PN, Sigman M, Collura B, et al. Diagnosis and treatment of infertility in men: AUA/ASRM guideline part I. *Fertil Steril.* 2021;115(1):54-61.

16. Dogra VS, Gottlieb RH, Oka M, Rubens DJ. Sonography of the scrotum. *Radiology.* 2003;227(1):18-36.

17. Dogra VS, Gottlieb RH, Rubens DJ, Liao L. Benign intratesticular cystic lesions: US features. *Radiographics.* 2001;21 Spec No:S273-281.

18. Spirnak JP, Resnick MI. *Ultrasound.* Philadelphia, PA: Lippincott, Williams, and Wilkins; 2002.

19. Middleton WD, Thorne DA, Melson GL. Color Doppler ultrasound of the normal testis. *AJR Am J Roentgenol.* 1989;152(2):293-297.

20. Practice Committee of the American Society for Reproductive Medicine, Society for Male Reproduction and Urology. Report on varicocele and infertility: a committee opinion. *Fertil Steril.* 2014;102(6):1556-1560.

21. Stahl P, Schlegel PN. Standardization and documentation of varicocele evaluation. *Curr Opin Urol.* 2011;21(6):500-505.

22. Hajek PC. [Magnetic resonance tomography (MRT) of the scrotum—initial results and comparison with sonography. II: Intratesticular pathology]. *Radiologe.* 1987; 27(11):529-536.

23. Eggener SE, Lotan Y, Cheng EY. Magnetic resonance angiography for the nonpalpable testis: a cost and cancer risk analysis. *J Urol.* 2005;173(5):1745-1749; discussion 1749-1750.

24. Puttemans T, Delvigne A, Murillo D. Normal and variant appearances of the adult epididymis and vas deferens on high-resolution sonography. *J Clin Ultrasound.* 2006;34(8):385-392.

25. Pezzella A, Barbonetti A, Micillo A, et al. Ultrasonographic determination of caput epididymis diameter is strongly predictive of obstruction in the genital tract in azoospermic men with normal serum FSH. *Andrology.* 2013;1(1):133-138.

26. Black JA, Patel A. Sonography of the normal extratesticular space. *AJR Am J Roentgenol.* 1996;167(2):503-506.

27. Keener TS, Winter TC, Nghiem HV, Schmiedl UP. Normal adult epididymis: evaluation with color Doppler US. *Radiology.* 1997;202(3):712-714.

28. Baker LL, Hajek PC, Burkhard TK, et al. MR imaging of the scrotum: normal anatomy. *Radiology.* 1987;163(1): 89-92.

29. Honig SC. New diagnostic techniques in the evaluation of anatomic abnormalities of the infertile male. *Urol Clin North Am.* 1994;21(3):417-432.

30. Ammar T, Sidhu PS, Wilkins CJ. Male infertility: the role of imaging in diagnosis and management. *Br J Radiol.* 2012;85 Spec No 1:S59-68.

31. Jarow JP. Transrectal ultrasonography in the diagnosis and management of ejaculatory duct obstruction. *J Androl.* 1996;17(5):467-472.

32. Silverman PM, Dunnick NR, Ford KK. Computed tomography of the normal seminal vesicles. *Comput Radiol.* 1985;9(6):379-385.

33. King BF, Hattery RR, Lieber MM, Williamson Jr B, Hartman GW, Berquist TH. Seminal vesicle imaging. *Radiographics.* 1989;9(4):653-676.

34. Secaf E, Nuruddin RN, Hricak H, McClure RD, Demas B. MR imaging of the seminal vesicles. *AJR Am J Roentgenol.* 1991;156(5):989-994.

35. Malvar T, Baron T, Clark SS. Assessment of potency with the Doppler flowmeter. *Urology.* 1973;2(4):396-400.

SECTION 4

Medical Treatment of Male Infertility

15

Hormonal Therapy of Male Infertility

Rossella Cannarella, Rosita A. Condorelli, Sandro La Vignera, and Aldo E. Calogero

KEY POINTS

- The hormonal treatments available for male infertility include the gonadotropin-releasing hormone (GnRH), the follicle-stimulating hormone (FSH), the human chorionic gonadotropin (hCG), the selective estrogen receptor modulators (SERMs), and the aromatase inhibitors (AIs).

- FSH and hCG are strongly recommended for the treatment of central hypogonadism.
- There is not a validated scheme for the treatment of central hypogonadism.
- FSH, SERMs, and AIs are used off-label for the treatment of idiopathic infertility.

INTRODUCTION

Treatment of male infertility includes nonhormonal and hormonal strategies. The nonhormonal therapeutic strategy includes antioxidants (e.g., carnitines, myoinositol, coenzyme Q10, vitamin C, vitamin E, lycopene, selenium, zinc, glutathione, N-acetyl-cysteine, arginine, taurine, ornithine, citrulline, magnesium, copper, etc.), fibrinolytic (e.g., bromelin, escin), and antibiotics (e.g., quinolones, tetracyclines, macrolides, penicillins). These drugs are available for the treatment of male accessory gland infection, inflammation, increased seminal oxidative stress, and idiopathic infertility. On the other hand, hormonal therapies include several molecules, such as gonadotropin-releasing hormone (GnRH), follicle-stimulating hormone (FSH), human chorionic gonadotropin (hCG), selective estrogen receptor modulators (SERMs), and aromatase inhibitors (AIs).[1]

In this chapter, we will discuss the hormonal therapies that are available for male infertility treatment, including GnRH, FSH, hCG, SERMs, and AIs. We will review their mechanisms of action and the evidence of their efficacy in male infertility.

HORMONAL THERAPY OF INFERTILE MALES

Gonadotropin-Releasing Hormone

GnRH is a decapeptide released by the hypothalamic GnRH neurons. It stimulates the pituitary gonadotropic cells to release luteinizing hormone (LH) and FSH. Physiologically, GnRH is secreted in pulses, whose frequency and amplitude are critical for normal gonadotropin release.[2]

Since the 1950s, GnRH has been used for male infertility treatment to improve conventional sperm parameters and pregnancy-related outcomes.[3] However, its use has been abandoned over time due to the route of administration. Indeed, treatment with GnRH requires a pulsatile administration that mimics the physiological pulses. A pattern of administration other than the physiological one is ineffective or results in inhibition of the hypothalamic-pituitary-testicular axis, as when GnRH superagonists (e.g., leuprolide, goserelin, triptorelin, and histrelin) are administered. Maintaining the frequency and amplitude of physiologic pulses can be achieved using specific devices for intravenous or subcutaneous administration. However, they can limit patient compliance. In patients with central hypogonadism and normal pituitary gonadotropic activity, spermatogenesis can be induced by long-term pulsatile GnRH administration, usually administered through a subcutaneous pump.[4] The therapeutic scheme used in the case of testicular volume less than 4 mL is 25 ng/kg every 2 h, titrated based on serum testosterone level.[5]

The 2022 European Association of Urology (EAU) guidelines include GnRH treatment via pump among the possible therapeutic options for patients with central hypogonadism (strong recommendation). However, the same panel of experts recognized that GnRH therapy is more expensive and does not offer any advantages when compared to gonadotropins in these patients (strong recommendation).[6] A recent clinical practice guideline endorsed by the European Society for Pediatric Endocrinology (ESPE), the European Society for Endocrinology (ESE), and the European Academy of Andrology (EAA) listed GnRH therapy among the possible available therapeutic schemes to be administered following FSH priming for induction of puberty in prepubertal patients with central hypogonadism.[7]

Follicle-Stimulating Hormone

FSH is a glycoprotein secreted by the anterior pituitary gland, mainly used in patients with pre- or postpubertal central hypogonadism.

The specific schemes and doses to be administered in prepubertal central hypogonadism are not standardized. The latest EAU guidelines, although they do not recommend a specific scheme, describe an approach that starts with hCG and suggest administering FSH after testosterone has reached its target values.[6] Conversely, ESPE, ESE, and EAA clinical practice guidelines mention the possible advantage of starting with FSH and adding hCG or GnRH only afterward.[7] This approach is supported by the FSH-induced Sertoli cell (SC) proliferation before puberty.

By triggering its receptor (FSHR) in SCs, FSH promotes their proliferation in the prepubertal phase. A marker of SC proliferation is the increasing anti-Müllerian hormone (AMH) serum levels. In turn, by secreting inhibin B, SCs are able to exert negative feedback on GnRH neurons, thereby decreasing FSH secretion (Fig. 15.1).

In vitro studies on prepubertal porcine SCs support the concept that FSH plays a role in combination with insulin-like growth factor 1, on SC proliferation, as incubation with these hormones leads to an increased proliferation rate detected by flow cytometry.[9] Furthermore, injection of FSH in prepubertal mice from birth to the 6th postnatal day increased levels of AMH measured on the 7th postnatal day.[10]

In healthy children, AMH rises and then decreases at puberty, thus indicating the pubertal shift of SCs from an immature and proliferative state to a mature one. The shift is mainly caused by an LH-dependent increase in intratubular testosterone levels. In this phase, SCs lose the capability to proliferate. Since each SC can support a specific number of germ cells, an abnormality of SC proliferation in the prepubertal phase could result in irreversible oligozoospermia.[11] On this basis, the recent ESPE, ESE, and EAA clinical practice guidelines on therapeutic management of central hypogonadism highlight the importance of FSH priming before administering GnRH or hCG in prepubertal male patients with central hypogonadism.[7] This would ensure the expansion of the immature Sertolian compartment before GnRH or hCG causes SC maturation.

A randomized controlled trial (RCT) compared the effects of FSH priming followed by GnRH or GnRH alone for puberty induction. The authors found that FSH priming is histologically able to induce SC and germ cell proliferation and SC/germ cell ratio reduction (from 0.74 to 0.35). Treatment with GnRH alone was instead associated with the appearance of Leydig cells and with signs of SC maturation. These changes result in increased inhibin B serum levels (a marker of testicular tubular health), which reached the normal values (>100 pg/mL) only in the patients who received the priming with FSH. On the other hand, those undergoing treatment with GnRH alone did not reach normal inhibin B levels. Furthermore, after a 24-month-long follow-up, the testicular volume, as well as the sperm output, were higher in the patients primed with FSH.[12] Although only a few prospective studies aimed at investigating the benefits of FSH as the first therapeutic option in prepubertal central hypogonadism for a better outcome on spermatogenesis, the preliminary available data encourage this approach, as the guidelines reported.[11] Still, further studies are needed.

FSH is recommended for induction of spermatogenesis in postpubertal patients with central hypogonadism, in combination with hCG. Even in this case, the therapeutic scheme is empirical. The latest EAU

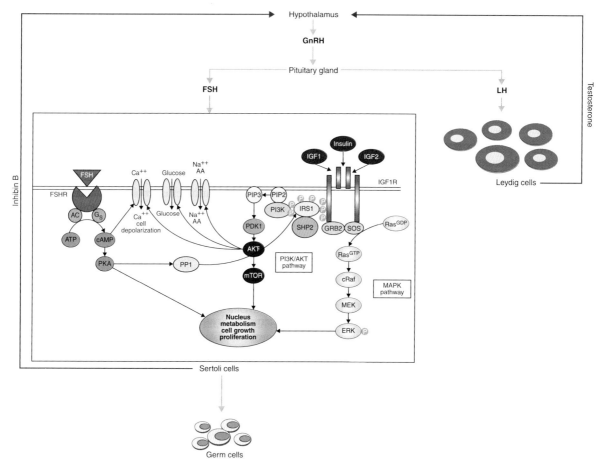

Fig. 15.1 Follicle-stimulating hormone *(FSH)* is produced by the pituitary gland following stimulation with the gonadotropin-releasing hormone *(GnRH)* secreted by the hypothalamus. By binding its receptors in Sertoli cells, FSH induces their proliferation, secretion of mitogens, and proliferation and differentiation of germ cells. In turn, Sertoli cells secrete inhibin B, which inhibits the release of hypothalamic GnRH, thus regulating FSH secretion. On the other hand, the pituitary gland also releases luteinizing hormone *(LH)*, which stimulates the secretion of testosterone from the Leydig cells. Testosterone exerts negative feedback at the hypothalamic level, thus inhibiting the release of GnRH. *Blue arrows*: stimulatory inputs; *Red arrows*: inhibitory inputs. (The pathway showed in the lower panel, on the right, is taken from Cannarella R, Condorelli RA, La Vignera S, et al. Effects of the insulin-like growth factor system on testicular differentiation and function: a review of the literature. *Andrology.* 2018;6(1):3-9.)

guidelines[6] suggest treatment with FSH at a dosage ranging from 75 to 150 IU subcutaneously three times weekly. This therapy can be started following hCG if the latter failed to induce spermatogenesis. However, FSH and hCG could be started also simultaneously.[6]

Another indication of FSH treatment with a level of evidence ranked from low to moderate (depending on the scientific society) is for patients with idiopathic oligozoospermia and FSH serum levels within the normal range (generally 1.5–8 mIU/mL), as suggested by the Italian Society of Andrology and Medical Sexology,[13] the EAA,[14] and the EAU.[6] Indeed, several RCTs have been performed over the years, with different therapeutic schemes, to understand whether the treatment with FSH is effective to improve conventional sperm parameters, sperm DNA fragmentation (SDF), and pregnancy rate in patients with idiopathic infertility[15] (Table 15.1[16–39]).

TABLE 15.1 Therapeutic Schemes and Weekly Follicle-Stimulating Hormone Dosages Administered to Oligozoospermic Males

Therapeutic Scheme	Reference	Weekly Dosage (IU)
hpFSH, 50 IU on alternate days for 3 months	Ding et al., 2015[16]	175
rhFSH, 50 IU on alternate days for 3 months	Foresta et al., 2002[17]	
hpFSH, 75 IU 3 times a week for 3 months	Radicioni et al., 1999[18]	225
	Merino et al., 1996[19]	
hpFSH, 75 IU on alternate days for 3 months	Zarilli et al., 2000[20]	
	Foresta et al., 1998[21], 2000[22]	262.5
	Casamonti et al., 2017[23]	
hpFSH, 100 IU on alternate days for 3 months	Ding et al., 2015[16]	
rhFSH, 100 IU on alternate days for 3 months	Foresta et al., 2002[17]	350
	Foresta et al., 2005[24]	
hpFSH, 150 IU 3 times a week for 3–6 months	Acosta et al., 1992[25]	
	Iacono et al., 1996[26]	
	Baccetti et al., 2004[27]	
	Arnaldi et al., 2000[28]	450
	Garolla et al., 2017[29]	
	Condorelli et al., 2014[30]	
rhFSH, 150 IU 3 times a week for 3–4 months	Caroppo et al., 2003[31]	
	Condorelli et al., 2014[30]	
hpFSH, 75 IU daily for 3 months	Dirnfeld et al., 2000[32]	
	Foresta et al., 2000[22]	
	Fernandez-Arjona et al., 2003[33]	525
hpFSH, 150 IU on alternate days for 3 months	Palomba et al., 2011[34]	
rhFSH, 150 IU on alternate days for 3 months	Colacurci et al., 2012[35]	
hpFSH, 200 IU on alternate days for 3 months	Ding et al., 2015[16]	700
hpFSH, 150 IU daily for 3 months	Strehler et al., 1997[36]	
	Baccetti et al., 2004[27]	
hpFSH, 300 IU on alternate days for 3 months	Ding et al. 2015[16]	1050
rhFSH, 150 IU daily for 3 months	Kamischke et al., 1998[37]	
rhFSH, 300 IU on alternate days for ≥4 months	Paradisi et al., 2006[38], 2014[39]	

hpFSH, Highly purified FSH; *IU*, international units; *rhFSH*, recombinant follicle-stimulating hormone.

Regarding the conventional sperm parameters, in the attempt to understand which therapeutic scheme is more effective in this kind of patient, a recent systematic review and metaanalysis collected all the available RCTs and compared the following dosages of FSH: low (175–262.5 IU per week), intermediate (350–525 IU per week), and high (700–1050 IU per week). The low dose was effective in improving only sperm motility. The intermediate dose improved sperm concentration and morphology, and the high dose improved sperm concentration, total sperm count, and progressive motility.[15] Therefore 150 IU/daily of 300 IU every other day resulted in the schemes with the best efficacy. Concerning the duration, only a few studies prolonged the treatment for more than 4 months. The RCTs by Ding and coworkers reported that both sperm concentration and total sperm count doubled at 5 months, compared to the values at 3 months, when a weekly dose of 1050 IU was administered. Progressive motility and morphology were further ameliorated in the 5th month of therapy. Therefore although many studies treated the patients for 3 to 4 months, a longer duration and a high dose seem to be more effective.[15]

Concerning the impact on SDF, the analysis of six studies showed the presence of a significant improvement in SDF following FSH therapy (mean difference [MD] 4.24%, 95% confidence interval [CI]: 0.24, 8.25) after 3 months of treatment.[40] A Cochrane systematic review on six RCTs, including 456 patients overall, reported significantly higher pregnancy and live birth rates compared to placebo or no treatment in patients with apparently idiopathic male infertility. On the other hand, when the impact on intracytoplasmic sperm injection (ICSI) or intrauterine insemination was analyzed, no difference was found.[41] More recently, a metaanalysis has assessed the effect of FSH on spontaneous pregnancy rate (on nine RCTs) and/or pregnancy after assisted reproductive technique (ART), reporting a significant increase in both cases (spontaneous pregnancy: odds ratio [OR] 4.5, 95% CI 2.17, 9.33; ART-induced pregnancy: OR 1.60, 95% CI 1.08, 2.37). Subdividing the studies based on the specific pharmaceutical preparations of FSH did not change the conclusions.[42]

Several FSH formulations are indeed available, including the human purified FSH (hpFSH), which is purified from the urine of postmenopausal females, and the in vitro synthesized, where the DNA recombinant technology (recombinant human FSH [rhFSH]) is used. The latter comprises the α and the β follitropin. Overall, the evidence suggests an equal efficacy of both hpFSH and rhFSH; hence both approaches are equally effective.[15]

Regarding the role of FSH treatment in azoospermic patients undergoing to testicular sperm extraction–ICSI, some evidence suggests that FSH treatment could increase the sperm retrieval rate as well as the pregnancy and fertilization rates compared to the untreated controls.[43] However, current data are weak, and more studies are needed to have clear recommendations on this. Indeed, if nonobstructive azoospermia (NOA) is due to a maturation arrest, FSH is generally not indicated, as the therapy cannot solve the spermatogenic failure,[44] since it is generally due to gene abnormalities.[9] In this regard, a placebo-controlled, double-blind, randomized study investigating the effects of FSH administration on sperm parameters and testicular cytology found that the treatment increased the spermatogonial population in all patients. However, the sperm concentration significantly increased only in patients with hypospermatogenesis (which is defined in the presence of a low number of germ cells within the seminiferous tubules). In contrast, patients with spermatogenic maturation arrest or with impaired germ cell maturation were defined as nonresponders, as FSH did not increase the sperm concentration.[21] Finally, other predictors of responsiveness to FSH therapy have been studied, such as *FSHβ* and *FSHR* polymorphisms. In greater detail, a metaanalysis on 3017 males explored the association between the *FSHB* -211G>T and *FSHR* 2039A>G on male reproductive parameters, including FSH levels and testis volume. The *FSHB* -211TT and the *FSHR* 2039GG were associated with the lowest testicular volume.[45] This was based on the fact that the TT polymorphism reduces the *FSH* gene transcription, and it is indeed associated with low FSH serum levels. The GG polymorphism was instead associated with a less efficient *FSHR* signal transduction in response to FSH.[46] Importantly, the *FSHB* -211TT allele is associated with the best response to FSH, in terms of sperm count and quality, compared to the response achieved in the GG carriers.[47] Another study assessed the effect of FSH on SDF, based on the *FSHR* 2039A>G allele. Among a cohort of 89 males with idiopathic infertility, FSH less than or equal to 8 IU/L and SDF greater than 15%, FSH treatment was able to significantly reduce the SDF only in the carriers of the A allele, which was associated with a more sensitive receptor.[48] However, despite predictors of FSH responsiveness in patients with idiopathic infertility that have been suggested (e.g., testicular histology, inhibin B, *FSHβ*, and *FSHR* polymorphisms), the evidence is still not robust enough to prompt scientific societies to formulate specific recommendations on this.

In conclusion, FSH is an important treatment for the infertile male that is mainly used in patients with central hypogonadism, although still without well-standardized protocols. Some evidence also assigns this hormone a role in the treatment of some patients with idiopathic oligozoospermia and normal but not high serum FSH levels. Again, protocols, as well as predictors of response to FSH administration, need to be further investigated.

Human Chorionic Gonadotropin

LH is secreted from the pituitary gland and enhances the production of testosterone by the Leydig cells in the testis (Fig. 15.1). Due to its very short half-life, this hormone cannot be used for the treatment of central hypogonadism. hCG has a longer half-life and an LH-similar function. It is extracted and purified from the urine of pregnant females or can be produced with recombinant technology. hCG is strongly recommended for the treatment of central hypogonadism.[6] Indeed, it has been developed to induce spermatogenesis in patients where central hypogonadism has arisen after the onset of puberty. On the other hand, in patients with central hypogonadism and a testicular volume less than 4 mL (suggesting that the patient is still prepubertal), hCG administration should be associated with FSH, since alone, it cannot enhance spermatogenesis.[6] hCG is usually given at a dose of 1000 IU twice weekly. The dose is titrated based on testosterone serum levels and can be increased to 2000, 3000, 4000, and 5000 IU two or three times a week until normal testosterone levels are achieved.[6] Although hCG is one of the therapies used for the medical treatment of cryptorchidism, evidence coming from metaanalyses shows a harmful effect on future spermatogenesis. This is the reason why the Nordic Consensus Statement on the treatment of cryptorchidism, as well as the EAU Guidelines on Pediatric Urology, do not recommend the use of hCG routinely for undescended testes.[6]

Selective Estrogen Receptor Modulators

SERMs represent a class of drugs that mimic or block the effect of estrogens in several tissues by interacting with the estrogen receptor. They include tamoxifen, raloxifene, lasofoxifene, bazedoxifene, and clomiphene citrate. Although SERMs are more classically used in female infertility, breast cancer, and osteoporosis, the evidence seems to place a low value on their use in male idiopathic infertility.[45] The rationale lies in their ability to interfere with the negative feedback that normally regulates the GnRH neuron function. This in turn increases the release of both LH and FSH from the pituitary gland, stimulating spermatogenesis.[49,50] Therefore the functional integrity of the hypothalamic-pituitary unit is an absolute prerequisite, but SERMs are not useful also in the case of primary hypogonadism.[6] However, some authors have suggested the possible occurrence of a direct effect of SERMS at the testicular level.[51] SERMs can ameliorate Leydig cells' sensitivity to LH, thus promoting testosterone production. Furthermore, they might interfere with xenoestrogens, which can be highly concentrated in the seminal plasma of infertile patients.[52,53] Furthermore, SERMs may increase the sex hormone–binding globulin levels by triggering its secretion from hepatocytes.[54] Several SERMs with no standardized therapeutic schemes are currently available for the off-label treatment of idiopathic infertility (Table 15.2[55–73]).[6,9]

A recent metaanalysis evaluated the efficacy of SERMs on conventional sperm parameters, finding that clomiphene (25 mg) and tamoxifen (20 or 30 mg)

TABLE 15.2 Main Therapeutic Schemes Reported in Literature

Drug	Therapeutic Scheme	Reference
Clomiphene citrate	25 mg on alternate days for 3–6 months	Homonai et al., 1988[55]
	25 mg daily for 3–6 months	Wang et al., 1983[56], 1985[57] Homonai et al., 1988[55] Moradi et al., 2010[58] ElSheikh et al., 2015[59]
	50 mg daily for 3–6 months	Rönnberg 1980[60] Wang et al., 1983,[56] 1985[57] Matsumiya et al., 1998[61]
Tamoxifen	10 mg twice a day for 3–6 months	Kotoulas et al., 1994[62] Kadioglu et al., 1999[63] Cakan et al., 2009[64] Guo et al., 2015[65]
	20 mg daily for 3–6 months	Buvat et al., 1983[66] Török, 1985[67] AinMelk et al., 1987[68] Sterzik et al., 1993[69] Kadioglu, 2009[63] Tsourdi et al., 2009[70]
	30 mg daily for 3–4 months	Höbarth et al., 1990[71] Krause et al., 1992[72]
Toremifene	60 mg daily for 3 months	Farmakiotis et al., 2007[73]
Raloxifene	60 mg daily for 3 months	Tsourdi et al., 2009[70]

administered once daily improved sperm concentration, total sperm count, and sperm motility but not morphology compared to baseline. At the dose of 50 mg, clomiphene was not effective, possibly due to the limited number of patients included in the subanalysis.[74]

Interestingly, SERMs may also have an antioxidant action. Accordingly, treatment with tamoxifen has been shown to decrease the production of sperm reactive oxygen species, and the total seminal antioxidant capacity, succinate dehydrogenase activity, mitochondrial membrane potential, and adenosine triphosphate levels following a 3-month-long treatment.[65] In line with this, another study reported a reduction in the malondialdehyde seminal levels, an index of lipid peroxidation, in patients with male infertility.[75] Although the molecular mechanisms are not clear, these studies indicate an antioxidant role of SERMs, which may explain the positive effect on pregnancy rate found in previous metaanalyses.[45] However, the studies included did not clarify the way through which the pregnancy is achieved (spontaneously or post ART).

To date, the last EAU guidelines allocate SERMs in the empirical treatment of male idiopathic infertility, with poor evidence.[6] Further RCTs are needed to confirm the benefit of SERMs on the pregnancy rate in patients with idiopathic infertility.

Aromatase Inhibitors

AIs act through the inhibition of aromatase, a cytochrome p450 enzyme, expressed in several tissues, such as testis, prostate, adipose tissue, brain, and bone. They block the conversion of androgens into estrogens. In turn, 17ß-estradiol inhibits the secretion of gonadotropins, by exerting negative feedback on the hypothalamus and pituitary. Therefore by reducing the levels of 17ß-estradiol, AIs augment GnRH pulses in terms of frequency and amplitude and, therefore increase the secretion of FSH.[76] For this reason, AIs represent a good choice for infertile patients having altered testosterone/17ß-estradiol ratios. AIs can be classified as steroidal (causing irreversible inhibition) or nonsteroidal (causing reversible inhibition and acting by competition with the endogenous substrates). They could also be classified as first-, second-, and third-generation. The last category includes anastrozole (Arimidex), letrozole (Femara), vorozole (Rivizor), and exemestane (Aromasin), which represent the most selective and potent AIs. Letrozole and anastrozole are the most frequently used AIs for the treatment of male infertility. In an experimental study, 140 patients with altered testosterone/17ß-estradiol ratio were treated with anastrozole, reporting a significant increase in sperm parameters.[77] The side effects were reported rarely and consisted of decreased libido in less than 5% of males, and altered liver function in 7.4% of males.[77] Another study using letrozole found a marked increase in FSH and testosterone serum levels in patients with NOA.[78] Other studies reported an

amelioration in sperm parameters.[76,79,80] The dosage can vary from 2.5 mg once a week to 2.5 daily.[77,81] Side effects include headache, decreased libido, and an increase in liver enzymes in less than 10% of patients.[77]

A recent systematic review/metaanalysis has reviewed the effect of AIs on the treatment of male infertility. By including a total of eight original articles, both steroidal (testolactone) and nonsteroidal (anastrozole and letrozole), AIs significantly improved the levels of testosterone and testosterone/17ß-estradiol ratio, sperm concentration, and sperm motility, in a safe and well-tolerated manner. However, the authors suggest the need for future randomized multicenter trials to better understand the effect of AIs on male infertility.[78] Indeed, according to the last EAU guidelines, no conclusive recommendations on the use of either steroidal (testolactone) or nonsteroidal (anastrozole and letrozole) AIs can be made in patients with idiopathic infertility, even before testis surgery (weak recommendation).[6]

CLINICAL CASE SCENARIOS

Example of Hormonal Treatment of a Patient with Central Hypogonadism

A patient searched for fertility with his wife for 2 years. He complained also of erectile dysfunction, fatigue, depression, and increase in body weight, and decided to ask for andrological counseling. At the physical examination, the androgenization was good, the testicular volume was 10 mL bilaterally, the epididymal consistency was normal, and there were no varices in the scrotum. The patient was asked for a semen analysis, which showed azoospermia. At the hormonal examination, he showed FSH of 0.1 IU/mL, LH of 0.2 IU/mL, total testosterone of 5 nmol/L, and prolactin within the normal range. The patient was therefore asked for a magnetic resonance of the pituitary gland, which did not show any abnormality. However, 1 year before, the patient was referred for a brain injury that led to hospitalization for 3 weeks. The other pituitary hormones once evaluated showed to be within the normal levels. Therefore the patient was diagnosed with central hypogonadism of postpubertal onset. The patient did not have obstructive apnea and had normal hemochrome, and his prostate was unremarkable. Combined therapy with FSH and hCG was then started. FSH was prescribed at a dose of 150 IU three times weekly subcutaneously, while hCG was prescribed at the dose of 1000 IU two times weekly subcutaneously. After 3 weeks the testosterone values, measured before the administration of hCG, resulted in 8 nmol/L. The dose of hCG was therefore increased to 2000 IU two times weekly and, 3 weeks later, the levels of testosterone reached the value of 16 nmol/L. He started referring to an amelioration of erectile dysfunction. At the semen analysis, 12 weeks after the therapy was begun, the patient showed a sperm concentration of 5 million/mL, a total sperm count of 12 million/ejaculate, progressive motility of 15%, a total motility of 40%, and a percentage of normal forms of 5%. After further 12 weeks, the patient repeated the semen analysis, showing a sperm concentration of 15 million/mL, a total sperm count of 30 million/ejaculate, progressive motility of 22%, total motility of 41%, and percentage of normal forms of 4%. At the blood testing, he had total testosterone of 18 nmol/L and a normal hemochrome, so the posology of the treatment was confirmed. After 8 months, his wife (26 years old) achieved a pregnancy spontaneously, and the patient was switched to testosterone replacement therapy for treatment of hypogonadism.

Example of Hormonal Treatment of a Patient with Idiopathic Oligozoospermia

A 32-year-old patient married to a 29-year-old female was searching for fertility. They had been trying to get pregnant for 2 years but without any result. The medical history and examinations of the female partner were unremarkable. At the sperm analysis, the patient showed a sperm concentration of 12 million/mL, total sperm count of 25 million/ejaculate, progressive motility of 25%, total motility of 43%, and percentage of normal forms of 5%. There were no germ cells and the seminal leukocyte concentration was less than 1 million/mL. The presence of oligozoospermia was confirmed in a second semen analysis. The patient did not refer to any symptoms. The physical examination showed a left testicular volume of 12 mL and a right testicular volume of 15 mL, the epididymis was of normal morphology and consistency, there were no scrotal varices, and the Valsalva maneuver was negative. The patient had a normal weight and was not exposed to cigarette smoke, drugs, alcohol, or chemicals. The blood testing showed an FSH of 1.9 IU/mL, an LH of 5 IU/mL, and total testosterone of 20 nmol/L. Therefore the diagnosis of idiopathic oligozoospermia was made. The patient was asked for an SDF test, which showed a result of 7% (normal values <4%). After counseling the patient, therapy with FSH was started at the empiric dose of 150 IU three times weekly, subcutaneously. After 12 weeks, the semen parameters were as follows: sperm concentration 20 million/mL, total sperm count 40 million/ejaculate, progressive motility 28%, total motility 41%, and percentage of normal forms 5%. The SDF showed a value of 4%. The therapy was confirmed and, after 6 months, his wife achieved a pregnancy. Therapy was then discontinued.

SUMMARY

Several hormone therapies are available for the treatment of male infertility. These include GnRH, FSH, hCG, SERMs, and AIs. All of these drugs act by directly or indirectly stimulating GnRH secretion, or by replacing the hormones that are not adequately produced and released (e.g., GnRH, FSH, and LH). GnRH has been used in the past for the treatment of central hypogonadism. However, its short half-life and the need for a pulsatile injection have led to the abandonment of this treatment in most countries. On the other hand, gonadotropins are strongly recommended in patients with central hypogonadism, as well as for the induction of puberty. However, some evidence supports the off-label use of FSH for the treatment of idiopathic infertility in patients with normal serum FSH levels. Since about half of patients respond to treatment, research is still ongoing to understand predictors of a positive response. Finally, SERMs and AIs are available as an empirical therapeutic strategy in infertile patients with altered testosterone/17ß-estradiol ratio (e.g., obesity). Although the evidence suggests the efficacy of these drugs on conventional sperm parameters and pregnancy rate in patients with idiopathic infertility, more robust data are needed to prompt scientific societies towards their recommendations for the treatment of male infertility.

REFERENCES

1. Duca Y, Calogero AE, Cannarella R, Condorelli RA, La Vignera S. Current and emerging medical therapeutic agents for idiopathic male infertility. *Expert Opin Pharmacother.* 2019;20(1):55-67.
2. Tsutsumi R, Webster NJ. GnRH pulsatility, the pituitary response and reproductive dysfunction. *Endocr J.* 2009; 56(6):729-737.

3. Turner D, Turner EA, Aparicio NJ, Schwarzstein L, Coy DH, Schally AV. Response of luteinizing hormone and follicle-stimulating hormone to different doses of D-leucine-6-LH-RH ethylamide in oligospermic patients. *Fertil Steril.* 1976;27(5):545-548.

4. Pitteloud N, Hayes FJ, Dwyer A, Boepple PA, Lee H, Crowley Jr WF. Predictors of outcome of long-term GnRH therapy in men with idiopathic hypogonado-tropic hypogonadism. *J Clin Endocrinol Metab.* 2002;87:4128-4136.

5. Boehm U, Bouloux PM, Dattani MT, et al. Expert consensus document: European Consensus Statement on congenital hypogonadotropic hypogonadism—pathogenesis, diagnosis and treatment. *Nat Rev Endocrinol.* 2015;11(9):547-564.

6. Salonia A, Bettocchi C, Boeri L, et al. European Associa-tion of Urology guidelines on sexual and reproductive health-2021 update: male sexual dysfunction. *Eur Urol.* 2021;80(3):333-357.

7. Nordenstrom A, Ahmed SF, van den Akker E, et al. Pubertal induction and transition to adult sex hormone replacement in patients with congenital pituitary or gonadal reproductive hormone deficiency. An Endo-ERN clinical practice guideline. *Eur J Endocrinol.* 2022;186(6):G9-G49. doi:10.1530/EJE-22-0073.

8. Cannarella R, Condorelli RA, La Vignera S, Calogero AE. Effects of the insulin-like growth factor system on testicu-lar differentiation and function: a review of the literature. *Andrology.* 2018;6(1):3-9. doi:10.1111/andr.12444.

9. Cannarella R, Mancuso F, Condorelli RA, et al. Effects of GH and IGF1 on basal and FSH-modulated porcine Sertoli cells in-vitro. *J Clin Med.* 2019;8(6):811.

10. Al-Attar L, No®l K, Dutertre M, et al. Hormonal and cellular regulation of Sertoli cell anti-Müllerian hormone production in the postnatal mouse. *J. Clin. Invest.* 1997; 100(6):1335-1343.

11. Condorelli RA, Cannarella R, Calogero AE, La Vignera S. Evaluation of testicular function in prepubertal children. *Endocrine.* 2018;62(2):274-280.

12. Dwyer AA, Sykiotis GP, Hayes FJ, et al. Trial of recombi-nant follicle-stimulating hormone pretreatment for GnRH-induced fertility in patients with congenital hypogonadotropic hypogonadism. *J Clin Endocrinol Metab.* 2013;98(11):E1790-E1795.

13. Ferlin A, Calogero AE, Krausz C, et al. Management of male factor infertility: position statement from the Italian Society of Andrology and Sexual Medicine (SIAMS): Endorsing Organization: Italian Society of Embryology, Reproduction, and Research (SIERR). *J Endocrinol Invest.* 2022;45(5):1085-1113.

14. Colpi GM, Francavilla S, Haidl G, et al. European Academy of Andrology guideline Management of

oligo-astheno-teratozoospermia. *Andrology.* 2018;6(4): 513-524.

15. Cannarella R, La Vignera S, Condorelli RA, Mongioì LM, Calogero AE. FSH dosage effect on conventional sperm parameters: a meta-analysis of randomized controlled studies. *Asian J Androl.* 2020;22(3):309-316.

16. Ding YM, Zhang XJ, Li JP, Chen SS, Zhang RT, Tan WL, Shi XJ. Treatment of idiopathic oligozoospermia with recombinant human follicle-stimulating hormone: a prospective, randomized, double-blind, placebo-controlled clinical study in Chinese population. *Clin Endocrinol (Oxf).* 2015;83(6):866-871.

17. Foresta C, Bettella A, Merico M, et al. Use of recombinant human follicle-stimulating hormone in the treatment of male factor infertility. *Fertil Steril.* 2002;77:238-244.

18. Radicioni A, Schwarzenberg TL. The use of FSH in adolescents and young adults with idiopathic, unilateral, left varicocele not undergoing surgical intervention. Preliminary study. *Minerva Endocrinol.* 1999;24: 63-68.

19. Merino G, Carranza-Lira S, Martínez-Chéquer JC, et al. Sperm characteristics and hormonal profile before and after treatment with follicle-stimulating hormone in infertile patients. *Arch Androl.* 1996;37(3):197-200.

20. Zarilli S, Paesano L, Colao A, et al. FSH treatment improves sperm function in patients after varicocelec-tomy. *J Endocrinol Invest.* 2000;23:68-73.

21. Foresta C, Bettella A, Ferlin A, Garolla A, Rossato M. Evidence for a stimulatory role of follicle stimulating hormone on the spermatogonial population in adult males. *Fertil Steril.* 1998;69:636-642.

22. Foresta C, Bettella A, Merico M, et al. FSH in the treat-ment of oligozoospermia. *Mol Cell Endocrinol.* 2000;161: 89-97.

23. Casamonti E, Vinci S, Serra E, et al. Short-term FSH treatment and sperm maturation: a prospective study in idiopathic infertile men. *Andrology.* 2017;5:414-422.

24. Foresta C, Bettella A, Garolla A, Ambrosini G, Ferlin A. Treatment of male idiopathic infertility with recombi-nant human follicle-stimulating hormone: a prospective, controlled, randomized clinical study. *Fertil Steril.* 2005; 84:654-661.

25. Acosta AA, Khalifa E, Oehninger S. Pure human follicle stimulating hormone has a role in the treatment of severe male infertility by assisted reproduction: Norfolk's total experience. *Hum Reprod.* 1992;7:1067-1072.

26. Iacono F, Barra S, Montano L, Lotti T. Value of high-dose pure FSH in the treatment of idiopathic male infertility. *J Urol (Paris).* 1996;102(2):81-84.

27. Baccetti B, Piomboni P, Bruni E, et al. Effect of follicle-stimulating hormone on sperm quality and pregnancy rate. *Asian J Androl.* 2004;6(2):133-137.

28. Arnaldi G, Balercia G, Barbatelli G, Mantero F. Effects of long-term treatment with human pure follicle-stimulating hormone on semen parameters and sperm-cell ultrastructure in idiopathic oligoteratoasthenozoospermia. *Andrologia*. 2000;32:155-161.

29. Garolla A, Ghezzi M, Cosci I, et al. FSH treatment in infertile males candidate to assisted reproduction improved sperm DNA fragmentation and pregnancy rate. *Endocrine*. 2017;56:416-425.

30. Condorelli RA, Calogero AE, Vicari E, et al. Reduced seminal concentration of CD45pos cells after follicle-stimulating hormone treatment in selected patients with idiopathic oligoasthenoteratozoospermia. *Int J Endocrinol*. 2014;2014:372060.

31. Caroppo E, Niederberger C, Vizziello GM, D'Amato G. Recombinant human follicle-stimulating hormone as a pretreatment for idiopathic oligoasthenoteratozoospermic patients undergoing intracytoplasmic sperm injection. *Fertil Steril*. 2003;80:1398-1403.

32. Dirnfeld M, Katz G, Calderon I, Abramovici H, Bider D. Pure follicle-stimulating hormone as an adjuvant therapy for selected cases in male infertility during in-vitro fertilization is beneficial. *Eur J Obstet Gynecol Reprod Biol*. 2000;93:105-108.

33. Fernández-Arjona M, Díaz J, Cortes I, González J, Rodríguez JM, Alvarez E. Relationship between gonadotrophin secretion, inhibin B and spermatogenesis in oligozoospermic men treated with highly purified urinary follicle-stimulating hormone (uFSH-HP): a preliminary report. *Eur J Obstet Gynecol Reprod Biol*. 2003;107(1):47-51.

34. Palomba S, Falbo A, Espinola S, et al. Effects of highly purified follicle-stimulating hormone on sperm DNA damage in men with male idiopathic subfertility: a pilot study. *J Endocrinol Invest*. 2011;34:747-752.

35. Colacurci N, Monti MG, Fornaro F, et al. Recombinant human FSH reduces sperm DNA fragmentation in men with idiopathic oligoasthenoteratozoospermia. *J Androl*. 2012;33:588-593.

36. Strehler E, Sterzik K, De Santo M, et al. The effect of follicle-stimulating hormone therapy on sperm quality: an ultrastructural mathematical evaluation. *J Androl*. 1997;18:439-447.

37. Kamischke A, Behre HM, Bergmann M, et al. Recombinant human follicle stimulating hormone for treatment of male idiopathic infertility: a randomized, double-blind, placebo-controlled, clinical trial. *Hum Reprod*. 1998;13:596-603.

38. Paradisi R, Busacchi P, Seracchioli R, Porcu E, Venturoli S. Effects of high doses of recombinant human follicle-stimulating hormone in the treatment of male factor infertility: results of a pilot study. *Fertil Steril*. 2006;86: 728-731.

39. Paradisi R, Natali F, Fabbri R, et al. Evidence for a stimulatory role of high doses of recombinant human follicle-stimulating hormone in the treatment of male-factor infertility. *Andrologia*. 2014;46:1067-1072.

40. Santi D, Spaggiari G, Simoni M. Sperm DNA fragmentation index as a promising predictive tool for male infertility diagnosis and treatment management - meta-analyses. *Reprod Biomed Online*. 2018;37(3):315-326.

41. Attia AM, Abou-Setta AM, Al-Inany HG. Gonadotrophins for idiopathic male factor subfertility. *Cochrane Database Syst Rev*. 2013;(8):CD005071.

42. Santi D, Granata AR, Simoni M. FSH treatment of male idiopathic infertility improves pregnancy rate: A meta-analysis. *Endocr Connect*. 2015;4(3):R46–R58.

43. Cocci A, Cito G, Russo GI, et al. Effectiveness of highly purified urofollitropin treatment in patients with idiopathic azoospermia before testicular sperm extraction. *Urologia*. 2018;85(1):19-21.

44. Valenti D, La Vignera S, Condorelli RA, et al. Follicle-stimulating hormone treatment in normogonadotropic infertile men. *Nat Rev Urol*. 2013;10(1):55-62.

45. Chua ME, Escusa KG, Luna S, Tapia LC, Dofitas B, Morales M. Revisiting oestrogen antagonists (clomiphene or tamoxifen) as medical empiric therapy for idiopathic male infertility: a meta-analysis. *Andrology*. 2013;1(5): 749-757.

46. Tüttelmann F, Laan M, Grigorova M, Punab M, Sõber S, Gromoll J. Combined effects of the variants FSHB -211G>T and FSHR 2039A>G on male reproductive parameters. *J Clin Endocrinol Metab*. 2012;97(10):3639-3647.

47. Ferlin A, Vinanzi C, Selice R, Garolla A, Frigo AC, Foresta C. Toward a pharmacogenetic approach to male infertility: polymorphism of follicle-stimulating hormone beta-subunit promoter. *Fertil Steril*. 2011;96(6):1344-1349.e2.

48. Simoni M, Santi D, Negri L, et al. Treatment with human, recombinant FSH improves sperm DNA fragmentation in idiopathic infertile men depending on the FSH receptor polymorphism p.N680S: a pharmacogenetic study. *Hum Reprod*. 2016;31(9):1960-1969.

49. Kumar R, Gautam G, Gupta NP. Drug therapy for idiopathic male infertility: rationale versus evidence. *J Urol*. 2006;176(4 Pt 1):1307-1312.

50. Cocuzza M, Agarwal A. Nonsurgical treatment of male infertility: specific and empiric therapy. *Biologics*. 2007; 1(3):259-269.

51. Damber JE, Abramsson L, Duchek M. Tamoxifen treatment of idiopathic oligozoospermia: effect on hCG-induced testicular steroidogenesis and semen variables. *Scand J Urol Nephrol*. 1989;23(4):241-246.

52. Vandekerckhove P, Lilford R, Vail A, Hughes E. Clomiphene or tamoxifen for idiopathic oligo/asthenospermia. *Cochrane Database Syst Rev*. 2000;(2):CD000151.

53. Rozati R, Reddy PP, Reddanna P, et al. Role of environmental estrogens in the deterioration of male factor fertility. *Fertil Steril.* 2002;78(6):1187-1194.

54. Riggs BL, Hartmann LC. Selective estrogen-receptor modulators — mechanisms of action and application to clinical practice. *N Engl J Med.* 2003;348(7):618-629.

55. Homonnai ZT, Yavetz H, Yogev L, Rotem R, Paz GF. Clomiphene citrate treatment in oligozoospermia: comparison between two regimens of low-dose treatment. *Fertil Steril.* 1988;50(5):801-804.

56. Wang C, Chan CW, Wong KK, Yeung KK. Comparison of the effectiveness of placebo, clomiphene citrate, mesterolone, pentoxifylline, and testosterone rebound therapy for the treatment of idiopathic oligospermia. *Fertil Steril.* 1983;40(3):358-365.

57. Wang C, Chan SY, Tang LC, Yeung KK. Clomiphene citrate does not improve spermatozoal fertilizing capacity in idiopathic oligospermia. *Fertil Steril.* 1985;44(1):102-105.

58. Moradi M, Moradi A, Alemi M, et al. Safety and efficacy of clomiphene citrate and L-carnitine in idiopathic male infertility: a comparative study. *Urol J.* 2010;7(3):188-193.

59. ElSheikh MG, Hosny MB, Elshenoufy A, Elghamrawi H, Fayad A, Abdelrahman S. Combination of vitamin E and clomiphene citrate in treating patients with idiopathic oligoasthenozoospermia: A prospective, randomized trial. *Andrology.* 2015;3(5):864-867.

60. Rönnberg L. The effect of clomiphene citrate on different sperm parameters and serum hormone levels in preselected infertile men: a controlled double-blind cross-over study. *Int J Androl.* 1980;3(5):479-486.

61. Matsumiya K, Kitamura M, Kishikawa H, et al. A prospective comparative trial of a gonadotropin-releasing hormone analogue with clomiphene citrate for the treatment of oligoasthenozoospermia. *Int J Urol.* 1998;5(4):361-363.

62. Kotoulas IG, Cardamakis E, Michopoulos J, Mitropoulos D, Dounis A. Tamoxifen treatment in male infertility. I. Effect on spermatozoa. *Fertil Steril.* 1994;61(5):911-914.

63. Kadioglu TC, Köksal IT, Tunç M, Nane I, Tellaloglu S. Treatment of idiopathic and postvaricocelectomy oligozoospermia with oral tamoxifen citrate. *BJU Int.* 1999;83(6):646-648.

64. Cakan M, Aldemir M, Topcuoglu M, Altuğ U. Role of testosterone/estradiol ratio in predicting the efficacy of tamoxifen citrate treatment in idiopathic oligoasthenoteratozoospermic men. *Urol Int.* 2009;83(4):446-451.

65. Guo L, Jing J, Feng YM, Yao B. Tamoxifen is a potent antioxidant modulator for sperm quality in patients with idiopathic oligoasthenospermia. *Int Urol Nephrol.* 2015;47(9):1463-1469.

66. Buvat J, Ardaens K, Lemaire A, Gauthier A, Gasnault JP, Buvat-Herbaut M. Increased sperm count in 25 cases of idiopathic normogonadotropic oligospermia following treatment with tamoxifen. *Fertil Steril.* 1983;39(5):700-703.

67. Török L. Treatment of oligozoospermia with tamoxifen (open and controlled studies). *Andrologia.* 1985;17(5):497-501.

68. AinMelk Y, Belisle S, Carmel M, Jean-Pierre T. Tamoxifen citrate therapy in male infertility. *Fertil Steril.* 1987;48(1):113-117.

69. Sterzik K, Rosenbusch B, Mogck J, Heyden M, Lichtenberger K. Tamoxifen treatment of oligozoospermia: a re-evaluation of its effects including additional sperm function tests. *Arch Gynecol Obstet.* 1993;252(3):143-147.

70. Tsourdi E, Kourtis A, Farmakiotis D, Katsikis I, Salmas M, Panidis D. The effect of selective estrogen receptor modulator administration on the hypothalamic-pituitary-testicular axis in men with idiopathic oligozoospermia. *Fertil Steril.* 2009;91(suppl 4):1427-1430.

71. Höbarth K, Lunglmayr G, Kratzik C. Effect of tamoxifen and kallikrein on sperm parameters including hypoosmotic swelling test in subfertile males. A retrospective analysis. *Andrologia.* 1990;22(6):513-517.

72. Krause W, Holland-Moritz H, Schramm P. Treatment of idiopathic oligozoospermia with tamoxifen—a randomized controlled study. *Int J Androl.* 1992;15(1):14-18.

73. Farmakiotis D, Farmakis C, Rousso D, Kourtis A, Katsikis I, Panidis D. The beneficial effects of toremifene administration on the hypothalamic-pituitary-testicular axis and sperm parameters in men with idiopathic oligozoospermia. *Fertil Steril.* 2007;88(4):847-853.

74. Cannarella R, Condorelli RA, Mongioì LM, Barbagallo F, Calogero AE, La Vignera S. Effects of the selective estrogen receptor modulators for the treatment of male infertility: a systematic review and meta-analysis. *Expert Opin Pharmacother.* 2019;20(12):1517-1525.

75. Nada EA, El Taieb MA, Ibrahim HM, Al Saied AE. Efficacy of tamoxifen and l-carnitine on sperm ultrastructure and seminal oxidative stress in patients with idiopathic oligoasthenoteratozoospermia. *Andrologia.* 2015;47(7):801-810.

76. Ring JD, Lwin AA, Köhler TS. Current medical management of endocrine-related male infertility. *Asian J Androl.* 2016;18(3):357-363.

77. Schlegel PN. Aromatase inhibitors for male infertility. *Fertil Steril.* 2012;98:1359-1362.

78. Del Giudice F, Busetto GM, De Berardinis E, et al. A systematic review and meta-analysis of clinical trials implementing aromatase inhibitors to treat male infertility. *Asian J Androl.* 2020;22(4):360-367.

79. Cavallini G, Ferraretti AP, Gianaroli L, Biagiotti G, Vitali G. Cinnoxicam and L-carnitine/acetyl-L-carnitine treatment for idiopathic and varicocele-associated oligoasthenospermia. *J Androl.* 2004;25:761-770.

80. Stephens SM, Polotsky AJ. Big enough for an aromatase inhibitor? How adiposity affects male fertility. *Semin Reprod Med.* 2013;31:251-257.

81. Gregoriou O, Bakas P, Grigoriadis C, et al. Changes in hormonal profile and seminal parameters with use of aromatase inhibitors in management of infertile men with low testosterone to estradiol ratios. *Fertil Steril.* 2012;98:48-51.

16

Antioxidants Therapy of Male Infertility

Ramadan Saleh and Ashok Agarwal

KEY POINTS

- Treatment with antioxidants (AOXs) to improve fertility potential in males by counteracting the effects of reactive oxygen species is theoretically feasible.
- An AOX is a substance that neutralizes or protects cells against the effects of oxidation and free radicals through different mechanisms.
- The supplementary AOXs that are predominantly used as therapeutic interventions of male infertility in clinical trials are vitamin E, vitamin C, carotenoids, carnitine, cysteine, coenzyme Q10, selenium, zinc, and folate.
- Recent systematic reviews and metaanalyses indicate a positive impact of AOX supplementation on basic sperm parameters and fertility potential of infertile males.

INTRODUCTION

Oxidative stress (OS) plays an important role in the pathogenesis of male infertility; hence antioxidant (AOX) supplementation to treat infertility is theoretically feasible. The large safety profile, together with the relatively low price of AOX products, encouraged their wide prescription by healthcare providers.[1] However, the outcome of AOX supplementation of infertile males is the subject of debate in the current research. In addition, the current guidelines of the European Association of Urology (EAU)[2] and the American Urological Association (AUA)/ American Society for Reproductive Medicine (ASRM)[3] do not provide a firm conclusion on the topic.

In this chapter, we discuss the efficacy of AOX therapy for male infertility based on the available literature. Additionally, we highlight the current practice patterns, professional societies' guidelines and limitations of AOX therapy of male infertility.

PROTECTIVE ACTION OF ANTIOXIDANTS

Naturally, there is a fine balance between reactive oxygen species (ROS) production and AOX capacity that enables the latter to protect cells against the effects of oxidation and free radicals.[4] The mechanisms of AOX protection in infertile males include scavenging and neutralizing of ROS, preserving sperm DNA integrity, and facilitating mitochondrial transport.[5] Several AOXs have been tested for their efficacy in treatment of male infertility, including carnitine, carotenoids, cysteine, coenzyme Q10, vitamin E, vitamin C, selenium, zinc, and folate.[6,7] These AOXs are available either individually or in various combinations of two or more.

IMPACT OF ANTIOXIDANT THERAPY OF INFERTILE MALES ON SEMEN PARAMETERS

The role of AOX therapy in infertile males has been extensively investigated in the last few decades. A recent systematic review indicated a positive impact of AOX therapy in cases of varicocele, unexplained infertility, and idiopathic infertility.[8] In another metaanalysis, a significant positive impact of AOX administration was found on basic sperm parameters following varicocele repair.[9] Significant improvement of sperm concentration, motility, and morphology was found in a metaanalysis investigating the impact of oral supplementation with vitamin E, vitamin C, N-acetyl cysteine (NAC), carnitines, CoQ10, lycopene, selenium, and zinc in infertile males.[10] Similarly, administration of L-carnitine or NAC resulted in significant improvement of basic sperm parameters.[11] Results of latest Cochrane review suggested improvement in sperm motility following therapy with carnitines and combined AOX, and improvement of sperm concentration following supplementation with polyunsaturated fats and zinc.[12] However, the authors of the latest Cochrane review stated that there was high heterogeneity in published studies and that reliable conclusions could not be drawn regarding the effect of AOX on sperm concentration, total motility, and progressive motility. Most recently, a metaanalysis by our group indicates significant positive effects of AOX therapy of infertile males on sperm concentration (mean difference (MD) 5.93 mil/mL; 95% confidence interval [CI]: 4.43, 7.43; $p < 0.01$), progressive motility (MD 7.21%; 95% CI: 3.66, 10.76; $p < 0.01$), total motility (MD 7.52%; 95% CI: 3.11, 11.94); $p < 0.01$), and sperm morphology (MD 3.28%; 95% CI: 2.40, 4.17; $p < 0.01$).[13] However, we were unable to find similar improvement in the sperm DNA fragmentation levels in infertile males following AOX supplementation, probably due to the limited number of studies testing this outcome. Our results also showed significantly higher levels of total AOX capacity in semen (MD 1.87; 95% CI: 1.26, 2.48; $p < 0.01$), and lower levels of malonaldehyde in infertile males following AOX therapy. Previous individual studies have also demonstrated improvement in seminal OS following therapy with several AOXs, such as vitamin C, vitamin E, beta-carotene, zinc, selenium, and NAC.[14–17]

IMPACT OF ANTIOXIDANT THERAPY OF INFERTILE MALES ON PREGNANCY OUTCOMES

The latest Cochrane review reported a significant positive impact of AOX supplementation in infertile males on pregnancy rate (odds ratio [OR] 2.97, 95% CI 1.91, 4.63), although the level of evidence was found to be low.[12] A similar finding was found in a recent metaanalysis by our

group (OR for spontaneous clinical pregnancy 1.97; 95% CI: 1.28, 3.04; $p < 0.01$).[13] Other older reviews also found increased clinical pregnancy rate following AOX therapy of infertile males under natural or assisted reproduction conditions.[10,18,19] However, the latest Cochrane review[12] and our recent metaanalysis[13] were unable to show improvement of live birth rate, possibly due to the low number of studies exploring this outcome. Similarly, neither study[12,13] found a significant correlation of AOX therapy of infertile males with miscarriage rates.

PRACTICE PATTERNS OF THE USE OF ANTIOXIDANT THERAPY IN MALE INFERTILITY

Currently, the use of AOXs therapy of male infertility continues to be a common practice, despite lack of strong scientific evidence and clear guidelines.[10] A recent global survey by our group to identify the practice patterns of 1327 reproductive physicians from around the world indicates that approximately half (43.7%) of clinicians routinely prescribe AOXs to all infertile males.[1] Another 41.9% of the survey participants reported that they recommend AOX therapy for selected categories of infertile males.

PROFESSIONAL SOCIETIES' GUIDELINES OF ANTIOXIDANT THERAPY IN MALE INFERTILITY

The major scientific societies, including the EAU[2] and the AUA/ASRM,[3] do not support the routine use of AOX therapy in infertile males, probably due to the heterogeneity of the current evidence. The latest recommendations by the EAU,[2] the AUA/ASRM,[3] the European Academy of Andrology,[20] and the Italian Society of Andrology and Sexual Medicine,[21] on AOX therapy for male infertility are shown in Table 16.1.

LIMITATIONS OF ANTIOXIDANT THERAPY IN MALE INFERTILITY

Currently, practitioners' pattern of the use of AOX therapy in male infertility is subject to great variability. This may reflect the lack of clinical practice guidelines

TABLE 16.1 Summary of the Societies' Recommendations on the Use of Antioxidants for the Treatment of Male Infertility

Society	Document	Recommendation
European Academy of Andrology (EAA)	Colpi et al., 2018[20]	• Recommendation 9. According to the current evidence, we cannot recommend either for or against antioxidants and for antiestrogens (tamoxifen or clomiphene) or aromatase inhibitors.
European Association of Urology (EAU)	Menhas et al., 2021[2]	• No clear recommendation can be made for the treatment of patients with idiopathic infertility using antioxidants, although antioxidant use may improve semen parameters (strength rating: weak).
American Urological Association (AUA)/ American Society for Reproductive Medicine (ASRM)	Schlegel et al., 2021[3]	• Recommendation 43. Clinicians should counsel patients that the benefits of supplements (e.g., antioxidants, vitamins) are of questionable clinical utility in treating male infertility. Existing data are inadequate to provide recommendation for specific agents to use for this purpose (*Conditional Recommendation; Evidence Level: Grade B*).
Italian Society of Andrology and Sexual Medicine (SIAMS)	Ferlin et al., 2021[21]	• We recommend against treatment with nutraceuticals/ antioxidants in unselected infertile males to increase sperm parameters (expert opinion). • We suggest considering the use of nutraceuticals/antioxidants in selected patients with idiopathic oligozoospermia and/or asthenozoospermia and/or clear signs of high oxidative stress, since in some cases they might improve sperm parameters. • We cannot recommend either for or against the use of nutraceuticals/antioxidants to increase the pregnancy rate (expert opinion).

Adapted from Agarwal A, Cannarella R, Saleh R, et al. Impact of antioxidant therapy on natural pregnancy outcomes and semen parameters in infertile males: a systematic review and meta-analysis of randomized controlled trials. *World J Mens Health.* 2023;41(1):14-48.

based on the topic. Also, information is lacking on the optimum dose, duration, or formulation of AOX that can be used in the treatment of infertile males. In addition, no tool is currently approved for assessment of seminal OS. The latter is an important step prior to starting therapy with AOXs, first, to determine the candidates that are most likely to benefit from treatment with AOXs, and second, to evaluate the direct impact of AOXs in lowering the OS status in semen.

in treatment of infertile males are controversial, and the current guidelines of major professional societies do not provide firm conclusions on the topic. Infertile males with high seminal OS may be good candidates for AOX therapy to overcome their OS status and improve fertility potential. Therefore future research should be focused on investigating the impact of AOX therapy in selected categories of infertile males with elevated seminal OS indices.

SUMMARY

Seminal OS has been established as a major contributor to the pathogenesis of male infertility. Several studies investigated the efficacy of AOX supplementation in treatment of infertile males. However, the results of published clinical trials on the impact of AOX therapy

REFERENCES

1. Agarwal A, Finelli R, Selvam MKP, et al. A global survey of reproductive specialists to determine the clinical utility of oxidative stress testing and antioxidant use in male infertility. *World J Mens Health.* 2021;39(3):470-488.

2. Minhas S, Bettocchi C, Boeri L, et al. European association of urology guidelines on male sexual and reproductive health: 2021 update on male infertility. *Eur Urol.* 2021; 80(5):603-620.

3. Schlegel PN, Sigman M, Collura B, et al. Diagnosis and treatment of infertility in men: AUA/ASRM guideline part II. *J Urol.* 2021;205(1):44-51.

4. Valko M, Rhodes CJ, Moncol J, Izakovic M, Mazur M. Free radicals, metals and antioxidants in oxidative stress-induced cancer. *Chem Biol Interact.* 2006;160(1):1-40.

5. Ali M, Martinez M, Parekh N. Are antioxidants a viable treatment option for male infertility? *Andrologia.* 2020; 53:e13644.

6. Majzoub A, Agarwal A. Antioxidant therapy in idiopathic oligoasthenoteratozoospermia. *Indian J Urol.* 2017;33(3): 207-214.

7. Barati E, Nikzad H, Karimian M. Oxidative stress and male infertility: current knowledge of pathophysiology and role of antioxidant therapy in disease management. *Cell Mol Life Sci.* 2020;77(1):93-113.

8. Agarwal A, Leisegang K, Majzoub A, et al. Utility of antioxidants in the treatment of male infertility: Clinical guidelines based on a systematic review and analysis of evidence. *World J Mens Health.* 2021;39:233-290.

9. Wang J, Wang T, Ding W, et al. Efficacy of antioxidant therapy on sperm quality measurements after varicocelectomy: a systematic review and meta-analysis. *Andrologia.* 2019;51:e13396.

10. Majzoub A, Agarwal A. Systematic review of antioxidant types and doses in male infertility: benefits on semen parameters, advanced sperm function, assisted reproduction and live-birth rate. *Arab J Urol.* 2018;16:113-124.

11. Zhou Z, Cui Y, Zhang X, Zhang Y. The role of N-acetyl-cysteine (NAC) orally daily on the sperm parameters and serum hormones in idiopathic infertile men: a systematic review and meta-analysis of randomised controlled trials. *Andrologia.* 2021;53:e13953.

12. Smits RM, Mackenzie-Proctor R, Yazdani A, Stankiewicz MT, Jordan V, Showell MG. Antioxidants for male subfertility. *Cochrane Database Syst Rev.* 2019;3(3): CD007411.

13. Agarwal A, Cannarella R, Saleh R, et al. Impact of antioxidant therapy on natural pregnancy outcomes and semen parameters in infertile men: a systematic review and meta-analysis of randomized controlled trials. *World J Mens Health.* 2023;41(1):14-48.

14. Ciftci H, Verit A, Savas M, Yeni E, Erel O. Effects of N-acetylcysteine on semen parameters and oxidative/antioxidant status. *Urology.* 2009;74:73-76.

15. Omu AE, Al-Azemi MK, Kehinde EO, Anim JT, Oriowo MA, Mathew TC. Indications of the mechanisms involved in improved sperm parameters by zinc therapy. *Med Princ Pract.* 2008;17:108-116.

16. Keskes-Ammar L, Feki-Chakroun N, Rebai T, et al. Sperm oxidative stress and the effect of an oral vitamin E and selenium supplement on semen quality in infertile men. *Arch Androl.* 2003;49:83-94.

17. Comhaire FH, Christophe AB, Zalata AA, Dhooge WS, Mahmoud AMA, Depuydt CE. The effects of combined conventional treatment, oral antioxidants and essential fatty acids on sperm biology in subfertile men. *Prostaglandins Leukot Essent Fat Acids.* 2000;63:59-165.

18. Imamovic Kumalic S, Pinter B. Review of clinical trials on effects of oral antioxidants on basic semen and other parameters in idiopathic oligoasthenoteratozoospermia. *Biomed Res Int.* 2014;2014:426951.

19. Ross C, Morriss A, Khairy M, et al. A systematic review of the effect of oral antioxidants on male infertility. *Reprod Biomed Online.* 2010;20:711-723.

20. Colpi GM, Francavilla S, Haidl G. European Academy of Andrology guideline Management of oligo-astheno-teratozoospermia. *Andrology.* 2018;6(4):513-524.

21. Ferlin A, Calogero AE, Krausz C, et al. Management of male factor infertility: position statement from the Italian Society of Andrology and Sexual Medicine (SIAMS). *J Endocrinol Invest.* 2022;45(5):1085-1113.

17

Antibiotic Therapy of Male Infertility

Taymour Mostafa, Ibrahim Abdel-Hamid, and Wael Zohdy

KEY POINTS

- Semen is not sterile, and the microbiome is a diverse community in both fertile and infertile males. Microbiota inhabiting the genital tract as well as gut microbiota may play important roles both in normal physiological symbiosis and in pathogenic dysbiosis.
- Males with genital tract infections may be asymptomatic or suffer from a diverse range of symptoms.
- Next-generation sequencing, which utilizes the 16S ribosomal RNA region of the bacterial genome as the target sequence, can detect 99% of human pathogenic bacteria missed with cultural methods or sexually transmitted infections.
- The four major urological and andrological international regulatory bodies vary in their approach in the diagnosis and management of leuckocytospermia. Therefore there is no consensus on how males with suspected genital tract infection and infertility should be evaluated or on the nature or duration of treatment.
- The most common antibiotic regimens used in treating infection-related male infertility include different combinations of trimethoprim-sulfamethoxazole, doxycycline, and/or ofloxacin.
- Probiotics may have a beneficial effect in infertile males due to their antimicrobial activity against certain pathogens, antiinflammatory effect, and antioxidant properties; however the limited number of studies represents a substantial barrier regarding their wide use in clinical practice.

INTRODUCTION

Approximately 15% of couples of the reproductive age could suffer from infertility, and male factor infertility contributes to at least 50% of these cases.[1,2] Infections and associated inflammation of the male genital tract have been perceived in 6% to 10% of cases.[3] Routes of infections of the genitourinary tract include sexual transmission, uropathogenic infection, or hematogenous spread.[4–6]

The pathogens, the products of inflammatory cells, and their mediators may result in irreversible damage to the testis or epididymis, or both.[7] Frequently, a significant number of males treated for acute genitourinary infection present later on with infertility and are asymptomatic, suggesting a chronic disease stage.[8,9] In this group of infertile males, the diagnosis depends on the identification of the pathogen, elevated white blood cells (WBCs), or the inflammatory markers in the urine, seminal plasma, and/or prostatic fluid. However, sorting out infection from inflammation is challenging, as inflammatory reactions may be observed but are not primarily related to a specific pathogen.[10,11] Some authors have claimed that seminal leukocytes may not be just a response to infection but rather, play a positive role in the surveillance and phagocytosis of abnormal and dead sperm.[12] Consequently, the potential effect of genital tract infections on male fertility and its management remains contentious.

In this context, several articles addressed the relationship between antibiotic therapy for male infertility from different aspects throughout the years (Fig. 17.1).

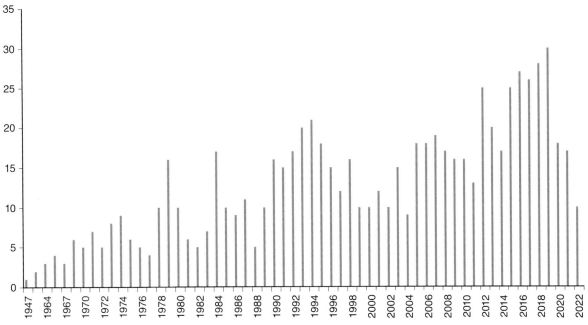

Fig. 17.1 Graphic presentation of the distribution of related studies (1947 to mid-2022).

This chapter aims to give an overview of the diagnosis and treatment of genital infections in males presenting with infertility.

SEMEN AND TESTICULAR MICROBIOMES

Nearly all tissues and organs within the human body previously thought to be sterile have been shown to harbor microbes that are present in unique communities (microbiota) that include bacteria, archaea, viruses, and fungi.[13] The term microbiome was originally defined by Whipps et al.[14] as "a characteristic microbial community occupying a reasonably well-defined habitat which has distinct physicochemical properties," and today, this definition is enriched by a dynamic consideration of the microbial activities that result in ecological niches.[15] Traditionally, microbiome studies were conducted with culture-based methods that were used to identify bacterial species, but the introduction of high-throughput DNA sequencing has overcome the limitations of the aforementioned approach. At present, the preferred methods for investigation are sequencing technologies with taxonomy-associated marker genes, such as the 16S rRNA or whole-genome sequences.[16,17]

The microbiome, which refers to the genetic collection of the microbiota, plays an important role both in normal physiological symbiosis and in pathogenic dysbiosis. Several concepts are emerging in microbiomes and male reproductive health, such as (1) impact of semen and testicular microbiomes on sperm function; (2) overlap between symptomatic and asymptomatic genital microbiota states; (3) interplay between reproductive tract microbiota and patients' immunological and/or metabolic pathways; and (4) the effect of using antibiotics on the microbiomes and male reproductive function.[18]

Diverse populations of abnormal microbiota were verified in both infertile and asymptomatic males, postulating that bacterial content of semen might not play a major role in male infertility.[19] Likewise, the microbiota inhabiting all parts of the genital tract may play different physiological roles that prevent the ascension of invading uropathogens and genitopathogens via the genital tract into the epididymis and testis.[20] In their study, Alfano et al.[21] observed small amounts of bacteria in the testis of normozoospermic males, with *Actinobacteria*, *Bacteroidetes*, *Firmicutes* *Proteobacteria* as dominating phyla, whereas increased amounts of bacteria were observed in the testes of nonobstructive azoospermia cases, with a predominance of *Actinobacteria* and *Firmicutes*.

Wang and Xie[22] revealed that gut microbiota could influence male reproduction through these possible mechanisms: (1) inducing immune system activation leading to testicular and epididymal inflammation through the release of microbial-associated molecular patterns such as lipopolysaccharides, lipoprotein acids, peptidoglycans, and lipoproteins entering the circulation via the hepatic portal vein or the lymphatic system causing testicular damage; and (2) playing a role in the formation and development of insulin resistance through disturbed production of leptin and ghrelin exerting inhibitory effects on testicular steroid production. Besides, metagenomics data showed significant alterations in the S-adenosyl-L-methionine cycle, suggesting a role in the pathogenesis of male infertility via DNA methylation, oxidative stress, and/or disruption of polyamine metabolism.[23]

Mechanistic studies exploring how seminal microbiome may impact fertility are rather few. These microorganisms may likely be able to change the concentration of seminal cytokines and increase the level of biofilm formation linked with minimal impairments of fertilizing ability participating in a complex crosstalk with the patient's immune system. In their study, Mashaly et al.[24] assessed seminal *Corynebacterium* strains in 60 infertile males with/without leukocytospermia by doing semen culture on Columbia agar medium confirmed by Gram-stained film and biochemical tests followed by analytical profile index biotyping and antibiotic susceptibility. Bacterial isolates were detected in 20/60 semen cultures (33.3%) as corynebacteria, staphylococci, alpha-hemolytic streptococci, and *Escherichia coli*, whereas 12/60 (20%) revealed *Corynebacterium*-positive semen culture, for which *C. seminal* was the major isolated species, followed by *C. amycolatum*, *C. jekium*, and *C. urealyticum*. In positive cultures, sperm motility was significantly lower compared with negative cultures. Antimicrobial sensitivity among corynebacteria strains was highest for vancomycin and rifampicin, then imipenem, ampicillin + sulbactam, and ciprofloxacin.

In a systematic review and metaanalysis that included 55 studies, Farahani et al.[25] showed that four studies only characterized seminal microbiome impact on male infertility (on small cohorts in China, Taiwan, and Europe). It was demonstrated that semen is not sterile, and that the microbiome is a diverse community in both fertile and infertile males. It has been revealed that *Ureaplasma urealyticum*, *Enterococcus faecalis*, *Mycoplasma hominis*, and *Prevotella* negatively impact semen parameters, whereas *Lactobacillus* appears to protect sperm quality.

Another study from the United States by Lundy et al.[23] pointed out that infertile males harbored increased seminal α-diversity and distinct ß-diversity, increased seminal *Aerococcus*, and decreased rectal *Anaerococcus*. These authors confirmed the previous finding that *Prevotella* abundance was inversely linked with sperm concentration and *Pseudomonas* was associated with total motile sperm count, whereas the anaerobes were overrepresented in the semen of infertile males with varicocele.

Lately, Bukharin et al.[26] assessed the levels of cytokine secretory inhibitors and the microbiota biofilms of 72 semen samples, showing that cell-free supernatants of *Staphylococcus* contained higher levels of secretory inhibitor of cytokines in fertile males compared with infertile patients. In infertile males, the ability to reduce cytokine levels was more characteristic of *Enterococcus* and *Corynebacterium*, whereas seminal *Staphylococcus*, *Corynebacterium*, and *Enterococcus* isolated from infertile subjects showed a greater ability to form biofilms than the same bacteria isolated from healthy fertile males. Besides, Yao et al.[27] showed that *Streptococcus*, *Lactobacillus*, *Burkholderia-Caballeronia-Paraburkholderia*, *Staphylococcus*, *Gardnerella*, *Ralstonia*, *Corynebacterium*, *Veillonella*, *Acinetobacter*, *Rhodococcus*, *Finegoldia*, *Peptoniphilus*, *Enterococcus*, *Prevotella*, and *Haemophilus* were frequently abundant in semen samples. These authors classified microbiota in the semen into two clustered groups: *Lactobacillus*-enriched and *Streptococcus*-enriched groups. Overall, 57.6% of the subjects with normal seminal leucocyte count were in the *Lactobacillus*-enriched group compared with those in the *Streptococcus*-enriched group.

SEMINAL MICROBIOME AND ASSISTED REPRODUCTIVE TECHNIQUE OUTCOME

Still, there is a paucity of data considering the impact of the semen microbiome on assisted reproductive technique (ART) outcome. Broadly speaking, ART procedures using either ejaculated or testicular sperm do not occur in a sterile environment.[28] In their research, Ricci et al.[29] included 164 couples undergoing ART, showing that leukocytospermia did not influence its outcome, mostly due to semen processing done before the sample was used. However, Štšepetova et al.[30] observed considerable bacterial microbiota in semen samples of males undergoing ART, with the prevalence of classes *Bacilli* in raw semen and embryo culture media, *Clostridia* in washed sperm, *Bacteroidia* in incubated sperm, and *Alphaproteobacteria* in both incubated sperm and culture media. Yet the prevalence of bacteria in these procedures was decreased during semen processing. These authors showed a positive correlation between low-quality embryos and higher counts of *Alphaproteobacteria* and *Gammaproteobacteria* in washed semen samples and *Corynebacterium spp.* in raw semen samples. In contrast, the mean proportion of *Enterobacteriaceae* group in raw semen was higher in couples with better embryo quality.

In a study, Vaughn et al.[31] demonstrated that diversity of semen microbiome does not affect fertilization but may affect blastocyst conversion rates in 52 couples who underwent in vitro fertilization (IVF)/intracytoplasmic sperm injection (ICSI) using freshly ejaculated sperm, suggesting that intrinsic testicular microbiome may interact with spermatogenesis. In their systematic review and metaanalysis on 28 case-controlled retrospective studies, Castellini et al.[32] reported that leukocytospermia samples displayed lower sperm concentrations and lower progressive motility, but the fertilization rate and pregnancy rate after ART were not significantly different. Lately, Okwelogu et al.[33] noted that semen samples with positive IVF were significantly colonized by *L. jensenii* and *Faecalibacterium*; significantly less colonized by *Proteobacteria*, *Prevotella*, and *Bacteroides*; and had a lower *Firmicutes/Bacteroidetes* ratio compared with semen samples with negative IVF procedure.

DIAGNOSIS OF GENITAL TRACT INFECTION

Males with genital tract infections suffer from a diverse range of symptoms in terms of quality and intensity. Therefore during history taking, physicians should pay attention to previous diseases such as sexually transmitted infections (STIs), urogenital infections, or systemic infections. Clinical examination of the genital organs is usually followed by ultrasonography of the scrotal compartment, as well as by transrectal ultrasonography.[34–36]

Leukocytospermia is an established indicator of infection in the male urogenital tract, although other microorganisms such as bacteria and viruses may also be contributors to the etiology of male infertility. Thereafter, the localization of the inflammation is of prime importance in patient management, whereas the four-glass test has been previously developed to detect the site of infection, with special attention to the prostate.[37] Three decades later, a simplified procedure has been evolved by Nickle[38] based on two glass tests instead of four, and shortly confirmed by other investigators.[39,40]

Assessment of Seminal Round Cells

Initial semen analysis is conducted for estimation of round cells on the wet preparation using a phase-contrast microscope with a green filter having a 10×10 ocular grid in the eyepiece. A 6-µL aliquot of the well-mixed semen sample is loaded onto the fixed cell chamber. Round cells in the semen can be leukocytes, immature germ cells, large anucleate residual cytoplasm, epithelial cells, or *Trichomonas vaginalis*. The number of round cells in all 100 squares of the grid using a 20× objective (high power field, HPF) is calculated as the average number of round cells/field multiplied with the microscope factor giving the concentration of round cells in 10^6/mL.[41] If greater than 5 round cells/HPF or a round cell concentration of greater than or equal to 1.0×10^6/mL is observed, a test for leukocytes is indicated.

Immunochemistry

Monoclonal antibodies against the common leukocyte antigen CD45 or CD53 have been demonstrated to distinguish granulocytes, lymphocytes, and macrophages concurrently.[42] By changing the nature of the primary antibody, this procedure can identify different types of leukocytes, such as macrophages, monocytes, neutrophils, B-cells, or T-cells. In a study, Ricci et al.[43] correlated positively between the flow cytometric immunocytological method using CD45 and CD53 with the simple peroxidase test. The American Society for Reproductive Medicine (ASRM) as well as the American Urological Association (AUA) recommended immunohistochemistry as a confirmatory diagnostic test for leucocytospermia.[44] However, the latest edition of the World Health Organization (WHO) laboratory manual has stated that there are no evidence-based reference values for CD45-positive cells in semen from fertile males.[45]

Seminal Granulocyte Elastase Test

Elastase is a protease released by polymorphonuclear leukocytes during the inflammatory process and is measured by an enzyme-linked immunosorbent immunoassay in seminal plasma, whereas Ela/α1-PI at a cut-off level of greater than 230 µg/mL can detect genital tract inflammation.[46] Elastase concentrations have been shown to negatively correlate with sperm motility, progressive motility, and sperm morphology.[47] Although this test affords information on the number of granulocytes and their inflammatory activation, its commercial use is expensive. Therefore the value of its routine use is limited when used as a single parameter to screen for subclinical infection/inflammation in males undergoing infertility investigation.[48]

Peroxidase Test

Peroxidase inside granulocytes catalyzes the reaction of orthotoluidine and hydrogen peroxide, whereas granulocytes stain brown as peroxidase-positive cells, and peroxidase-negative cells remain unstained. Since peroxidase-positive cells are a portion of the leukocytes identified in the ejaculate, the suggested threshold value of 1.0×10^6 cells/mL denotes a higher concentration of total leukocytes. The number of peroxidase-positive cells has been determined as a marker of inflammation in the ejaculate by multiplying the concentration of peroxidase-positive cells by the ejaculate volume.[3,49] However, this test cannot detect lymphocytes, macrophages, or monocytes that do not contain peroxidase, or identify polymorphonuclear leukocytes that have released their granules. These cells can be detected by immunocytochemical tests, which are more expensive and time consuming.[45]

In their study, Cumming and Carrell[50] analyzed 17,142 consecutive semen samples, in which 4.7% had leukocytospermia, but significant bacterial colonies had been isolated in 12.7% of them. These authors pointed out that those urogenital samples can get contaminated by the normal microbiota of the urethra, including bacteria such as *Streptococcus viridans* and *S. epidermidis* nonpathogenic flora. On the other side, obligatory pathogenic bacteria, such as *Neisseria gonorrhea* and *Chlamydia trachomatis*, beside the facultative pathogenic bacteria, such as enterobacteria (*E. coli, Klebsiella spp., Proteus spp.*), enterococci, ureaplasma, mycoplasms, and *Staphylococcus saprophyticus* can infect the host.[51] Therefore the proper sampling technique, transport, and processing time are critical, as the lack of cleaning of the urethral orifice and its surrounding before microbiological analysis of the ejaculate should be performed before urination.[45]

For pathogens that are difficult to grow in culture media or a case of very sensitive bacteria, the culture-independent nucleic acid amplification techniques (e.g., STI polymerase chain reaction [PCR]) could be of choice.[52,53] In case of negative culture and negative STI

PCR, an additional universal bacterial PCR can be performed using the next-generation sequencing (NGS), which utilizes the 16S ribosomal RNA region of the bacterial genome as the target sequence is highly conserved in all bacteria that could detect 99% of human pathogenic bacteria missed with cultural methods and STI.[54,55] Besides, shotgun metagenomics provides additional insight into the functional metabolic aberrations underpinning the taxonomic microbial differences.[23]

IMPACT OF LEUKOCYTOSPERMIA ON MALE FERTILITY

Leukocytes are present in the ejaculates of almost all males. The majority of seminal fluid leukocytes originate from the testis and the epididymis, playing a key role in both immune surveillance and phagocytosis of abnormal sperm cells. Overall, 50% to 60% of leukocytes in the semen are granulocytes, followed by macrophages (20%–30%), then T lymphocytes (2%–5%).[55–58] Collectively, genital tract infection could affect male fertility by disturbing sperm quality by pathogens, inflammation molecular products, ROS release, antisperm antibodies, accessory sex gland dysfunction, ductal obstruction, and pathogen-induced epigenetic changes.[7,59–62] Therefore leukocytospermia has been considered as a risk factor for altered semen quality. Besides, high concentrations of seminal leukocytes and infectious agents could affect sperm function, resulting in clumping of motile sperm and decreased acrosomal function. Average ROS production was found to be 77 times greater in samples with greater than 0.1×10^6 WBCs/mL, suggesting that the WHO's threshold of 1×10^6 WBCs/mL is far too high.[63,64] Interestingly, some investigators advocate that at moderate levels of seminal leukocytic count ($<10^6$/mL), leukocytospermia appears to be physiologically linked with improved sperm fertilization ability.[65]

In their work, Hou et al.[66] reported no significant differences among infertile males and the controls but showed a negative correlation between the presence of the *Anaerococcus* and low sperm quality. Monteiro et al.[67] correlated between seminal hyperviscosity and oligoasthenoteratozoospermia with increased *Neisseria, Klebsiella,* and *Pseudomonas* pathogens, with a concomitant reduction in *Lactobacillus* probiotic agent. Weng et al.[68] analyzed 96 seminal fluids from infertile males and observed three major clusters:—*Lactobacillus*-predominant, *Pseudomonas*-predominant, and *Prevotella*-predominant—with a link between the *Prevotella*-predominant cluster and low semen quality. Chen et al.[69] observed a significant reduction in the biodiversity of seminal fluid microbiota and an increased *Firmicutes* and *Bacteroidetes* in azoospermic males compared with fertile males. Lately, Yao et al.[27] confirmed that males with leukocytospermia have worse sperm parameters and different semen microbiota composition compared to males with normal seminal leukocyte count.

ANTIBIOTICS THERAPY OF MALE INFERTILITY

Treatment of Leukocytospermia: Pros and Cons

Still, leuckocytospermia continues to be a controversial issue in the field of male infertility, without a consensus on either clinical significance or treatment. However, it remains to be determined whether such changes compromise male reproductive function or not.[70]

Yamamoto et al.[71] conducted a placebo-controlled study using trimethoprim-sulfamethoxazole (TMP/SMX, co-trimoxazole) two times a day for a month with/without frequent ejaculation, demonstrating that 76% of males in the combination therapy group experienced resolution of pyospermia compared with 56% of males in the antibiotic-alone group and 6.7% of the males in the placebo group. In contrast, Hamada et al.[72] found no significant improvement in the semen parameters in infertile males treated with doxycycline (100 mg twice daily for 3 weeks) that could be attributed to their definition of pyospermia ($\geq 0.2 \times 10^6$ WBCs/mL); but interestingly, the pregnancy rate was higher in patients receiving treatment compared with that in untreated controls (47% vs. 20%, respectively). In an attempt to solve this mystery, Brunner et al.[43] conducted a literature review of 11 studies, evaluating pyospermia therapies and their outcomes. In three papers, significant resolution of pyospermia was observed in patients treated with antibiotics compared with those observed in controls, and in three, no difference was found. One study randomized patients to four pyospermia treatment groups: doxycycline (100 mg twice daily for the first week, then 100 mg daily for the following 3 weeks), placebo, frequent ejaculation (at least every 3 days), and doxycycline plus frequent ejaculation. The combination therapy of antibiotics with frequent ejaculation was the most successful, with the effects persisting at a 3-month follow-up. Frequent ejaculation was thought to clear stored secretions, which may facilitate antibiotic effectiveness and minimize inflammation.

In summary, the most common antibiotic regimens used in the literature are as follows:
- Trimethoprim (TMP)/Sulfamethoxazole (SMX) (80 mg/400 mg daily twice orally for 4 weeks)
- Doxycycline (100 mg daily for 3–4 weeks)
- Ofloxacin (200 mg by mouth every 12 h for 2 to 4 weeks)

The abovementioned combination with/without frequent ejaculation (every 3 days).

Nevertheless, the negative effects of antimicrobial medications are confounded with improvements due to drug administration, as some antibiotics might harm testicular functions. A literature search revealed that the majority of studies on the possible adverse effects of administered antibiotics on spermatogenesis as well as sperm functions, were carried out on experimental animals whereas few studies were carried out in humans that are represented at this juncture.

Aminoglycosides

Generally, aminoglycosides appear to negatively affect spermatogenesis but have negligible, if any, effects on mature sperm. Previously, Timmermans[73] showed that males treated with gentamicin before prostatic surgery developed a cessation of meiosis at the stage of primary spermatocytes, with an increase of normal and abnormal primary spermatocytes on testis biopsy. Neomycin was found to hurt sperm concentration, total sperm count, and sperm motility in males with chronic inflammatory urologic conditions.[74] In contrast to the adverse effects of aminoglycosides on spermatogenesis, this class of antibiotics has virtually no direct effects on either sperm viability or motility in vitro. Hence the lack of adverse effects of streptomycin on human sperm at concentrations up to 5 mg/mL has led to its acceptance as a component in semen extenders for cryopreservation of human sperm.[75]

Trimethoprim/Sulfamethoxazole

Sulfasalazine is used in the treatment of inflammatory bowel disease and has been in clinical use since the 1940s. It is metabolized to a sulfa moicty, sulfapyridine, as well as 5-aminosalicylic acid, and is absorbed from the colon after oral administration. The active agent against bowel disease is salicylate; however, it was demonstrated that the antifertility effect of sulfasalazine is most likely mediated by sulfapyridine.[76] Despite the long period of administration to a significant number of patients, the alterations in fertility of males treated with this drug also appear to be independent of general health or severity of inflammatory bowel disease, as evidenced by the rapid improvement of semen quality after discontinuation of the drug, despite worsening of bowel symptoms. The reinstitution of sulfasalazine therapy in patients without symptoms has been shown by Cosentino et al.,[77] resulting in deterioration of semen quality. However, the effects of sulfasalazine on semen parameters appear to be fully reversible, as many pregnancies have been reported in couples after the male has stopped taking the drug despite treatment for up to 11 years. The time of full reversibility would be consistent with a toxic effect on the testis, probably early in the process of spermatogenesis, and a possible secondary effect on later stages of spermiogenesis implied by the partial response of semen parameters within 2 weeks after drug withdrawal.

Previously, Lange and Schirren[78] indicated a possible effect of co-trimoxazole on semen parameters in their study on 45 patients who underwent semen analysis before, during, and after 7 to 80 days of treatment with 160 mg of trimethoprim and 800 mg of sulfamethoxazole daily orally. The adverse effects on total sperm count, sperm motility, and morphology were not seen during the treatment period but only 4 weeks after the combination drug. Besides, Murdia et al.[79] reported a drop in sperm count in 15/40 infertile males (37%) treated with TMP/SMX for 2 weeks, although an increase in sperm count has been observed in 42% of the cohort. These results suggest that transient disruption of spermatogenesis is a possible risk facing males receiving TMP/SMX.

Tetracycline

Tetracycline is an inhibitor of mitochondrial translation and is known to cause hepatic oxidative stress. Pulkkinen and Mäenpää[80] investigated serum testosterone in nine young males receiving tetracycline to treat acne vulgaris. Both total and free testosterone were decreased significantly on day 3 of treatment (initial means of 599 ng/dL and 496 ng/dL, respectively), falling below normal in eight subjects (89%), and returned to the normal range the first day after drug cessation, with no change in sex hormone-binding globulin levels.

Fluoroquinolones

Fluoroquinolones are broad-spectrum antibiotics that are extensively prescribed in genitourinary infections or for pathogens resistant to other antibiotics. Fluroquinolones can target topoisomerase II in eukaryotic cells due to this enzyme's similarity to the bacterial target, DNA gyrase. At high doses, fluoroquinolones might exhibit a negative impact on male infertility.[81] Ciprofloxacin has been linked to an increase in abnormal sperm forms, whereas a temporary reduction in sperm motility has been observed in males receiving ofloxacin for 20 days.[82,83] In a study, Abd-Allah et al.[84] demonstrated that after using ofloxacin, ciprofloxacin, and pefloxacin, sperm count and motility, as well as testicular lactate dehydrogenase activity, were decreased significantly in a dose-dependent manner.

In their systematic review on 25 randomized controlled trials, Khaki[85] focused on the effects of aminoglycosides and fluoroquinolones on male infertility, reporting that streptomycin has fewer negative effects on cell apoptosis and sperm cell parameters compared to other drugs. On the other hand, gentamicin has more harmful effects, and lower doses and duration are advised. Fluoroquinolones showed a negative impact on testicular tissue and sperm parameters, whereas ciprofloxacin has fewer adverse effects than gentamicin in intrauterine insemination.

OVERVIEW OF THE CURRENT GUIDELINES

The four major urological and andrological international professional societies vary in their approach in the diagnosis and management of leucocytospermia. The AUA, as well as the ASRM, recommends that patients with greater than 1 million WBCs/mL semen be evaluated for an underlying genital tract infection or inflammation. However, there is no formal consensus on how males with suspected genital tract infection and infertility should be evaluated (i.e., based on symptoms, signs of inflammation, urine or prostatic fluid cultures, semen culture, etc.) or on the nature or duration of treatment.[86]

The Canadian Urological Association does not reference pyospermia in their guideline *Workup of Azoospermic Males*, but rather references it in the *Prostatitis* guideline, in which semen culture is not recommended.[87] The European Association of Urology reported that the impact of urethritis, prostatitis, orchitis, and epididymitis on sperm quality and overall fertility is unclear.

Leukocytospermia may be a marker of inflammation rather than a sign of an underlying pathogenic infection.[87] The key decision points of the four major urological and andrological international governing bodies are illustrated in Fig. 17.2.

ANTIBIOTICS AS ADJUVANTS IN ASSISTED REPRODUCTIVE TECHNIQUE

Empirical use of antibiotics has been summoned to improve the fertility potential in both males and females before the starting of the ART cycle or before embryo transfer. Antibiotics use in males before ART could be discussed at the following levels: treating leucocytospermia before ART, using antibiotics in culture media during sperm processing procedures, and using antibiotics in the embryo culture media.

Whether leukocytospermia in the semen on the day of oocyte retrieval does influence the outcomes in IVF or ICSI is still a controversial issue. Although antimicrobial treatment decreased the incidence of pathogens in semen by 16.3% in one study,[88] a systematic review and metaanalysis included 28 case-controlled retrospective studies comparing fertility outcomes after ART in males

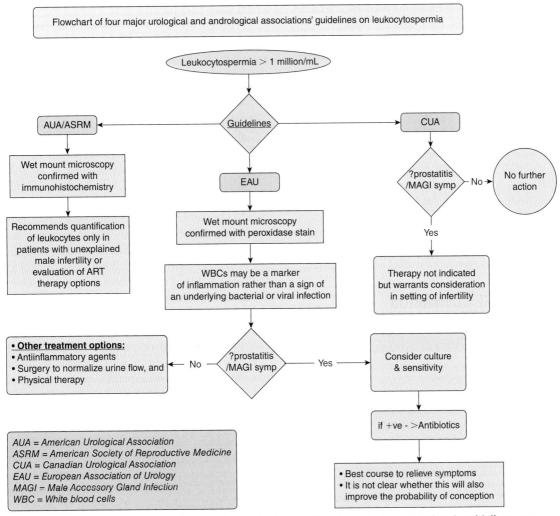

Fig. 17.2 Flowchart of the four major urological and andrological associations' guidelines on leukocytospermia.

with/without leukocytospermia showed that leukocytospermia is not linked with reduced fertility after ART.[31] These findings may suggest that the clinical criteria for the definition of leukocytospermia should be reassessed in infertile heterosexual couples attending the ART clinic. Interestingly, some studies demonstrated that moderate leukocyte concentration (<1 million/mL) has been associated with increased fertilization and pregnancy rates.[64,89]

Several authors revealed that semen processing methods such as density gradient centrifugation and swim-up method significantly reduced bacteria in semen by more than 50%, but total clearance was not achieved. However, it has been demonstrated that washing and swim-up of semen samples in an antibiotic (penicillin and streptomycin)-rich culture medium effectively eliminates greater than 95% of the organisms.[90,91] Unfortunately, adding antibiotics to culture media does not translate into improvement of pregnancy rate since pregnancy rate was comparable between semen samples washed in antibiotic-supplemented culture medium and those without.[89] In this context, Lin et al.[92] reported 12 cases of contaminations in ART culture dishes caused by bacterial strains emanating from semen which were resistant to the antibiotics (gentamicin) used in the medium system. These bacterial strains were *E. coli* (83%), followed by *K. pneumonia*, *E. faecalis*, and *Morganella morganii*.

Collectively, although antibiotics might have a positive effect on the ART process, new technologies such as microfluidics, electrophoresis, motile sperm organelle morphology examination, and birefringence may help these cases.[93,94] However, more studies are warranted.

CLINICAL CASE SCENARIOS

CASE SCENARIO

A 36-year-old male, whose sperm concentration was 7.3 million/mL (total motility 38% and normal forms of spermatozoa 8%), was coming to the infertility clinic for care. Serum follicle-stimulating hormone, luteinizing hormone, and testosterone levels were within normal levels, and the patient had 46,XY (normal karyotypes with no microdeletion in the Y chromosome. His wife (29 years old) showed normal ovulatory cycles, with no gross pelvic lesions. The couple was exposed to two IVF cycles with recurrent failure. Microbial contamination of semen was raised as one of the causes of IVF

failure. NGS testing for seminal plasma revealed *E. coli*, *Bacteroidetes*, *Aerococcaceae*, and *Candida* species. The couple received ofloxacin (200 mg by mouth every 12 h for 2 weeks), followed by azithromycin (500 mg daily for 9 days) plus tinidazole (1000 mg daily for 2 days), and was treated with ICSI, with a successful live birth delivery.

ANTIBIOTIC ALTERNATIVES

Attention is being directed towards using antibiotic alternatives (such as probiotics, prebiotics, and synbiotics) as modalities in treating several disorders, including male infertility. Probiotics are defined as "live microorganisms, which when administered in adequate amounts, confer a health benefit on the host.[95]" Prebiotics are nondigestible carbohydrates such as fructooligosaccharides and inulin, among many others that promote the growth of beneficial bacteria over harmful ones. The combination of probiotics and prebiotics is termed symbiotic and gives a synergistic effect.

In their pilot placebo-controlled study, Maretti and Cavallini[96] evaluated the effect of a 6-month course of probiotics linked with prebiotics (Flortec, Bracco; one sachet contains: *L. paracasei* B21060 5×10^9 cells + arabinogalctan 1243 mg + oligofructosaccharides 700 mg + L-glutamine 500 mg) on sperm parameters in 41 idiopathic oligoasthenoteratospermia, showed significant improvements in semen volume, median sperm concentration, progressive motility, and percentage of typical form compared with the control group. Moreover, Valcarce et al.[97] observed a 6-week course of two selected probiotic strains (*L. rhamnosus* CECT8361 and *Bifidobacterium longum* CECT7347) significantly improved sperm motility and sperm DNA fragmentation in nine asthenozoospermic males. Lately, Abbasi et al.[98] revealed that FamiLact (probiotic + prebiotic) administration improved sperm concentration, motility, and abnormal morphology, and decreased sperm DNA damage in 56 idiopathic infertile males compared with the controls.

Collectively, the beneficial effects of probiotics in infertile males appear to be due to antimicrobial activity against certain pathogens, antiinflammatory effect, modulation of sex hormones, and antioxidant properties.[99,100] Due to the limited number of studies, more trials are still needed to address many aspects, such as proper administration, exact functional strains, dosage, application method, duration of treatment, and the kind of infertile males who could respond.

SUMMARY

In this chapter, we discussed how antimicrobial therapy might be used for a variety of indications in male infertility, including leuckocytospermia and ART. Although urogenital infections have been demonstrated to contribute significantly to male infertility, males with genital tract infections may be asymptomatic or suffer from a diverse range of symptoms. For these reasons, the use of NGS could detect 99% of human pathogenic bacteria missed with cultural methods or STIs. The most common antibiotic regimens used in treating infection-related male infertility include different combinations of TMP/SMX, doxycycline, and/or ofloxacin. However, there is no consensus among the four major urological and andrological international regulatory bodies regarding the approach in the diagnosis and management of leuckocytospermia. The adverse effects of antimicrobials are infrequent and usually not serious, but follow-up is needed. As a rule, semen is not sterile. Research on the role of genital and gut microbiota, as well as the use of antibiotic alternatives (such as probiotics), is ongoing. Further research is required before it is widely applied.

REFERENCES

1. Mascarenhas MN, Flaxman SR, Boerma T, et al. National, regional, and global trends in infertility prevalence since 1990: a systematic analysis of 277 health surveys. *PLoS Med.* 2012;9(12):e1001356.
2. Agarwal A, Mulgund A, Hamada A, et al. A unique view on male infertility around the globe. *Reprod Biol Endocrinol.* 2015;13:37.
3. Weidner W, Pilatz A, Diemer T, et al. Male urogenital infections: impact of infection and inflammation on ejaculate parameters. *World J Urol.* 2013;31(4):717-723.
4. Schuppe HC, Meinhardt A, Allam JP, et al. Chronic orchitis: a neglected cause of male infertility? *Andrologia.* 2008; 40(2):84-91.
5. Haidl G, Allam JP, Schuppe HC. Chronic epididymitis: impact on semen parameters and therapeutic options. *Andrologia.* 2008;40(2):92-96.
6. Davis NF, McGuire BB, Mahon JA, et al. The increasing incidence of mumps orchitis: a comprehensive review. *BJU Int.* 2010;105(8):1060-1065.
7. Rusz A, Pilatz A, Wagenlehner F, et al. Influence of urogenital infections and inflammation on semen quality and male fertility. *World J Urol.* 2012;30(1):23-30.
8. Liu KS, Mao XD, Pan F, et al. Application of leukocyte subsets and sperm DNA fragment rate in infertile men with asymptomatic infection of genital tract. *Ann Palliat Med.* 2021;10(2):1021.
9. Veiga E, Treviño M, Romay AB, et al. Colonisation of the male reproductive tract in asymptomatic infertile men: effects on semen quality. *Andrologia.* 2020;52(7):e13637.
10. Fraczek M, Kurpisz M. Mechanisms of the harmful effects of bacterial semen infection on ejaculated human spermatozoa: potential inflammatory markers in semen. *Folia Histochem Cytobiol.* 2015;53(3):201-217.
11. Sharma R, Gupta S, Agarwal A, et al. Relevance of leukocytospermia and semen culture and its true place in diagnosing and treating male infertility. *World J Mens Health.* 2022;40(2):191-207.
12. Jung JH, Kim MH, Kim J, et al. Treatment of leukocytospermia in male infertility: a systematic review. *World J Men's Health.* 2016;34(3):165-172.
13. Lundy SD, Vij SC, Rezk AH, et al. The microbiome of the infertile male. *Curr Opin Urol.* 2020;30(3):355-362.
14. Whipps JM, Lewis K, Cooke RC. Mycoparasitism and plant disease control 161-187. In: Burge NM, ed. *Fungi in Biological Control Systems.* Manchester, UK: Manchester University Press; 1988:176.
15. Prescott SL. History of medicine: origin of the term microbiome and why it matters. *Hum. Microbiome J.* 2017;4:24-25.
16. Moreno I, Simon C. Relevance of assessing the uterine microbiota in infertility. *Fertil Steril.* 2018;110(3):337-343.
17. Vitale SG, Ferrari F, Ciebiera M, et al. The role of genital tract microbiome in fertility: a systematic review. *Int J Mol Sci.* 2021;23(1):180.
18. Brandão P, Gonçalves-Henriques M, et al. Seminal and testicular microbiome and male fertility: a systematic review. *Porto Biomed J.* 2021;6(6):e151.
19. Baud D, Pattaroni C, Vulliemoz N, et al. Sperm microbiota and its impact on semen parameters. *Front Microbiol.* 2019;10:234.
20. Altmäe S, Franasiak JM, Mändar R. The seminal microbiome in health and disease. *Nat Rev Urol.* 2019;16(12): 703-721.
21. Alfano M, Ferrarese R, Locatelli I, et al. Testicular microbiome in azoospermic men-first evidence of the impact of an altered microenvironment. *Hum Reprod.* 2018; 33(7):1212-1217.
22. Wang Y, Xie Z. Exploring the role of gut microbiome in male reproduction. Andrology. 2022;10(3):441-450.
23. Lundy SD, Sangwan N, Parekh NV, et al. Functional and taxonomic dysbiosis of the gut, urine, and semen microbiomes in male infertility. *Eur Urol.* 2021;79(6):826-836.

24. Mashaly M, Masallat DT, Elkholy AA, et al. Seminal Corynebacterium strains in infertile men with and without leucocytospermia. *Andrologia*. 2016;48(3):355-359.

25. Farahani L, Tharakan T, Yap T, et al. The semen microbiome and its impact on sperm function and male fertility: a systematic review and meta-analysis. *Andrology*. 2021;9(1):115-144.

26. Bukharin OV, Perunova NB, Ivanova EV, et al. Semen microbiota and cytokines of healthy and infertile men. *Asian J Androl*. 24(4):353-358.

27. Yao Y, Qiu XJ, Wang DS, et al. Semen microbiota in normal and leukocytospermic males. *Asian J Androl*. 2022;24(4):398-405.

28. Molina NM, Plaza-Díaz J, Vilchez-Vargas R, et al. Assessing the testicular sperm microbiome: a low-biomass site with abundant contamination. *Reprod Biomed Online*. 2021;43(3):523-531.

29. Ricci G, Granzotto M, Luppi S, et al. Effect of seminal leukocytes on in vitro fertilization and intracytoplasmic sperm injection outcomes. *Fertil Steril*. 2015;104(1):87-93.

30. Štšepetova J, Baranova J, Simm J, et al. The complex microbiome from native semen to embryo culture environment in human in vitro fertilization procedure. *Reprod Biol Endocrinol*. 2020;18(1):3.

31. Vaughn, SJ, Badamjav O, Vaughn, DV, et al. The semen microbiome in assisted reproductive technology: lower species diversity predicts higher blastocyst conversion rate. *Fertil Steril*. 2020;113(4):e14-e15.

32. Castellini C, D'Andrea S, Martorella A, et al. Relationship between leukocytospermia, reproductive potential after assisted reproductive technology, and sperm parameters: a systematic review and meta-analysis of case-control studies. *Andrology*. 2020;8(1):125-135.

33. Okwelogu SI, Ikechebelu JI, Agbakoba NR, et al. Microbiome compositions from infertile couples seeking in vitro fertilization, using 16S rRNA gene sequencing methods: any correlation to clinical outcomes? *Front Cell Infect Microbiol*. 2021;11:709372.

34. Benelli A, Hossain H, Pilatz A, et al. Prostatitis and its management. *Eur Urol Suppl*. 2017;16(4):132-137.

35. McAdams CR, Del Gaizo AJ. The utility of scrotal ultrasonography in the emergent setting: beyond epididymitis versus torsion. *Emerg Radiol*. 2018;25(4):341-348.

36. Shakur A, Hames K, O'Shea A, et al. Prostatitis: imaging appearances and diagnostic considerations. Clin Radiol. 2021;76(6):416-426.

37. Meares EM, Stamey TA. Bacteriologic localization patterns in bacterial prostatitis and urethritis. Invest Urol. 1968;5(5):492-518.

38. Nickel JC. The pre and post massage test (PPMT): a simple screen for prostatitis. *Techniques Urol*. 1997;3(1):38-43.

39. Nickel JC, Shoskes D, Wang Y, et al. How does the pre-massage and post-massage 2-glass test compare to the Meares-Stamey 4-glass test in men with chronic prostatitis/chronic pelvic pain syndrome? *J Urol*. 2006;176(1):119-124.

40. Wagenlehner FME, Naber KG, Bschleipfer T, et al. Prostatitis and male pelvic pain syndrome: diagnosis and treatment. *Dtsch Arztebl Int*. 2009;106(11):175-183.

41. Agarwal A, Gupta S, Sharma R. Leukocytospermia quantitation (ENDTZ) test. In: Agarwal A, Gupta S, Sharma R, eds. *Andrological Evaluation of Male Infertility*. Cham: Springer; 2016:69-72.

42. Villegas J, Schulz M, Vallejos V, et al. Indirect immunofluorescence using monoclonal antibodies for the detection of leukocytospermia: comparison with peroxidase staining. *Andrologia*. 2002;34(2):69-73.

43. Ricci G, Presani G, Guaschino S, et al. Leukocyte detection in human semen using flow cytometry. *Hum Reprod*. 2000;15(6):1329-1337.

44. World Health Organization. *WHO Laboratory Manual for the Examination and Processing of Human Semen*. 6th ed. Geneva: WHO Press; 2021.

45. Zorn B, Sesek-Briski A, Osredkar J, et al. Semen polymorphonuclear neutrophil leukocyte elastase as a diagnostic and prognostic marker of genital tract inflammation-a review. *Clin Chem Lab Med*. 2003;41(1):2-12.

46. Kopa Z, Wenzel J, Papp GK, Haidl G. Role of granulocyte elastase and interleukin-6 in the diagnosis of male genital tract inflammation. *Andrologia*. 2005;37(5):188-194.

47. Brunner RJ, Demeter JH, Sindhwani P. Review of guidelines for the evaluation and treatment of leukocytospermia in male infertility. *World J Mens Health*. 2019;37(2):128-137.

48. Eggert-Kruse W, Zimmermann K, Geissler W, et al. Clinical relevance of polymorphonuclear (PMN-) elastase determination in semen and serum during infertility investigation. *Int J Androl*. 2009;32(4):317-329.

49. Wolff H. The biologic significance of white blood cells in semen. *Fertil Steril*. 1995;63(6):1143-1157.

50. Cumming JA, Carrell DT. Utility of reflexive semen cultures for detecting bacterial infections in patients with infertility and leukocytospermia. *Fertil Steril*. 2009;91(suppl 4):1486-1488.

51. Schiefer HG. Microbiology of male urethroadnexitis: diagnostic procedures and criteria for aetiologic classification. *Andrologia*. 1998;30(suppl 1):7-13.

52. Van Der Pol B, Ferrero D, Buck-Barrington L, et al. Multicenter evaluation of the BDProbeTec ET system for the detection of *Chlamydia trachomatis* and *Neisseria gonorrhoeae* in urine specimens, female endocervical swabs, and male urethral swabs. *J Clin Microbiol*. 2001;39(3):1008-1016.

53. Gaydos CA, Quinn TC. Urine nucleic acid amplification tests for the diagnosis of sexually transmitted infections in clinical practice. *Curr Opin Infect Dis*. 2005;18(1):55-66.

54. Pilatz A, Hossain H, Kaiser R, et al. Acute epididymitis revisited: impact of molecular diagnostics on etiology

and contemporary guide line recommendations. *Eur Urol.* 2015;68(3):428-435.

55. Chen JZ, Gratrix J, Brandley J, et al. Retrospective review of gonococcal and chlamydial cases of epididymitis at 2 Canadian sexually transmitted infection clinics, 2004-2014. *Sex Transm Dis.* 2017;44(6):359-361.

56. Kiessling AA, Lamparelli N, Yin HZ, et al. Semen leukocytes: friends or foes? *Fertil Steril* 1995;64(1):196-198.

57. Aitken RJ, Buckingham DW, Brindle J, et al. Analysis of sperm movement in relation to the oxidative stress created by leukocytes in washed sperm preparations and seminal plasma. *Hum Reprod.* 1995;10(8):2061-2071.

58. Haidl F, Haidl G, Oltermann I, et al. Seminal parameters of chronic male genital inflammation are associated with disturbed sperm DNA integrity. *Andrologia.* 2015;47(4):464-469.

59. Fraczek M, Kurpisz M. Mechanisms of the harmful effects of bacterial semen infection on ejaculated human spermatozoa: potential inflammatory markers in semen. *Folia Histochem Cytobiol.* 2015;53(3):201-217.

60. Akgul A, Kadioglu A, Koksal MO, et al. Sexually transmitted agents and their association with leucocytospermia in infertility clinic patients. *Andrologia.* 2018;50(10):e13127.

61. Schagdarsurengin U, Teuchert LM, Hagenkoetter C, et al. Chronic prostatitis affects male reproductive health and associates with systemic and local epigenetic inactivation of CXCL12 receptor CXCR4. *Urologia Int.* 2017;98(1):89-101.

62. Eini F, Kutenaei MA, Zareei F, et al. Effect of bacterial infection on sperm quality and DNA fragmentation in subfertile men with leukocytospermia. *BMC Mol Cell Biol.* 2021;22(1):42.

63. Henkel R, Kierspel E, Stalf T, et al. Effect of reactive oxygen species produced by spermatozoa and leukocytes on sperm functions in non-leukocytospermic patients. *Fertil Steril.* 2005;83(3):635-642.

64. Domes T, Lo KC, Grober ED, et al. The incidence and effect of bacteriospermia and elevated seminal leukocytes on semen parameters. *Fertil Steril.* 2012;97(5):1050-1055.

65. Barraud-Lange V, Pont JC, Ziyyat A, et al. Seminal leukocytes are good Samaritans for spermatozoa. *Fertil Steril.* 2011;96(6):1315-1319.

66. Hou D, Zhou X, Zhong X, et al. Microbiota of the seminal fluid from healthy and infertile men. *Fertil. Steril.* 2013;100(5):1261-1269.

67. Monteiro C, Marques PI, Cavadas B, et al. Characterization of microbiota in male infertility cases uncovers differences in seminal hyperviscosity and oligoasthenoteratozoospermia possibly correlated with increased prevalence of infectious bacteria. *Am J Reprod Immunol.* 2018;79(6):e12838.

68. Weng SL, Chiu C, Lin F, et al. Bacterial communities in semen from men of infertile couples: metagenomic sequencing reveals relationships of seminal microbiota to semen quality. *PLoS One.* 2014;9(10):e110152.

69. Chen H, Luo T, Chen T, et al. Seminal bacterial composition in patients with obstructive and non-obstructive azoospermia. *Exp Ther Med.* 2018;15(3):2884-2890.

70. Rosenfeld CS, Javurek AB, Johnson SA, et al. Seminal fluid metabolome and epididymal changes after antibiotic treatment in mice. *Reproduction.* 2018;156(1):1-10.

71. Yamamoto M, Hibi H, Katsuno S, et al. Antibiotic and ejaculation treatments improve resolution rate of leukocytospermia in infertile men with prostatitis. *Nagoya J Med Sci.* 1995;58(1-2):41-45.

72. Hamada A, Agarwal A, Sharma R, et al. Empirical treatment of low-level leukocytospermia with doxycycline in male infertility patients. *Urology.* 2011;78(6):1320-1325.

73. Timmermans L. Influence of antibiotics on spermatogenesis. *J Urol.* 1974;112(3):348.

74. Yunda IF, Kushniruk YI. Neomycin effect on testicle function. *Antibiot Med Biotekhnol.* 1973;18(1):43-48.

75. Schlegel PN, Chang TS, Marshall FF. Antibiotics: potential hazards to male fertility. *Fertil Steril.* 1991;55(2):235-242.

76. O'Morain CO, Smethurst P, Dore CJ, et al. Reversible male infertility due to sulphasalazine: studies in man and rat. *Gut.* 1984;25(10):1078-1084.

77. Cosentino MJ, Chey WY, Takihara H, et al. The effects of sulfasalazine on human male fertility and seminal prostaglandins. *J Urol.* 1984;32(4):682-686.

78. Lange D, Schirren C. Untersuchungen uber den einflub von trimethoprim/sulfamethoxazol auf die qualitat des spermas bei andrologischen patienten-zugleich ein beitrag zur pharmakologischen prufung eines medikamentes auf die spermatogenetische aktivitat des hodens. *Z Hautkr.* 1974;49(20):863-878.

79. Murdia A, Mathur V, Kothari LK, et al. Sulpha-trimethoprim combinations and male fertility. *Lancet.* 1978;2(8085):375-376.

80. Pulkkinen MO, Mäenpää J. Decrease in serum testosterone concentration during treatment with tetracycline. *Acta Endocrinol (Copenh).* 1983;103(2):269-272.

81. Drobnis EZ, Nangia AK. Antimicrobials and male reproduction. *Adv Exp Med Biol.* 2017;1034:131-161.

82. Andreessen R, Sudhoff F, Borgmann V, et al. Results of ofloxacin therapy in andrologic patients suffering from therapy-requiring asymptomatic infections. *Andrologia.* 1993;25(6):377-383.

83. Carranza-Lira S, Tserotas K, Morán C, et al. Effect of antibiotic therapy in asthenozoospermic men associated with increased agglutination and minimal leukospermia. *Arch Androl.* 1998;40(2):159-162.

84. Abd-Allah AR, Aly HA, Moustafa AM, et al. Adverse testicular effects of some quinolone members in rats. *Pharmacol Res.* 2000;41(2):211-219.

85. Khaki A. Assessment on the adverse effects of amino-glycosides and flouroquinolone on sperm parameters and male reproductive tissue: a systematic review. *Iran J Reprod Med.* 2015;13(3):125-134.

86. Velez D, Ohlander S, Niederberger C. Pyospermia: background and controversies. *F S Rep.* 2021;2(1):2-6.

87. Jungwirth A, Giwercman A, Tournaye H, et al. European Association of Urology guidelines on male infertility: the 2012 update. *Eur Urol.* 2012;62(2):324-332.

88. Huyser C, Fourie FL, Oosthuizen M, et al. Microbial flora in semen during in vitro fertilization. *J In Vitro Fert Embryo Transf.* 1991;8(5):260-264.

89. Palermo GD, Neri QV, Cozzubbo T, et al. Shedding light on the nature of seminal round cells. *PLoS One.* 2016;11(3):e0151640.

90. Dissanayake DM, Amaranath KA, Perera RR, et al. Antibiotics supplemented culture media can eliminate non-specific bacteria from human semen during sperm preparation for intra uterine insemination. *J Hum Reprod Sci.* 2014;7(1):58-62.

91. Palini S, Primiterra M, De Stefani S, et al. A new micro swim-up procedure for sperm preparation in ICSI treatments: preliminary microbiological testing. *JBRA Assist Reprod.* 2016;20(3):94-98.

92. Lin LL, Guu HF, Yi YC, et al. Contamination of ART culture media-the role of semen and strategies for prevention. *Taiwan J Obstet Gynecol.* 2021;60(3):523-525.

93. Rappa KL, Rodriguez HF, Hakkarainen GC, et al. Sperm processing for advanced reproductive technologies: where are we today? *Biotechnol Adv.* 2016;34(5):578-587.

94. Jue JS, Ramasamy R. Significance of positive semen culture in relation to male infertility and the assisted reproductive technology process. *Transl Androl Urol.* 2017;6(5):916-922.

95. Gibson GR, Probert HM, Van Loo J, Rastall RA, Roberfroid MB. Dietary modulation of the human colonic microbiota: updating the concept of prebiotics. *Nutr Res Rev.* 2004;17:259-275.

96. Maretti C, Cavallini G. The association of a probiotic with a prebiotic (Flortec, Bracco) to improve the quality/quantity of spermatozoa in infertile patients with idiopathic oligoasthenoteratospermia: a pilot study. *Andrology.* 2017;5(3):439-444.

97. Valcarce DG, Genovés S, Riesco MF, et al. Probiotic administration improves sperm quality in asthenozoospermic human donors. *Benef Microbes.* 2017;8(3):193-206.

98. Abbasi B, Abbasi H, Niroumand H. Synbiotic (FamiLact) administration in idiopathic male infertility enhances sperm quality, DNA integrity, and chromatin status: a triple-blinded randomized clinical trial. *Int J Reprod Biomed.* 2021;19(3):235-244.

99. Younis N, Mahasneh A. Probiotics and the envisaged role in treating human infertility. *Middle East Fertil Soc J.* 2020;25:33.

100. Corbett GA, Crosby DA, McAuliffe FM. Probiotic therapy in couples with infertility: a systematic review. *Eur J Obstet Gynecol Reprod Biol.* 2021;256:95-100.

18

Alternative Therapy of Male Infertility

Tan V. Le, Phu V. Pham, and Hoang P.C. Nguyen

KEY POINTS

- The possibility of finding and treating modifiable risk factors for male infertility remains a significant subject for continuous research, even though the actual frequency of infertility and its change over time remains unknown.
- Herbal medicines have been entrusted for use in the treatment of male infertility since ancient times and in recent decades, they are regaining popularity. However, research regarding the efficacy of herbal medicine seems to be a rediscovery of old traditional medicines.
- Although exercising reduces the risk of developing diseases and promotes many health benefits, exhaustive exercise and overtraining may alter male fertility and the hypothalamic-pituitary-gonadal axis.
- Counseling and behavioral therapy are unquestionably essential in managing psychological-related male infertility.

INTRODUCTION

Nowadays, the treatment of infertility is increasingly focused on male factors. A person is said to be healthy only when their mind and body are healthy. Similarly, a male's reproductive health is beneficial only when he is physically strong and mentally fit. Since ancient times, people have begun to treat male infertility by herbs, with insufficient evidence. To this day, treating male infertility has been an art with many factors that need to be brought together. Besides formal treatment methods, many alternative treatment options are also available, such as nutrition, herbs, and exercise, as well as psychobehavioral therapy. In this chapter, we focus on reviewing the level of evidence as well as a brief overview of these alternative treatment options (Fig. 18.1).

NUTRITION AND MALE FERTILITY

Male factor fertility problems are a relatively prevalent condition that impacts up to one in every 20 males globally and contributes to approximately 80 million

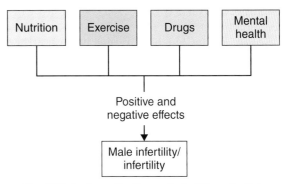

Fig. 18.1 Factors affecting male fertility potential.

instances.[1,2] As a result of the numerous cultural changes that happened over this period, including environmental, dietary, and lifestyle changes, some researchers have looked for links between these factors. Although the actual frequency of infertility and how it has changed over time is unknown, the possibility of discovering and treating modifiable risk factors for male infertility is still a hot topic for research.

The findings of Antoine Aoun and colleagues' review were reported in terms of pregnancy outcomes and sperm characteristics, with most studies indicating that the experimental group improved on at least one of these outcome measures.[3] Some research that looked at the impact of dietary intake found a link between specific macronutrient(s) or micronutrient(s) and the risk of infertility, while others found mixed results.[3]

A few studies have found links between poor male factor fertility and eating habits. In a survey of 701 young Danish males undergoing standard screening before enlisting in the military, those who consumed more saturated fat had lower sperm counts, with the highest quartile having a 41% lower count than the lowest quartile.[4] Gaskin and colleagues, who studied 188 males aged 18 to 22 years at the University of Rochester, backed this finding.[5] The scientists found a link between a "prudent" diet (high consumption of fish, poultry, fruit, vegetables, legumes, and whole grains) and gradually motile sperm in patients with a "Western" diet (high intake of red meat, refined grains, pizza, snacks, high-energy beverages, and sweets).[5] More research has found a link between intake of fruits, vegetables, poultry, skim milk, and seafood with an increased risk of asthenospermia in individuals who consume the most processed meats and sweets (odds ratio [OR] 2.0, 95% confidence interval [CI] 1.7, 2.4 and OR 2.1, 95% CI 1.1, 2.3, respectively).[6,7]

Semen quality has been related to overall body mass index (BMI) and specific diets. High BMI was found to have a deleterious impact on sperm motility and concentration in a study of 250 spouses who had intracytoplasmic sperm injection. Those on a weight-loss program, on the other hand, had better sperm counts. Overconsumption of grains and legumes had a beneficial effect on sperm parameters.[8]

Salas-Huetos and colleagues discovered that the quality of males's diets in heterosexual couples undergoing assisted reproductive technology (ART), as measured by a priori determined healthy dietary scores, has no bearing on the chance of ART success.[9] Their findings also show that food quality is unrelated to semen quality in these males. However, the directionality of this relationship may not be reflected effectively by these specific findings. Importantly, their results may not apply to couples trying to conceive without medical assistance. They may reflect the success of ART in selecting a population of sperm that is minimally affected by environmental factors, such as diet, rather than the actual biologic effect of diet and other environmental factors on the male's contributions to a couple's fertility.[9]

An empirical dietary score quantifying the total impact of nutrition on semen quality was not associated with infertility treatment outcomes with ART, according to Makiko Mitsunami and colleagues.[10] Given that ART includes rigorous sperm selection processes, it is feasible that these therapies, mediated through semen quality, will counteract the effects of environmental factors on a couple's ability to conceive. As a result, it is unclear how far these findings may be applied to couples who try to conceive without medical help. Furthermore, these findings underscore the limitations of semen quality measures as a predictor of fertility in a couple.[10] More research is needed to learn how males's food, environment, and behaviors affect a couple's fertility naturally and with medical assistance, and how males's reproductive potential may be measured using biomarkers other than bulk semen characteristics.

MALNUTRITION/NUTRIENT DEFICIENCIES AND MALE INFERTILITY

Proper diet is expected to have a critical role in ensuring healthy fertility (Fig. 18.2). Despite the lack of data, several observational studies have identified associations between subfertility/infertility and lower vitamin/mineral concentrations.[11–14] Reduced levels of numerous vitamins and minerals, which have decisive indirect or direct antioxidant action, may cause an alteration in the reactive oxygen species to antioxidant ratio, resulting in a decrease in total antioxidant capacity.[11]

Several studies have shown an optimal value for specific vitamin/mineral delivery, with both under- and oversupplementation causing reproductive problems. Two studies on the effect of selenium in mice found that animals receiving either under- or oversupplementation had lower fertility, with oxidative stress (OS) triggering germ cell death.[15,16] Other investigations have found optimal vitamin D ranges, with reproductive problems at high and low serum levels.[14,17]

Even though there is limited research on the toxicity of oversupplementation, all nutrients are likely to have a cut-off beyond which their influence is nullified or deleterious. This is especially important because many studies utilize different vitamin/mineral doses and/or combinations in their patient cohorts. Furthermore,

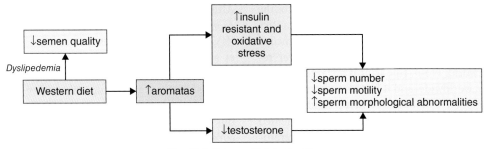

Fig. 18.2 Diet and Male Fertility.

because different communities are likely to have different dietary shortages, some groups may benefit more than others from supplementing. This could also explain (in part) the inconsistent results of research looking at the effects of certain nutrients.

HERBAL TREATMENT FOR MALE INFERTILITY

Herbal medicine refers to herbs, herbal materials, and drugs containing plant parts or mixtures of plant parts as active substances. Plant elements such as leaves, bark, flowers, roots, fruits, and seeds make these herbs. Traditional medicine (including herbal medications) is described by the World Health Organization (WHO) as therapeutic interventions that have existed for many years before the advent and extension of modern medicine but are still used today. Herbal remedies are traditional medicines that primarily treat patients with medicinal plant extracts.[18]

It is hard to calculate the total number of medicinal plants on the planet; according to one estimate, roughly 35,000 to 70,000 plant species are utilized in human healthcare services globally, and the Indian pharmacopeia alone contains around 3000 medications.[19]

Despite the rapid growth of mass-produced, chemically manufactured pharmaceuticals, herbal medicine is still widely used.[20] People in nations like China, India, and Peru, where ancient cultures previously thrived, still rely on traditional medicine for their primary healthcare. Herbal medicine is so widely used in many nations that hospitals have traditional medicine units (China and Peru are two examples).[20] Fertility is one of the topics where individuals turn to herbal treatments the most[21] since conventional therapy is expensive and may be out of reach for a significant percentage of the population.

Many infertile males have turned to herbal treatments as an effective treatment.[22]

Because OS has been shown to play an essential role in male infertility in dozens of studies, it is probable that many situations of "idiopathic male infertility" are caused by changes in OS, particularly methylation status.[23,24] Medicinal plants have shown to be effective in treating idiopathic male infertility in clinical trials, and they may be an essential source for treating male infertility.[25]

HERBS WITH POSITIVE EFFECTS ON SPERM QUALITY

Panax quinquefolius (American ginseng) is a perennial herb in the Araliaceae family that grows in North America. It is among the world's eight ginseng species and one of only three with therapeutic benefits. However, Asian ginseng (*P. ginseng*) is better renowned for its male health benefits. Evidence suggests that *P. quinquefolius* may provide andrological benefits to its users.[26]

Once male rats were given diluted American ginseng in saline for 6 weeks, their sperm count rose compared to the control group. Additionally, the extract may be able to reverse cyclophosphamide's harmful effects on sperm cells.[27] The active molecules that exert these qualities could be ginsenosides, triterpenoid saponins found only in the genus *Panax*. Ginsenosides are divided into two groups: 20(S)-protopanaxatriol and 20(S)-protopanaxadiol.[26] Ginsenoside Re, together with ginsenosides Rg1, Rg2, and Rb3, belongs to the 20(S)-protopanaxatriol group, whereas Rb1, Rb2, Rc, and Rd belong to the 20(S) protopanaxadiol group.[26] Low-Rg1 and high-Re ginsenosides are seen in most American ginseng populations.[28] Re has been shown to increase sperm motility in viable and infertile sperm by activating nitric oxide synthase.[26]

The papaya tree (*Carica papaya*) belongs to the Caricaceae family. It was originally found in Costa Rica and Mexico in Central America, but has been cultivated throughout North and South America and other regions of the world. Fresh, ripe fruit is a staple of many people's diets worldwide, and it has been shown to protect against oxidative damage.[29] When provided alongside vitamin C and E, lactoferrin, and glucan, fermented papaya fruit improves sperm quality in asthenoteratozoospermic males.[30] The benefit of ripe fruit alone has not been thoroughly studied.

Nonetheless, papaya seeds and leaves contain proteolytic enzymes, primarily papain and chemopapain,[31] exhibiting antispermatogenic and spermicidal activity in animal models and males.[32] The seed extract of *C. papaya* has a significant effect on sperm motility characteristics, essential for fertilization.[21] According to several experts, papain's capacity to lower seminal viscosity is a surprising characteristic of considerable economic value for ART in animals. These researchers found that combining papain with its inhibitor E64 lowered viscosity in alpacas without compromising sperm integrity.[22] On the other hand, others have hypothesized that it could be a good option for male contraception.[21]

Bertholletia excelsa, or Brazil nuts, are touted as sexual enhancers. Even though there have been no in vitro or in vivo investigations utilizing plant extracts, the nuts are known for their excellent selenium content.[32] In vitro studies have shown that this inorganic element protects the sperm of asthenoteratozoospermic males from reactive oxygen species (ROS) damage.[33] Squalene, an organic component with apparent sperm quality–enhancing properties, is also abundant in these nuts.[34] *Lepidium meyenii* is a prolific crop found only in Peru's Central Andean region, specifically the Junin highlands. It was widely used among ancient Peruvians for medicinal purposes. They knew about its fertility-boosting qualities, so when the Spanish arrived in these places and could not conceive, native Peruvians prescribed this plant. Fortunately, various chronicles have retained this knowledge. *L. meyenii*, sometimes known as "maca," is undoubtedly Peru's most studied plant, with its impacts on male fertility being the first to be scientifically confirmed. The hypocotyl is the edible component of the plant, which comes in a variety of phenotypes that can be distinguished by color.[35]

In animal studies, the enhancement in sperm quality exhibited following maca therapy has been documented.

After dosing male rats with an aqueous extract of *L. meyenii*, the duration and incidence of stages IX to XIV of spermatogenesis increased.[24] Valdivia Cuya et al. found that maca can cure the negative consequences of chemically and physically produced testicular dysfunction, including subfertility and impaired seminal parameters.[25] Similarly, when cyclophosphamide caused subfertility in mice, maca therapy corrected gonadal insufficiency and testicular morphology.[36] Maca improved in vitro fertilization rates by inducing an acrosome reaction and increasing sperm motility.[37]

HERBS WITH NEGATIVE EFFECTS ON SPERM QUALITY

Some plants harm sperm parameters, which is something worth exploring further. Yarrow (*Achillea millefolium* subspecies lanulosa [Nutt.]) is a native North American herb that was frequently used by populations that historically lived in boreal Canada to cure wounds and other health conditions such as respiratory and digestive difficulties.[38] Despite this, Montanari et al. found that ethanolic and hydroalcoholic extracts of yarrow flowers significantly affected spermatogenesis in mice.[39]

Locals believe that *Tropaeolum tuberosum* (mashua), an Andean food crop, has fertility-reducing effects. Mashua made soldiers "forget" their ladies, according to ancient chroniclers such as Father Bernabé Cobo and Inca Garcilaso de la Vega.[40] Research in rats has backed up these anecdotal claims. Mashua reduced sperm production daily while increasing the percentage of aberrant sperm morphology and postponement. This benefit was reversed 24 hours after the medication was stopped.[41]

PHYSICAL EXERCISE AND MALE FERTILITY

The benefits and drawbacks of physical activity and sports on reproductive success are poorly understood. While numerous studies have shown that prolonged intense exercise can negatively affect physiological systems, particularly the reproductive system and fertility, others have not.[42,43] Others feel that frequent exercise impacts one's overall health and happiness. The negative impact of exercise on male reproductive functioning has been highlighted by researchers.[44,45] Extremely strenuous endurance exercise has been shown to have a deleterious impact on reproductive hormones[43,45] and semen parameters.[43,43,45] Intense exercise has recently been shown to promote OS and DNA damage in the spermatozoa of male athletes.[46,47]

While exercise quantity was initially thought to be the most crucial factor in reproduction, subsequent research suggested that the effects of exercise intensity on male fertility were at least similar in terms of the negative consequences.[45,48] Other elements, like bike saddle friction, may be added to this equation based on the exercise modality.[49] Others appear to believe that exercise can be hazardous in the case of a preexisting disorder affecting the reproductive system.[50,51] Nevertheless, from a scientific point of view, establishing a clear and obvious affirmation of this connection is quite tricky because male reproductive characteristics are per se subject to a great deal of variation. Without a doubt, the reproductive system is a complicated system influenced by various circumstances.[52] As a result, the well-known lack of agreement on the aforementioned interdependent relationship is most likely because different criteria were employed during the athletes' training sessions.

Nonetheless, there has been some research into the possible benefits of physical training on reproduction. In this regard, Vaamonde and associates recently demonstrated that physically active people have better semen parameters and hormone levels than inactive people.[53]

THE POSITIVE IMPACT OF EXERCISE ON MALE FERTILITY

Regular exercise has long been known to positively impact the cardiorespiratory system, immune system, endocrine system, brain, muscle, and other organs and to protect against diseases like obesity, cardiovascular disease, diabetes, osteoporosis, and chronic systemic inflammation. Exercising appears to be beneficial to the reproductive system as well.

Manipulation of circulating anabolic hormone concentrations and the anabolic–catabolic hormone balance in males could be advantageous. An increase in anabolic-androgenic hormones can help athletes perform better by reducing body fat and boosting lean body mass and physical strength.[54] Anabolic endocrine hormones and local load-sensitive autocrine/paracrine growth factors play a significant role in exercising muscle tolerance. Because they increase protein production, growth hormone (GH), insulin-like growth factor 1 (IGF-1), and testosterone are directly implicated in muscle response to exercise. On the other hand, testosterone and locally produced IGF-1 have stimulated muscle stem cells. Testosterone increases lean body mass and maximum voluntary strength.[55]

Heavy resistance training can boost testosterone levels, affecting other hormones involved in male fertility. The acute testosterone response to resistance exercise is marked by a transitory increase accompanied by a return to resting (or even lower) levels.[56]

Most studies on the impact of exercise on androgens have been limited to acute effects in short-term exercise protocols. Most of them show that exercise bouts are linked to an initial burst in testosterone, followed by a drop to or less than baseline levels, with varying effects on other androgens when tested.[57,58] Long-term moderate-intensity aerobic exercise has not been adequately investigated in males's hormone levels. In conclusion, it may be necessary to distinguish between exercise's acute and chronic effects as acute changes may be more related to muscle development and tissue regeneration. On the other hand, chronic alterations may mediate the effects of exercise on long-term health.[56] Some cross-sectional investigations in middle-aged and older males suggest that males who exercise regularly have higher circulating testosterone concentrations.[59] Resistance training over a few weeks either boosted testosterone or did not, in prospective, nonrandomized investigations.[60,61]

On the other hand, one study found that daily aerobic exercise and a low-fat diet raised sex hormone–binding globulin (SHBG), which could offset testosterone's biological activity.[62] Males who have engaged in long-term exercise have been found to have higher SHBG levels than those who have not.[63] Compared to the control group, randomized clinical research of a 12-month moderate-intensity aerobic exercise intervention on serum hormones in sedentary males found an increase in serum dihydrotestosterone and SHBG levels at 3 and 12 months during the exercise intervention.[64] Vaamonde and associates found that physically active males have greater levels of follicle-stimulating hormone (FSH), luteinizing hormone (LH), testosterone, and the T/C ratio (an indication of anabolic vs. catabolic status) than inactive males, supporting the likelihood of a better hormonal environment.[53]

There has not been much evidence that exercise or physical activity improves seminal parameters in males who engage in sports or other physical activity. However, according to a new study by Vaamonde and colleagues, physically active males have better semen parameters than sedentary males.[53] Several semen measures, such as total progressive motility (physically active: 60.94 5.03; sedentary: 56.07 4.55) and morphology (physically active: 15.54 1.38, sedentary: 14.40 1.15), showed statistically significant variations. Differences in hormones backed up the seminal values obtained.[53] Palmer and colleagues found that 8 weeks of swimming improved sperm motility (1.2-fold) and morphology (1.1-fold, $p < 0.05$) in C57BL6 male mice.[65]

THE NEGATIVE IMPACT OF EXERCISE ON MALE FERTILITY

It should be mentioned that this type of training is closely linked to anabolic steroid use and, as a result, caution should be exercised. Anabolic steroids are utilized in resistance training, whereas many other doping agents are used by athletes and persons exercising to improve performance, physical fitness, and appearance. Muscle strength and size are the goals of this form of exercise. Steroids' anabolic and androgenic effects are inextricably connected.[66]

Resistance exercise has an anabolic influence on hormonal markers, increasing testosterone, as expected. Testosterone mediates anabolic reactions via two pathways: one that directly stimulates protein synthesis and muscle growth, and the other (indirect) that increases GH release and muscle force via interactions with the neurological system.[67] A single session of resistance exercise typically results in a rise in testosterone. Resistance exercise appears to increase testosterone production frequency and amplitude.[67] The recruitment and activation of major muscle groups and moderate- to high-volume training are associated with increases in testosterone.[56] Unless training becomes extreme, there is a rise in testosterone as part of chronic adaptations, and this increase is associated with more significant muscle and strength development.[68]

Even though most research shows an increase in testosterone secretion after resistance training, Arce and colleagues found lower levels of total and free testosterone in both stamina and resistance-trained athletes once compared to sedentary controls, suggesting that both training types have similar effects on male reproductive hormones.[69]

Whenever anabolic steroids (e.g., oxandrolone, methandienone, stanozolol, nandrolone decanoate, and boldenone undecylenate) are used, the outcome is a reduction in endogenous testosterone release. This is due to the negative feedback that governs the reproductive hormones.[70]

Even though only one study reports sperm quality as a result of resistance training under physiological (non–steroid-taking) conditions, to our expertise, there are some findings on the effect of concomitant use of androgenic-anabolic steroids (AASs) and resistance training. In contrast to endurance athletes, no changes in sperm density, motility, or morphology, as well as in vitro cervical mucus sperm penetration, were found by Arce and associates.[69]

To begin, we must recognize that many AAS abusers do not reveal their use and that they frequently combine AAS with other substances (aromatase inhibitors, antiestrogens, and human chorionic gonadotropin [hCG]) in the expectation of reducing the adverse effects of AAS abuse, such as hypogonadotropic hypogonadism and gynecomastia, and avoiding detection of their use.[65] In addition, hCG and clomiphene are occasionally administered together to boost endogenous testosterone production and prevent testicular atrophy.[71]

However, when AAS intake reaches supraphysiologic levels, they cause a drop in FSH, LH, and endogenous testosterone due to negative feedback on the hypothalamic-pituitary-gonadal (HPG) axis. As a response, changes in the testes (atrophy, hypogonadotropic hypogonadism) and spermatogenesis (azoospermia, oligozoospermia, motility changes, and an increasing amount of morphological defects, particularly in the head and midpiece) may occur.[69] When nandrolone decanoate was given to rats and made to exercise, testis weights and other sperm parameters dropped, but apoptosis in male germline cells improved.[72] Although the exercise model used was swimming, an everyday endurance activity, the study should be included in this area because endurance athletes rarely use AAS in supraphysiologic dosages, which would be required for a detrimental effect.

Both hypothalamus and testicular endocrine activities are inhibited during acute and sustained physical exercise. Exercise-induced serum testosterone reduction is linked to reduced endogenous gonadotropin-releasing hormone stimulation of gonadotropin release during exercise. Normal spermatogenesis is qualitatively and quantitatively based on an intact HPG axis as androgens are required to begin and maintain normal spermatogenesis.[73]

It is essential to understand how different exercise training conditions may have distinct effects on hormonal activity. As a result, we will start talking about the various research on workload. First, we will look at studies in which athletes covered a low to medium training load.

In the case of running, several of the research examining hormonal behavior in endurance sports found no significant changes in either free testosterone or total testosterone.[44,74] Another line of research, on the other side, discovered a considerable drop in total testosterone and free testosterone.[73,75]

In terms of sperm, there is no firm agreement on the benefits of endurance exercise on sperm production. However, there are data that show it can affect spermatogenesis and sperm output. Long-term strenuous activity harms sperm quality and reproductive capacity.[43]

A few studies in runners report changes in seminal quality, with up to 10% of the subjects exhibiting severe oligospermia; on the other hand, other authors argue that there is no distinction or that, if there is, it will not achieve clinical significance even though there is a difference between runners and control subjects.[44,68,73,74] A rise in non–sperm cell components, such as round cells,[68] has been recorded by certain researchers, indicating infection and/or inflammation. Compared to control participants, subjects who received a higher training volume showed more significant differences than those who received a lesser amount.[44] A minimum weekly running amount of 100 km has been proposed for athletes to show differences in semen parameters.[68] Nonetheless, several studies have found that 6 weeks of intense training (gradual rise to 186% of regular exercise) followed by 2 weeks of detraining (50% of regular training) does not affect sperm count, motility, or morphology.[76] Changes in sperm density, motility, and morphology and the in vitro cervical mucus sperm penetration test were observed in another study.[68] Safarinejad and associates consistently decreased semen parameters in the high-intensity exercise group compared to the moderate-intensity training groups. Surprisingly, all of the above markers returned to their preexercise levels.[43]

Both intensity and volume can influence the hormonal and seminal response. Furthermore, various training-related features and traits may have a role. Accordingly, the outcome will be determined by the participants' features and how their adaptive systems are prepared for the task. Because exercise might promote or exacerbate preexisting reproductive profile disorders, such as hormonal and seminal changes, it is essential to investigate this association further.

PSYCHOLOGICAL AND BEHAVIORAL THERAPY

Infertility is a complex issue that affects each individual differently. It is a thorny issue for males, making many hesitant to seek medical help.[77] Previously, treating female infertility has emphasized more than treating male component issues. Infertile males have been the subject of a small number of studies in the last decade, beginning in 2001. From 1927 to 2000, there was not a single report on male infertility in the Psychoanalytic Electronic Publishing archives of the seven critical psychoanalytic magazines.[77]

Despite the scarcity of psychological studies on male infertility, it is widely accepted that a considerable percentage of infertile males suffer from psychological trauma.[78,79] In males with infertility, the signs and effects of psychological stress are numerous and variable. Mental trauma can express itself in various ways, including changes in emotional behavior, sexual dysfunction, and decreased fertility.[78] In any infertile male, though, psychological stress's systemic and reproductive impacts are intertwined and negatively complementary.[78,79]

Psychological stress plays a crucial impact on male infertility, which is often underestimated. According to Morrow,[80] every sixth couple is infertile, and 40% of infertile people endure substantial emotional and psychological pain, which could have long-term consequences. At the annual meeting of the American Urological Association in 2008, Smith presented findings from a study demonstrating that infertile males incur emotional and social distress, confirming that the male partner in an infertile couple feels severe mental distress. Psychological stress has emotional consequences and hurts reproduction.[81]

EFFECTS OF PSYCHOLOGICAL STRESS ON REPRODUCTIVE FUNCTION

Psychological stress is one source of anxiety that can impact male fertility and reproductive outcomes. Human reproductive function is disrupted by chronic psychological stress, which can have a deleterious impact on spermatozoa count, motility, and morphology, as well as couples' fecundity. Furthermore, it increases the frequency of male sexual problems.[79]

Sexual desire is inextricably linked to emotions, and sex is more than just a bodily response. Stress is a prevalent side effect of today's fast-paced lifestyle, in which material performance is measured by accomplishment. Desire, arousal, orgasm, and resolution are the four interactive, nonlinear stages of typical male sexual arousal.[77] Orgasm is a different cognitive and emotional cerebral experience that frequently occurs with ejaculation. Any disturbance to this regular cycle can result in various sexual problems.

The most prevalent difficulties among infertile males are psychosexual diseases such as diminished libido, ejaculatory and erectile dysfunction, orgasmic failure, and deterioration of sperm parameters. Furthermore, an unsatisfactory pattern of sexual engagement among partners may result in common dissatisfaction.[82]

Stress has been shown to harm libido. It works cyclically. Stress causes a decrease in libido, which results in decreased sexual activity. Anxiety also inhibits libido and the desire for sexual engagement by suppressing positive sentiments and emotions. During stress, most males have experienced a decrease in libido or an inability to sustain an erection. However, these episodes are usually brief, and regular sexual function returns as the stressors are removed.[77]

Ejaculation is the most critical subvent in a male's erectile response. Ejaculation needs neuronal, physiologic, anatomic, and psychological coordination and collaboration. Ejaculatory difficulties can result from a failure in the synchronization of these events. Premature ejaculation, retrograde ejaculation, delayed ejaculation, and anejaculation are all examples of irregular ejaculation. Psychological trauma could be to blame for some of the ejaculatory issues.[83]

Stress does affect sperm production, but it is not always stable and does not follow a predictable pattern. Individual males react to stimuli in various ways, and their sperm production systems are also variable. Stress appears to cause meiotic and structural changes in spermatozoa, among other things.[84]

Stress has been shown to affect spermatozoa motility and limit their capacity to reach the egg. Stress makes it difficult for sperm to reach the ovum in the first place. Stress was one of the elements that adversely

linked with semen characteristics in a study of 225 infertile males.[84]

The study participants had aberrant morphology and reduced viability of their spermatozoa, with 80% admitting to being in a stressful personal or professional circumstance. Eskiocak et al. confirmed this observation of negative sperm parameters, showing that mental stress negatively affected sperm quality, most likely due to damaging components of enhanced superoxide dismutase activities operating on ROS.[85,86] At the time of semen analysis, a survey was used to examine psychological aspects such as exposure to acute stress, coping with stress, the WHO Well-Being Index, and the Zung's Anxiety Scale Inventory scores in 1076 males from infertile couples. According to regression tests, sperm concentration and the WHO Well-Being Index score have a substantial positive connection. Each subsequent score number accounts for a 7.3% rise in sperm concentration.[87]

TREATMENT OF PSYCHOLOGICAL STRESS–RELATED DISEASE

Treating psychological stress-related diseases takes on a different viewpoint than treating organic stress-related diseases because the target is metaphysical, and there is no identifiable organ to target. Only a few medical professionals and psychologists have the necessary training and expertise to deal with the complicated phenomenon of psychological stress in infertility. Its successful management necessitates identifying and controlling both acute and chronic stress.

Psychotherapy is likely an essential step in developing a treatment plan for mental stress in infertile couples.[88] Infertility is a problem that affects both members of a sexually active couple. As a result, both partners must be involved in treating psychological stress-related infertility. Infertility counseling is typically a practical solution since problematic relationship communication is a significant predictor of psychological stress in males.[89,90]

In the past, psychological and behavioral therapy has played an essential role in treating premature ejaculation (PE). Many medications, including tricyclic antidepressants (clomipramine) and serotonergic (selective serotonin reuptake inhibitors [SSRIs]) medicines such as paroxetine, sertraline, and others, have demonstrated varying degrees of efficacy. In PE, new medications such as dapoxetine, prilocaine-lidocaine cream, and aerosol spray have shown promise. Various antioxidants and anxiolytic drugs effectively reduce anxiety in all forms of psychological stress.[91]

By suppressing serotonin reuptake into presynaptic cells, SSRI medications increase extracellular levels of the neurotransmitter serotonin (5-hydroxytryptamine [5-HT]). This increases its amount in the synaptic cleft that can bind to the postsynaptic 5-HT2 and 5-HT3 receptors in the spinal cord. As a result, serotonin lingers in the synaptic gap for more extended periods, stimulating the receptors of the recipient cell. Increased extracellular serotonin concentrations in the brain reduce dopamine and norepinephrine release from the substantia nigra, resulting in sexual dysfunction.[92] Simultaneously, the SSRIs' ability to reduce sexual stimulation is sensibly harnessed to treat PE.[93]

Infertility has psychological effects on marriage, as well as societal implications. According to human psychosomatic beliefs, every somatic problem has an emotional component. In general, it is in just the last two decades that the psychological stress of infertile males has been brought to light. In determining treatment, the societal construction of infertility and the roles of both parties in a heterosexual couple must be considered. Counseling, a vital therapy modality, requires both partners' engagement to be effective.

CLINICAL/LABORATORY CASE SCENARIO

CASE

Treatment of psychological stress–related male fertility

A 44-year-old male was referred by a colleague due to infertility for 2 years. His wife's reproductive function was normal. He was so stressed with his business due to the COVID-19 pandemic. Physical examination revealed no palpable varicocele and normal-sized testes. His semen parameters were: (1) volume, 2.5 mL; (2) concentration, 5×10^6 per mL; (3) total motility, 5%. He was diagnosed with psychological stress-related male fertility. He was referred to a psychologist. Six months later, he came back to our clinic without stress. His second semen parameters were: (1) volume, 3 mL; (2) concentration, 84×10^6 per mL; (3) total motility, 58%. His wife had a spontaneous pregnancy 6 months later.

SUMMARY

Male infertility is a common condition, and its causes are increasingly diverse. Therefore male infertility treatment is becoming more and more like an art, requiring a harmonious combination of drugs, lifestyle, a healthy mind, and other factors. Knowledge of these aspects will help clinicians to have a better treatment plan, increasing the success rate of male infertility treatment.

REFERENCES

1. Vander Borght M, Wyns C. Fertility and infertility: definition and epidemiology. *Clin Biochem*. 2018;62:2-10.
2. Agarwal A, Mulgund A, Hamada A, et al. A unique view on male infertility around the globe. *Reprod Biol Endocrinol*. 2015;13:37.
3. Aoun A, Khoury VE, Malakieh R. Can nutrition help in the treatment of infertility? *Prev Nutr Food Sci*. 2021; 26(2):109-120.
4. Jensen TK, Heitmann BL, Blomberg Jensen M, et al. High dietary intake of saturated fat is associated with reduced semen quality among 701 young Danish men from the general population. *Am J Clin Nutr*. 2013; 97(2):411-418. doi:10.3945/ajcn.112.042432.
5. Gaskins AJ, Colaci DS, Mendiola J, Swan SH, Chavarro JE. Dietary patterns and semen quality in young men. *Hum Reprod*. 2012;27(10):2899-2907.
6. Eslamian G, Amirjannati N, Rashidkhani B, Sadeghi MR, Hekmatdoost A. Intake of food groups and idiopathic asthenozoospermia: a case-control study. *Hum Reprod*. 2012;27(11):3328-3336.
7. Mendiola J, Torres-Cantero AM, Moreno-Grau JM, et al. Food intake and its relationship with semen quality: a case-control study. *Fertil Steril*. 2009;91(3):812-818.
8. Braga DP, Halpern G, Figueira Rde C, Setti AS, Iaconelli Jr A, Borges Jr E. Food intake and social habits in male patients and its relationship to intracytoplasmic sperm injection outcomes. *Fertil Steril*. 2012;97(1):53-59.
9. Salas-Huetos A, Mínguez-Alarcón L, Mitsunami M, et al. Paternal adherence to healthy dietary patterns in relation to sperm parameters and outcomes of assisted reproductive technologies. *Fertil Steril*. 2022;117(2): 298-312.
10. Mitsunami M, Salas-Huetos A, Mínguez-Alarcón L, et al. A dietary score representing the overall relation of men's diet with semen quality in relation to outcomes of infertility treatment with assisted reproduction. *F S Rep*. 2021;2(4):396-404.
11. Benedetti S, Tagliamonte MC, Catalani S, et al. Differences in blood and semen oxidative status in fertile and infertile

men, and their relationship with sperm quality. *Reprod Biomed Online.* 2012;25(3):300-306.

12. Murphy LE, Mills JL, Molloy AM, et al. Folate and vitamin B12 in idiopathic male infertility. *Asian J Androl.* 2011; 13(6):856-861.

13. Clagett-Dame M, Knutson D. Vitamin A in reproduction and development. *Nutrients.* 2011;3(4):385-428.

14. Hammoud AO, Meikle AW, Peterson CM, Stanford J, Gibson M, Carrell DT. Association of 25-hydroxy-vitamin D levels with semen and hormonal parameters. *Asian J Androl.* 2012;14(6):855-859. doi:10.1038/aja.2012.77.

15. Kaushal N, Bansal MP. Diminished reproductive potential of male mice in response to selenium-induced oxidative stress: involvement of HSP70, HSP70-2, and MSJ-1. *J Biochem Mol Toxicol.* 2009;23(2):125-136.

16. Kaushal N, Bansal MP. Dietary selenium variation-induced oxidative stress modulates CDC2/cyclin B1 expression and apoptosis of germ cells in mice testis. *J Nutr Biochem.* 2007; 18(8):553-564.

17. Ramlau-Hansen CH, Moeller UK, Bonde JP, Olsen J, Thulstrup AM. Are serum levels of vitamin D associated with semen quality? Results from a cross-sectional study in young healthy men. *Fertil Steril.* 2011;95(3):1000-1004.

18. Goswami S, Mishra KN, Singh RP, Singh P, Singh P. Sesbaniasesban, a plant with diverse therapeutic benefits: an overview. *SGVU J Pharm Res Educ.* 2016;1:111-121.

19. Safarinejad MR, Shafiei N, Safarinejad S. A prospective double-blind randomized placebo-controlled study of the effect of saffron (Crocus sativus Linn.) on semen parameters and seminal plasma antioxidant capacity in infertile men with idiopathic oligoasthenoteratozoo-spermia. *Phytother Res.* 2011;25(4):508-516.

20. Lohiya NK, Kothari LK, Manivannan B, Mishra PK, Pathak N. Human sperm immobilization effect of Carica papaya seed extracts: an in vitro study. *Asian J Androl.* 2000;2(2):103-109.

21. Ghaffarilaleh V, Fisher D, Henkel R. Carica papaya seed extract slows human sperm. *J Ethnopharmacol.* 2019; 241:111972.

22. Kershaw CM, Evans G, Rodney R, Maxwell WMC. Papain and its inhibitor E-64 reduce camelid semen viscosity without impairing sperm function and improve post-thaw motility rates. *Reprod Fertil Dev.* 2017;29(6):1107-1114.

23. Strunz CC, Oliveira TV, Vinagre JCM, Lima A, Cozzolino S, Maranhão RC. Brazil nut ingestion increased plasma selenium but had minimal effects on lipids, apolipopro-teins, and high-density lipoprotein function in human subjects. *Nutr Res.* 2008;28(3):151-155.

24. Gonzales GF, Ruiz A, Gonzales C, Villegas L, Cordova A. Effect of Lepidium meyenii (maca) roots on spermato-genesis of male rats. *Asian J Androl.* 2001;3(3):231-233.

25. Valdivia Cuya M, Yarasca De La Vega K, Lévano Sánchez G, et al. Effect of Lepidium meyenii (maca) on testicular function of mice with chemically and physically induced subfertility. *Andrologia.* 2016;48(8):927-934.

26. Peng D, Wang H, Qu C, Xie L, Wicks SM, Xie J. Ginsenoside Re: its chemistry, metabolism and pharmacokinetics. *Chin Med.* 2012;7:2. doi:10.1186/1749-8546-7-2.

27. Akram H, Ghaderi Pakdel F, Ahmadi A, Zare S. Beneficial effects of American ginseng on epididymal sperm analyses in cyclophosphamide treated rats. *Cell J.* 2012;14(2):116-121.

28. Qi LW, Wang CZ, Yuan CS. Ginsenosides from American ginseng: chemical and pharmacological diversity. *Phyto-chemistry.* 2011;72(8):689-699.

29. Aruoma OI, Colognato R, Fontana I, et al. Molecular effects of fermented papaya preparation on oxidative damage, MAP kinase activation and modulation of the benzopyrene mediated genotoxicity. *Biofactors.* 2006; 26(2):147-159.

30. Piomboni P, Gambera L, Serafini F, Campanella G, Morgante G, De Leo V. Sperm quality improvement after natural anti-oxidant treatment of asthenoteratospermic men with leukocytospermia. *Asian J Androl.* 2008; 10(2):201-206.

31. Chávez-Quintal P, González-Flores T, Rodríguez-Buenfil I, Gallegos-Tintoré S. Antifungal activity in ethanolic extracts of Carica papaya L. cv. maradol leaves and seeds. *Indian J Microbiol.* 2011;51(1):54-60.

32. Lohiya NK, Kothari LK, Manivannan B, Mishra PK, Pathak N. Human sperm immobilization effect of Carica papaya seed extracts: an in vitro study. *Asian J Androl.* 2000;2(2):103-109.

33. Ghafarizadeh AA, Vaezi G, Shariatzadeh MA, Malekirad AA. Effect of in vitro selenium supplementation on sperm quality in asthenoteratozoospermic men. *Andrologia.* 2018;50(2). doi:10.1111/and.12869.

34. Awolu OO, Osemeke RO, Ifesan BOT. Antioxidant, func-tional and rheological properties of optimized composite flour, consisting wheat and amaranth seed, brewers' spent grain and apple pomace. *J Food Sci Technol.* 2016; 53(2):1151-1163.

35. Gonzales GF, Alarcón-Yaquetto DE. Maca, a nutraceutical from the Andean highlands. *Therapeut Foods.* 2017; 373-396.

36. Onaolapo AY, Oladipo BP, Onaolapo OJ. Cyclophospha-mide-induced male subfertility in mice: an assessment of the potential benefits of Maca supplement. *Andrologia.* 2018;50(3). doi:10.1111/and.12911.

37. Aoki Y, Tsujimura A, Nagashima Y, et al. Effect of Lepidium meyenii on in vitro fertilization via improvement in acro-some reaction and motility of mouse and human sperm. *Reprod Med Biol.* 2019;18(1):57-64.

38. Applequist WL, Moerman DE. Yarrow (Achillea millefolium L.): a neglected panacea? A review of ethnobotany, bioactivity, and biomedical research. *Econ Bot.* 2011;65(2):209-225.

39. Montanari T, de Carvalho JE, Dolder H. Antispermatogenic effect of Achillea millefolium L. in mice. *Contraception.* 1998;58(5):309-313.

40. Johns T, Kitts WD, Newsome F, Towers GH. Antireproductive and other medicinal effects of Tropaeolum tuberosum. *J Ethnopharmacol.* 1982;5(2):149-161.

41. Leiva-Revilla J, Cárdenas-Valencia I, Rubio J, et al. Evaluation of different doses of mashua (Tropaeolum tuberosum) on the reduction of sperm production, motility and morphology in adult male rats. *Andrologia.* 2012;44:205-212.

42. Vaamonde D, Da Silva-Grigoletto ME, Garcia-Manso JM, Vaamonde-Lemos R, Swanson RJ, Oehninger SC. Response of semen parameters to three training modalities. *Fertil Steril.* 2009;92:1941-1946.

43. Safarinejad MR, Azma K, Kolahi AA. The effects of intensive, long-term treadmill running on reproductive hormones, hypothalamus-pituitary-testis axis, and semen quality: a randomized controlled study. *J Endocrinol.* 2009;20:259-271.

44. De Souza MJ, Arce JC, Pescatello LS, Scherzer HS, Luciano AA. Gonadal hormones and semen quality in male runners. A volume threshold effect of endurance training. *Int J Sports Med.* 1994;15:383-391.

45. Vaamonde D, Da Silva ME, Poblador MS, Lancho JL. Reproductive profile of physically active men after exhaustive endurance exercise. *Int J Sports Med.* 2006;27:680-689.

46. Vaamonde D, Da Silva-Grigoletto ME, Garcia-Manso JM, Vaamonde-Lemos R. Differences in sperm DNA fragmentation between high- and low-cycling volume triathletes: preliminary results. *Fertil Steril.* 2012;98 (suppl 3):S85.

47. Tartibian B, Maleki BH. Correlation between seminal oxidative stress biomarkers and antioxidants with sperm DNA damage in elite athletes and recreationally active men. *Clin J Sport Med.* 2012;22:132-139.

48. Jensen CE, Wiswedel K, McLoughlin J, van der Spuy Z. Prospective study of hormonal and semen profiles in marathon runners. *Fertil Steril.* 1995;64:1189-1196.

49. Brock G. Erectile function of bike patrol officers. *J Androl.* 2002;23:758-759.

50. Di Luigi L, Gentile V, Pigozzi F, Parisi A, Giannetti D, Romanelli F. Physical activity as a possible aggravating factor for athletes with varicocele: impact on the semen profile. *Hum Reprod.* 2001;16:1180-1184.

51. Naessens G, De Slypere JP, Dijs H, Driessens M. Hypogonadism as a cause of recurrent muscle injury in a high level soccer player. A case report. *Int J Sports Med.* 1995; 16:413-417.

52. WHO. *WHO Laboratory Manual for the Examination of Human Semen and Sperm-Cervical Mucus Interaction.*

4th ed. Cambridge, UK: Cambridge University Press; 1999.

53. Vaamonde D, Da Silva-Grigoletto ME, García-Manso JM, Barrera N, Vaamonde-Lemos R. Physically active men show better semen parameters and hormone values than sedentary men. *Eur J Appl Physiol.* 2012;112:3267-3273.

54. Myhal M, Lamb DR. Hormones as performance enhancing drugs. In: Warren MP, Constantini NW, eds. *Sport Endocrinology.* Totowa, NJ: Humana; 2000:433-476.

55. Giannoulis MG, Martin FC, Nair KS, Umpleby AM, Sonksen P. Hormone replacement therapy and physical function in healthy older men. Time to talk hormones? *Endocr Rev.* 2012;33:314-377.

56. Kraemer WJ, Ratamess NA. Hormonal responses and adaptations to resistance exercise and training. *Sports Med.* 2005;35:339-361.

57. Hackney AC, Premo MC, McMurray RG. Influence of aerobic versus anaerobic exercise on the relationship between reproductive hormones in men. *J Sports Sci.* 1995;13:305-311.

58. Willoughby DS, Taylor L. Effects of sequential bouts of resistance exercise on androgen receptor expression. *Med Sci Sports Exerc.* 2004;36:1499-1506.

59. Ari Z, Kutlu N, Uyanik BS, Taneli F, Buyukyazi G, Tavli T. Serum testosterone, growth hormone, and insulin-like growth factor-1 levels, mental reaction time, and maximal aerobic exercise in sedentary and long-term physically trained elderly males. *Int J Neurosci.* 2004;114:623-637.

60. Izquierdo M, Hakkinen K, Ibanez J, et al. Effects of strength training on muscle power and serum hormones in middle-aged and older men. *J Appl Physiol.* 2001; 90:1497-1507.

61. Nicklas BJ, Ryan AJ, Treuth MM, et al. Testosterone, growth hormone and IGF-I responses to acute and chronic resistive exercise in men aged 55–70 years. *Int J Sports Med.* 1995;16:445-450.

62. Tymchuk CN, Tessler SB, Aronson WJ, Barnard RJ. Effects of diet and exercise on insulin, sex hormone-binding globulin, and prostate-specific antigen. *Nutr Cancer.* 1998;31:127-131.

63. Cooper CS, Taaffe DR, Guido D, Packer E, Holloway L, Marcus R. Relationship of chronic endurance exercise to the somatotropic and sex hormone status of older men. *Eur J Endocrinol.* 1998;138:517-523.

64. Hawkins VN, Foster-Schubert K, Chubak J, et al. Effect of exercise on serum sex hormones in men: a 12-month randomized clinical trial. *Med Sci Sports Exerc.* 2008; 40:223-233.

65. Palmer NO, Bakos HW, Owens JA, Setchell BP, Lane M. Diet and exercise in an obese mouse fed a high-fat diet improve metabolic health and reverse perturbed sperm

function. *Am J Physiol Endocrinol Metab*. 2012;302: E768-E780.

66. Kanayama G, Brower KJ, Wood RI, Hudson JI, Pope Jr HG. Anabolic-androgenic steroid dependence: an emerging disorder. *Addiction*. 2009;104:1966-1978.

67. McArdle WD, Katch FI, Katch VL. *Essentials of Exercise Physiology*. 3rd ed. Philadelphia, PA: Williams and Wilkins; 2006.

68. Hakkinen K, Pakarinen A, Kraemer WJ, Newton RU, Alen M. Basal concentrations and acute responses of serum hormones and strength development during heavy resistance training in middle-aged and elderly men and women. *J Gerontol A Biol Sci Med Sci*. 2000; 55:B95-B105.

69. Arce JC, De Souza MJ, Pescatello LS, Luciano AA. Sub-clinical alterations in hormone and semen profile in athletes. *Fertil Steril*. 1993;59:398-404.

70. Fronczak CM, Kim ED, Barqawi AB. The insults of illicit drug use on male fertility. *J Androl*. 2012;33:515-528.

71. Hoffman JR, Kraemer WJ, Bhasin S, et al. Position stand on androgen and human growth hormone use. *J Strength Cond Res*. 2009;23(suppl. 5):S1-59.

72. Shokri S, Aitken RJ, Abdolvahhabi M, et al. Exercise and supraphysiological dose of nandrolone decanoate increase apoptosis in spermatogenic cells. *Basic Clin Pharmacol Toxicol*. 2010;106:324-330.

73. Griffith RO, Dressendorfer RH, Fullbright CD, Wade CE. Testicular function during exhaustive endurance training. *Phys Sports Med*. 1990;18:54-64.

74. Bagatell CJ, Bremner WJ. Sperm counts and reproductive hormones in male marathoners and lean controls. *Fertil Steril*. 1990;53:688-692.

75. Wheeler GD, Singh M, Pierce WD, Epling WF, Cumming DC. Endurance training decreases serum testosterone levels in men without change in luteinizing hormone pulsation release. *J Clin Endocrinol Metab*. 1991;72:422-425.

76. Hall HL, Flynn MG, Carroll KK, Brolinson PG, Shapiro S, Bushman BA. Effects of intensified training and detraining on testicular function. *Clin J Sport Med*. 1999;9:203-208.

77. Du Plessis SS, Agarwal A, Sabanegh ES, eds. *Male Infertility: A Complete Guide to Lifestyle and Environmental Factors*. New York: Springer; 2014:141-145.

78. Fenster L, Katz DF, Wyrobek AJ, et al. Effects of psychological stress on human semen quality. *Andrology*. 1997;18:194-202.

79. Hjollund NH, Bonde JP, Henriksen TB, Giwercman A, Olsen J, Danish First Pregnancy Planner Study Team. Reproductive effects of male psychologic stress. *Epidemiology*. 2004;15(1):21-27.

80. Morrow KA, Thoreson RW, Penney LL. Predictors of psychological distress among infertility clinic patients. *Clin Psychol*. 1995;63(1):163-167.

81. Smith JF. *Emotional, Psychological, and Marital Stress in Male Factor Infertility. The Annual Meeting of the American Urological Association (AUA)*. Orlando, FL: Orange County Convention Center; 2008.

82. Sand MS, Fisher W, Rosen R, Heiman J, Eardley I. Erectile dysfunction and constructs of masculinity and quality of life in the multinational Men's Attitudes to Life Events and Sexuality (MALES) study. *J Sex Med*. 2008;5(3):583-594.

83. Araujo AB, Johannes CB, Feldman HA, Derby CA, McKinlay JB. Relation between psychosocial risk factors and incident erectile dysfunction: prospective results from the Massachusetts Male Aging Study. *Am J Epidemiol*. 2000;152(6):533-541.

84. Gerhard I, Lenhard K, Eggert-Kruse W, et al. Clinical data which influence semen parameters in infertile men. *Hum Reprod*. 1992;7:830-837.

85. Eskiocak S, Gozen AS, Kilic AS, Molla S. Association between mental stress & some antioxidant enzymes of seminal plasma. *Indian J Med Res*. 2005;122(6):491-496.

86. Eskiocak S, Gozen AS, Taskiran A, Kilic AS, Eskiocak M, Gulen S. Effect of psychological stress on the L-arginine-nitric oxide pathway and semen quality. *Braz J Med Biol Res*. 2006;39(5):581-588.

87. Zorn B, Auger J, Velikonja V, Kolbezen M, Meden-Vrtovec H. Psychological factors in male partners of infertile couples: relationship with semen quality and early miscarriage. *Int J Androl*. 2008;31(6):557-564.

88. Boivin J. A review of psychosocial interventions in infertility. *Soc Sci Med*. 2003;57(12):2325-2341.

89. Van den Broeck U, Emery M, Wischmann T, Thorn P. Counselling in infertility: individual, couple and group interventions. *Patient Educ Couns*. 2010;81(3):422-428.

90. Wischmann T. Implications of psychosocial support in infertility—a critical appraisal. *J Psychosom Obstet Gynaecol*. 2008;29(2):83-90.

91. Kefer JC, Agarwal A, Sabanegh E. Role of antioxidants in the treatment of male infertility. *Int J Urol*. 2009; 16(5):449-457.

92. Dording CM, Fisher L, Papakostas G, et al. A double-blind, randomized, pilot dose-finding study of maca root (L. meyenii) for the management of SSRI-induced sexual dysfunction. *CNS Neurosci Ther*. 2008;14(3):182-191.

93. Waldinger MD, Olivier B. Utility of selective serotonin reuptake inhibitors in premature ejaculation. *Curr Opin Investig Drugs*. 2004;5(7):743-747.

Surgical Treatment of Male Infertility

19

Varicocele Repair in Infertile Males

Kanha Charudutt Shete, Megan McMurray, Edmund Yuey Kun Ko, and Nicholas N. Tadros

KEY POINTS

- Varicocele is a common cause of male factor infertility, found in almost one-quarter of males presenting for evaluation.
- Varicocele can have a negative impact on semen parameters, including count, motility, morphology, or sperm DNA, by increasing oxidative stress.
- Current society guidelines recommend repairing palpable varicoceles in infertile males, unless they have azoospermia, to improve their chances of conceiving.
- Varicoceles can be repaired percutaneously or surgically, with varying rates of success and complications.
- There is evidence to show improved semen analysis and pregnancy rates in infertile males after varicocele repair.

INTRODUCTION

Varicocele is characterized as an abnormal dilatation of the pampiniform plexus, a network of veins within the spermatic cord that provides vascular drainage of the testicles. It is usually asymptomatic but may also present as a dull, throbbing scrotal pain.[1] Varicoceles are thought to be the most common attributable cause of male factor infertility, accounting for up to 26.6% of final diagnoses in male infertility evaluation.[2] They can also negatively impact testicular volume.[3] Varicoceles can be found in approximately 15% to 20% of males in the general population. Varicoceles are much more common in males with primary (35%–44%) and secondary (45%–81%) infertility.[4,5]

In the current chapter, we discuss different aspects of varicocele repair in the context of male infertility management.

PATHOGENESIS OF VARICOCELE

Varicocele develops as the result of increased pressure in the gonadal vein(s). Turbulent blood flow may result in increased venous pressure, particularly on the left. In contrast to the right gonadal vein, which drains obliquely into the inferior vena cava, the left gonadal vein drains into the left renal vein at a right angle. Furthermore, the insertion of the left gonadal vein is approximately 8 to 10 cm superior to the insertion of the right gonadal vein. This results in more turbulence and back pressure. This is thought to be the reason that almost 90% of varicoceles are found on the left side. Additionally, absence or incompetence of venous valves results in increased retrograde blood flow. Less commonly, compression of the left renal vein between the superior mesenteric artery and aorta, known as nutcracker syndrome, can also lead to increased pressure transmitted to the left gonadal vein.[2,6,7]

DIAGNOSIS AND GRADING OF VARICOCELE

Varicocele is primarily a clinical diagnosis. On physical exam, varicoceles are classically described as feeling like a "bag of worms," which becomes more prominent with standing and with Valsalva maneuvers. Grading criteria

TABLE 19.1	**Varicocele Grading**
Subclinical	Varicocele only detected on imaging studies, not on physical exam
Grade 1	On physical exam, varicocele is palpable only with Valsalva
Grade 2	On physical exam, varicocele is palpable only without Valsalva
Grade 3	Varicocele is visible through scrotal skin

(Table 19.1) were first introduced in 1970 by Dubin and Amelar. Grade 1 varicoceles are palpable only during Valsalva maneuver. Grade 2 varicoceles are palpable without Valsalva. Grade 3 varicoceles are visible through the scrotal skin.[8] Varicoceles that are only detected on imaging studies such as ultrasound are deemed grade 0 or subclinical.[2]

Additional imaging may be considered when the exam is inconclusive.[1] Scrotal ultrasound with gray scale and color Doppler can be used to identify the presence of venous reflux and/or dilated pampiniform plexus veins (>2–3 mm is considered diagnostic).[9] Testicular volume calculations may be useful and generally, single testicular volume of 12 to 15 mL is considered normal.[9] Testicular venography can be used to visualize reflux of contrast into the gonadal vein and is the gold standard for varicocele diagnosis. However, due to its invasive nature, venography is typically only used clinically in the setting of varicocele embolization.[9] Because unilateral right-sided varicocele is uncommon, traditionally, it warrants further work-up to rule out retroperitoneal pathology; however, some studies suggest this may not be necessary.[10,11]

IMPACT OF VARICOCELE ON MALE FERTILITY

Mechanisms of Varicocele-Induced Male Infertility

There are several proposed mechanisms of varicocele-induced male infertility; however, oxidative stress appears to play a central role. Males with varicocele have a higher production of reactive oxygen species and lower levels of antioxidants. This imbalance of reactive oxygen species and antioxidants leads to sperm membrane and DNA damage, as well as dysfunction of spermatogenesis and spermatozoa.[12–14] The pathophysiology of increased

oxidative stress is likely related to increased intrascrotal temperature from venous pooling. Testicular hyperthermia stimulates the production of reactive oxygen species by spermatozoa and leukocytes.[13] Additionally, reflux of renal and adrenal metabolites and testicular hypoxia due to impaired venous blood flow may play a role.[1]

Impact on Sperm Parameters and Sperm DNA Integrity

Males with varicoceles are known to have poorer sperm parameters and sperm DNA integrity. Varicoceles are associated with reduced sperm count, decreased sperm motility, and abnormal sperm morphology.[14–16] Sperm concentrations in males with grade 3 varicoceles are less than 50% of those in males without varicoceles, indicating that higher grades are associated with poorer semen quality.[17] Sperm DNA fragmentation rates are significantly higher in males with varicoceles than in those without.[18]

SOCIETY GUIDELINES

Multiple professional bodies, including the American Urological Association (AUA), American Society of Reproductive Medicine (ASRM), and European Association of Urology (EAU), have published guidelines for indications and intervention for varicoceles as subsections within their male infertility guidelines. Currently, the AUA, in collaboration with the ASRM, recommends the following:[19]

Surgical varicocelectomy should be considered in males attempting to conceive who have palpable varicocele(s), infertility, and abnormal semen parameters, except for azoospermic males (Moderate Recommendation; Evidence Level: Grade C).

Clinicians should not recommend varicocelectomy for males with nonpalpable varicoceles detected solely by imaging (Strong Recommendation; Evidence Level: Grade C).

For males with clinical varicocele and NOA [nonobstructive azoospermia], the couple should be informed of the absence of definitive evidence supporting varicocele repair prior to ART [Assisted Reproductive Technologies] (Expert Opinion).

Guidelines as outlined by the EAU are presented below[20] and show some differences in comparison to the above-described AUA/ASRM guidelines, as follows:

Treat varicoceles in adolescents with ipsilateral reduction in testicular volume and evidence of progression of testicular dysfunction (Strength rating: weak).

Do not treat varicocele in infertile males who have normal semen analysis and in males with a sub-clinical varicocele (Strength rating: weak).

Treat infertile males with a clinical varicocele, abnormal semen parameters, and otherwise unexplained infertility in a couple where the female partner has good ovarian reserve to improve fertility rates (Strength rating: strong).

Varicocelectomy may be considered in males with raised DNA fragmentation with otherwise unexplained infertility or who have suffered from failure of assisted reproductive techniques, including recurrent pregnancy loss, failure of embryogenesis, and implantation (Strength rating: weak).

TYPES OF INTERVENTION

Broadly, varicocele repairs can be divided into two overarching categories: percutaneous treatment and surgical treatment. Surgical repair of varicoceles can be further divided into inguinal, subinguinal, retroperitoneal, and laparoscopic, of which microsurgical techniques have classically been utilized for both the inguinal and subinguinal approaches.

Percutaneous Repair

Percutaneous treatment of varicoceles has evolved over the last five decades. Lima et al. were the first team to describe a novel percutaneous approach to sclerose the testicular vein in 1978.[21] This involved the use of hypertonic glucose and ethanolamine as the sclerosing agent. With time, agents and techniques have changed to include venous embolization with balloons and coils.[22,23] Most modern percutaneous embolization techniques continue to require venous access, with embolization performed with a sclerosing or glue agent versus coils. Recurrence rates for percutaneous embolization are as high as 11%, and so currently, this modality has a stronger role in treating persistent or recurrent varicoceles after prior surgical repair.[24–26]

A more novel sclerosing technique is antegrade scrotal sclerotherapy, initially described in 1994 by Tauber et al.[27] This technique involves a small high scrotal incision, followed by spermatic cord and more specifically pampiniform plexus isolation, dilated vein cannulization with consideration of phlebography, and antegrade injection of the sclerosing agent. More recent publications show about a 5% varicocele recurrence rate with antegrade scrotal sclerotherapy.[28]

Surgical Repair

Surgical varicocele repair has been described in a variety of different methods, of which we will focus on retroperitoneal, laparoscopic, inguinal, and subinguinal. The decision to choose a particular approach varies based on operative surgeon preference, patient anatomy, success rates, and complication rates. Accordingly, we present a decision tree for choice of surgical approach in Fig. 19.1.

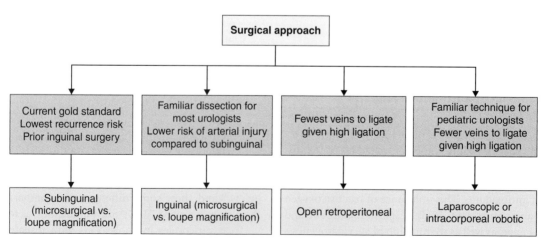

Fig. 19.1 Decision Tree for Surgical Approach.

Currently, surgical varicocele ligation is the most commonly performed procedure for the management of male factor infertility, with varicoceles initially being described with this intent by Tulloch in 1955.[29,30]

A retroperitoneal varicocelectomy can be performed both open and laparoscopically, with different points of access. The open retroperitoneal approach was first described by Palomo in 1949.[31] This involves high ligation of the spermatic vein and necessitates incision at the level of the internal ring, dissection down to and through the external oblique aponeurosis, blunt splitting of the internal oblique muscle, and identification of the gonadal vessels in the retroperitoneum. Palomo initially described ligating both gonadal artery and vein, although current attempts are made to preserve the artery. The advantage of the retroperitoneal approach is the high ligation, resulting in typically needing to ligate only one to two veins for a successful outcome as opposed to the inguinal approach, which usually requires ligation of many more veins for successful outcomes. The drawback of this approach is the high recurrence rate, described as being around 15%, likely due to unidentified but dilated scrotal or cremasteric veins or veins adherent to the gonadal artery that are not ligated in an attempt to preserve the artery.[32–35]

Laparoscopic varicocelectomy attempts to emulate a retroperitoneal varicocelectomy, although it does so in a minimally invasively and transperitoneal fashion while allowing the inherent magnification of the laparoscope to allow better visualization of the critical structures. In doing so, there is an attempt to better view the veins, artery, and potentially even lymphatics as a means to decrease complications that may be seen with the open retroperitoneal approach.[36] Laparoscopic varicocelectomy entails gaining access to the intrabdominal cavity with insufflation; identifying the internal ring at the confluence of the critical structures of dissection; medializing the colonic segment, which may impede the view of the gonadal vessels; incising the peritoneum over the gonadal vessels as to expose them; isolating the dilated veins; and then ligating the veins while preserving the artery. Inherent to it being an intrabdominal laparoscopic surgery come added risks not seen in the other surgical techniques, including complications of insufflation and port placement, bowel injury, and great vessel injury, as well as CO_2 air embolism and pulmonary compromise secondary to insufflation. Laparoscopic varicocelectomy remains the mainstay of treatment among pediatric urologists at tertiary care facilities, likely due to similarity in procedural steps to laparoscopic orchiopexy.[37] Furthermore, while inguinal and subinguinal approaches remain the current gold standard of varicocelectomy, laparoscopic varicocelectomy continues to prove beneficial and increasingly efficient in surgical management of bilateral varicocelectomies.[38] Currently, publications show variance in recurrence rates of laparoscopic varicocelectomy between a low of 2% and a high of 17%.[39,40]

Advances have been made with both open retroperitoneal varicocelectomy and laparoscopic varicocelectomy in the last decade and a half. A microsurgical approach to retroperitoneal varicocelectomy has been described in both adult and pediatric patients but warrants further investigation of efficacy due to small study sizes.[41,42] Robotic varicocelectomy has also been described, both for extracorporeal techniques replacing an operating microscope as well as intracorporeal techniques, which are similar operatively to the traditional laparoscopic varicocelectomy. Currently, there are a lack of robust data to change practice patterns; however, a single institution has published their retrospective findings of an extracorporeal robotic varicocelectomy, with their outcomes being similar to microscopic varicocelectomies. The advocates for the robotic approaches comment on less surgeon fatigue, improved identification of lymphatics so as to minimize hydroceles, no tremor during operation, and three-dimensional visualization as reasons to consider pursuing this technique.[43–45]

The inguinal approach to a varicocelectomy can be performed under standard vision or microsurgical technique, be it loupe magnification or under an operating microscope. An incision is made over the inguinal canal, similar to the incision for a radical orchiectomy. Dissection is taken down until the external oblique aponeurosis is encountered and opened. The spermatic cord is then readily identified, encircled, and brought up, at which point the cord is dissected. This allows visualization of the dilated veins, the gonadal artery and the vas deferens, and with it, arteries, veins, and lymphatics.

The subinguinal approach was first described in 1985 by Marmar et al., with the goal of providing a technique that did not violate the external oblique fascia and reduced postoperative pain.[46] With this technique, the incision is made below the level of the external ring (Fig. 19.2), at which point the spermatic cord is identified and pulled extracorporeally. A Penrose drain alone or a Penrose with

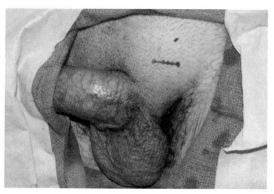

Fig. 19.2 Incision location below the level of the external ring for a subinguinal varicocelectomy.

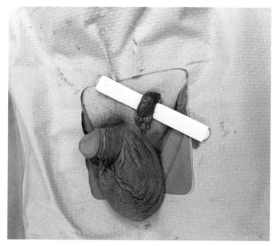

Fig. 19.3 Subinguinal varicocelectomy with spermatic cord dissected and placed on tongue depressor surgical platform.

a tongue depressor inside are placed under the cord as a means of providing a small surgical platform (Fig. 19.3). The cord is then dissected in order to identify the critical structures as a means to ligate the dilatated veins while preserving the gonadal artery, vas deferens, and lymphatics. A handheld Doppler can be used to help identify the arterial structures to be preserved. Dr. Goldstein and his team popularized the microsurgical technique of varicocelectomy in 1992 and also further described delivery of the testes and ligation of all dilated scrotal veins (including the gubernaculum) for an increased rate of successful outcomes.[47]

In comparing the inguinal versus subinguinal approaches, there are some relative indications for one over the other. The inguinal approach is preferred when minimizing arterial injury is warranted in the case of adults with a solitary testis or in children and adolescents where the artery is slightly larger and less branched within the inguinal canal. The subinguinal approach is favored in patients whose prior inguinal surgery has resulted in scarring of the external aponeurosis and in obese patients or cases of recurrent varicoceles, as branched venous structures are more readily identifiable.[48]

OUTCOMES OF INTERVENTION

Impact on Semen Analysis Parameters

Over the last few decades, there has been much debate over the outcomes of semen parameters on infertile males after varicocelectomy. With an increasing number of retrospective analyses and metaanalyses, the pendulum has swung to support the concept of varicocele repair improving semen parameters.

Agarwal et al. published a metaanalysis in 2007 that was highly persuasive in describing the specific semen parameters with improvements after varicocelectomy.[49] In this metaanalysis, microsurgical repair was seen to result in a sperm count increase of 9.71×10^6/mL, motility increase of 9.92%, and, for both microsurgical and high ligation techniques, a World Health Organization sperm morphology improvement of 3.16%. Similar findings have been echoed in more recent studies, including a 2020 metaanalysis by Birowo et al., which also further suggests using DNA fragmentation index as a guide to proceed with varicocele repair.[50] With respect to the pediatric population, there is evidence showing increased testes volume with varicocelectomy but conflicting evidence as to whether there is a statistically significant improvement in semen parameters.[51,52] No study to date has been able to directly correlate fertility outcomes of this same pediatric population.

While the AUA/ASRM guidelines advise against varicocelectomy in the setting of azoospermia, new data are challenging this statement, showing there may be a role for varicocelectomy in males with severe oligospermia or nonobstructive azoospermia (NOA). A number of small series have demonstrated improvement in semen parameters and spontaneous pregnancies for this patient population. Rates of motile sperm count vary between 26.2% and 55% after varicocelectomy in these case series for NOA.[53–55] A recent metaanalysis with 78 patients showed a statistically significant increase in total motile sperm count (TMSC) to over 5 million and a 27.5% natural pregnancy rate after varicocelectomy in patients with severe oligospermia.[56]

Impact on Reproductive Hormones

A large cross-sectional multicenter study performed across six European nations was undertaken in order to investigate semen parameters and reproductive hormone levels in their general population.[17] While there was evidence supporting no significant decrease in testosterone level in the general population, this same patient population showed decreased sperm quality as well as changes in other reproductive hormones such as higher follicle stimulating hormone (FSH) levels, higher luteinizing hormone levels, and lower inhibin B levels. In trying to assess determinates of worsening semen parameters, Chen and Chen were able to show that those individuals with varicoceles and impaired semen quality also had lower testosterone levels and increased FSH levels as well as progressively worsening semen quality parameters compared to those initially seen with varicoceles and normal semen quality parameters.[57] Similar findings were seen by Van Batavia et al., who investigated reproductive hormone levels in adolescents with varicoceles comparing those with a TMSC below 9 million sperm/ejaculate versus those with a TMSC greater than 9 million sperm/ejaculate.[58] They demonstrated that a TMSC below 9 million sperm/ejaculate is correlated with higher FSH and lower inhibin B levels, although testosterone levels were not statistically significantly different between groups. Infertile males have previously been shown to have significant increases in their testosterone levels after varicocelectomy, although direct relationships to semen quality or pregnancy rates were not evaluated in these studies.[59,60] Newer studies provide more conflicting evidence, with some continuing to show improvement in testosterone levels after varicocelectomy while others show no significant increase.[61,62]

Impact on Spontaneous Pregnancy Rates

Currently, the general consensus is that varicocelectomy in males with clinically significant varicoceles increases spontaneous pregnancy rates. The published rates of spontaneous pregnancy vary among sources and surgical techniques used, and further vary depending on status as an infertile male versus patients with severe oligospermia versus those with azoospermia. Per a metaanalysis comparing surgical technique including

data from 36 studies between 1980 and 2008, pregnancy rates varied between 30% (laparoscopic varicocelectomy) to 42% (microsurgical varicocelectomy).[63] A separate metaanalysis investigating infertile males undergoing varicocelectomy compared to medical therapy demonstrated an odds ratio of 2.87 in favor of surgical management of varicoceles to increase spontaneous pregnancy rates.[64] A prospective randomized trial found a six-fold increase in pregnancy rates after varicocelectomy. In the same study, subsequent varicocelectomy in the control group resulted in a four-fold increase in pregnancy rates.[65] In two separate contemporary systematic reviews of the literature of males with severe oligospermia, Mazjoub et al. were able to identify a spontaneous pregnancy rate of 27.5% after microsurgical varicocelectomy,[56] while Jensen and Ko were able to elucidate an average spontaneous pregnancy rate of 5.24% postvaricocelectomy in their systematic review of the literature for males with NOA.[66]

Impact on Assisted Reproductive Technology Outcomes

In line with increased spontaneous pregnancy rates for males with clinically significant varicoceles, there is growing evidence of the increased success of assisted reproductive technology (ART) for this same patient population.[66–70] Specifically, in males with NOA, microscopic testicular sperm extraction rates were seen to be 48.9% in those who had previously had a varicocelectomy versus 32.1% in those who had not had varicocele repair.[66] This same systematic review showed average pregnancy rates of 65.2% post intracytoplasmic sperm injection (ICSI) in those who had varicocele repairs compared to an average pregnancy rate of 39.5% for those undergoing ICSI without varicocele repair. Furthermore, a metaanalysis using studies and data from 1989 through 2013 showed that in this same NOA patient population, there were significantly higher odds of sperm retrieval after varicocele repair, with an odds ratio of 2.51, as well as higher pregnancy rates in this NOA population after varicocelectomy undergoing ICSI or in vitro fertilization (IVF), with an odds ratio of 1.76.[67] In looking at nonazoospermic males, Esteves et al. were able to demonstrate statistically significant increases in pregnancy rates (odds ratio 1.59) and live birth rates (odds ratio 2.17) for males undergoing varicocelectomy prior to ICSI compared to those without varicocele repair prior to ICSI in their metaanalysis.[71]

With regard to the impact of varicocelectomy on intra-uterine insemination (IUI) outcomes, the data are less conclusive, with older studies showing no significant impact on pregnancy rates, while newer studies have data supporting higher IUI pregnancy rates after varicocelectomy.[69]

Cayan and colleagues studied a cohort of 540 couples to determine if varicocele repair would change patient candidacy for ART.[72] They divided the patients into four groups based on their TMSC: ICSI candidates (<1.5 million), IVF candidates (1.5–5 million), IUI candidates (5–20 million), and natural birth candidates (>20 million). All patients underwent either a bilateral (73%) or unilateral (27%) microscopic varicocelectomy. Postoperatively, half of the patients had a greater than 50% increase in their TMSC, 31% of couples moved from the ICSI and IVF groups to the IUI and natural birth groups, and 42% of IUI candidates were upgraded to natural birth candidates.

COMPLICATIONS OF VARICOCELECTOMY

Complications of all approaches to varicocelectomy include testicular artery injury and subsequent testes atrophy, hydrocele formation, and recurrence of varicocele. Specifically, laparoscopic and robotic techniques have additional potential complications inherent to them, being intrabdominal procedures with insufflation as described previously.

With the use of microsurgical techniques, subinguinal approaches rarely have issues with hydrocele formation as the lymphatics are generally preserved. However, due to the more challenging delineation of the lymphatic vessels, lymphatic compromise and subsequent hydrocele is more common in inguinal, laparoscopic, and retroperitoneal repairs, and the incidence ranges from 0% to 29%.[73,74]

Testes atrophy remains a concern for varicocele treatment due to the potential for ligation of the testicular artery. True data on testes atrophy are very limited, but akin to decreasing hydrocele rates with the operating microscope, testicular artery injury and consequential testes atrophy appear to be lowest with operating microscope utilization.[74,75]

The incidence of recurrence rates also variesy greatly in the literature, with microsurgical techniques consistently demonstrating the lowest rates, and open and

laparoscopic techniques demonstrating higher rates of recurrence. Current published data indicate that recurrence rates for subinguinal microsurgical approaches are about 0.4% to 1.1 %.[74,76] The literature continues to show variance within the laparoscopic data, with a recent 15-year retrospective single academic institution showing a 21% recurrence rate in their pediatric population, while another institution retrospectively showed an 11.9% recurrence rate in their adult population.[77,78] Furthermore, a recent metaanalysis challenges the concept of testicle delivery to maximize identification and ligation of dilated veins as this study showed no significant difference in recurrence rates between varicocelectomy with versus without testes delivery.[79]

SUMMARY

Varicocele is a common cause of male infertility. Diagnosis of varicocele is through a thorough physical examination. Ultrasound can be used to confirm the diagnosis in males with difficult anatomy. There are many different methods of treating a clinical or palpable varicocele. Treatment of clinical varicoceles can result in improvement in semen analysis parameters and ultimately, spontaneous conception and ART pregnancy rates.

CLINICAL CASE SCENARIOS

CASE 1

A 32 year-old male has been referred to your clinic for further evaluation and work-up. The patient states that he and his 30-year-old wife have been attempting to have a child for 2 years now. The patient's wife previously completed a negative fertility work-up with her gynecologist. Your patient denies any significant past medical or surgical history. His wife's gynecologist has already ordered a semen analysis for him, which he has brought, showing a TMSC of 9 million and normal morphology. On examination, you note a left-sided grade 3 varicocele. The patient has been aware of this for many years from routine physicals but is asymptomatic from it, and so he never sought out further treatment. The patient would like to know what further steps could be taken to help his family to conceive a child.

REFERENCES

1. Su JS, Farber NJ, Vij SC. Pathophysiology and treatment options of varicocele: an overview. *Andrologia*. 2021; 53(1):1-9. doi:10.1111/and.13576.

2. Sigman M, Lipshultz LI, Howards SS. Office evaluation of the subfertile male. In: Lipshultz LI, Howards SS, Niederberger CS, eds. *Infertility in the Male*. 4th ed. New York: Cambridge University Press; 2009:153-176.

3. Lipshultz LI, Corriere JN. Progressive testicular atrophy in the varicocele patient. *J Urol*. 1977;117(2):175-176. doi:10.1016/S0022-5347(17)58387-1.

4. Gorelick JI, Goldstein M. Loss of fertility in men with varicocele. *Fertil Steril*. 1993;59(3):613-616. doi:10.1016/s0015-0282(16)55809-9.

5. Jarow JP, Coburn M. Incidence of varicoceles in men with primary and secondary infertility. *Urology*. 1995; 47(I):73-76.

6. Braedel HU, Steffens J, Ziegler M, Polsky MS, Platt ML. A possible ontogenic etiology for idiopathic left varicocele. *J Urol*. 1994;151(1):62-66. doi:10.1016/S0022-5347(17) 34872-3.

7. Agarwal A, Hamada A, Esteves SC. Insight into oxidative stress in varicocele-associated male infertility: part 1. *Nat Rev Urol*. 2012;9(12):678-690. doi:10.1038/nrurol.2012.197.

8. Dubin L, Amelar RD. Varicocele size and results of varicocelectomy in selected. *Fertil Steril*. 1970;21(8):606-609.

9. Ammar T, Sidhu PS, Wilkins CJ. Male infertility: the role of imaging in diagnosis and management. *Br J Radiol*. 2012;85(Spec Iss 1):S59-S68. doi:10.1259/bjr/31818161.

10. Itani M, Kipper B, Corwin MT, Burgan CM, Fetzer DT. Right-sided scrotal varicocele and its association with

malignancy : a multi-institutional study. *Abdom Radiol (NY)*. 2021;46(5):2140-2145. doi:10.1007/s00261-020-02840-9.

11. Elmer DeWitt M, Greene DJ, Gill B, Nyame Y, Haywood S, Sabanegh Jr E. Isolated right varicocele and incidence of associated cancer. *Urology*. 2018;117:82-85. doi:10.1016/j.urology.2018.03.047.

12. Agarwal A, Sharma RK, Desai NR, Prabakaran S, Tavares A, Sabanegh E. Role of oxidative stress in pathogenesis of varicocele and infertility. *Urology*. 2009;73(3):461-469. doi:10.1016/j.urology.2008.07.053.

13. Ko EY, Sabanegh ES, Agarwal A. Male infertility testing: reactive oxygen species and antioxidant capacity. *Fertil Steril*. 2014;102(6):1518-1527.

14. Agarwal A, Sharma R, Harlev A, Esteves S. Effect of varicocele on semen characteristics according to the new 2010 World Health Organization criteria: a systematic review and meta-analysis. *Asian J Androl*. 2016;18(2):163-170. doi:10.4103/1008-682X.172638.

15. Buggio L, Barbara G, Facchin F, Frattaruolo MP, Aimi G, Berlanda N. Self-management and psychological-sexological interventions in patients with endometriosis: strategies, outcomes, and integration into clinical care. *Int J Womens Health*. 2017;9:281-293. Available at: http://dx.doi.org/10.2147/IJWH.S119724.

16. Sofikitis N, Miyagawa I. Effects of surgical repair of experimental left varicocele on testicular temperature, spermatogenesis, sperm maturation, endocrine function, and fertility in rabbits. *Syst Biol Reprod Med*. 1992; 29(2):163-175. doi:10.3109/01485019208987721.

17. Damsgaard J, Joensen UN, Carlsen E, et al. Varicocele is associated with impaired semen quality and reproductive hormone levels: a study of 7035 healthy young men from six European countries. *Eur Urol*. 2016;70(6):1019-1029.

18. Wang Y, Zhang R, Lin Y, Zhang R, Zhang W. Relationship between varicocele and sperm DNA damage and the effect of varicocele repair : a meta- analysis. *Reprod Biomed Online*. 2012;25(3):307-314. doi:10.1016/j.rbmo.2012.05.002.

19. Schlegel PN, Sigman M, Collura B, et al. Diagnosis and treatment of infertility in men: AUA/ASRM guideline Part II. *J Urol*. 2021;205(1):44-51.

20. Salonia A, Bettocchi C, Boeri L, et al. European Association of Urology Guidelines on Sexual and Reproductive Health-2021 Update: Male Sexual Dysfunction. *Eur Urol*. 2021;80(3):333-357.

21. Lima SS, Castro MP, Costa OF. A new method for the treatment of varicocele. *Andrologia*. 1978;10:103-106.

22. Walsh PC, White RI. Balloon occlusion of the internal spermatic vein for the treatment of varicoceles. *JAMA*. 1981;246:1701-1702.

23. Weissbach L, Thelen M, Adolphs HD. Treatment of idiopathic varicoceles by transfemoral testicular vein occlusion. *J Urol.* 1981;126:354-356.

24. Khera M, Lipshultz LI. Evolving approach to the varicocele. *Urol Clin North Am.* 2008;35:183-189, viii.

25. Kaufman SL, Kadir S, Barth KH, Smyth JW, Walsh PC, White RI. Mechanisms of recurrent varicocele after balloon occlusion or surgical ligation of the internal spermatic vein. *Radiology.* 1983;147:435-440.

26. Punekar SV, Prem AR, Ridhorkar VR, Deshmukh HL, Kelkar AR. Post-surgical recurrent varicocele: efficacy of internal spermatic venography and steel-coil embolization. *Br J Urol.* 1996;77:124-128.

27. Tauber R, Johnsen N. Antegrade scrotal sclerotherapy for the treatment of varicocele: technique and late results. *J Urol.* 1994;151:386-390.

28. Crestani A, Giannarini G, Calandriello M, et al. Antegrade scrotal sclerotherapy of internal spermatic veins for varicocele treatment: technique, complications, and results. *Asian J Androl.* 2016;18(2):292-295.

29. Goldstein M. Surgical management of male infertility. In: Partin AW, Dmochowski RR, Kavoussi LR, Peters CA eds. *Campbell-Walsh-Wein Urology.* Philadelphia, PA: Elsevier; 2021:1453-1483.

30. Tulloch WS. Varicocele in subfertility; results of treatment. *Br Med J.* 1955;2:356-358.

31. Palomo A. Radical cure of varicocele by a new technique: preliminary report. *J Urol.* 1949;61(3):604-607.

32. Homonnai ZT, Fainman N, Engelhard Y, Rudberg Z, David MP, Paz G. Varicocelectomy and male fertility: comparison of semen quality and recurrence of varicocele following varicocelectomy by two techniques. *Int J Androl.* 1980;3:447-458.

33. Rothman CM, Newmark H, Karson RA. The recurrent varicocele—a poorly recognized problem. *Fertil Steril.* 1981;35:552-556.

34. Watanabe M, Nagai A, Kusumi N, Tsuboi H, Nasu Y, Kumon H. Minimal invasiveness and effectivity of subinguinal microscopic varicocelectomy: a comparative study with retroperitoneal high and laparoscopic approaches. *Int J Urol.* 2005;12:892-898.

35. Sayfan J, Adam YG, Soffer Y. A new entity in varicocele subfertility: the "cremasteric reflux." *Fertil Steril.* 1980;33:88-90.

36. Glassberg KI, Poon SA, Gjertson CK, DeCastro GJ, Misseri R. Laparoscopic lymphatic sparing varicocelectomy in adolescents. *J Urol.* 2008;180:326-331.

37. Harel M, Herbst KW, Nelson E. Practice patterns in the surgical approach for adolescent varicocelectomy. *Springerplus.* 2015;4:772.

38. Méndez-Gallart R, Bautista-Casasnovas A, Estevez-Martínez E, Varela-Cives R. Laparoscopic Palomo varicocele surgery: lessons learned after 10 years' follow

39. Sun HB, Liu Y, Yan MB, Li ZD, Gui XG. Comparing three different surgical techniques used in adult bilateral varicocele. *Asian J Endosc Surg.* 2012;5:12-16.

40. Al-Said S, Al-Naimi A, Al-Ansari A, et al. Varicocelectomy for male infertility: a comparative study of open, laparoscopic and microsurgical approaches. *J Urol.* 2008; 180:266-270.

41. Zhang H, Li H, Hou Y, et al. Microscopic retroperitoneal varicocelectomy with artery and lymphatic sparing: an alternative treatment for varicocele in infertile men. *Urology.* 2015;86:511-515.

42. Silveri M, Bassani F, Adorisio O. Changing concepts in microsurgical pediatric varicocelectomy: is retroperitoneal approach better than subinguinal one? *Urol J.* 2015;12(1):2032-2035.

43. Esposito C, Settimi A, Del Conte F, et al. Image-guided pediatric surgery using indocyanine green (ICG) fluorescence in laparoscopic and robotic surgery. *Front Pediatr.* 2020;8:314.

44. McCullough A, Elebyjian L, Ellen J, Mechlin C. A retrospective review of single-institution outcomes with robotic-assisted microsurgical varicocelectomy. *Asian J Androl.* 2018;20(2):189-194.

45. Darves-Bornoz A, Panken E, Brannigan RE, Halpern JA. Robotic surgery for male infertility. *Urol Clin North Am.* 2021;48(1):127-135.

46. Marmar JL, DeBenedictis TJ, Praiss D. The management of varicoceles by microdissection of the spermatic cord at the external inguinal ring. *Fertil Steril.* 1985;43:583-588.

47. Goldstein M, Gilbert BR, Dicker AP, Dwosh J, Gnecco C. Microsurgical inguinal varicocelectomy with delivery of the testis: an artery and lymphatic sparing technique. *J Urol.* 1992;148(6):1808-1811.

48. Demirdögen ŞO, Özkaya F, Cinislioğlu AE, et al. A comparison between the efficacy and safety of microscopic inguinal and subinguinal varicocelectomy. *Turk J Urol.* 2019;45(4):254-260. doi:10.5152/tud.2019.7254.

49. Agarwal A, Deepinder F, Cocuzza M, et al. Efficacy of varicocelectomy in improving semen parameters: new meta-analytical approach. *Urology.* 2007;70(3):532-538.

50. Birowo P, Rahendra Wijaya J, Atmoko W, Rasyid N. The effects of varicocelectomy on the DNA fragmentation index and other sperm parameters: a meta-analysis. *Basic Clin Androl.* 2020;30:15.

51. Zhou T, Zhang W, Chen Q, et al. Effect of varicocelectomy on testis volume and semen parameters in adolescents: a meta-analysis. *Asian J Androl.* 2015;17:1012-1016.

52. Locke JA, Noparast M, Afshar K. Treatment of varicocele in children and adolescents: a systematic review and meta-analysis of randomized controlled trials. *J Pediatr Urol.* 2017;13(5):437-445.

up of 156 consecutive pediatric patients. *J Pediatr Urol.* 2009;5:126-131.

53. Elbardisi H, El Ansari W, Majzoub A, Arafa M. Does varicocelectomy improve semen in men with azoospermia and clinically palpable varicocele? *Andrologia*. 2020;52(2):e13486.
54. Kiraç M, Deniz N, Biri H. The effect of microsurgical varicocelectomy on semen parameters in men with nonobstructive azoospermia. *Curr Urol*. 2013;6(3):136-140.
55. Matthews GJ, Matthews ED, Goldstein M. Induction of spermatogenesis and achievement of pregnancy after microsurgical varicocelectomy in men with azoospermia and severe oligoasthenospermia. *Fertil Steril*. 1998;70:71-75.
56. Majzoub A, ElBardisi H, Covarrubias S, et al. Effect of microsurgical varicocelectomy on fertility outcome and treatment plans of patients with severe oligozoospermia: an original report and meta-analysis. *Andrologia*. 2021;53(6):e14059.
57. Chen SS, Chen LK. Risk factors for progressive deterioration of semen quality in patients with varicocele. *Urology*. 2012;79(1):128-132.
58. Van Batavia JP, Lawton E, Frazier JR, et al. Total motile sperm count in adolescent boys with varicocele is associated with hormone levels and total testicular volume. *J Urol*. 2021;205(3):888-894.
59. Su LM, Goldstein M, Schlegel PN. The effect of varicocelectomy on serum testosterone levels in infertile men with varicoceles. *J Urol*. 1995;154(5):1752-1755.
60. Hsiao W, Rosoff JS, Pale JR, Powell JL, Goldstein M. Varicocelectomy is associated with increases in serum testosterone independent of clinical grade. *Urology*. 2013;81(6):1213-1217.
61. Abdel-Meguid TA, Farsi HM, Al-Sayyad A, Tayib A, Mosli HA, Halawani AH. Effects of varicocele on serum testosterone and changes of testosterone after varicocelectomy: a prospective controlled study. *Urology*. 2014;84(5):1081-1087.
62. Jangkhah M, Farrahi F, Sadighi Gilani MA, et al. Effects of varicocelectomy on serum testosterone levels among infertile men with varicocele. *Int J Fertil Steril*. 2018;12(2):169-172.
63. Cayan S, Shavakhabov S, Kadıoğlu A. Treatment of palpable varicocele in infertile men: a meta-analysis to define the best technique. *J Androl*. 2009;30(1):33-40.
64. Marmar JL, Agarwal A, Prabakaran S, et al. Reassessing the value of varicocelectomy as a treatment for male subfertility with a new meta-analysis. *Fertil Steril*. 2007;88(3):639-648.
65. Madgar I, Weissenberg R, Lunenfeld B, Karasik A, Goldwasser B. Controlled trial of high spermatic vein ligation for varicocele in infertile men. *Fertil Steril*. 1995;63(1):120-124. doi:10.1016/s0015-0282(16)57306-3.
66. Jensen S, Ko EY. Varicocele treatment in non-obstructive azoospermia: a systematic review. *Arab J Urol*. 2021;19(3):221-226.
67. Kirby EW, Wiener LE, Rajanahally S, Crowell K, Coward RM. Undergoing varicocele repair before assisted reproduction improves pregnancy rate and live birth rate in azoospermic and oligospermic men with a varicocele: a systematic review and meta-analysis. *Fertil Steril*. 2016;106(6):1338-1343.
68. Esteves SC, Roque M, Agarwal A. Outcome of assisted reproductive technology in men with treated and untreated varicocele: systematic review and meta-analysis. *Asian J Androl*. 2016;18(2):254-258. doi:10.4103/1008-682X.163269.
69. Kohn JR, Haney NM, Nichols PE, Rodriguez KM, Kohn TP. Varicocele repair prior to assisted reproductive technology: patient selection and special considerations. *Res Rep Urol*. 2020;12:149-156.
70. Samplaski MK, Lo KC, Grober ED, Zini A, Jarvi KA. Varicocelectomy to "upgrade" semen quality to allow couples to use less invasive forms of assisted reproductive technology. *Fertil Steril*. 2017;108(4):609-612.
71. Esteves SC, Miyaoka R, Roque M, Agarwal A. Outcome of varicocele repair in men with nonobstructive azoospermia: systematic review and meta-analysis. *Asian J Androl*. 2016;18(2):246-253. doi:10.4103/1008-682X.169562.
72. Cayan S, Erdemir F, Ozbey I, Turek PJ, Kadıoğlu A, Tellaloğlu S. Can varicocelectomy significantly change the way couples use assisted reproductive technologies? *J Urol*. 2002;167:1749-1752.
73. Nees SN, Glassberg KI. Observations on hydroceles following adolescent varicocelectomy. *J Urol*. 2011;186(6):2402-2407.
74. Yuan R, Zhuo H, Cao D, Wei Q. Efficacy and safety of varicocelectomies: a meta-analysis. *Syst Biol Reprod Med*. 2017;63(2):120-129.
75. Ding H, Tian J, Du W, Zhang L, Wang H, Wang Z. Open non-microsurgical, laparoscopic or open microsurgical varicocelectomy for male infertility: a meta-analysis of randomized controlled trials. *BJU Int*. 2012;110:1536-1542.
76. Persad E, O'Loughlin CA, Kaur S, et al. Surgical or radiological treatment for varicoceles in subfertile men. *Cochrane Database Syst Rev*. 2021;4(4):CD000479.
77. Soares-Aquino C, Vasconcelos-Castro S, Campos JM, Soares-Oliveira M. 15-year varicocelectomy outcomes in pediatric age: beware of genitofemoral nerve injury. *J Pediatr Urol*. 2021;17(4):537.e1-537.e5.
78. Lv JX, Wang LL, Wei XD, et al. Comparison of treatment outcomes of different spermatic vein ligation procedures in varicocele treatment. *Am J Ther*. 2016;23(6):e1329-e1334.
79. Song Y, Lu Y, Xu Y, Yang Y, Liu X. Comparison between microsurgical varicocelectomy with and without testicular delivery for treatment of varicocele: a systematic review and meta-analysis. *Andrologia*. 2019;51(9):e13363.

20

Management of Ejaculatory Duct Obstruction

Taha Abo-Almagd Abdel-Meguid Hamoda,
Hassan Mohammed Aljifri, and Mahmoud Fareed Qutub

KEY POINTS

- Ejaculatory duct obstruction (EDO) is uncommon condition but should be considered in the differential diagnosis of male infertility.
- The seminal vesicles secretions contribute to about 80% of seminal volume.
- EDO can be classified as congenital or acquired, unilateral or bilateral, partial or complete, and functional.
- Congenital cysts are known causes of EDO.
- EDO has no pathognomonic criteria, but the characteristic seminal features of EDO are thought to be azoospermia or oligospermia, low volume, low pH, and absent or low fructose.

- Transrectal ultrasound (TRUS) has revolutionized the diagnosis of EDO and, together with endorectal MRI, has supplanted the historical vasography in diagnosing EDO.
- Almost half of patients with TRUS findings suggestive of EDO are not truly obstructed.
- Additional adjunct diagnostic tests were proposed to refine the diagnosis of EDO and to improve the outcomes of treatment.
- The disease is usually surgically correctable.
- Transurethral resection of the ejaculatory duct is the mainstay treatment in most cases.

INTRODUCTION

EDO was described by Gutierrez in 1942.[1] EDO is an uncommon etiology of males presenting with reproductive health problems. However, it should be considered in the differential diagnosis of male infertility.[2,3] Patients usually present with low ejaculate volume associated with oligospermia or azoospermia. Although vasography has been historically considered the mainstay of diagnosis, currently TRUS and endorectal magnetic resonance imaging (MRI) have revolutionized the diagnosis of EDO and have supplanted the usage of vasography in this setting. The disease is usually surgically correctable. Transurethral resection of the ejaculatory ducts (TURED) is the mainstay treatment in most cases.[2–4]

The process of diagnosis and treatment of EDO in the "typical" patient is usually straightforward. Even so, in

occasional cases, this process is problematic, and prediction of treatment outcomes is a challenge. The aim of this chapter is to provide reproductive specialists with an overview on the fundamentals of EDO and an update on contemporary methods of diagnosis and treatment.

EPIDEMIOLOGY OF OBSTRUCTION OF MALE REPRODUCTIVE TRACT

Obstruction of reproductive ducts is a relatively less common cause of azoospermia compared to primary testicular failure, with as many as 40% of males with azoospermia diagnosed with obstructive etiologies. The obstruction can occur at different anatomical levels of the reproductive ducts, such as rete testis, efferent ductules, epididymis, vas deferens, or ejaculatory duct.[5] Among these sites, EDO accounts for 1% to

5% of all males with azoospermia. The rare, "classic" complete bilateral EDO is reported in less than 1% of azoospermic males.[3,6]

ANATOMICAL CONSIDERATIONS

Understanding the embryology and anatomy of the ejaculatory ducts and seminal vesicles is fundamental for further understanding of the pathophysiology of EDO and, consequently, for understanding the basis of any proposed treatment. The ejaculatory duct shares the same embryological background of the seminal vesicle, vas deferens, and epididymis, which all originate from the Wolffian (mesonephric) duct, unlike the prostate, which originates from the endoderm.[7–12]

The ejaculatory ducts are paired tubular structures, with each duct being approximately 1 to 2 cm in length and 0.45 to 1.31 mm in diameter. Each ejaculatory duct is anatomically divided into three segments: proximal extraprostatic, middle intraprostatic, and distal verumontanum segments.[7–9] The ejaculatory duct begins at the junction of the cystic duct of the seminal vesicle with the ampulla of the ipsilateral vas and terminates at the verumontanum of the prostatic urethra (Fig. 20.1).[7] The ducts enter the prostate gland by an oblique angle at its base and course anteromedially in almost a straight line until they open into the verumontanum of the prostatic urethra at an acute angle (Figs. 20.2 and 20.3).[12] Between both openings of the ejaculatory ducts at the level of verumontanum lies the prostatic utricle, which is a Müllerian duct remnant. During autopsy studies, the anatomical relationships between these structures have showed that the ejaculatory ducts open as slitlike orifices anterolateral to the prostatic utricle opening.[7–9]

Histologically, each duct consists of three layers: an inner pseudostratified columnar epithelium, a middle collagenous layer, and an outer longitudinal muscular coat the outer muscle layer in the distal segment of the duct, where they open into the verumontanum at an acute angle (see Fig. 20.2). Nguyen et al., in a 1996 study on cadaveric and surgical specimens, proposed that these characteristic anatomical and histological configurations help maintain the ejaculatory ducts, continence and prevent urinary reflux into the ducts.[7] However, in 2019, Li et al. described a functioning one-way valve mechanism at the terminal portion of each ejaculatory duct, precluding reflux into the duct.[13]

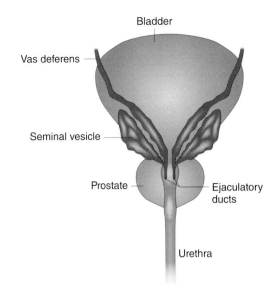

Fig. 20.1 Ejaculatory Duct Anatomy. The ejaculatory duct begins at the junction of the cystic duct of the seminal vesicle with the ampulla of the vas and terminates at the verumontanum of the prostatic urethra. (From Modgil V, Rai S, Ralph DJ, Muneer A. An update on the diagnosis and management of ejaculatory duct obstruction. *Nat Rev Urol.* 2016;13(1):13-20.)

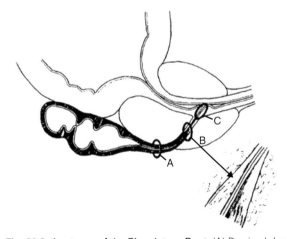

Fig. 20.2 Anatomy of the Ejaculatory Duct. (A) Proximal duct segment, (B) middle intraprostatic duct segment, and (C) distal segment. The figure shows that the muscle wall thins at the level of the intraprostatic segment, whereas it thickens more proximally at the seminal vesicle level. (From Nguyen HT, Etzell J, Turek PJ. Normal human ejaculatory duct anatomy: a study of cadaveric and surgical specimens. *J Urol.* 1996;155(5): 1639-1642.)

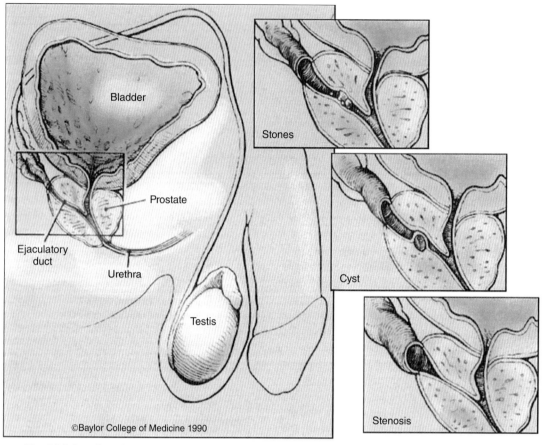

Fig. 20.3 Drawing of ejaculatory duct obstruction due to stones, cysts, and stenosis. (From Avellino GJ, Lipshultz LI, Sigman M, Hwang K. Transurethral resection of the ejaculatory ducts: etiology of obstruction and surgical treatment options. *Fertil Steril.* 2019;111(3):427-443.)

FUNCTIONAL CONSIDERATIONS

The seminal vesicles' secretions are responsible for the bulk of volume of semen, as they alone contribute to as much as 80% to 85% of volume of the semen. The prostatic secretions add about 15% to the seminal volume, while all other components comprise less than 1% of the volume (e.g., sperm, testicular, and epidydimal fluids, and Cowper and urethral glands secretions).[4,14] The seminal vesicles function under influence of testosterone, which enhances their secretions.[4] The seminal vesicles are compliant reservoirs that can accommodate their secreted fluids. They also have properties of contractility of their smooth muscles to eject and evacuate these fluids via the ejaculatory ducts into the prostatic urethra during ejaculation.[2]

The seminal vesicles secretions are alkaline in nature. As their fluids dominate the ejaculate volume, they are responsible for the alkalinity of semen, which protects the sperm by buffering the acidic environment of the vagina. Additionally, the seminal vesicles are responsible for the initial "coagulum" consistency of the ejaculate, which will later liquefy by action of proteolytic enzymes of prostatic secretions to provide the sperm with a medium of abundant fluid to move through and help ease their motility. Further, the seminal vesicles are also the major source of the seminal fructose.[4]

The ejaculatory duct serves as a conduit to transport the seminal fluid and sperm from seminal vesicle and vas deferens to the prostatic urethra during ejaculation.[15] As discussed before, the ejaculatory ducts, structural and functional characteristics help keep them continent and prevent reflux of urine into the ducts.[7,13]

ETIOLOGY AND PATHOPHYSIOLOGY OF EJACULATORY DUCT OBSTRUCTION

According to the etiology, site, and degree of obstruction, EDO can be classified as congenital or acquired, unilateral or bilateral, partial or complete, and functional. Complete obstruction usually denotes complete bilateral EDO, whereas incomplete obstruction may refer to one obstructed duct or bilaterally partially obstructed ducts. Pryor and Hendry,[16] in a study on 87 infertile males with EDO, have identified the etiologies of Müllerian, utricular, and Wolffian duct congenital malformations (41%), traumatic causes (17%), postinfectious causes (22%), tuberculosis (9%), megavesicles (9%), and neoplasm (1%); with some overlapping etiologies. The obstruction can be localized to the terminal ends of the ducts or may extend to involve as proximal as the distal parts of the vasa deferentia.[4] Such a wide variety of classification will consequently result in widely variable manifestations and seminal characteristics. For instance, complete bilateral obstruction is usually associated with low ejaculate volume, whereas partial or unilateral obstruction may be associated with low or average ejaculate volume.[3] As well, the site, length, and etiology of the obstruction determine the possible treatment options and the expected outcomes. Generally, the treatment outcomes of congenital noninfectious obstruction tend to be better than those of acquired or infectious obstruction.[3,4,6,17]

Congenital causes of EDO are various (Tables 20.1 and 20.2). Midline utricular, Müllerian, and Wolffian duct cysts are located in the midline behind the prostatic urethra and are known causes of congenital obstruction. Although it is difficult to differentiate among them, midline cysts can be categorized into two types. The first type (median cysts) includes utricle and Müllerian cysts, which originate from the Müllerian duct and do not contain sperm. Utricle cysts can be found in the midline near the utricle of verumontanum and do not extend proximal to prostate base, while Müllerian cysts are usually extending above the prostate base. The second, less common type (paramedian cysts) includes Wolffian and ejaculatory duct cysts, which contain sperm and fructose. These cysts originate from the Wolffian duct and tend to locate more laterally but close to the midline (paramedian).[3,4,10,18] EDO may also result from congenital atresia or stenosis of the ejaculatory ducts. Occasionally, an ectopic ureteral orifice terminating into the ejaculatory duct may lead to EDO. Renal agenesis may also be associated with cystic obstruction of ejaculatory duct.[11,19,20] The very rare Zinner syndrome, first described in 1914, entails a triad of unilateral renal agenesis, ipsilateral seminal vesicle cyst, and obstruction of ejaculatory duct, and is due to Wolffian duct anomaly.[21]

Acquired causes of EDO are less frequent than congenital causes (see Table 20.2 and Fig. 20.3). Acquired EDO is usually secondary to prolonged urethral catheterization and infectious causes (e.g., genitourinary tuberculosis or prostatic abscess), where the ejaculatory duct is stenosed or completely obstructed by fibrosis.

TABLE 20.1 **Characteristics of Congenital Prostatic Cysts Causing Ejaculatory Duct Obstruction**

	Embryological Origin	Type	Location	Content	Other Content
Utricle cyst	Müllerian duct	Median	Midline, near utricle of verumontanum, below prostate base	No sperm	Possible in all cysts: calculi blood pus
Müllerian duct cyst	Müllerian duct	Median	Midline, may extend above prostate base	No sperm	
Ejaculatory duct cyst	Wolffian duct	Paramedian	Just lateral to midline	Sperm and fructose	

TABLE 20.2 Congenital, Acquired, and Functional Etiologies of Ejaculatory Duct Obstruction

Congenital	Acquired	Functional
Utricle cyst	Prolonged indwelling urethral catheter	MS
Müllerian duct cyst	Infectious and inflammatory conditions (e.g., tuberculous prostatoseminal vesiculitis, etc.)	SCI
Wolffian duct cyst		DM
		RPLND
Ejaculatory duct atresia		Pelvic surgery
Ejaculatory duct stenosis	Iatrogenic urethral trauma (e.g., post-TURP)	Medications
	External urethral trauma	
	Calculi of the seminal vesicles	

DM, Diabetes mellitus; *EDO*, ejaculatory duct obstruction; *MS*, multiple sclerosis; *RPLND*, retroperitoneal lymph node dissection; *SCI*, spinal cord injury; *TURP*, transurethral resection of the prostate.

Genitourinary trauma is another cause of acquired EDO, which can occur after surgical procedures such as previous transurethral resection of the prostate (TURP).[3] Penetrating injury to the perineal body caused by bullets in military patients was also reported to cause EDO when complicated by infection, as described by Pryor and Hendry.[16] Calculus formation in the seminal vesicles has also been described to cause EDO (see Fig. 20.3).[3]

Functional EDO is an infrequent condition caused by neurological functional abnormalities of the seminal vesicles and vasa deferentia, resulting in hypocontractility and failure of peristalsis of their smooth muscles, with subsequent failure of emission and dilatation of the seminal vesicles (megavesicles). The neurological deficit may be caused by multiple sclerosis, spinal cord injury, diabetes mellitus, pelvic surgery, or retroperitoneal lymph node dissection. Functional obstruction may manifest with low semen volume or azoospermia, similar to complete obstruction. Nevertheless, with the absence of physical obstruction, the diagnosis of functional obstruction is primarily made by exclusion. Of note, functional obstruction is not amenable to surgical correction.[19]

Several medications such as α-adrenergic antagonists, tricyclic antidepressant agents, antipsychotic drugs, thiazide diuretics, and antihypertensives are also associated with impaired contractility of the seminal vesicles and can reduce ejaculate volume.[2,15,19]

EVALUATION OF EJACULATORY DUCT OBSTRUCTION

Although EDO is an uncommon diagnosis and has no pathognomonic criteria, the characteristic seminal features of EDO are thought to be azoospermia or oligospermia, low volume, low pH, and absent or low fructose (Table 20.3), along with bilaterally normal vas deferens, epididymis, and testicles on physical examination, and dilated or normal-sized seminal vesicles in imaging studies.[3–6,22]

History and Physical Examination

The presentations of EDO are widely variable. While some patients are asymptomatic, most patients present with infertility complaints. Other patients may present with symptoms of low-volume ejaculate, hemospermia, painful ejaculation, postejaculatory pain, perineal pain, suprapubic pain, low back pain, chronic scrotal pain, dysuria, and/or other urinary symptoms, which may eventually affect their psychological integrity and sexual health.[2,6,23] The clinician should also identify the predisposing factors for EDO. Thus a detailed history includes previous genitourinary infections (e.g., prostatitis or epididymitis), previous genitourinary trauma (e.g., urethral trauma), or history of prolonged catheterization.

TABLE 20.3 Usual Semen Characteristics of Different Categories of Ejaculatory Duct Obstruction

Semen Variable	TYPE OF OBSTRUCTION		
	Complete	Partial	Functional
Volume	Low	Low or normal	Low
pH	Low	Low or normal	Low or normal
Sperm count	Azoospermia	Oligospermia or normal	Azoospermia or oligospermia
Sperm motility	No sperm	Impaired	No sperm or impaired
Fructose	Absent	Absent or low	Absent or low

Past surgical history is also essential, as patients who had a history of TURP or posterior urethral valve ablation may develop EDO.[23] Furthermore, the patients should be asked about any medications that might impair the ejaculation.[2,4,19]

On physical examination, the patients with suspected EDO usually demonstrate normal testis size, normal or full epididymis, and palpable vas deferens. However, a digital rectal examination may occasionally identify a midline prostatic cyst (MPC) or dilated seminal vesicle(s).[2–6]

Laboratory Testing

Semen analysis is a key tool in the evaluation of males with infertility. Important semen parameters to consider for the assessment of EDO are the ejaculate volume, pH, and fructose content (see Table 20.3). As discussed previously, the seminal volume is the contribution of multiple reproductive organ secretions, such as seminal vesicles, the prostate gland, bulbourethral glands, and other organs. The seminal vesicles produce the majority of ejaculate volume. According to the World Health Organization (WHO) manual, the lower limit of ejaculate volume is 1.5 mL.[24] However, the most frequently used value for initiating evaluation of seminal hypovolemia is 1.0 mL.[25] The different causes of low semen volume are discussed later in this chapter (Box 20.1). The seminal pH is another important parameter in semen analysis during evaluation of patients with suspected EDO. The semen pH represents the

secretion balance between the reproductive organs. The seminal vesicles secret alkaline fluids, while in contrast, the prostate gland secretes acidic fluid. The WHO manual has determined 7.2 as the lower limit of semen pH.[24] Lastly, seminal vesicles secrete fructose; therefore low or absent fructose in semen may suggest EDO as well.[23] In summary, although semen analysis is not diagnostic for EDO, it may show low ejaculate volume associated with decreased sperm count or azoospermia, low pH, and absent or low fructose.[2,3,6]

Hormonal profiles in EDO patients should be within normal ranges, similar to other causes of obstruction of reproductive tract.[5] FSH and testosterone should be within the normal ranges in males presenting with EDO.[2] Inhibin B should also be within the normal range in obstructive azoospermia, whereas it is decreased in nonobstructive azoospermia patients.[5]

Imaging Studies and Other Diagnostic Procedures

Historically, vasography has been used as the diagnostic modality of choice for EDO. However, due to the invasiveness of the procedure, the potential complication of development of vasal stricture, the need for anesthesia, and the exposure to radiation, vasography has been supplanted by other diagnostic modalities. Currently, the key tool adopted in evaluating a patient with suspected EDO is TRUS. TRUS has revolutionized the diagnosis of EDO and can also help diagnosis of other seminal vesicle abnormalities such as agenesis, hypoplasia, or atrophy.[17,26] Although TRUS is an attractive, noninvasive initial diagnostic tool, it has some drawbacks, including low specificity and operator-dependent outcome. Because of TRUS's limitations, some additional diagnostic tools were proposed to improve the diagnosis and treatment outcomes. The additional diagnostic algorithm includes endorectal MRI, TRUS-guided aspiration of seminal vesicles, seminal vesicle chromotubation, and seminal vesiculography.[3,6,27,28] Despite this armamentarium of diagnostic tools, the definitive diagnostic test for EDO that can precisely predict successful outcome of treatment has not been defined yet (Table 20.4).[29]

Transrectal Ultrasound

The high-resolution TRUS has been established during the recent years as a method of choice imaging study in initial evaluation of patients with suspected EDO. It is considered

---

BOX 20.1   Causes of Low Volume of Semen

- Incomplete collection of semen
- Short abstinence period
- Retrograde ejaculation
- Congenital agenesis or hypoplasia of seminal vesicles (as in congenitally absent vas deferens and cystic fibrosis)
- Hypogonadism (leading to seminal vesicles' hypoplasia or hypofunction)
- Inflammation of seminal vesicles (seminal vesicle atrophy or hypofunction)
- Medications
- Functional ejaculatory duct obstruction
- Ejaculatory duct obstruction (physical: classic form and other varieties)

TABLE 20.4 **Characteristics of Different Diagnostic Modalities for Ejaculatory Duct Obstruction**

Characteristics	TRUS	MRI	SVA	Chromotubation	Vesiculography	Manometry
Invasive	Minimal	Minimal or no	Yes	Yes	Yes	Yes
Radiation exposure	No	No	No	No	Yes	No
Nonionic contrast injection	No	No	No	No	Yes	No
Colored dye injection	No	No	No	Yes	No	Yes
Overdiagnosis	Yes	Yes	Unusual	No	No	Undetermined
Underdiagnosis	Unusual	Unusual	Unusual	Yes	Yes	Undetermined

MRI, Magnetic resonance imaging; *SVA*, seminal vesicle aspiration; *TRUS*, transrectal ultrasound.

a simple and less invasive tool for evaluation than other modalities. It also provides good anatomical information for reproductive ducts and demonstrates accurate measurements of the dimensions of seminal vesicles and ejaculatory ducts. Seminal vesicle dilatation (transverse diameter >15 mm), ejaculatory duct dilatation (diameter >2.3 mm), midline cystic structure in the prostate, or prostatic calcifications are all TRUS findings suggestive of EDO.[17,29] Moreover, if TRUS shows variability in size between the right and left ejaculatory ducts and/or seminal vesicles, this may suggest unilateral EDO.[2]

However, the anatomical findings in TRUS do not always correspond to the presence of EDO. While not all patients with dilated seminal vesicles in TRUS have actual EDO, on the contrary, the absence of seminal vesicle dilatation does not rule out the presence of EDO. For instance, in a study by Purohit et al. in males with suspected EDO, the investigators performed TRUS, seminal vesicle aspiration, chromotubation of the duct, and seminal vesiculography. The authors observed only 48% of patients with findings suggestive of EDO on TRUS having actual obstruction confirmed by the other modalities.[29] Engin et al.[28] have also reported comparable results, where only 49.1% of patients with evidence of EDO in TRUS were proved to have confirmed obstruction using seminal vesicle aspiration.

Thus TRUS may not be the most accurate test for EDO evaluation, given its poor specificity compared to other modalities. The clinician should appreciate that almost half of patients with TRUS findings suggestive of EDO are not truly obstructed. Therefore the use of TRUS as the sole test for diagnosing EDO may lead to overdiagnosis

and to an unnecessary and unsuccessful TURED surgery. Additional adjunct diagnostic tests were proposed to refine the diagnosis of EDO—particularly when suspecting partial or functional obstruction—and consequently to improve the outcomes of treatment.[29]

Magnetic Resonance Imaging

Endorectal MRI provides multiplanar high-resolution images of the prostate gland, ejaculatory ducts, seminal vesicles, and surrounding structures. T2-weighted MRI provides invaluable information to assess cystic soft tissue lesions and their location and relationship to adjacent structures. T2-weighted images indicate EDO with the finding of ejaculatory duct diameter greater than 2 mm and duct wall thickness and enhancement.[6,26,30] The effectiveness of endorectal MRI, as compared to TRUS, in diagnosing suspected partial and complete EDO among infertile males was investigated by Engin et al.[26] TRUS was initially done on all studied 218 infertile males with low-volume ejaculate. Then, out of the 218 patients, 62 were randomly selected for endorectal MRI examination. Among males with azoospermia, pathologic findings were detected in 75% and 61% on TRUS and endorectal MRI, respectively. Of males without azoospermia, TRUS and MRI did not detect the diagnosis in 65% and 59% of patients, respectively. Thus the authors suggested that in males with suspected EDO, endorectal MRI is to be reserved for cases where TRUS findings are equivocal.[26] Similar to TRUS, endorectal MRI might lead to overdiagnosis and unjustified treatment of EDO if used alone.[6,26] Additionally, MRI is not widely available, is time consuming and costly, and can miss calcifications.

Seminal Vesicle Aspiration

TRUS-guided fine-needle aspiration (FNA) of seminal vesicle fluid provides an important adjunct to the diagnosis of EDO. Notably, among normal fertile males, aspirate of seminal vesicles in a 24-hour abstinence period should reveal no sperm or only rare sperm (<3 sperm per high-power field [HPF]; ×400). However, greater numbers of sperm may be found if 5 days of abstinence elapse before aspiration.[31] In patients with partial or unilateral EDO—similar to normal fertile males—sperm are present in the ejaculate, and also, some sperm may be identified in the seminal vesicle aspirate. So, to minimize any confusion, if partial EDO is suspected, it is advisable to perform the FNA on the day of ejaculation. Nevertheless, if many sperm (>3 per HPF) are detected in the aspirate, partial EDO should be presumed.[31,32] On the other hand, in the case of azoospermia and suspected complete obstruction, any sperm identified in the aspirated fluid should strongly suggest EDO. In fact, most cases of EDO demonstrate large numbers of sperm in the aspirated fluid, making the diagnosis more obvious.[33] Aspiration is considerably more likely to reveal sperm—and thus is more advisable—in patients with midline prostatic or ejaculatory duct cysts, or with dilated seminal vesicles on TRUS.[28]

FNA has some advantages and limitations.[3,6,27,28] Aspiration is a simple procedure that does not require anesthesia or radiation exposure and can be performed in an office setting. Detection of sperm in the aspirate confirms intact spermatogenesis and rules out more proximal obstruction, thus obviating the need for further assessment of proximal reproductive tracts or testicular biopsy. FNA can also be performed in conjunction with seminal vesicle chromotubation or seminal vesiculography, as discussed later.

Aspiration has some limitations and carries some risks. FNA cannot localize the site of obstruction and is unable to distinguish between anatomical and functional obstructions. Potential complications of invasiveness include hemospermia, pelvic hematoma, infection, and sepsis.[27]

Seminal Vesicle Chromotubation

Seminal vesicle chromotubation is a dual TRUS-cystoscopic guided technique done during TURED, where a diluted dye (e.g., methylene blue or indigo carmine) is injected into the seminal vesicle after FNA; meanwhile, the efflux of dye from the ejaculatory duct orifice is visually observed using a cystourethroscope. This technique can help guide the depth of resection, assesses ejaculatory duct patency, and ensure the relief of obstruction during TURED.[3,6]

Seminal Vesiculography

Seminal vesiculography is similar to chromotubation but, instead of the dye, a nonionic contrast is injected into the seminal vesicle, and fluoroscopy or X-ray is used to assess for obstruction. If contrast is not visualized passing to the urethra or the bladder, then the diagnosis of EDO can be made. This technique can be performed concurrent with seminal vesicle aspiration and under TRUS guidance.[3,6]

Similar to other modalities, vesiculography has advantages and limitations. Advantageously, it can help determine the location of obstruction and can be used in conjunction with TURED. However, it carries the risks of needle invasiveness as well as contrast and radiation exposure. Importantly, vesiculography, like vasography and chromotubation, can overlook partial obstruction. The forceful manual injection of the contrast material or dye can forcibly pass through the partial obstruction, giving false-negative findings.[3,6,27,28]

Manometry

In a study published in 2008 by Eisenberg et al.,[34] manometry was suggested to refine the diagnosis of EDO; to better categorize complete, partial, or functional EDO; and to assess the success of TURED. The technique entails a modification of chromotubation via measuring the seminal vesicle pressure at which the dye starts to egress from the ejaculatory ducts to the prostatic urethra. The authors have termed that pressure as the "open pressure." In a control group of males without evidence of EDO, the authors reported an open pressure of 33 cm H_2O. In a group of nine males with suspected EDO who underwent TURED, the mean open pressure significantly decreased from 116 cm H_2O (range 80–150 cm H_2O) to 54 cm H_2O (range 10–82 cm H_2O), before and after TURED, respectively. The measured post-TURED pressures were comparable to those of the control group, with nonsignificant differences. No other studies trying to replicate the work of Eisenberg et al. have been published to date.

DIFFERENTIAL DIAGNOSIS OF EJACULATORY DUCT OBSTRUCTION

Since EDO has no pathognomonic findings during a presentation, proper and precise evaluation is necessary for a better outcome. A careful evaluation is essential to help differentiate EDO from more proximal reproductive duct obstructions such as epidydimal obstruction and congenital bilateral absence of the vas deferens, and also from nonobstructive azoospermia. The symptoms associated with EDO, such as painful ejaculation and scrotal pain, may be confused with prostatitis, chronic pelvic pain syndrome, epididymitis, and other causes of orchialgia.[2–6] Functional EDO and medications impairing the ejaculation and reducing semen volume should be considered in the differential diagnosis.[3,6,19] More details on differentiating EDO from these conditions are discussed in the previous sections of this chapter.

Causes of Low-Volume Ejaculate

Of particular importance and deserving a special discussion is the differentiation of EDO from other causes of low-volume ejaculate.[2–6,19] Since the seminal vesicles are the major contributors to the seminal fluid volume, disorders of the seminal vesicles (e.g., hypofunction) or their draining ejaculatory ducts (i.e., obstruction) should be considered in males with low-volume ejaculate after ruling out other more common causes of low volume such as incomplete collection of semen, a short abstinence period, retrograde ejaculation, or medications (Box 20.1). EDO should particularly be suspected in males with azoospermia or severe oligospermia.[2,5,15,19] Proper work-up, as described earlier in this chapter, can help distinguish EDO from other seminal vesicle disorders such as agenesis/hypoplasia or hypofunction.

"Taha's Lows" in Seminal Vesicle Hypofunction Disorders

The senior author of this chapter (TAAH) proposed a group of "lows" in males with low-volume ejaculate due to seminal vesicle hypofunction disorders that may be caused by agenesis, hypoplasia, or hypogonadism. The group of lows includes combinations of but not necessarily all of the following:
- Low volume (semen)
- Low pH (semen)
- Low fructose (semen)
- Low sperm count or azoospermia (semen)
- Low serum testosterone (hypogonadism)
- Low libido (hypogonadism)
- Low volume or absence of seminal vesicles (imaging)

TREATMENT OF EJACULATORY DUCT OBSTRUCTION

Treatment of EDO is usually offered to infertile males to reverse the obstruction, improve the semen quality, and eventually enable them to achieve spontaneous conception with a female partner, or to lessen their need for assisted reproduction. Treatment is also occasionally indicated to alleviate the symptoms of postejaculatory pain and/or hemospermia.

The mainstay of EDO treatment is TURED, which was first described by Farley and Barnes in 1973 and still remains the gold standard treatment method.[35] Several minor technical modifications were proposed to decrease the complications of TURED and improve the outcomes, such as using a smaller monopolar cutting loop, bipolar electrocautery, holmium laser, and balloon dilatation of the ducts.[3,6]

Transurethral Resection of Ejaculatory Duct
Technique

TURED can be done under either spinal or general anesthesia, with surgical settings similar to that of TURP. Urethrocystoscopy is initially done to evaluate the urethra and bladder, to identify the verumontanum and other landmarks, and to examine for midline cysts at prostatic urethra. Using a 24-Fr resectoscope, a cutting loop, and pure cutting electric current, the ejaculatory ducts are resected in the midline just proximal to the verumontanum (Fig. 20.4). Typically, one or two cuts may suffice to relieve the obstruction. A usual sign of successful treatment of obstruction is the appearance of efflux of milky, cottonlike, or cloudy fluid from the site of the resected ejaculatory ducts. A finger in the rectum applying mild pressure on seminal vesicles can help expression of the efflux. Additionally, intraoperative chromotubation or seminovesiculography can also be used to assess the patency of the ducts and adequacy of resection depth, as described in previous sections of this chapter. Resection lateral to the verumontanum is not necessary, as the ejaculatory ducts are midline structures at

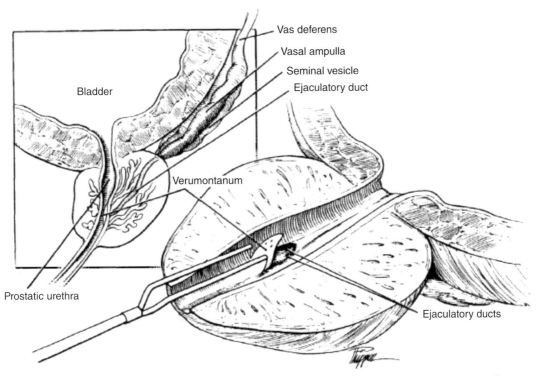

Fig. 20.4 Transurethral resection of ejaculatory ducts using cutting loop at the verumontanum. (From Meacham RB, Hellerstein DK, Lipshultz LI. Evaluation and treatment of ejaculatory duct obstruction in the infertile male. *Fertil Steril.* 1993;59(2):393-397.)

this level. Lateral resection of the ejaculatory ducts may be considered for unilateral EDO. At the end of the procedure, an indwelling Foley urethral catheter is placed for up to 24 hours.[3,6,35]

It is prudent to use only pure cutting current and to avoid excessive coagulation to minimize scarring at the resection site, with later development of secondary EDO. If bleeding is encountered, pinpoint coagulation of the bleeder is recommended, without overzealous coagulation. Considering that most patients undergoing TURED are infertile young adults with normal prostatic size, care should be taken not to resect too deeply, so to avoid rectal injury, nor too proximally or too distally, so to avoid bladder neck injury and external striated sphincter injury, respectively.[3,6,35]

Patients are instructed to abstain from ejaculation for at least 1 to 2 weeks after TURED.[36] Semen analysis can be performed 6 weeks post TURED and repeated at regular intervals every 3 months until semen parameters stabilize.

Transurethral Resection of the Ejaculatory Duct Outcomes

TURED can considerably improve the semen parameters and spontaneous pregnancy rates and decrease the need for assisted reproductive techniques (ART). However, the treatment outcomes vary, depending on several characteristics of the obstruction, such as the etiology, partial or complete, unilateral or bilateral, the methods of diagnosis and treatment, etc. Generally, treatment of congenital obstruction yields better outcomes than acquired causes associated with scarring or calcifications. The same applies to partial EDO, which tends to respond to treatment better than the complete form.[3,37] The characteristic features predicting the treatment outcomes of TURED are summarized in Table 20.5.

Semen variables improve in 63% to 83% of patients overall after TURED,[3,6,17,38] with better improvements being reported in partial versus complete obstructions (94% vs. 59% of patients, respectively).[37] Semen volume[39] increased significantly in 90.5% of treated

TABLE 20.5 Prediction of Treatment Outcomes According to the Characteristics of Ejaculatory Duct Obstruction

Characteristic	Better Outcome	Less Outcome
Etiology	Congenital	Acquired
Degree of obstruction	partial	complete
Laterality	Unilateral	Bilateral
Cystic obstruction	Yes	No
Seminal vesicle dilatation	Yes	No
Sperm in SVA	Yes	No
Scarring or calcification	No	Yes
Concomitant proximal obstruction	No	Yes

SVA, Seminal vesicle aspiration.

patients, while increased sperm count[17] and motility[40] have been shown in 50% of patients post TURED. Notably, about 60% of males with azoospermia can benefit from TURED, with recovery of sperm in their ejaculate. As many as 38% of males with azoospermia or oligospermia have acquired normal semen quality after TURED.[39] The spontaneous pregnancy rates—the ultimate goal—vary between 12.5% and 31% according to the etiology of treated EDO.[3,17,36–40]

Better TURED outcomes were noted in patients with midline or eccentric cystic obstruction, while obstruction caused by calcifications showed the lowest successful response rate to TURED. A study by Kadioglu et al. was conducted to examine differences in TURED outcomes among 38 EDO patients with different pathologies.[37] All patients involved in the study were potential candidates for in vitro fertilization–intracytoplasmic sperm injection (IVF-ICSI). However, post TURED, 32% of males with azoospermia and 81% of males with oligospermia achieved spontaneous pregnancy or were referred for intrauterine insemination instead of IVF-ICSI. Similar findings were reported by El-Assmy et al., who examined the outcomes of TURED in 23 infertile males with EDO.[36] Semen parameters were improved in all patients with partial obstruction as compared to only 23.5% with complete obstruction. Of patients with midline cysts as a cause of EDO, 71.5% showed an increase in sperm count

compared to 31% with noncystic causes. Spontaneous pregnancy rates post TURED were higher in cases of partial EDO compared to complete obstruction, with percentages of 33.3% and 5.9%, respectively. They concluded that partial EDO would result in the best outcomes of TURED, regardless of the etiology.[36]

Complications of Transurethral Resection of the Ejaculatory Duct

TURED is a relatively simple procedure, with complication rates varying between 4% and 26%, with most studies reporting lower rates.[3,17] Early postoperative complications include gross hematuria, acute urinary retention, urinary tract infection, and acute epididymoorchitis.

Urinary incontinence may result from injury to the external urinary sphincter, while retrograde ejaculation can follow injury to the bladder neck. Rectal injury due to undue deep resection has been reported.

Excessive use of coagulation can lead to scarring and development of secondary recurrent ductal obstruction, even if initial ductal patency was documented post TURED (Table 20.6). Some patients with partial EDO who underwent TURED may develop dire and frustrating secondary complete EDO due to fibrosis. If such complication is evident, repeat TURED can be performed, with satisfactory results.[16] Approximately 4% of patients with partial EDO treated with TURED develop azoospermia due to fibrosis.[38] Thus patients should be counseled about sperm cryopreservation and should be monitored on a regular basis postoperatively until their fertility goal is achieved.[3]

Significant and bothersome terminal dribbling can develop post TURED due to urinary reflux into the ejaculatory ducts and seminal vesicles. Males with watery high-volume ejaculates are suspected to have such urinary reflux, which can be confirmed by the presence of high creatinine levels in the semen. Having urine in the ejaculate has a profound negative impact on sexual relationships between partners. For such a complaint, instructing patients to stand for an extended period of time after urination is possibly helpful, as described by Goluboff et al.[41]

Other Procedures

Although TURED is the standard treatment of EDO, other procedures have been proposed, including retrograde seminal vesiculoscopy, TRUS- or MRI-guided antegrade balloon dilation of ejaculatory ducts, laser incision, and TRUS-guided aspiration of MPCs causing EDO.[3,6]

TABLE 20.6 Transurethral Resection of the Ejaculatory Duct Complications, Causes, and Avoidance

Complication	Cause	Prevention
Urinary incontinence	Injury to external urinary sphincter	Avoid resection distal to verumontanum
Retrograde ejaculation	Injury to bladder neck	Avoid resection at bladder neck level
Rectal perforation	Undue deep resection	Perform careful, meticulous resection
		Avoid unnecessary deep resection
		Use adjunctive techniques to assess for relief of obstruction and adequacy of resection depth (e.g., chromotubation or seminovesiculography)
Recurrent/secondary ejaculatory duct obstruction	Undue coagulation at resection site, with scar formation	Use cutting electric current only
		Avoid excessive undue coagulation

Seminal Vesiculoscopy

Seminal vesiculoscopy is performed via a retrograde transurethral transutricular route, by inserting a 6-Fr or 9-Fr vesiculoscope into the natural orifice and lumen of the ejaculatory duct using saline irrigation. Occasionally, puncture of the presumptive duct orifice and using holmium laser incision at the wall of the prostatic utricle is required. However, due to the ejaculatory duct's anatomical complexity, in cases where the duct orifice is not identified, TURED should be the treatment of choice. The rationale of seminal vesiculoscopy is to passively dilate the ejaculatory ducts and to visually identify and treat the causes of obstruction such as calculi, blood clots, or debris.[42,43] Success of this method to treat EDO is questionable, and no compelling evidence exists to support its effectiveness in terms of improvement of semen parameters or pregnancy rates.

Balloon Dilation

Balloon dilation of the ejaculatory duct is another novel method to treat EDO. TRUS-guided antegrade access to the duct is done via the seminal vesicle; then the duct is cannulated with a guidewire and angiographic catheter that reach the urethra. The guidewire is then retrieved from the urethra with the use of a urethroscope. A balloon dilator is inserted retrograde over the retrieved guidewire and inflated to dilate the ejaculatory duct. The success of surgery is confirmed by visualizing fluid efflux from the duct.[44] However, replication of this procedure was attempted by Kayser et al., but they failed to reproduce it.[45]

Aspiration of Midline Prostatic Cysts

In a study by Lotti et al.[46] including 648 infertile patients and 103 control fertile males, MPCs were reported with a prevalence of 10.2% and 5.8% among infertile and fertile males, respectively. Larger cysts, with volumes greater than 0.117 mL, were identified in infertile patients with severe oligospermia or azoospermia. Aiming to provide a simple and less invasive treatment, the authors have proposed a technique of TRUS-guided cyst aspiration (TRUCA), performed in a limited number of eleven infertile males with impaired semen quality and large MPC volume greater than 0.25 mL.

At 1 month after TRUCA, semen volume, sperm count, and MPC volume improved significantly in all patients. However, at 3 months' follow-up, significantly lower sperm counts and higher MPC volumes were observed, compared to the 1-month follow up, although still significantly better than the baseline. At 1 year after TRUCA, the authors reported natural pregnancy in four couples, albeit they did not report on the semen quality. Notably, the rapid increase in MPC volume and quick decline in sperm parameters during the short follow-up period raise the concern of cyst recurrence and nondurable efficacy of TRUCA, and thus necessitates considering sperm cryopreservation.[46]

Treatment of Functional Ejaculatory Duct Obstruction

Functional EDO does not respond to endoscopic treatment modalities, as the problem does not lie in mechanical obstruction, and surgical treatment should not be offered to this subset of patients with neurological functional obstruction.[3] In fact, there is a lack of evidence supporting any intervention to treat functional obstruction. Thus a sperm retrieval technique and IVF-ICSI may be a valid option for these patients.[3] However, some investigators have reported the use of oral phosphodiesterase inhibitors in diabetic patients with functional obstruction and suggest it may improve seminal vesicles, ejection fraction.[19] Importantly, before offering surgical treatment, the use of medications causing functional EDO should be checked and discontinued or substituted accordingly. Medications that may cause functional EDO include thiazide diuretics, adrenergic blockers (e.g., phentolamine and prazosin), antipsychotics (haloperidol, thioridazine), antidepressants (amitriptyline and imipramine), antiandrogens, and alpha blockers.[19]

Sperm Retrieval and Assisted Reproduction Techniques

As previously discussed, because the improvements of semen parameters and spontaneous pregnancy rates are not universal after treatment of EDO, sperm retrieval, sperm cryopreservation, and ART often required in some couples. Additionally, some patients may sustain recurrent obstruction after initial documented patent ejaculatory ducts. Further, functional neurological EDO may not respond to treatment and requires ART. Moreover, occasional couples may prefer ART rather than treatment of EDO. Such cases can be offered diverse options for sperm retrieval such as epididymal sperm aspiration, microsurgical epididymal sperm aspiration, testicular sperm aspiration, or testicular sperm extraction (TESE) with or without microscopic assistance (micro-TESE), along with IVF-ICSI.[2-6]

Infrequently, EDO can occur in combination with more proximal obstruction, such as epididymal obstruction. In such patients, vasoepididymostomy and TURED may be performed concomitantly. However, the success rates of concomitant TURED and vasal reconstructive surgeries are low, and such patients may be offered sperm retrieval and ICSI.[16,47] Patients who undergo EDO treatment or reconstructive surgeries for infertility such as vasoepididymostomy should have concomitant intraoperative sperm retrieval and cryopreservation. This recommendation stems from the unpredictable spontaneous pregnancy rates post treatment and the possibility of EDO recurrence due to scaring of the ejaculatory ducts or restenosis of the vasoepididymostomy anastomosis site and obviates the need for future procedure for sperm retrieval.[16,47] The use of cryopreserved sperm for IVF-ICSI has conception rates similar to that of fresh sperm.[47] Nevertheless, a redo sperm retrieval procedure is a valid option for patients

with obstructive azoospermia, with quite high successful sperm retrieval rates exceeding 96% of cases.[3]

More details on sperm retrieval procedures and ART are discussed in other parts in this book.

CLINICAL CASE SCENARIO

CASE

A 35-year-old male with secondary infertility is married to a 29-year-old healthy female whom her gynecologist has cleared. The patient had a history of trauma 5 years ago that required prolonged indwelling urethral catheterization. Since then, they have been seeking conception with no success. He mentioned that he noticed a decrease in his seminal volume. His semen analysis revealed decreased ejaculate volume, semen pH of 7.0, and no sperm in the ejaculate. Serum testosterone and follicle-stimulating hormone (FSH) were within normal ranges, and postejaculate urinalysis showed no sperm. The patient underwent transrectal ultrasound (TRUS) examination, which showed dilated seminal vesicles with a transverse diameter of 17 mm.

How should the data be interpreted?
The patient presented with secondary infertility and decreased ejaculate volume. He has a history of previous trauma requiring prolonged indwelling urethral catheterization. As an initial next step in his evaluation, semen analysis was carried out, which revealed decreased ejaculate volume, low semen pH of 7.0, and no sperm in the ejaculate. Furthermore, testosterone and FSH were within normal ranges. To rule out retrograde ejaculation, postejaculate urine analysis was requested which, in his scenario, showed no sperm. These findings suggest that the patient is likely experiencing ejaculatory duct obstruction (EDO). Since the imaging study of choice in the evaluation of patients with suspected EDO is TRUS, this imaging study was then performed and showed dilated seminal vesicles (17 mm in transverse diameter), which indicates the diagnosis of EDO.

Solution: Males who are infertile due to EDO who seek treatment typically do so in an effort to resolve the obstruction, improve the quality of their semen, and ultimately improve the chances of achieving spontaneous conception or to minimize their need for assisted reproductive techniques (ART). The standard of care in the majority of EDO patients, with generally positive outcomes, is transurethral resection of the ejaculatory duct (TURED). In some heterosexual couples, however, sperm retrieval and ART are valid alternatives.

SUMMARY

EDO is an uncommon cause of male infertility, with variable clinical presentations. The patients usually present with low ejaculate volume associated with oligospermia or azoospermia. Postejaculatory pain and/or hemospermia may manifest in some patients. Currently, TRUS is the mainstay in EDO diagnosis, although a variety of equivocal cases may require further work-up, including MRI, seminal vesicle aspiration, and other investigations to help improve diagnosis. TURED is the standard treatment, with good outcomes in most cases. Yet, the outcomes are variable, depending on many etiological, anatomical, and functional features, which underline the importance of proper evaluation and diagnosis. Sperm retrieval and/or ART are valid options in some couples.

REFERENCES

1. Gutierrez R. Surgery of seminal vesicles, ampullae, vas deferentia and spermatic cord. In: Lowsly OS, Hinman F, Smith R, eds. *The Sexual Glands of the Male*. New York: Oxford University Press; 1942.
2. Smith JF, Walsh TJ, Turek PJ. Ejaculatory duct obstruction. *Urol Clin North Am*. 2008;35(2):221-227. doi:10.1016/j.ucl.2008.01.011.
3. Avellino GJ, Lipshultz LI, Sigman M, Hwang K. Transurethral resection of the ejaculatory ducts: etiology of obstruction and surgical treatment options. *Fertil Steril*. 2019;111(3):427-443. doi:10.1016/j.fertnstert.2019.01.001.
4. Modgil V, Rai S, Ralph DJ, Muneer A. An update on the diagnosis and management of ejaculatory duct obstruction. *Nat Rev Urol*. 2016;13(1):13-20. doi:10.1038/nrurol.2015.276.
5. Wosnitzer MS, Goldstein M. Obstructive azoospermia. *Urol Clin North Am*. 2014;41(1):83-95. doi:10.1016/j.ucl.2013.08.013.
6. Achermann APP, Esteves SC. Diagnosis and management of infertility due to ejaculatory duct obstruction: summary evidence. *Int Braz J Urol*. 2021;47(4):868-881. doi:10.1590/S1677-5538.IBJU.2020.0536.
7. Nguyen HT, Etzell J, Turek PJ. Normal human ejaculatory duct anatomy: a study of cadaveric and surgical specimens. *J Urol*. 1996;155(5):1639-1642. doi:10.1016/s0022-5347(01)66150-0.
8. McMahon S. An anatomical study by injection technique of the ejaculatory ducts and their relations. *J Anat*. 1938;72(Pt 4):556-574.
9. McCarthy JF, Bitter JS, Klemperer, P. Anatomical and histological study of the verumontanum with especial reference to the ejaculatory ducts. *J Urol*. 1927;17(1):1-16. doi:10.1016/s0022-5347(17)73322-8.
10. Shebel HM, Farg HM, Kolokythas O, El-Diasty T. Cysts of the lower male genitourinary tract: embryologic and anatomic considerations and differential diagnosis. *Radiographics*. 2013;33(4):1125-1143. doi:10.1148/rg.334125129.
11. Vohra S, Morgentaler A. Congenital anomalies of the vas deferens, epididymis, and seminal vesicles. *Urology*. 1997;49(3):313-321. doi:10.1016/S0090-4295(96)00433-5.
12. Stifelman MD, Tanaka K, Jones JG, Amin H, Fisch H. Transurethral resection of ejaculatory ducts: anatomy and pathology. *Fertil Steril*. 1993;60:S55-S56 (Abstract O-117).
13. Li ZY, Xu Y, Liu C, et al. Anatomical study of the seminal vesicle system for transurethral seminal vesiculoscopy. *Clin Anat*. 2019;32(2):244-252. doi:10.1002/ca.23293.
14. Tauber PF, Zaneveld LJ, Propping D, Schumacher GF. Components of human split ejaculates. I. Spermatozoa, fructose, immunoglobulins, albumin, lactoferrin, transferrin and other plasma proteins. *J Reprod Fertil*. 1975;43(2):249-267. doi:10.1530/jrf.0.0430249.
15. Master VA, Turek PJ. Ejaculatory physiology and dysfunction. *Urol Clin North Am*. 2001;28(2):363-375, x. doi:10.1016/s0094-0143(05)70145-2.
16. Pryor JP, Hendry WF. Ejaculatory duct obstruction in subfertile males: analysis of 87 patients. *Fertil Steril*. 1991;56(4):725-730. doi:10.1016/s0015-0282(16)54606-8.
17. Schroeder-Printzen I, Ludwig M, Köhn F, Weidner W. Surgical therapy in infertile men with ejaculatory duct obstruction: technique and outcome of a standardized surgical approach. *Hum Reprod*. 2000;15(6):1364-1368. doi:10.1093/humrep/15.6.1364.
18. Ozgök Y, Tan MO, Killer M, Tahmaz L, Kibar Y. Diagnosis and treatment of ejaculatory duct obstruction in male infertility. *Eur Urol*. 2001;39(1):24-29. doi:10.1159/000052408.
19. Font MD, Pastuszak AW, Case JR, Lipshultz LI. An infertile male with dilated seminal vesicles due to functional obstruction. *Asian J Androl*. 2017;19(2):256-257. doi:10.4103/1008-682X.179858.
20. Sandlow JI. Seminal vesicle and ejaculatory duct surgery. In: Goldstein M, ed. *Glenn's Urologic Surgery*. 7th ed. Philadelphia: Lippincott Williams & Wilkins; 2008:369.
21. Zinner A. Ein fall von intravesikaler Samenblasenzyste. *Wien Med Wochenschr*. 1914;64:605.
22. Du J, Li FH, Guo YF, et al. Differential diagnosis of azoospermia and etiologic classification of obstructive

azoospermia: role of scrotal and transrectal US. *Radiology*. 2010;256(2):493-503. doi:10.1148/radiol.10091578.

23. McQuaid JW, Tanrikut C. Ejaculatory duct obstruction: current diagnosis and treatment. *Curr Urol Rep*. 2013;14(4):291-297. doi:10.1007/s11934-013-0340-y.

24. World Health Organization. *WHO Laboratory Manual for the Examination and Processing of Human Semen*. 5th ed. Geneva: WHO Press; 2010.

25. Niederberger CS. Clinical evaluation of the male. In: Niederberger CS, ed. *An Introduction to Male Reproductive Medicine*. New York: Cambridge University Press; 2011:29-57.

26. Engin G, Kadioğlu A, Orhan I, Akdöl S, Rozanes I. Transrectal US and endorectal MR imaging in partial and complete obstruction of the seminal duct system. A comparative study. *Acta Radiol*. 2000;41(3):288-295. doi:10.1080/028418500127345271.

27. Engin G. Transrectal US-guided seminal vesicle aspiration in the diagnosis of partial ejaculatory duct obstruction. *Diagn Interv Radiol*. 2012;18(5):488-495. doi:10.4261/1305-3825.DIR.5528-11.1.

28. Engin G, Celtik M, Sanli O, Aytac O, Muradov Z, Kadioglu A. Comparison of transrectal ultrasonography and transrectal ultrasonography-guided seminal vesicle aspiration in the diagnosis of the ejaculatory duct obstruction. *Fertil Steril*. 2009;92(3):964-970. doi:10.1016/j.fertnstert.2008.07.1749.

29. Purohit RS, Wu DS, Shinohara K, Turek PJ. A prospective comparison of 3 diagnostic methods to evaluate ejaculatory duct obstruction. *J Urol*. 2004;171(1):232-236. doi:10.1097/01.ju.0000101909.70651.d1.

30. Cho IR, Lee MS, Rha KH, Hong SJ, Park SS, Kim MJ. Magnetic resonance imaging in hemospermia. *J Urol*. 1997;157(1):258-262.

31. Jarow JP. Seminal vesicle aspiration of fertile men. *J Urol*. 1996;156(3):1005-1007.

32. Jarow JP. Seminal vesicle aspiration in the management of patients with ejaculatory duct obstruction. *J Urol*. 1994;152(3):899-901. doi:10.1016/s0022-5347(17)32603-4.

33. Orhan I, Onur R, Cayan S, Koksal IT, Kadio«ßlu A. Seminal vesicle sperm aspiration in the diagnosis of ejaculatory duct obstruction. *BJU Int*. 1999;84(9):1050-1053. doi:10.1046/j.1464-410x.1999.00379.x.

34. Eisenberg ML, Walsh TJ, Garcia MM, Shinohara K, Turek PJ. Ejaculatory duct manometry in normal men and in patients with ejaculatory duct obstruction. *J Urol*. 2008;180(1):255-260. doi:10.1016/j.juro.2008.03.019.

35. Farley S, Barnes R. Stenosis of ejaculatory ducts treated by endoscopic resection. *J Urol*. 1973;109(4):664-666. doi:10.1016/s0022-5347(17)60510-x.

36. El-Assmy A, El-Tholoth H, Abouelkheir RT, Abou-El-Ghar ME. Transurethral resection of ejaculatory duct in infertile men: outcome and predictors of success. *Int Urol Nephrol*. 2012;44(6):1623-1630. doi:10.1007/s11255-012-0253-6.

37. Kadioglu A, Cayan S, Tefekli A, Orhan I, Engin G, Turek PJ. Does response to treatment of ejaculatory duct obstruction in infertile men vary with pathology? *Fertil Steril*. 2001;76(1):138-142. doi:10.1016/s0015-0282(01)01817-9.

38. Turek PJ, Magana JO, Lipshultz LI. Semen parameters before and after transurethral surgery for ejaculatory duct obstruction. *J Urol*. 1996;155(4):1291-1293.

39. Tu XA, Zhuang JT, Zhao L, et al. Transurethral bipolar plasma kinetic resection of ejaculatory duct for treatment of ejaculatory duct obstruction. *J Xray Sci Technol*. 2013;21(2):293-302. doi:10.3233/XST-130377.

40. Meacham RB, Hellerstein DK, Lipshultz LI. Evaluation and treatment of ejaculatory duct obstruction in the infertile male. *Fertil Steril*. 1993;59(2):393-397. doi:10.1016/s0015-0282(16)55683-0.

41. Goluboff ET, Kaplan SA, Fisch H. Seminal vesicle urinary reflux as a complication of transurethral resection of ejaculatory ducts. *J Urol*. 1995;153(4):1234-1235.

42. Yang SC, Rha KH, Byon SK, Kim JH. Transutricular seminal vesiculoscopy. *J Endourol*. 2002;16(6):343-345. doi:10.1089/089277902760261347.

43. Xu B, Niu X, Wang Z, et al. Novel methods for the diagnosis and treatment of ejaculatory duct obstruction. *BJU Int*. 2011;108(2):263-266. doi:10.1111/j.1464-410X.2010.09775.x.

44. Jarow JP, Zagoria RJ. Antegrade ejaculatory duct recanalization and dilation. *Urology*. 1995;46(5):743-746. doi:10.1016/S0090-4295(99)80316-1.

45. Kayser O, Osmonov D, Harde J, Girolami G, Wedel T, Schäfer P. Less invasive causal treatment of ejaculatory duct obstruction by balloon dilation: a case report, literature review and suggestion of a CT- or MRI-guided intervention. *Ger Med Sci*. 2012;10:Doc06. doi:10.3205/000157.

46. Lotti F, Corona G, Cocci A, et al. The prevalence of midline prostatic cysts and the relationship between cyst size and semen parameters among infertile and fertile men. *Hum Reprod*. 2018;33(11):2023-2034. doi:10.1093/humrep/dey298.

47. Anger JT, Gilbert BR, Goldstein M. Cryopreservation of sperm: indications, methods and results. *J Urol*. 2003;170(4 Pt 1):1079-1084. doi:10.1097/01.ju.0000084820.98430.b8.

21

Surgical Sperm Retrieval and Processing for Assisted Reproductive Technology

Edson Borges Jr., Amanda Souza Setti, and Daniela Paes de Almeida Ferreira Braga

KEY POINTS

- This chapter covers topics such as surgical sperm retrieval methods, discussing different surgical methods such as percutaneous epididymal sperm aspiration, microsurgical epididymal sperm aspiration, testicular sperm aspiration, testicular sperm extraction, and microdissection testicular sperm extraction for the retrieval of spermatozoa from either the epididymis or the testis according to the type of azoospermia (obstructive or nonobstructive).

- Timing of sperm retrieval and the most appropriate types of sperm preparation techniques in cases of epidydimal- or testicular-retrieved spermatozoa, and low or high numbers of retrieved spermatozoa, are discussed.
- Methods for handling of immotile testicular spermatozoa and the use of artificial oocyte activation are also reviewed.

INTRODUCTION

Azoospermia, defined as the absence of sperm in ejaculated semen, is the most severe form of male factor infertility and is observed in 1% of the general population and in 10% to 15% of infertile males. In 1992, intracytoplasmic sperm injection (ICSI) was introduced in the field of assisted reproduction, allowing the treatment of this type of male factor infertility. Sperm can be retrieved for ICSI from either the epididymis or the testis, depending on the type of azoospermia: obstructive azoospermia (OA) or nonobstructive azoospermia (NOA).[1]

Successful rates of sperm retrieval are possible both in OA and NOA patients, using techniques that capture spermatozoa directly from the epididymis or testes: percutaneous epididymal sperm aspiration (PESA), microsurgical epididymal sperm aspiration (MESA), testicular sperm aspiration (TESA), testicular sperm extraction (TESE), and microdissection testicular sperm extraction (micro-TESE).[2] Despite epididymal sperm rendering higher fertilization rates, similar clinical pregnancy and implantation rates are obtained with testicular or epididymal spermatozoa, regardless of the type of azoospermia.[3]

Successful retrieval of sperm is only the initial step towards the achievement of pregnancy with ICSI. The mere use of ejaculated sperm for ICSI already made us question about the circumvention of natural sperm selection. Therefore, methods to aid in the selection of not only the "best-looking" but also the most functional sperm, as well as methods to compensate for lack of oocyte activation, are in order.

This chapter summarizes surgical sperm retrieval methods, processing, and selection of surgically retrieved sperm, and the use of oocyte activation in heterosexual couples in which the male partner has azoospermia.

NARRATIVE REVIEW

Surgical Sperm Retrieval Methods

The type of azoospermia will guide the choice of sperm retrieval method. In males with OA, sperm may be harvested from the epididymis and/or testis, while in males with NOA, only testicular sperm retrieval procedures are effective. The use of preoperative diagnostic tools (such as clinical history, physical examination, and assessment of serum follicle-stimulating hormone and testosterone levels) is recommended, providing almost 90% prediction of the azoospermia type.[4] Table 21.1 summarizes the most used techniques to harvest sperm and their indications.

Percutaneous Epididymal Sperm Aspiration[5]

After cleaning the scrotum with antiseptic and washing with saline, the head of the epididymis is palpated and punctured through the scrotal skin with a 26-G needle attached to a syringe containing 0.1 mL of sperm-washing medium, or with a large butterfly needle and a 20-mL syringe. In OA, better-quality sperm are obtained from the head of the epididymis rather than from the distal body or tail. A suction force is created by pulling the plunger all the way to the top of the syringe. The needle is slowly inserted through the epididymal

ductule, rotated 180 degrees, and partially withdrawn. It is then reinserted in a different direction. Only then the suction is partially released and the needle withdrawn from the epididymis (Fig. 21.1). The content of the syringe is poured into a dish and analyzed for the presence of sperm. The procedure is repeated at a slightly different location on the epididymis if motile sperm are not identified.

This is a less invasive technique for sperm retrieval that can be performed on an outpatient basis under local anesthesia. The advantages of PESA in relation to MESA for patients with OA are minimal discomfort and a lower complication rate. In addition, PESA does not need microsurgical instruments, thus being a low-cost, simple technique. Cryopreservation of surplus sperm is feasible for most patients, avoiding the necessity of additional retrieval procedures.

Microsurgical Epididymal Sperm Aspiration[6]

An incision is performed in the scrotum for the exposure of the epididymis. Using an operating microscope, the epididymal tunica is incised, and an epididymal ductule is dissected so the spermatic fluid is aspirated and examined for the presence of sperm. The ductule is sutured. If no sperm are found, another ductule is mobilized and opened. The MESA technique allows for accurate, blood-free aspiration of multiple ductules and consequently, many motile sperm can be harvested and frozen for future ICSI cycles. However, it is a time-consuming, expensive procedure that demands an operating microscope and a highly skilled microsurgeon.

TABLE 21.1 Sperm Retrieval Techniques and Their Indications	
Technique	Indication
Percutaneous epididymal sperm aspiration (PESA)	Obstructive azoospermia exclusively
Microsurgical epididymal sperm aspiration	Obstructive azoospermia exclusively
Testicular sperm aspiration (TESA)	• Nonobstructive azoospermia with favorable testicular histopathology • Epididymal agenesis • Failed PESA in obstructive azoospermia
Testicular sperm extraction	• Failed PESA or TESA in obstructive azoospermia • Nonobstructive azoospermia
Microsurgical testicular sperm extraction	Nonobstructive azoospermia exclusively

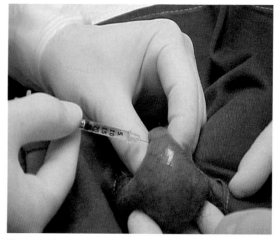

Fig. 21.1 Percutaneous Epididymal Sperm Aspiration.

Testicular Sperm Aspiration[7]

This procedure can be performed under local or general anesthesia. While applying suction with a 20-mL syringe, the testicular body is punctured with a 22-G butterfly needle (Fig. 21.2). The aspirated fluid is examined for the presence of sperm. Color Doppler ultrasonography guidance can be used to avoid blood vessels and reduce hematoma formation.[8]

Testicular Sperm Extraction[9]

A local anesthetic is injected in to the spermatic cord. A small incision is made through the skin over the scrotum, exposing the testis. The tunica is incised, and small pieces of testicular tissue are removed from the incision. The tunica is sutured, and the incision is closed with self-dissolving suture. A portion of the recovered tissue is examined under microscope by an andrology specialist, and the remnant of the tissue can be either incubated until the moment of ICSI or frozen. This is a sperm retrieval method that can be easily performed by any surgeon, yielding a fair quantity of tissue. Nevertheless, it is an open surgery, and damage to testicular vessels can occur. In addition, in males with testicular failure, repeated biopsies can impair testicular function.[10]

Microdissection Testicular Sperm Extraction[11]

An incision is made on the front of the scrotum, exposing the testis. A long incision is made in outer tunical layer of the testicle, and the testicle is bivalved to expose the parenchyma. The seminiferous tubules are separated and examined under an operating microscope, which

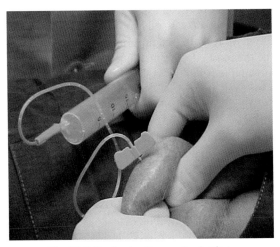

Fig. 21.2 Testicular Sperm Aspiration.

aids the identification of healthy-appearing tubules that are more likely to contain sperm[12] (Fig. 21.3A–C). Dissection and biopsy continue until sufficient sperm are harvested. The tunica is closed with a running suture. This technique results in less testicular damage since the seminiferous tubule biopsy is selective. The chances of finding sperm are much improved in cases of focal spermatogenesis since a large area of testicular tissue can be identified and excised.

Timing of Sperm Retrieval

Sperm retrieval can be performed before oocyte retrieval or the day of female partner's oocyte retrieval. Both method schedules come with limitations and benefits and generally, the decision relies on the in vitro fertilization (IVF) center's practice.

As most IVF centers prefer handling fresh surgically retrieved sperm rather than frozen samples, sperm retrieval is most frequently performed in conjunction with egg retrieval. This practice is even more usual in the presence of OA, in which sperm retrieval is believed to be a simple procedure. Nevertheless, the disadvantage of this schedule relates to the availability of staff (surgeons and embryologists) and infrastructure (operating and recovery rooms, especially in the busy morning hours) and the fact that sometimes, egg retrieval is not performed on the date originally scheduled. In addition, some couples may be unwilling to have surgery on the same day because of lack of home assistance and transportation, among other personal reasons. These limitations can be obviated by harvesting sperm prior to oocyte retrieval.

When the chances of successful sperm retrieval are low, the best option is to harvest and freeze sperm in advance. Should the sperm retrieval fail, the couple must choose between freezing all retrieved oocytes until another sperm retrieval attempt is performed or using donor sperm. The use of freeze-thawed or fresh, testicular or epididymal spermatozoa yields similar ICSI outcomes, especially when several spermatozoa are retrieved.[13] By virtue of the procedure's complexity, micro-TESE is usually performed the day before oocyte retrieval.[14]

When appropriately incubated in culture media, sperm retrieved from epididymis and testes can survive for up to 3 days. In fact, it may take a while for sperm extracted from the tubules of the testicular tissue to acquire motility. In the worst-case scenario, motility

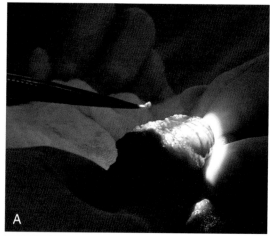

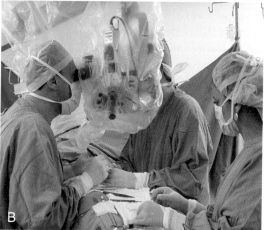

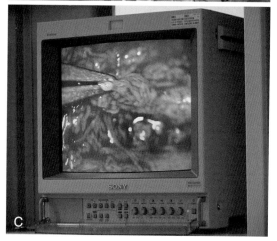

Fig. 21.3 Microsurgical Testicular Sperm Extraction. Seminiferous tubules are separated (A) and examined under an operating microscope (B and C).

enhancers can be used for the selection of viable sperm for injection.

Processing Surgically Retrieved Sperm for Intracytoplasmic Sperm Injection

Epididymal sperm samples such as PESA and MESA are usually combined with buffered culture medium prior to assessment of count, motility, and morphology. Samples presenting with high sperm count can be prepared using density gradient centrifugation followed by double washing, while those aspirates presenting with low sperm count are generally prepared using double washing and centrifugation (reviewed by Verheyen et al.[15]). An aliquot of the prepared sample covered with mineral oil is laid on a petri dish until sperm selection for ICSI. Surplus sperm can be frozen for usage in subsequent ICSI cycles.

Testicular aspirated sperm are dispensed in droplets of culture medium covered with mineral oil or in a dry tube until the moment of ICSI. Different processing methods have been described for sperm retrieved by TESE, such as mechanical processing, as well as the use of enzymes or erythrocyte-lysing buffer to improve sperm recovery.

The most used processing method for testicular tissue is rupture of seminiferous tubules by shredding and fine mincing. In a petri dish containing buffered culture medium, the testicular tissue is shredded with needles, microscope slides, or scissors, thereby releasing sperm into the medium. Upon the identification of sperm under an inverted or a phase-contrast microscope, the sample is allowed to rest, and then the supernatant is centrifuged, removed, and resuspended. The sample is poured on a petri dish overlaid with oil from which the sperm will be selected for ICSI. In fact, fine mincing was demonstrated to be the most effective method regarding motile sperm count and morphology among the other three mechanical methods to retrieve testicular spermatozoa—rough shredding, vortexing, and crushing in a grinder with a pestle.[16]

A frequent feature in the testicular tissue sample that may hinder visualization of sperm cells is red blood cell contamination. Exposition of tissue samples, after shredding, to an erythrocyte-lysing buffer may be useful in those cases, improving sperm recovery and selection in a reduced interval of time.[17]

In males presenting with reduced sperm production, sperm recovery can be improved by using enzymatic

TESE instead of mechanical sperm extraction. Enzymatic digestion is routinely used after failure of sperm identification with mechanical shredding. In fact, it has been demonstrated that, after sperm recover failure post mechanical shredding, the use of enzymes was successful in the recovery of sperm in nearly 26% of males undergoing ICSI.[17] Collagenases type IA and IV are the most conventional enzymes used to digest the collagen from membranes and the extracellular matrix of testicular tissue. Nevertheless, the mechanical approaches are more prevalent and routinely employed.

The management of infertility in males with NOA is still hampered by several factors, at both the clinical and the laboratory level. Clinically, the development of diagnostic tests for the prediction of testicular sperm retrieval success is needed. On the other hand, some methods have already been developed at the laboratory level to enhance sperm selection in NOA patients.

Selection of Surgically Retrieved Sperm for Intracytoplasmic Sperm Injection

Successful retrieval of sperm is only the initial step towards the achievement of pregnancy with ICSI. The mere use of ejaculated sperm for ICSI already made us question about the circumvention of natural sperm selection. This matter is much more pressing when ICSI is performed with testicular sperm. That said, the use of methods to assist in the selection of sperm that are not only morphologically normal but also functional is necessary.

As previously cited, several centers choose to collect spermatozoa the day before oocyte collection since the prolonged culture of surgically recovered spermatozoa until ICSI can allow their maturation and the achievement of motility, regardless of type of azoospermia. Despite improvements in harvested sperm peak within 48 hours of extended culture, incubation of sperm for more than 2 days is associated with increased DNA damage and chromosomal abnormalities, which suggests sperm aging.[18]

In some cases, however, surgically retrieved spermatozoa fail to acquire motility even after extended culture, so the use of add-on sperm selection techniques is recommended (reviewed by Verheyen et al.[15]).

Mechanical Touch Technique

Previously described as the sperm tail flexibility test, the mechanical touch technique has been used for identification of viable immotile sperm before ICSI. Its principle is the fact that tail flexibility of immotile vital and nonvital sperm differs when handled with the microinjection pipette. Vital sperm are flexible; thus the sperm head will not move along with the tail, and the tail returns to its initial position. Nonvital sperm are rigid and when the tail is touched with the pipette, the sperm head will also move and the tail will not recover its initial position.

Similar clinical outcomes (pregnancy and delivery rates) have been demonstrated when ICSI cycles using immotile testicular sperm selected with mechanical touch technique were compared to those using motile testicular sperm.[19] The mechanical touch technique is a real-time technique that is free of dyes and chemicals, allowing the examined sperm to be used for ICSI, which is a major advantage. On the other hand, it is a subjective test resulting in inter- and intraobserver variability, and it can be time consuming to access sperm cell by sperm cell prior to ICSI.

Hypoosmotic Swelling Test

The test is based on the principle that live sperm cells possess undamaged and functional membranes, able to react to hypoosmotic media. Live sperm exposed to hypotonic solution will allow water influx and present tail swelling or curling, while dead sperm with damaged, nonfunctional membranes will not respond.[15,20,21]

Chemical Motility Enhancers

Pentoxifylline and theophylline are phosphodiesterase inhibitors that increase levels of cyclic adenosine monophosphate which, in turn, participates in sperm motility. Both the achievement of sperm motility and successful clinical outcomes post ICSI have been demonstrated with the addition of pentoxifylline and theophylline to epididymal- and testicular-retrieved sperm.

A reason for concern could be the toxicity of these chemical compounds, even though the sperm is washed post treatment; yet there is no evidence of offspring abnormalities. The addition of pentoxifylline and theophylline may shorten sperm selection without harming the outcomes of pregnancy.[15,22]

Laser-Assisted Immotile Sperm Selection

Introduced in 2004 by Aktan et al.,[23] laser-assisted immotile sperm selection (LAISS) distinguishes between viable and dead immotile sperm by examining sperm tail reaction when hit by a single laser shot. Live sperm will demonstrate tail curling, while dead sperm will not show tail dislocation. LAISS is a chemical-free, fast sperm selection technique that safely provides immediate response on sperm viability. The main limitation of the technique is the high cost of the equipment, which is a disappointment since increased fertilization potential has been shown when testicular sperm selected via this technique were used for ICSI.[24]

Birefringence-Polarization Microscopy

The analysis of double reflection or birefringence in spermatozoa is an indicator of structural normalcy, as corroborated by transmission electron microscopy.[25] Positive birefringence is associated with an organized and compact structure which, in turn, indicates normal sperm nucleus, acrosome, and flagellum, whereas sperm cells lacking birefringence are considered nonvital because of their distinct consistency. Sperm selection using this technique was shown to be beneficial for ejaculated sperm sample from males with severe male factor and for testicular-retrieved sperm.[26]

The effectiveness of sperm selection using sperm head birefringence is somewhat controversial (reviewed by Henkel[27]). Polarization microscopy is a high-priced acquisition to the IVF laboratory, reliable cut-off values are not established, and cheaper sperm selection methods are available, which preclude a more extensive use of the technique.

Artificial intelligence

Artificial intelligence (AI) is a very broad term that conglomerates processes that mimic intelligence or behavioral archetypes of any living entity. Artificial neural networks (ANNs), computational models developed to mimic the way the human brain processes data,[28] can learn and make decisions based on this training.

Regarding male infertility, Samli and Dogan[29] developed an ANN model showing significantly higher sensitivity than the logistic regression one and able to correctly predict outcomes and reach clinically acceptable sensitivity in nearly 81% of NOA patients in the test set, using variables such as age, duration of infertility, serum hormone levels, and testicular volume. Ramasamy et al.[30] used a different way to predict the chance of identifying sperm with micro-TESE in males with NOA consisting of a retrospective investigation of males who underwent micro-TESE using readily available clinical features to model, showing 59.4% success in correctly predicting the outcome of sperm retrieval based on preexisting clinical evidence.

Nevertheless, the main challenges, which are predicting the presence of sperm cells, identifying them during biopsy, and classifying sperm integrity after extraction, remain. These processes are currently andrologist dependent, but there is a possibility that they will soon be automated with the help of AI systems.

Artificial Oocyte Activation

In mammals, fertilization involves a series of physiological and biochemical events that starts with the recognition and fusion of sperm and oocyte membranes. This event triggers a pathway that induces persistent cytosolic calcium (Ca^{2+}) oscillations, the starting point of a developmental program leading to the intricate embryonic development process to form a new individual, the oocyte activation.[31,32]

The intracellular Ca^{2+} oscillations last for several hours[12,33] and orchestrate a series of further key events, such as cortical granule material exocytosis, prevention of polyspermy, polar body extrusion, cytoskeletal rearrangements, resumption of meiosis, formation of pronuclei, initiation of the first mitotic division in the new zygote, recruitment of maternal mRNA, and regulation of gene expression.[34]

For quite some time, sperm have been considered mere vectors that carry the paternal genetic component to the oocyte. However, the contribution of sperm to the embryo has recently been better elucidated, with accumulating evidence suggesting that various spermatozoa components actively participate in early human development. The sperm cell contributes both its DNA and its entire structure to embryo formation.[33] Upon fertilization, sperm-specific proteins and factors trigger Ca^{2+} oscillations to activate the oocyte. While the sperm centriole guides both oocyte and sperm nuclei to form the zygote nucleus and sperm DNA structures, chromatin and free RNAs can be modified to activate/deactivate gene expression involved in embryo development.[35] These interactions demonstrate that the spermatozoon has an active role in both oocyte activation and zygote formation, affecting the embryo's phenotype directly.

The exact mechanism responsible for oocyte activation has been a matter of debate for decades. Accumulating evidence has suggested that the sperm oocyte-activator factor, phospholipase C zeta (PLCζ), present in the sperm head and released in the ooplasm following gamete fusion, is involved in oocyte activation, promoting metaphase II resumption and pronuclear formation through the inositol-1,4,5-triphosphate pathway.[36,37]

A pivotal goal is to identify specific receptors within the oocyte that interact with these factors, triggering Ca^{2+} oscillations and oocyte activation upon fertilization.

ICSI was introduced to overcome severe male infertility and at present, is widely used in assisted reproductive technology. The aim of ICSI is to achieve fertilization by directly injecting the sperm into the oocyte, bypassing the many biological barriers in the process.[38] Continuous improvement in this technique has allowed severe infertility cases to be successful, even when recurrent fertilization failures occur after conventional IVF. Although the procedure results in an average fertilization rate of 70%, in rare cases, fertilization fails due to the lack of oocyte activation. The total fertilization failure occurs when all the oocytes collected within one cycle of stimulation fail to form pronuclei, with oocyte activation deficiency as the primary cause of such failures.[39]

It has been postulated that fertile males present a significantly higher proportion of sperm exhibiting PLCζ than infertile males. Reduced levels, abnormal localization, reduced activity/expression, or mutations in PLCζ have been associated with oocyte activation deficiency and therefore ICSI failure,[40] even in patients with normal sperm parameters.[41]

It has been reported that up to 70% of unfertilized metaphase II oocytes after ICSI contain a swollen sperm head, indicating that the oocyte may have been correctly injected but failed to become activated to complete the second meiotic division.[42]

Oocyte activation failure can be compensated by artificially increasing Ca^{2+} in the oocyte, the so-called artificial oocyte activation (AOA). Protocols used for AOA can be classified based on whether the mechanism evoking the Ca^{2+} trigger that promotes fertilization is mechanical, electrical, or chemical. For cases in which AOAs have failed, modifications of reproductive technologies such as ICSI followed by microinjections of PLCζ mRNA and recombinant active PLCζ protein have been developed.[39] However, there is a need to establish reference clinical ranges to apply this treatment to infertile patients.[43]

Mechanical Activation

Mechanical oocyte activation entails a modified ICSI technique in which the microinjection pipette is advanced during the ICSI procedure and peripheral cytoplasm is aspirated. Subsequently, the aspirated cytoplasm and the spermatozoon are deposited into the center of the oocyte.

Tesarik et al.[44] reported an ICSI technique primarily based on the repeated dislocation of the central ooplasm to the periphery, which increases the intracellular concentration of free Ca^{2+} either by creating an influx of Ca^{2+} or by inducing the release of stored Ca^{2+} from cell organelles. It was suggested that this mechanical oocyte activation may have an immediate clinical application in patients with repeated fertilization failures after ICSI, suspected to be caused by insufficiency of PLCζ or by a defective oocyte response to this sperm factor.[44] This technique may represent an alternative to the use of Ca^{2+} ionophores. The possibility of using a simple modification of the standard ICSI micromanipulation technique instead of ionophores alleviates concerns about the possible harmful effects on human embryos.

Considering a possible negative effect of this rather vigorous injection technique on further preimplantation development, Ebner et al.[45] developed a modified ICSI technique based on the hypothetical accumulation of highly polarized mitochondria. The cytoplasm in the periphery of the oocyte is thought to be rich in mitochondria, with high inner membrane potential and high metabolic adenosine triphosphate activity. Therefore this method aims to accumulate peripheral mitochondria and thus increase energy sources at the site of subsequent pronuclear formation.[45] The authors suggested that the modified ICSI possibly accumulates mitochondria with a higher inner mitochondrial membrane potential and may be a reliable and safe alternative to conventional ICSI, leading to comparable rates of blastocyst formation, implantation, and clinical pregnancy. In particular, this technology was proven to be useful in cases of previous failure of fertilization in ICSI cycles.[45]

Electrical Activation

An electrical field can generate micropores in the cell membrane of gametes to induce sufficient Ca^{2+} influx through the pores to activate cytoplasm through a Ca^{2+}-dependent mechanism.[9] In animal models, oocytes injected with secondary spermatocytes or spermatids were fertilized when stimulated by electroporation and developed into normal offspring when the resultant embryos were transferred to a recipient uterus.[46]

Yanagida et al. was the first to use ICSI followed by electrical oocyte activation for human oocyte activation, which resulted in healthy twins for a couple with previously failed fertilization after ICSI.[47] This study was followed by others with different experimental designs and different situations (i.e., previous fertilization failure, severe oligoasthenospermia, or NOA with total teratospermia).

Mansour et al.[48] evaluated the electroactivation of oocytes after ICSI in 241 cycles with either severe oligoasthenoteratospermia or azoospermia. For this trial, sibling oocytes for each patient were randomly divided after ICSI into two groups: the study group (electroactivation) and the control group (without electroactivation). Electrical activation resulted in a significant improvement in the fertilization rate after ICSI.

Oocyte electrical activation was also assessed in infertile couples having a history of total fertilization failure in previous ICSI cycles. For this study, a significantly increased fertilization rate and high-quality embryo rate was noted.[49]

Some studies evaluated the effectiveness of oocyte electrical activation in nonfertilized oocytes after ICSI (rescue oocyte activation). Traditionally, oocyte electrical activation is performed, on average, 30 minutes after ICSI. For the rescue oocyte activation, oocytes showing no evidence of fertilization by 16 to 24 hours after ICSI are electroactivated.

Zhang et al.[50] demonstrated that electrical stimulation can "rescue" oocytes that fail to fertilize by 24 hours after ICSI and stimulate them to complete the second meiotic division, form pronuclei, and undergo early embryonic development. One hundred failed-to-fertilize oocytes after ICSI were randomly assigned by stratified allocation according to oocyte grading before ICSI. Fifty unfertilized oocytes were electroactivated, and the remaining 50 unfertilized oocytes were treated in the same way but without electrical activation. The embryo formation rates in the electrically activated group were 80% compared to 16% in the control group, suggesting once again that failed-to-fertilize oocytes after ICSI seem to be able to resume embryonic development after electrical activation.

It has been demonstrated that electroactivation results in a rapid rise in Ca^{2+} inside the oocyte, which gradually decreases to the original level in about 300 seconds. The aforementioned studies suggested that the oocyte electrical activation soon after ICSI or in unfertilized oocytes may be a promising approach for the treatment of patients with the risk of fertilization failure or those with high fertilization failure rates in previous cycles. However, electrical oocyte activation has not yet been proven to be the most efficient and safest method for oocyte activation in humans. Moreover, there is insufficient evidence available from randomized controlled trials to judge the efficacy and safety of this method in couples undergoing assisted reproduction cycles, and long-term follow-up studies are needed to ensure safety.

Chemical Activation

The potential of Ca^{2+} ionophores to support AOA and yield high fertilization rates was shown at the beginning of the ICSI era.[51] Since that time, a number of studies have been conducted to assess the value of Ca^{2+} ionophores and others chemical agents as methods of AOA in humans. The chemical oocyte activation remained the most common method for AOA.

Chemical activation agents are classified based on the Ca^{2+} response they elicit in mammalian oocytes: (1) single Ca^{2+} transients, (2) dynamic Ca^{2+} oscillations, and (3) oocyte activation independent of the initial Ca^{2+} trigger.

Agents Inducing Single Calcium Transients

Calcium ionophores. Calcium ionophores, such as ionomycin and calcimycin, confer high permeability to cell membranes, allowing Ca^{2+} ions to penetrate through. Oocytes exposed to Ca^{2+} ionophores experience an increase of free intracytoplasmic Ca^{2+}, which results from Ca^{2+} influx, as well as Ca^{2+} release from the intracellular stores, particularly the endoplasmic reticulum.

When poor ICSI oocyte activation rates are observed, Ca^{2+} ionophores are the most commonly used treatment option. Ca^{2+} ionophores have been used in many cases of complete activation failure or previous high rates of fertilization failure.

The effect of AOA with a Ca^{2+} ionophore on ICSI cycles using surgically retrieved sperm was also suggested. Borges at al.[52] demonstrated that AOA might be useful in improving ICSI outcomes in azoospermic patients when epididymal but not testicular spermatozoa are injected.[52] It was also proven that AOA may be a useful tool to improve ICSI outcomes when ejaculated or epididymal spermatozoa are used in younger but not older female partners.[53] These findings highlight the theory that both sperm maturity and oocyte quality play roles in oocyte activation.

A previously published metaanalysis suggested that the use of Ca^{2+} ionophores after ICSI treatment increases the overall pregnancy rate per embryo transfer and the live birth rate per both embryo transfer and treatment cycle. It has also been demonstrated that the use of Ca^{2+} ionophores after ICSI increases the multiple pregnancy rate.[54]

The results after analysis of secondary outcomes were also encouraging: the fertilization, cleavage, blastocyst formation, and implantation rates were all increased after the use of Ca^{2+} ionophores.[54]

In a large series of patients with a history of total fertilization failure or low fertilization (<33%) after ICSI, for whom the oocyte-activating capacity of the sperm was examined by means of mouse oocyte activation test, it was demonstrated that AOA with the use of $CaCl_2$ injection in combination with a two-fold ionomycin exposure resulted in significantly higher fertilization, pregnancy, and live birth rates compared with previous ICSI cycles.[55]

More recently, a retrospective cohort study involving 796 couples undergoing oocyte activation with calcimycin after ICSI suggested that AOA is able to "rescue" the poor reproductive outcomes in certain types of infertile couples with history of failure to achieve pregnancy.[56]

In a prospective sibling oocyte approach, 78 ICSI patients with suspected fertilization problems had half of their metaphase II oocytes treated with a ready-to-use Ca^{2+} ionophore (calcimycin) immediately following ICSI (study group), while untreated ICSI eggs served as the control group. The authors evaluated the effect of AOA on embryo on morphokinetics and it was concluded that Ca^{2+} oonophore application does not negatively affect cleavage timing nor is it associated with irregular cleavage.[57]

Although they can give rise to live births in cycles that would otherwise fail, Ca^{2+} ionophores can only cause one or, in some protocols, two large Ca^{2+} increases, which fails to mimic the multiple Ca^{2+} oscillations that occur at fertilization.

The importance of Ca^{2+} oscillation in embryo development and pregnancy outcome has been highlighted. In contrast, the aberrant induced Ca^{2+} rise, which includes a single surge without subsequent oscillations when chemical and electrical methods of AOA are used, raises concerns regarding the safety and physiological relevance of AOA and requires further clinical evaluation.

Indeed, concern still exists regarding the potentially deleterious effects of these substances on embryogenesis.[58] Vanden Meerschaut et al.[59] conducted a study on neonatal and neurodevelopmental outcomes in 21 children born after an ICSI-AOA treatment, and no severe effects in the offspring were reported. However, the high response rate and the robustness of the test used in this study are still considered preliminary because the sample size was small.

A recently published report evaluated whether ionomycin-AOA treatment would affect individual normal developmental by disturbing subsequent gene expression at different embryonic development stages in mouse. The study demonstrated that ionomycin-AOA treatment affects imprinted gene *Igf2r* expression and methylation states in mouse pre- and postimplantation embryos, which is regulated by the imprinted *Airn*. Nevertheless, no significant differences were found in postnatal growth of the pups in the study.[60]

Moreover, a recently published metaanalysis evaluating the risk of birth defects (chromosomal and nonchromosomal aberrations) in children conceived by ICSI-AOA indicated that ICSI-AOA represents no significant difference in the prevalence of major birth defects or types of birth defects (chromosomal and nonchromosomal aberrations) compared with conventional ICSI.[61]

Nevertheless, accumulating evidence supports the biosafety of ionomycin as an activating agent. First, high oocyte survival rates are observed following chemical AOA in mouse and human oocytes. Moreover, ionomycin did not increase the incidence of meiotic errors of maternal origin in human oocytes.

Most importantly, the follow-up studies of children born after AOA support the safety of this methodology. Together, these data endorse the use of AOA for clinical applications. Defining a proper indication, however, requires further investigation. Diagnostic tools to identify cases that could benefit from AOA are needed to guide clinicians.

Nevertheless, the use of ionophores remains experimental. The knowledge concerning their potential cytotoxic, teratogenic, and mutagenic effects on embryos and offspring is still insufficient. No long-term follow-up studies of children born after chemical ICSI-AOA are yet available.

Agents Inducing Oscillatory Calcium Signaling

Thimerosal. Thimerosal has the capacity to induce Ca^{2+}-induced Ca^{2+} oscillations by oxidizing protein thiol groups at the inositol trisphosphate receptors. As a consequence, the receptors become sensitized to the cytosolic concentration of inositol trisphosphate, a key component determining intracellular Ca^{2+} oscillations and oocyte activation.

Strontium. Strontium (Sr^{2+}) is able to replace Ca^{2+} for triggering somatic cellular responses and eliciting Ca^{2+} oscillations, not just a single surge like Ca^{2+} ionophores. Treatment with Sr^{2+} has been proposed previously as a strategy to "rescue" human oocytes that failed to fertilize after ICSI.[62]

Even though Sr^{2+} is the most efficient method for mouse oocyte activation, leading to high blastocyst formation rates, its efficiency in activating human oocytes is still under debate.[62,63]

Recombinant phospholipase Cζ. Accumulating evidence favors the idea that Ca^{2+} oscillations are triggered after entry of PLCζ into the oocyte cytoplasm. The activation of mammalian oocytes at fertilization involves an extensive series of Ca^{2+} oscillations.

Each Ca^{2+} spike lasts about 1 minute, and the Ca^{2+} transients occur at intervals of 5 to 30 minutes. AOA to overcome failed fertilization after ICSI in human oocytes typically employs Ca^{2+} ionophores to produce a single cytosolic Ca^{2+} increase. In contrast, recombinant PLCζ causes Ca^{2+} oscillations indistinguishable from those occurring during fertilization and subsequent development of embryos up to the blastocyst stage at rates similar to those seen after fertilization.

PLCζ remains the only physiological agent that has been repeatedly shown to produce a prolonged series of Ca^{2+} oscillations in all mammalian oocytes studied, including human oocytes. In this regard, the use of PLCζ as an oocyte activation agent seems promising, particularly in cases where sperm is devoid of PLCζ, such as in globozoospermia or in patients carrying punctual mutations in the PLCζ gene.

It has been demonstrated that both recombinant PLCζ protein and PLCζ RNA trigger intracellular Ca^{2+} oscillations in both mouse and human oocytes.[64–68]

Sanusi et al.[69] tested the efficacy of AOA with recombinant PLCζ in a scenario of ICSI fertilization failure. The authors compared PLCζ with other activation stimuli (Ca^{2+} ionophore or with Sr^{2+} media) in a mouse model of failed oocyte activation after ICSI. All tested treatments rescued oocyte activation, although Sr^{2+} and PLCζ gave the highest rates of development to blastocyst.

When recombinant PLCζ was given to oocytes previously injected with control sperm, they developed normally to the blastocyst stage at rates similar to that after control ICSI, suggesting that recombinant human PLCζ is an efficient means of rescuing oocyte activation after ICSI failure and that it can be effectively used even if the sperm already contains endogenous Ca^{2+}-releasing activity.

However, the introduction of genetic material into the oocyte is forbidden for human medicine in most parts of the world. In contrast, recombinant PLCζ could be synthesized in bacteria as a fusion protein. This resolves the problem of varying PLCζ expression but gives rise to PLCζ diminishing its activity quickly. Therefore, recombinant PLCζ protein must be stabilized and calibrated before its application.[70] Still, its application in IVF clinics is limited because of commercial availability.[43]

Oocyte Activation Independent of the Initial Calcium Trigger

Puromycin. Puromycin is known to inhibit mitogen-activating protein kinase (MAPK), which is a component of cytostatic factor in mammal's oocytes. MAPK possibly activates a positive regulator of the maturation-promoting factor (MPF) or inhibits negative regulators. Therefore, puromycin may decrease MPF activity via suppression of MAPK, resulting in the formation of a pronucleus.

It has been reported that puromycin induces parthenogenetic activation in about 90% of human oocytes, and the combination of puromycin and a Ca^{2+} ionophore could effectively produce human and mouse haploid parthenogenones.

This combination has been tested for activating unfertilized oocytes after ICSI. It was demonstrated that

Ca^{2+} ionophores with puromycin can stimulate unfertilized oocytes 20 to 68 hours after ICSI to complete the second meiosis, to form pronuclei, and to undergo early embryonic development. Furthermore, nearly all embryos had a normal set of sex chromosomes and could develop normally. All these findings suggested that the chemical approach has the potential to "rescue" unfertilized oocytes after ICSI.[71]

Sperm Selection Methods

Since PLCζ has been defined as the main sperm factor-inducing oocyte, researchers have focused on novel sperm selection procedures based on cellular characteristics of spermatozoa such as surface electrical charge (zeta potential) to isolate normal sperm subpopulations with intact chromatin.

In this regard, Kashir et al.[72] suggested density gradient centrifugation as a routine procedure of sperm preparation before assisted reproduction techniques could select high percentage of spermatozoa expressing PLCζ.

During epididymal maturation, human spermatozoa obtain three forms of the sialylated glycoproteins, which are liable for membrane negative charge by means of epididymosomes and prostasomes. This electrical charge of the sperm plasma membrane, called zeta potential, is acquired during spermatogenesis and passage through the epididymis (reviewed by Henkel[27]). Considering it, Chan et al. proposed a method based on zeta-potential selection according to the electric charge that could produce a higher percentage of normal sperm morphology with intact chromatin.[73] In accordance, Khakpour et al.[74] suggested a noninvasive method based on zeta potential along with the density-gradient selection method, which improved the intact chromatin and membrane selection of a morphologically normal spermatozoon with a high amount of PLCζ.

SUMMARY

Several surgical methods such as PESA, MESA, TESA, TESE, and micro-TESE have been developed to retrieve sperm from either the epididymis or the testis, depending on to the type of azoospermia, and may be used for ICSI and/or cryopreservation. The removal of contaminants, cellular debris, and red blood cells may be performed after collection of the epididymal fluid or testicular tissue using different laboratory techniques. Numerous tests for

the selection of viable immotile spermatozoa for ICSI are available, and the choice of the most suitable will vary according to the expertise of the laboratory personnel, equipment availability, and weighing the pros and cons intrinsic to each method. There is evidence that the use of sperm selection methods improves fertilization and pregnancy rates in couples undergoing ICSI using testicular-retrieved spermatozoa. Consequently, the use of at least one of these sperm selection methods is recommended when handling harvested immotile sperm.

Although the efficiency of AOA in terms of increased fertilization rate has been largely reported, it is worth noting that AOA does not benefit all infertile males. These approaches benefit patients with problems related to the spermatozoon, such as globozoospermia or recurrent ICSI cycle failure because of oocyte activation deficiency. Not all cases are similar, so treatment could differ among patients. Additionally, one should keep in mind that although it has been previously reported that ICSI-AOA represents no risks in terms of increased incidence of major birth defects or types of birth defects comparing with conventional ICSI, AOA is still an experimental technique. It is important to highlight that AOA includes additional manipulations on the injected oocyte and incubation in activating agents that may interfere the cell metabolism or embryo development; therefore, AOA should be carefully considered.

REFERENCES

1. Male Infertility Best Practice Policy Committee of the American Urological Association Practice Committee of the American Society for Reproductive Medicine, Report on evaluation of the azoospermic male. *Fertil Steril.* 2006;86(5 suppl 1):S210-S215.
2. Proctor M, Johnson N, van Peperstraten AM, Phillipson G. Techniques for surgical retrieval of sperm prior to intra-cytoplasmic sperm injection (ICSI) for azoospermia. *Cochrane Database Syst Rev.* 2008;(2):CD002807.
3. Semiao-Francisco L, Braga DP, Figueira Rde C, et al. Assisted reproductive technology outcomes in azoospermic men: 10 years of experience with surgical sperm retrieval. *Aging Male.* 2010;13(1):44-50.
4. Schlegel PN. Causes of azoospermia and their management. *Reprod Fertil Dev.* 2004;16(5):561-572.
5. Shrivastav P, Nadkarni P, Wensvoort S, Craft I. Percutaneous epididymal sperm aspiration for obstructive azoospermia. *Hum Reprod.* 1994;9(11):2058-2061.

6. Girardi SK, Schlegel PN. Microsurgical epididymal sperm aspiration: review of techniques, preoperative considerations, and results. *J Androl.* 1996;17(1):5-9.

7. Craft I, Tsirigotis M. Simplified recovery, preparation and cryopreservation of testicular spermatozoa. *Hum Reprod.* 1995;10(7):1623-1626.

8. Belenky A, Avrech OM, Bachar GN, et al. Ultrasound-guided testicular sperm aspiration in azoospermic patients: a new sperm retrieval method for intracytoplasmic sperm injection. *J Clin Ultrasound.* 2001;29(6):339-343.

9. Esteves SC, Miyaoka R, Agarwal A. Sperm retrieval techniques for assisted reproduction. *Int Braz J Urol.* 2011;37(5):570-583.

10. Schlegel PN, Su LM. Physiological consequences of testicular sperm extraction. *Hum Reprod.* 1997;12(8):1688-1692.

11. Schlegel PN. Nonobstructive azoospermia: a revolutionary surgical approach and results. *Semin Reprod Med.* 2009;27(2):165-170.

12. Kashir J, Jones C, Mounce G, et al. Variance in total levels of phospholipase C zeta (PLC-ζ) in human sperm may limit the applicability of quantitative immunofluorescent analysis as a diagnostic indicator of oocyte activation capability. *Fertil Steril.* 2013;99(1):107-117.e3.

13. Urman B, Alatas C, Aksoy S, Nuhoglu A, Sertac A, Balaban B. Performing testicular or epididymal sperm retrieval prior to the injection of hCG. *J Assist Reprod Genet.* 1998;15(3):125-128.

14. Levran D, Ginath S, Farhi J, Nahum H, Glezerman M, Weissman A. Timing of testicular sperm retrieval procedures and in vitro fertilization-intracytoplasmic sperm injection outcome. *Fertil Steril.* 2001;76(2):380-383.

15. Verheyen G, Popovic-Todorovic B, Tournaye H. Processing and selection of surgically-retrieved sperm for ICSI: a review. *Basic Clin Androl.* 2017;27(1):6.

16. Verheyen G, De Croo I, Tournaye H, Pletincx I, Devroey P, Van Steirteghem A. Comparison of four mechanical methods to retrieve spermatozoa from testicular tissue. *Hum Reprod.* 1995;10(11):2956-2959.

17. Crabbé E, Verheyen G, Silber S, et al. Enzymatic digestion of testicular tissue may rescue the intracytoplasmic sperm injection cycle in some patients with nonobstructive azoospermia. *Hum Reprod.* 1998;13(10):2791-2796.

18. Dalzell LH, McVicar CM, McClure N, Lutton D, Lewis SE. Effects of short and long incubations on DNA fragmentation of testicular sperm. *Fertil Steril.* 2004;82(5):1443-1445.

19. de Oliveira NM, Vaca Sanchez R, Rodriguez Fiesta S, et al. Pregnancy with frozen-thawed and fresh testicular biopsy after motile and immotile sperm microinjection,

using the mechanical touch technique to assess viability. *Hum Reprod.* 2004;19(2):262-265.

20. Sallam H, Farrag A, Agameya A, Ezzeldin F, Eid A, Sallam A. The use of a modified hypo-osmotic swelling test for the selection of viable ejaculated and testicular immotile spermatozoa in ICSI. *Hum Reprod.* 2001;16(2):272-276.

21. Sallam HN, Farrag A, Agameya AF, El-Garem Y, Ezzeldin F. The use of the modified hypo-osmotic swelling test for the selection of immotile testicular spermatozoa in patients treated with ICSI: a randomized controlled study. *Hum Reprod.* 2005;20(12):3435-3440.

22. Loughlin KR, Agarwal A. Use of theophylline to enhance sperm function. *Arch Androl.* 1992;28(2):99-103.

23. Aktan TM, Montag M, Duman S, Gorkemli H, Rink K, Yurdakul T. Use of a laser to detect viable but immotile spermatozoa. *Andrologia.* 2004;36(6):366-369.

24. Nordhoff V, Schuring AN, Krallmann C, et al. Optimizing TESE-ICSI by laser-assisted selection of immotile spermatozoa and polarization microscopy for selection of oocytes. *Andrology.* 2013;1(1):67-74.

25. Baccetti B. Microscopical advances in assisted reproduction. *J Submicrosc Cytol Pathol.* 2004;36(3-4):333-339.

26. Tournaye H, Verheyen G, Nagy P, et al. Are there any predictive factors for successful testicular sperm recovery in azoospermic patients? *Hum Reprod.* 1997;12(1):80-86.

27. Henkel R. Novel sperm tests and their importance. In: Agarwal A, Borges Jr E, Setti A, eds. *Non-Invasive Sperm Selection for In Vitro Fertilization.* Springer: New York, NY; 2015:23-40.

28. Ramesh AN, Kambhampati C, Monson JR, Drew PJ. Artificial intelligence in medicine. *Ann R Coll Surg Engl.* 2004;86(5):334-338.

29. Samli MM, Dogan I. An artificial neural network for predicting the presence of spermatozoa in the testes of men with nonobstructive azoospermia. *J Urol.* 2004;171(6 Pt 1):2354-2357.

30. Ramasamy R, Padilla WO, Osterberg EC, et al. A comparison of models for predicting sperm retrieval before microdissection testicular sperm extraction in men with nonobstructive azoospermia. *J Urol.* 2013;189(2):638-642.

31. Ciapa B, Chiri S. Egg activation: upstream of the fertilization calcium signal. *Biol Cell.* 2000;92(3-4):215-233.

32. Nomikos M, Kashir J, Swann K, Lai FA. Sperm PLCζ: from structure to Ca2+ oscillations, egg activation and therapeutic potential. *FEBS Lett.* 2013;587(22):3609-3616.

33. Ostermeier GC, Miller D, Huntriss JD, Diamond MP, Krawetz SA. Reproductive biology: delivering spermatozoan RNA to the oocyte. *Nature.* 2004;429(6988):154.

34. Malcuit C, Kurokawa M, Fissore RA. Calcium oscillations and mammalian egg activation. *J Cell Physiol.* 2006;206(3):565-573.

35. Gòdia M, Swanson G, Krawetz SA. A history of why fathers' RNA matters. *Biol Reprod*. 2018;99(1):147-159.

36. Yeste M, Jones C, Amdani SN, Patel S, Coward K. Oocyte activation deficiency: a role for an oocyte contribution? *Hum Reprod Update*. 2016;22(1):23-47.

37. Wu AT, Sutovsky P, Manandhar G, et al. PAWP, a sperm-specific WW domain-binding protein, promotes meiotic resumption and pronuclear development during fertilization. *J Biol Chem*. 2007;282(16):12164-12175.

38. Palermo GD, Neri QV, Schlegel PN, Rosenwaks Z. Intracytoplasmic sperm injection (ICSI) in extreme cases of male infertility. *PLoS One*. 2014;9(12):e113671.

39. Meerschaut FV, Nikiforaki D, Heindryckx B, De Sutter P. Assisted oocyte activation following ICSI fertilization failure. *Reprod Biomed Online*. 2014;28(5):560-571.

40. Yelumalai S, Yeste M, Jones C, et al. Total levels, localization patterns, and proportions of sperm exhibiting phospholipase C zeta are significantly correlated with fertilization rates after intracytoplasmic sperm injection. *Fertil Steril*. 2015;104(3):561-568.e4.

41. Lee HC, Arny M, Grow D, Dumesic D, Fissore RA, Jellerette-Nolan T. Protein phospholipase C Zeta1 expression in patients with failed ICSI but with normal sperm parameters. *J Assist Reprod Genet*. 2014;31(6):749-756.

42. Mahutte NG, Arici A. Failed fertilization: is it predictable? *Curr Opin Obstet Gynecol*. 2003;15(3):211-218.

43. Zafar MI, Lu S, Li H. Sperm-oocyte interplay: an overview of spermatozoon's role in oocyte activation and current perspectives in diagnosis and fertility treatment. *Cell Biosci*. 2021;11(1):1-15.

44. Tesarik J, Rienzi L, Ubaldi F, Mendoza C, Greco E. Use of a modified intracytoplasmic sperm injection technique to overcome sperm-borne and oocyte-borne oocyte activation failures. *Fertil Steril*. 2002;78(3):619-624.

45. Ebner T, Moser M, Sommergruber M, Jesacher K, Tews G. Complete oocyte activation failure after ICSI can be overcome by a modified injection technique. *Hum Reprod*. 2004;19(8):1837-1841.

46. Sasagawa I, Yanagimachi R. Comparison of methods for activating mouse oocytes for spermatid nucleus transfer. *Zygote*. 1996;4(4):269-274.

47. Yanagida K, Katayose H, Yazawa H, et al. Successful fertilization and pregnancy following ICSI and electrical oocyte activation. *Hum Reprod*. 1999;14(5):1307-1311.

48. Mansour R, Fahmy I, Tawab NA, et al. Electrical activation of oocytes after intracytoplasmic sperm injection: a controlled randomized study. *Fertil Steril*. 2009;91(1):133-139.

49. Baltaci V, Ayvaz OU, Unsal E, et al. The effectiveness of intracytoplasmic sperm injection combined with piezoelectric stimulation in infertile couples with total fertilization failure. *Fertil Steril*. 2010;94(3):900-904.

50. Zhang J, Wang CW, Blaszcyzk A, et al. Electrical activation and in vitro development of human oocytes that fail to fertilize after intracytoplasmic sperm injection. *Fertil Steril*. 1999;72(3):509-512.

51. Tesarik J, Sousa M, Mendoza C. Sperm-induced calcium oscillations of human oocytes show distinct features in oocyte center and periphery. *Mol Reprod Dev*. 1995;41(2):257-263.

52. Borges Jr E, de Almeida Ferreira Braga DP, de Sousa Bonetti TC, Iaconelli Jr A, Franco Jr JG. Artificial oocyte activation with calcium ionophore A23187 in intracytoplasmic sperm injection cycles using surgically retrieved spermatozoa. *Fertil Steril*. 2009;92(1):131-136.

53. Borges Jr E, de Almeida Ferreira Braga DP, de Sousa Bonetti TC, Iaconelli Jr A, Franco Jr JG. Artificial oocyte activation using calcium ionophore in ICSI cycles with spermatozoa from different sources. *Reprod Biomed Online*. 2009;18(1):45-52.

54. Murugesu S, Saso S, Jones BP, et al. Does the use of calcium ionophore during artificial oocyte activation demonstrate an effect on pregnancy rate? A meta-analysis. *Fertil Steril*. 2017;108(3):468-482.e3.

55. Bonte D, Ferrer-Buitrago M, Dhaenens L, et al. Assisted oocyte activation significantly increases fertilization and pregnancy outcome in patients with low and total failed fertilization after intracytoplasmic sperm injection: a 17-year retrospective study. *Fertil Steril*. 2019;112(2):266-274.

56. Lv M, Zhang D, He X, et al. Artificial oocyte activation to improve reproductive outcomes in couples with various causes of infertility: a retrospective cohort study. *Reprod Biomed Online*. 2020;40(4):501-509.

57. Shebl O, Trautner PS, Enengl S, et al. Ionophore application for artificial oocyte activation and its potential effect on morphokinetics: a sibling oocyte study. *J Assist Reprod Genet*. 2021;38(12):3125-3133.

58. Nasr-Esfahani MH, Deemeh MR, Tavalaee M. Artificial oocyte activation and intracytoplasmic sperm injection. *Fertil Steril*. 2010;94(2):520-526.

59. Meerschaut FV, D'Haeseleer E, Gysels H, et al. Neonatal and neurodevelopmental outcome of children aged 3–10 years born following assisted oocyte activation. *Reprod Biomed Online*. 2014;28(1):54-63.

60. Yin M, Yu W, Li W, et al. DNA methylation and gene expression changes in mouse pre-and post-implantation embryos generated by intracytoplasmic sperm injection with artificial oocyte activation. *Reprod Biol Endocrinol*. 2021;19(1):1-14.

61. Long R, Wang M, Yang QY, Hu SQ, Zhu LX, Jin L. Risk of birth defects in children conceived by artificial oocyte activation and intracytoplasmic sperm injection: a meta-analysis. *Reprod Biol Endocrinol*. 2020;18(1):1-9.

62. Kim JW, Kim SD, Yang SH, Yoon SH, Jung JH, Lim JH. Successful pregnancy after SrCl2 oocyte activation in couples with repeated low fertilization rates following calcium ionophore treatment. *Syst Biol Reprod Med.* 2014;60(3):177-182.

63. Yanagida K, Morozumi K, Katayose H, Hayashi S, Sato A. Successful pregnancy after ICSI with strontium oocyte activation in low rates of fertilization. *Reprod Biomed Online.* 2006;13(6):801-806.

64. Yoon SY, Eum JH, Lee JE, et al. Recombinant human phospholipase C zeta 1 induces intracellular calcium oscillations and oocyte activation in mouse and human oocytes. *Hum Reprod.* 2012;27(6):1768-1780.

65. Sanusi R, Yu Y, Nomikos M, Lai FA, Swann K. Rescue of failed oocyte activation after ICSI in a mouse model of male factor infertility by recombinant phospholipase Cζ. *Mol Hum Reprod.* 2015;21(10):783-791.

66. Rogers N, Hobson E, Pickering S, Lai FA, Braude P, Swann K. Phospholipase Cζ causes Ca2+ oscillations and parthenogenetic activation of human oocytes. *Reproduction.* 2004;128(6):697-702.

67. Yamaguchi T, Ito M, Kuroda K, Takeda S, Tanaka A. The establishment of appropriate methods for egg-activation by human PLCZ1 RNA injection into human oocyte. *Cell Calcium.* 2017;65:22-30.

68. Nomikos M, Yu Y, Elgmati K, et al. Phospholipase Cζ rescues failed oocyte activation in a prototype of male factor infertility. *Fertil Steril.* 2013;99(1):76-85.

69. Sanusi R, Yu Y, Nomikos M, Lai FA, Swann K. Rescue of failed oocyte activation after ICSI in a mouse model of male factor infertility by recombinant phospholipase Czeta. *Mol Hum Reprod.* 2015;21(10):783-791.

70. Swann K. The role of Ca2+ in oocyte activation during in vitro fertilization: insights into potential therapies for rescuing failed fertilization. *Biochim Biophys Acta Mol Cell Res.* 2018;1865(11):1830-1837.

71. Lu Q, Zhao Y, Gao X, et al. Combination of calcium ionophore A23187 with puromycin salvages human unfertilized oocytes after ICSI. *Eur J Obstet Gynecol Reprod Biol.* 2006;126(1):72-76.

72. Kashir J, Heynen A, Jones C, et al. Effects of cryopreservation and density-gradient washing on phospholipase C zeta concentrations in human spermatozoa. *Reprod Biomed Online.* 2011;23(2):263-267.

73. Chan PJ, Jacobson JD, Corselli JU, Patton WC. A simple zeta method for sperm selection based on membrane charge. *Fertil Steril.* 2006;85(2):481-486.

74. Khakpour S, Sadeghi E, Tavalaee M, Bahadorani M, Nasr-Esfahani MH. Zeta method: a noninvasive method based on membrane charge for selecting spermatozoa expressing high level of phospholipaseCζ. *Andrologia.* 2019;51(5):e13249.

Assisted Reproduction

22

Intrauterine Insemination With Homologous Semen

Willem Ombelet and Hassan Sallam

KEY POINTS

- Indications of intrauterine insemination (IUI) include retrograde ejaculation, cervical factor infertility, mild and moderate male factor infertility, immunological infertility, mild and moderate endometriosis, and unexplained infertility.
- Other indications for IUI are human immunodeficiency virus– or hepatitis C virus–discordant couples and gender preselection.
- Inseminating motile count and sperm morphology are the most valuable sperm parameters to predict IUI outcome.
- Many studies have shown that 5% normal forms and 1 million motile spermatozoa after sperm

preparation are potential cut-off values to select couples for IUI treatment, but more detailed studies are needed to confirm these findings.
- Factors affecting the outcome of IUI include age of the female partner, stimulation protocol, quality of the semen and presence of oxidative stress, timing and technique of insemination, and the sperm preparation technique.
- According to a prospective multicenter trial, IUI–controlled ovarian stimulation is the most cost-effective strategy for mild and moderate male factor or unexplained infertility.

INTRODUCTION

Over the last centuries, the popularity of artificial insemination has varied tremendously,[1] although this history goes back to much earlier times (Fig. 22.1). In 1770, John Hunter described the first case of human intravaginal insemination because of severe hypospadias. In the mid-1800s, James Marion Sims reported on 55 intravaginal inseminations. Only one pregnancy occurred, which is probably explained by the fact that Sims believed that ovulation occurred during menstruation.

The first reports on human artificial insemination originated from Guttmacher and Kohlberg.[2,3] For many years, homologous artificial insemination was only performed in case of physiologic and psychological dysfunction, such as retrograde ejaculation, vaginismus, hypospadias, and impotence.

In the early days, the ejaculate of the male was inseminated without preparation, resulting in uterine cramps and increasing the probability of tubal infections in female partners. With the arrival of in vitro fertilization (IVF), semen preparation techniques were developed, and intrauterine insemination (IUI) became popular, being safer and generally painless. The introduction of various sperm processing techniques able to remove prostaglandins, infectious agents, nonmotile spermatozoa, leukocytes, and immature germ cells, subsequently enhancing sperm quality by decreasing the release of lymphokines and/or cytokines and also a reduction in the formation of free oxygen radicals, was an undeniable breakthrough in the history of artificial insemination. These techniques significantly improved the fertilizing capacity of the sperm sample.

The renewed interest in sperm washing procedures owing to the introduction of IVF could be regarded as

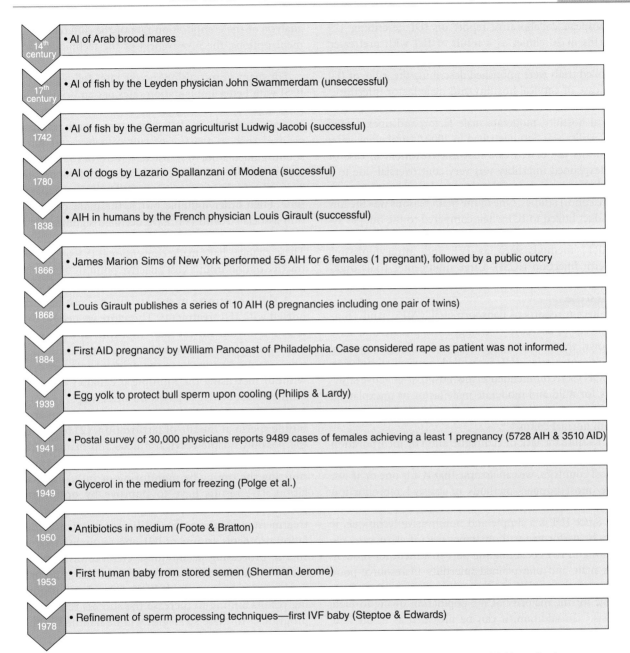

14th century	• AI of Arab brood mares
17th century	• AI of fish by the Leyden physician John Swammerdam (unseccessful)
1742	• AI of fish by the German agriculturist Ludwig Jacobi (successful)
1780	• AI of dogs by Lazario Spallanzani of Modena (successful)
1838	• AIH in humans by the French physician Louis Girault (successful)
1866	• James Marion Sims of New York performed 55 AIH for 6 females (1 pregnant), followed by a public outcry
1868	• Louis Girault publishes a series of 10 AIH (8 pregnancies including one pair of twins)
1884	• First AID pregnancy by William Pancoast of Philadelphia. Case considered rape as patient was not informed.
1939	• Egg yolk to protect bull sperm upon cooling (Philips & Lardy)
1941	• Postal survey of 30,000 physicians reports 9489 cases of females achieving a least 1 pregnancy (5728 AIH & 3510 AID)
1949	• Glycerol in the medium for freezing (Polge et al.)
1950	• Antibiotics in medium (Foote & Bratton)
1953	• First human baby from stored semen (Sherman Jerome)
1978	• Refinement of sperm processing techniques—first IVF baby (Steptoe & Edwards)

Fig. 22.1 Most Important Milestones in the History of Artificial Insemination (AI). *AID*, Artificial insemination with donor semen; *AIH*, artificial insemination with homologous semen; *IVF*, in vitro fertilization.

one of the most important milestones in the history of IUI.[4] The results of the first randomized clinical trial of IUI were published in 1984 by Kerin et al.[5] This trial included males with poor semen quality and compared the effectiveness of IUI on the day of the luteinizing hormone (LH) surge with intercourse in which timing was based on the basal body temperature, and with intercourse in which timing was based on the LH surge. IUI was significantly more successful than the two other treatment policies. Sunde et al.[6] reported the data of a

European collaborative report on IUI describing 127 births in 20 clinics as a result of IUI with pretreated sperm. In 1989, the results of the first prospective controlled trials were published describing the value of IUI in case of cervical hostility and male factor infertility.[7] The evidence-based value of IUI as a treatment for cervical hostility, moderate male factor, and unexplained infertility was first described in 2000.[8] Until a few years ago, the use of IUI as a first-line treatment in case of unexplained infertility was very controversial due to a lack of prospective randomized trials and large prospective cohort studies. One of the main reasons was the low budget linked to IUI when compared to the budget associated with other assisted reproductive technology (ART) methods such as IVF and intracytoplasmic sperm injection (ICSI). Large multicenter trials organized by the pharmaceutical industry are scarce in the IUI scene.

Recent reports of Bensdorp et al. (2015)[9] and Tjon-Kon-Fat et al. (2015)[10] changed the picture and have shown that according to the results of a prospective multicenter trial, IUI–controlled ovarian stimulation (COH) is recommended as the most cost-effective strategy for mild and moderate male factor or unexplained infertility with a poor prognosis of becoming pregnant with normal coitus.[9,10]

Despite the lack of IUI registration or incorporation of IUI procedures reported within IVF/ICSI registries in most countries, we can assume that IUI is one of, if not the, most popular methods of assisted reproduction worldwide, for different reasons.

Since IUI is a simple and noninvasive technique, it can be performed without expensive infrastructure, resulting in IUI becoming the only treatment for moderate male and unexplained infertility in resource-poor countries where IVF is either not available or not accessible for the majority of the population owing to high costs.[11] In addition, it can be provided as a safe and simple treatment with minimal risks when appropriately monitored. These factors are responsible for high couple compliance in IUI programs compared to IVF programs.

Considering the future of artificial insemination with a partner's semen, IUI has to be weighed against expectant management, timed coitus, IVF, and ICSI. This comparison should not only involve success rates but should also include a cost-benefit analysis and an analysis of the complication rate of the different treatment options, the invasiveness of the techniques, and patient compliance.

For many years, raising success rates following IVF/ICSI with better implantation rates per embryo are reported, partly caused by better air quality and quality control programs in IVF laboratories and technical changes such as the use of soft catheters and ultrasound-guided embryo transfers.[12] Most of the previous cohort studies on cost effectiveness tend to become "dated," as both costs and outcome results changed over time. High-order multiple births, the main complication associated with IVF, have declined significantly in many countries because fewer embryos are transferred. These changes have made conventional IVF a more attractive option from a cost effective point of view compared to IUI.

A similar increase in success rate has not been reported with IUI treatments. Therefore we believe that if IUI is to remain the best first-line option in selected cases of moderate male and unexplained infertility, we need to increase the delivery rate per cycle without increasing the multiple pregnancy rate. The quintessence of IUI is based on three steps: (1) processing semen, resulting in an increasing number of motile sperm at the site of fertilization, (2) bypassing the possibly hostile cervical mucus and bringing the semen in closer proximity of the oocyte, and (3) optimizing the timing by monitoring or inducing ovulation. IUI results have to improve by optimizing patient selection and refining the techniques and treatment strategies such as different ovarian stimulation protocols, timing of IUI, sperm quality factors, sperm processing techniques, etc. Prewashing the catheter with culture medium prior to IUI[13] and performing slow-release IUI (SRI)[14,15] also show promising results aiming to increase the success rate in IUI programs. All these strategies will be handled in this chapter.

Fig. 22.2 gives an overview of the different factors that may influence success rates after IUI. Evidence-based data from 2023 clearly indicate that in cases of unexplained or mild/moderate male infertility, three to six cycles of IUI with ovarian stimulation should be recommended as a first-line therapy for females below 40 years of age, provided a strict cancellation strategy is followed to avoid multiple pregnancies.

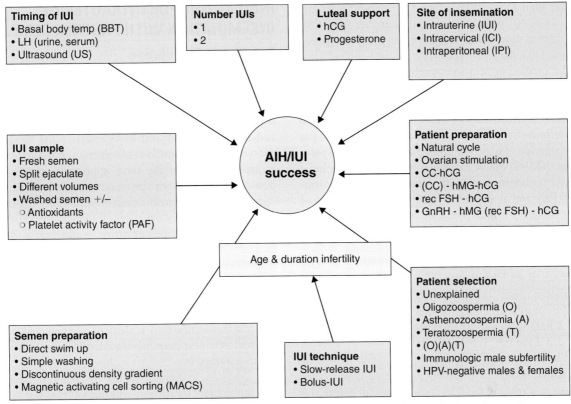

Fig. 22.2 Overview of different factors that may influence success rates after intrauterine insemination (IUI). *CC*, Clomiphene citrate; *FSH*, follicle-stimulating hormone; *GnRH*, gonadotropin-releasing hormone; *hCG*, human chorionic gonadotropin; *hMG*, human menopausal gonadotropin; *HPV*, human papillomavirus; *LH*, luteinizing hormone.

DIAGNOSTIC WORK-UP BEFORE INTRAUTERINE INSEMINATION AND WHEN TO START WITH INTRAUTERINE INSEMINATION

The diagnostic work-up of a heterosexual couple before IUI should be limited to tests that contribute to the prediction of effectiveness of IUI. In general, the indications for IUI are moderate male or longstanding unexplained subfertility.

All females should have a gynecological examination and an ultrasound as part of their general diagnostic work-up. Causes for ovulatory problems should be investigated and corrected if possible. Ultrasound may reveal visible hydrosalpinges or ovarian pathology. In order for IUI to be successful, fallopian tubes should be patent.

Patient characteristics and the chlamydia antibody test (CAT) can help to differentiate between females who have a low or a high risk of bilateral tubal pathology. Traditionally, hysterosalpingography (HSG), hysterosalpingo-foam sonography (HyFoSy), and/or diagnostic laparoscopy (DL) are performed, HSG being the first line test and DL the so-called reference test. An alternative for DL is transvaginal hydrolaparoscopy, which has a comparable diagnostic accuracy to DL but can be performed in an outpatient setting, without general anesthesia.[16] Identification of those females at highest risk for bilateral tubal pathology is best obtained by combining the patient characteristics with CAT and HSG or HyFoSy findings.

According to the 2010 World Health Organization (WHO) criteria, a semen analysis is considered normal when the volume is greater than 1.5 mL, concentration is greater than 15×10^6/mL, total sperm count is greater than 39×10^6, percentage motility is greater than 40%, and normal morphology is greater than 4%.[17] It has been reported that the 2010 WHO criteria have a limited value in the prediction of a spontaneous pregnancy and no value in the prediction of a pregnancy after IUI.[18] Semen quality can differ considerably within one male over time, so a second semen analysis with 1-month interval should be performed if the first semen analysis is abnormal. For the diagnosis of male subfertility, the total motile sperm count (TMSC) can be calculated by multiplying volume (mL) $\times$ concentration (million/mL) $\times$ progressive motility (%) and is helpful in identifying two groups of male subfertility: mild/moderate male subfertility with a TMSC 5 to 10 million and severe male subfertility with a TMSC less than 5 million.[19] If male subfertility is diagnosed, semen processing should be part of the fertility work-up to establish the postwash TMSC or inseminating motile count (IMC). Most studies indicate that IUI can be considered if the postwash IMC lies between 0.8 and 5 million motile spermatozoa.[20] IUI is not recommended if the IMC is below 0.8 million.

Whether testing for antisperm antibodies (ASAs) in the semen should be routinely performed is not clear. However, screening for ASA could be useful before the start of IUI because in the presence of ASA ($>50\%$), semen preparation with an additional medium can elute the antibodies from the acrosome region and lead to a better fertilization capacity of spermatozoa.[21]

Beside the outcome results of the infertility investigation, female age and duration of subfertility should also be taken into account in the decision making of whether IUI is a feasible option or not.

IUI with controlled ovarian hyperstimulation (COH) has not been shown to be effective in heterosexual couples with (1) cervical factor subfertility and (2) unexplained subfertility with a good prognosis, according to prognostic models such as the Hunault score.[22] Couples with an intermediate to good prognosis of a treatment-independent pregnancy may be encouraged with expectant management and to postpone IUI for a while.

It is essential to identify those couples that will benefit from IUI and those that will not; the exact cut-off point for the prognosis to treat or not to treat has not been assessed in a randomized clinical trial yet. Therefore randomized clinical trials on the effectiveness of IUI in heterosexual couples with a poor prognosis or male subfertility are needed.

INDICATIONS FOR INTRAUTERINE INSEMINATION WITH PARTNER SEMEN

Retrograde Ejaculation

Retrograde ejaculation is an uncommon cause of infertility. Retrograde ejaculation is due to a problem with the bladder muscle and can be caused by blood pressure and depression medications, urethral and prostate surgery, and nerve damage. Controversy exists in the literature concerning the best method of treating this disorder. The controversies involve the most appropriate method of obtaining the sperm, with proposals ranging from bladder catheterization to centrifugation of urine after orgasm.[23]

A postejaculatory urine specimen can be obtained after alkalinization of the urine using oral sodium bicarbonate. The postejaculatory urine specimen is suspended in medium, centrifuged, and resuspended before use for IUI, with good results.[24]

Cervical Factor Infertility

Cervical factor infertility is defined as a repeated negative postcoital test despite adequate timing and normal sperm parameters.

A Cochrane systematic review by Helmerhorst et al. concluded that IUI with or without COH is not an effective treatment of cervical factor infertility.[25] Although more recent studies were published on this subject, most clinicians no longer support performing postcoital testing as part of a fertility check-up. Therefore cervical factor is less often diagnosed. On the other hand, Steures et al. performed a randomized study in subfertile couples with an isolated cervical factor showing that the ongoing pregnancy rate was significantly higher when IUI was performed for 6 months when compared to expectant management for 6 months. The same group found that in case of a cervical factor, adding ovarian hyperstimulation does not improve pregnancy rates.[26]

Male Factor Infertility

Whether IUI can be used in case of male infertility is still under debate. One of the major problems in male subfertility is the lack of validated definitions and strict cut-off values of sperm parameters to make a clear distinction among mild, moderate, and severe male infertility. A Cochrane systematic review by Bensdorp et al. analyzed IUI (with or without COH) in patients with male infertility according to the WHO criteria.[27]

Because of the lack of a harmonized definition, all studies with various definitions of male infertility were included. It was concluded that there was insufficient evidence to recommend for or against IUI (with or without COH) in male infertility, mainly because large, high-quality randomized trials are lacking.[27] In a Cochrane review, Cohlen et al.[8] concluded that IUI is superior to timed intercourse both in natural cycles and in cycles with COH. According to this review, IUI in natural cycles should be the treatment of choice in cases of moderate to severe male subfertility, providing an IMC of more than 1 million can be obtained after sperm preparation.

Another systematic review and metaanalysis clearly reported on the lack of evidence for clear lower cut-off levels of sperm parameters in IUI treatment. Based on very low quality of evidence, a TMSC greater than 1 million and a morphology greater than 4% are of possible prognostic value, in such a case that below these cut-off levels, IUI should be withheld.[20] Van Waart et al. found the postwash TMSC to be predictive for nonpregnancy but the lower cut-off levels varied tremendously, between 0.8 and 5 million.[28]

According to the results of a large, randomized controlled trial (RCT) of Bensdorp et al.[9] IUI-COH is noninferior to IVF in heterosexual couples with mild male infertility, defined as a TMSC of 3 to 10 million. These findings are very encouraging in performing IUI as a first-line treatment in case of mild male infertility, although up till now, it is almost impossible to define clear lower cut-off levels of pre- or postwash sperm parameters below which IUI should not be performed.

Immunologic Male Infertility

In Western countries, the most important origin of ASAs is probably vasectomy. More than 80% of vasectomized males develop ASAs during the first year following their operation. In most cases, it concerns IgGs, which are considered to be less harmful. Nevertheless, even IgAs are frequently found in these males. Other clinical situations causing immunologic male infertility are torsion of the testis, varicocele, testicular trauma, and orchitis.[29]

The most obvious way ASAs are responsible for male infertility is by agglutination of the sperm cells after ejaculation. This results in lowering of their motility and their ability to penetrate the cervical mucus. If more than 50% of sperm are bound to antibodies,

reduced cervical mucus penetration can result. In particular, IgA antibodies are more harmful for fertilization than IgGs. Other mechanisms by which ASAs are interfering with conception are disturbances of sperm transport, disruptions in gamete interaction and zona binding, and penetration problems.[29]

The clinical significance of ASAs in male subfertility remains unclear, and the importance of circulating ASAs is probably low. However, most studies demonstrate a clear association between sperm surface antibodies and the fertility potential of the male. In 1997, we published a prospective study comparing the effectiveness of the first-line IUI approach versus IVF for male immunological subfertility.[30] In a prospective study, we compared success rates after two different treatment protocols, COH-IUI versus IVF. In this selected group of patients with longstanding subfertility due to sperm surface antibodies, both IUI and IVF yielded unexpectedly high pregnancy rates. Since a cost-benefit analysis comparing COH-IUI with IVF may favor a course of four IUI cycles, we concluded that IUI could be promoted as the first-line therapy in male immunological subfertility.

Nowadays, it is widely accepted that in severe cases of immunologic male infertility in which more than 80% of spermatozoa are antibody coated, ICSI has to be recommended.

Although most fertility centers use ICSI in case of immunological male subfertility, we believe that a well-organized prospective study is mandatory to examine the real value of IUI for this specific indication. The postwash TMSC or IMC may have a unique value as a prognostic tool since it reflects the motile sperm available for insemination.

Unexplained Infertility

If an infertility work-up fails to identify a plausible explanation for heterosexual couples with a history of subfertility of at least 1 year, we use the term "unexplained infertility." Because it is a diagnosis of exclusion and a good explanation for the subfertility is lacking, the treatment is often empiric and the reported prevalence varies widely.

Clinical management for unexplained infertility includes expectant management as well as active treatments such as COH, IUI, COH-IUI, and IVF, with or without ICSI.

In a 2020 Cochrane systematic review,[31] it was found that due to insufficient data, it remains uncertain whether treatment with IUI compared to timed intercourse with or without COH or expectant management with or without COH improves cumulative live birth rates (CLBRs) with acceptable multiple pregnancy rates in heterosexual couples with unexplained subfertility. On the other hand, IUI with COH probably results in a higher CLBR compared to expectant management without COH in heterosexual couples with a low prediction score of natural conception, according to prognostic models. Treatment with IUI in a stimulated cycle may result in a higher CLBR compared to treatment with IUI in a natural cycle.[31]

In a network metaanalysis, based on low to moderate quality of evidence, IUI with gonadotrophins ranked highest on live birth/ongoing pregnancy rates, taking into account an increased risk for multiple pregnancies.[32,33] By using a protocol with adherence to strict cancellation criteria, gonadotrophins seem to improve live birth/ongoing pregnancy rates, compared to clomiphene citrate (CC).

Minimal and Mild Endometriosis

Guidelines of the European Society of Human Reproduction and Embryology[34] state that IU treatment is only recommended in subfertile females with minimal-to-mild endometriosis. Werbrouck et al.[35] reported no difference in cycle pregnancy rate between females with surgically treated minimal to mild endometriosis and females with unexplained infertility after COH and IUI program. The CLBR within four cycles of IUI was also comparable in females with minimal endometriosis, mild endometriosis, and unexplained infertility. In patients with endometriosis American Fertility Society grade 1 or 2, the exact mechanism of declined fertility remains unknown. When adhesions are present, one can understand a declined pick-up mechanism, but when only small spots of endometriosis are present, an explanation is more difficult to give. It has been assumed that in cases of mild endometriosis, heterosexual couples should be treated as those with unexplained subfertility and that patients might benefit from IUI in combination with mild ovarian hyperstimulation. On the other hand, there is evidence that during laparoscopy, ablation of endometriotic lesions plus adhesiolysis is effective in enhancing spontaneous pregnancy compared to diagnostic DL alone.[36] In a retrospective matched cohort study, Cai et al.[37] recently showed that per-cycle pregnancy rate was comparable between females with unexplained infertility and females with endometrioma-associated subfertility and no other identifiable infertility factors.

Human Immunodeficiency Virus and Hepatitis C Virus in Discordant Couples

According to the Joint United Nations Program on HIV/AIDS, there were 37.7 million people living with acquired immunodeficiency syndrome in 2020, of whom over 80% were of childbearing age.[38] Couples including a human immunodeficiency virus (HIV)-infected male living with a noninfected female are strongly advised to use condoms during sexual intercourse to prevent of transmitting the infection, although the per-coital probability of HIV transmission is around 0.1%.[39] Obviously, this prevents the couple from having children, but IUI with washed sperm offers an opportunity for these heterosexual couples to safely start a family.

Various methods of sperm preparation are used for IUI in HIV-discordant couples, but most laboratories use the method first described by Semprini et al., which entails gradient centrifugation followed by a swim-up procedure.[40] In this study, 29 uninfected female partners were treated by IUI using prepared semen from their HIV-positive partners, with none of the females being HIV seroconverted.[40] In 2004, Englert et al. used this method of sperm preparation and found no viral load in the semen unless the blood viral load was greater than 10,000 copies/mL.[41] These early studies were subsequently repeated in many heterosexual couples, with satisfactory results. A metaanalysis of 11,585 assisted reproduction cycles (including IUI, IVF, and ICSI) in 3994 females found no single HIV transmission in the treated patients.[42] In addition, there were no cases of vertical transmission and all the infants born were HIV-negative.[42] The technique is also associated with acceptable clinical outcomes. In a recent study by Cavalho et al., 69 HIV-discordant couples were treated for 180 cycles with IUI using washed semen, resulting in 16 clinical pregnancies, a clinical pregnancy rate (CPR) of 9.0% per cycle and 23.2% per patient, with no seroconversion detected in the patients or the newborns.[43]

Similar results were reported in hepatitis C virus (HCV)-discordant couples. For example, in 2012, an Italian group treated 85 HCV-discordant couples with assisted reproduction, including 47 couples with IUI. The semen was prepared by the method of Semprini mentioned above. The CPR for IUI was similar to the rate reported by the Italian ART register, and no mother or baby was infected by HCV.[44] It seems therefore that sperm washing followed by IUI is a safe and effective treatment option for HIV- and HCV-serodiscordant couples wishing to conceive.

Sex Preselection

IUI has also been suggested and used for sex preselection after separating spermatozoa carrying an X chromosome from those carrying a Y chromosome. This was originally suggested as a method for the prevention of X-linked genetic diseases, although the method can also be used for so-called "family balancing." Various methods of sperm separation have been used. In 1991, Jaffe et al. retrospectively compared the gender outcome of pregnancies of 46 heterosexual couples who conceived spontaneously with 48 heterosexual couples who conceived secondary to an insemination with separated semen using serum albumin density separation gradient. They found that this method enriched the proportion of Y-bearing sperm.[45]

High-speed flow cytometry can also be used as a sperm-sorting method of gender selection. The method is based upon the detection of differential fluorescence emitted by fluorescently stained X and Y chromosome–bearing spermatozoa and results in shifting the 50:50 X:Y ratio in the unsorted spermatozoa to 90% X or 75% Y after sorting. The method was found to be safe and effective, with no increase in miscarriage rates or congenital anomalies in the offspring.[46] A simpler method of sperm sorting using the swim-up preparation method was described by Khatamee et al., who used the bottom 0.5 mL of the separated semen to inseminate patients desiring a female child and the top 0.5 mL for those wishing to have a male child. They found the method to be 86.7% effective in heterosexual couples seeking a female child (p = 0.002) and 89.2% effective in those seeking a male child (p = 0.0002) compared to controls.[47]

FACTORS INFLUENCING INTRAUTERINE INSEMINATION OUTCOME

Duration of Infertility

A few studies demonstrated that IUI is less effective with increasing duration of infertility,[48,49] but most studies did not reveal differences in pregnancy rate according to the duration of infertility.[50,51]

Male and Female Age

Female age is the most relevant predictor of the probability of pregnancy in IUI treatment. A sharp decline of IUI success rate is observed in females over the age of 40 years, presumably related to oocyte quality. The benefit of COH in IUI treatment remains unclear in older females. In addition to chronological age, ovarian reserve tests are of poor predictive value for nonpregnancy, suggesting that these tests may only be useful to exclude older females from treatment if levels are significantly abnormal, and the only effective treatment may be oocyte donation.[52]

Declining reproductive function with aging at the level of the testis has been proven in rodent models. In humans, effects of aging demonstrated a reduction in testicular volume only in the 8th decade of life. When analyzing the effect of male age on sperm analysis by motile sperm organelle morphology examination, a consistent decline in semen quality with increasing age was observed.[53]

Semen Quality and Oxidative Stress

Increasing evidence suggests that oxidative stress (OS) plays an important role in the etiology of male infertility. Male OS infertility has been proposed as a descriptor for infertile males with abnormal semen characteristics and OS, including many patients who were previously classified as having unexplained male infertility.[54] Actual treatment protocols for OS, including the use of antioxidants, have not yet been supported by randomized studies, as excessive use of antioxidants may lead to reductive stress, which may also be harmful.[55]

Sperm Preparation Techniques

Currently, there are three semen preparation techniques that are routinely used worldwide: a simple dilution and washing technique, a swim-up technique, and a density gradient centrifugation technique (Fig. 22.3). Whether one of these techniques is preferable was the subject of a Cochrane systematic review.[56] It was concluded that there is insufficient evidence to recommend any specific semen preparation technique. Considering the very low quality of evidence, they are uncertain whether there is a difference in CPRs, ongoing pregnancy rates, multiple pregnancy rates, or miscarriage rates per couple among the three sperm preparation techniques. Large, high-quality RCTs comparing the effectiveness of a gradient and/or a swim-up and/or wash and centrifugation

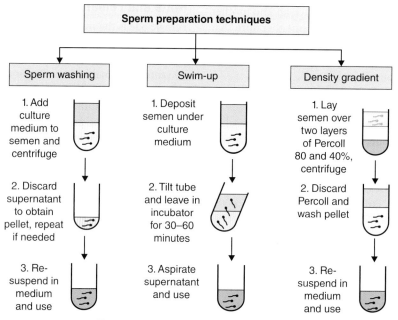

Fig. 22.3 Sperm Preparation Techniques.

technique on clinical outcome are lacking. Results from studies comparing semen parameters may suggest a preference for gradient technique, but firm conclusions cannot be drawn and the limitations should be taken into consideration. Further randomized trials that report live birth data are warranted.[56]

Ovarian Hyperstimulation or Natural Cycle

The rationale behind the use of ovarian hyperstimulation in artificial insemination is to increase of the number of oocytes available for fertilization and to correct subtle, unpredictable ovulatory dysfunction. Other advantages of superovulation with human menopausal gonadotropins are the enhanced opportunity for oocyte capture, fertilization, and implantation.

Cohlen et al.[57] conducted an RCT comparing IUI with or without OS in male infertility. In heterosexual couples with a TMSC less than 10 million, COH did not improve pregnancy outcome, while it did in couples with a TMSC greater than 10 million. It was concluded that, in male subfertility cases, ovarian stimulation only improved the success rate in moderate cases (IMC >10 million).

Ten years later, and according to a systematic review of Cohlen et al.[58] and based on reasonable evidence, it was concluded that (1) in couples with unexplained infertility with a prognosis of becoming pregnant without assistance within the next 12 months (estimate >30%), IUI could be postponed for at least 6 months, (2) in couples with unexplained infertility and males with a TMSC above 10 million, IUI should be combined with OS to improve live birth rates, and (3) in couples with unexplained infertility and males with a TMSC greater than 10 million and a prognosis of spontaneous pregnancy < 30% within a year, it is recommended that IUI plus OS are the treatments of first choice.

To prevent high rates of multiple gestation pregnancies in IUI-COH, IUI should be withheld when more than two dominant follicles greater than 15 mm or more than 5 follicles greater than 10 mm at the time of human chorionic gonadotropin (hCG) injection or surge are present.[58] Starting dose with gonadotrophins should be 75 IU because higher doses have similar pregnancy rates but increase multiple pregnancy rates. Clomiphene citrate and tamoxifen are acceptable alternatives to low-dose gonadotrophins, although at a lower live birth rate than with gonadotrophins.[58]

Luteal Phase Support

Luteal phase is the important period of the menstrual cycle in which embryonic implantation occurs. A good quality luteal phase is characterized by an adequate progesterone secretion from the corpus luteum and endometrial secretory transformation. Optimum follicular development followed by adequate LH surge for ovulation and persistent LH secretion are required for adequate luteal phase function. Any factors altering the follicular and hormonal dynamics may have a deleterious effect on luteal phase functions. The supraphysiological hormonal environment caused by COH for multiple follicular development may influence corpus luteum function and endometrial receptivity for implantation. In a prospective randomized study, Erdem et al.[59] demonstrated that luteal phase support with progesterone gel increases live birth rates in IUI cycles mildly stimulated with recombinant gonadotropins. In another prospective randomized study, luteal phase support with vaginal progesterone affected the success of gonadotropin-stimulated IUI cycles with multifollicular response but not with monofollicular response.[60] The results of the one RCT do not show any benefit of luteal phase support with vaginal progesterone to improve pregnancy rates in CC-stimulated IUI cycles of normoovulatory females.[61] The effectiveness of luteal support in gonadotropin IUI cycles is well documented in heterosexual couples with unexplained subfertility; there are yet no data in the subgroup of mild male factor infertility. Further studies are needed for different progesterone forms and doses, different routes of administration, and the necessity to continue supplementation after pregnancy occurs.

Lifestyle

Awareness and recognition of the possible impact of lifestyle factors are important among heterosexual couples seeking conception. Smoking and body mass index (BMI) are the most examined lifestyle factors influencing success rates after assisted reproduction. In a prospective cohort study, Huyghe et al.[62] examined the influence of smoking and BMI in 1401 IUI cycles with partner semen, primary outcome being CPR. Multivariate analysis through generalized estimating equations (GEE) could not confirm a significant influence of female BMI on fecundity. For smoking, univariate statistical analysis revealed male smoking to be a negative influence for the CPR (10.9% CPR in couples with male nonsmokers vs. 5.9% with male partners smoking 1–14 cigarettes/day, p = 0.017). After multivariate GEE analysis, this result remained significant. They also found a trend to a decreased CPR with both partners being smokers compared to the group where both partners are nonsmokers. A detrimental effect of smoking on sperm parameters is based on the biological finding that smoking increases the presence of reactive oxygen species, thereby resulting in OS, though the complete effect of smoking on fertility remains inconclusive.[63]

Site of Insemination

Artificial inseminations can be intravaginal, intracervical, pericervical using a cap, intrauterine, transcervical intrafallopian, or intraperitoneal. Most studies refer to IUI, which seems to be an easy and better way of treatment. Studies comparing pregnancy outcome after IUI versus cervical cap insemination and transuterotubal insemination favored the intrauterine method.[64]

Timing and Number of Intrauterine Insemination Cycles

Exact timing is probably crucial in IUI treatment cycles. On the other hand, conflicting data on which methodology is to be used are reported in the literature. Ultrasound and hormonal monitoring with hCG induction probably allows the most exact timing but is relatively expensive and time consuming. Urinary LH-timed IUI is commonly used but has the disadvantage that the LH surge can last for up to 2 days before ovulation in some patients.

There is no evidence to recommend one or another method of triggering in IUI stimulated with gonadotrophins, and the same counts for timing IUI in natural cycles.[58] If an hCG injection is used, single IUI can be performed any time between 24 and 40 hours after hCG injection without compromising pregnancy rates. When using a natural cycle, IUI should be performed 1 day after LH rise.

Theoretically, improved chances for conception may be expected when two consecutive inseminations are performed since ovulation of oocytes does not occur in a synchronized pattern, but rather in waves of release after hCG administration. Another appeal to double IUI is the attrition phenomenon by which IUI bypasses the cervical mucus. In the natural cycle, the cervical mucus acts as a reservoir for sperm at midcycle, and a single IUI might miss later released cohorts of oocytes. According to a metaanalysis and structured review, there is no clear benefit in the overall CPR in heterosexual couples with unexplained infertility, and the available evidence regarding the use of double IUI in couples with male factor infertility is fragmentary and weak, although there may be a trend towards higher pregnancy rates when the number of IUIs per cycle is increased.[65,66]

In a recent Cochrane review, it was concluded that due to low quality evidence, it remains uncertain if double IUI improves live birth and reduces miscarriage compared to single IUI. Clinical pregnancy rate may increase in the double IUI group, but this should be interpreted with caution due to the low quality evidence.[67]

Immobilization after Intrauterine Insemination

Studies on the intrauterine behavior of spermatozoa have shown that spermatozoa already reach the fallopian tubes within 5 to 10 minutes after insemination.[68] After vaginal intercourse, a large percentage of the semen is lost by "flowback," and no more than 1% of the spermatozoa are retained in the female reproductive tract. An assumed hypothesis is that immobilization in the supine position after IUI could prevent direct loss of a large percentage of the spermatozoa and that this action will improve fertility outcomes. A systematic search resulted in the identification of two relevant articles. Saleh et al.[69] randomized 95 heterosexual couples to either direct mobilization after IUI or immobilization in the supine position for 10 minutes. After three cycles, pregnancy rates per couple were significantly higher in the immobilization group. Custers et al. performed a well-designed RCT in 391 heterosexual couples. Live birth rates after three cycles were significantly higher in the immobilization group.[70] In a follow-up study, the same authors compared the long-term effectiveness of immobilization subsequent to IUI. They confirmed a persistent significant difference in ongoing pregnancy rates in favor of immobilization.[71]

The Effect of the Abstinence Period

Prolonged abstinence time increases ejaculate volume, sperm count, sperm concentration, and total number of motile spermatozoa, although the effect on sperm concentration is only small for oligozoospermic males. In a prospective study we performed in Genk, abstinence did not influence pH, viability, morphology, total or grade A motility, or sperm DNA fragmentation. A short (24-hour) abstinence period negatively influenced chromatin quality.[72] It seems that looking for the optimal time of abstinence is not very important in IUI programs and is probably only valuable in selected male subfertility cases.

Human Papilloma Virus

Although HPV infection is one of the most common viral infections worldwide, it is almost exclusively linked with the pathogenesis of cancer. More recent studies have shown that male and couple subfertility may result from an HPV virion producing infection in one or both of the partners. A significant negative effect of HPV positivity in males and/or females is observed on CPRs following IUI.[73] In a prospective multicenter study, it was shown that females inseminated with HPV-positive sperm had four times fewer clinical pregnancies compared with females who had HPV-negative partners. If an increased DNA fragmentation index greater than 26% is associated with HPV positivity in semen, the pregnancy rate can be expected to be very low or even zero.[74] Detection of HPV virions in sperm is associated with a negative IUI outcome and should be part of routine examination and counseling of infertile couples. Therefore HPV-positive males should not receive IUI as a first-line treatment and a waiting period of 6 months can be recommended, as HPV is a transient infection, clearing spontaneously within 6 to 12 months in most cases.[75]

Insemination Technique

Lavie et al.[76] compared the results after IUI using two different catheters. Although one catheter was significantly less traumatic (objectified by ultrasound), only a trend towards increase in the chance of conception was found. According to the results of another prospective randomized study comparing two different catheters, the catheter type does not affect the outcome after IUI.[77]

The preceding reports showed that SRI might improve the pregnancy rate compared to bolus IUI. The rationale underlying SRI is that the inseminated motile spermatozoa are released into the uterus during an extended period of time, with fewer spermatozoa expelled through the fallopian tube into the peritoneum.

In a randomized crossover study with a Grasby-type MS16 pump for 3 hours, the CPR per cycle and cumulative pregnancy rate after 4 cycles improved from 6.1% to 22% and from 15.0% to 63.1%, respectively.[78] The authors hypothesized that the period of potential fertilization might increase by injecting a persistent low concentration of spermatozoa.

Marschalek et al.[79] published data from two pilot randomized controlled crossover studies, indicating a statistically significant advantage of SRI over conventional bolus IUI. To perform the slow-release injection, they used a disposable EVIE syringe pump and a customized HSG catheter with an inflatable anchor balloon at the tip.

Moreover, results of a multicenter RCT comparing bolus IUI with SRI with a duration of 4 hours were recently reported by the same authors, using the same EVIE device.[80] Pregnancy rates following SRI and IUI showed a nonsignificant difference of 13.2% and 10.0%, respectively. In a subgroup of females aged less than 35 years, the pregnancy rate with SRI was 17% compared to 7% with bolus IUI, a significant difference. These results support the hypothesis that pregnancy rates might be improved with SRI compared to bolus IUI, especially in females aged less than 35 years.

In a prospective cohort study, we recently found that the application of modified slow release of processed semen appears to significantly increase the CPR from 9.0% to 13.5 % per cycle after IUI with homologous semen.[81] In this study, a slow release sperm injection of at least 45 to 60 seconds was compared to a bolus injection of less than 10 seconds.

PERINATAL OUTCOME AFTER INTRAUTERINE INSEMINATION/ PREVENTION OF MULTIPLE PREGNANCIES

Only a few papers have been published reporting the obstetric and perinatal outcome after IUI. According to Nuojua-Huttunen[82] and using the data obtained from the Finnish Medical Birth Register, IUI treatment did not increase obstetric or perinatal risks compared with matched spontaneous or IVF pregnancies. On the other hand, Wang et al.[83] examined preterm birth in 1015 IUI/ artificial insemination by donor (AID) singleton births compared to 1019 IVF/ICSI and 1019 naturally conceived births. Singleton IUI/AID births were about 1.5 times more likely to be born preterm than naturally conceived singletons, whereas the IVF/ICSI group were 2.4 times more likely to be born preterm than the naturally conceived group. In a retrospective cohort study, Gaudoin et al.[84] described a poorer perinatal outcome of singletons born to subfertile mothers conceived

through COH-IUI compared to matched natural conceptions within the Scottish national cohort. This was caused by a higher incidence of prematurity and low birth weight infants. In Belgium, we also performed a study to investigate differences in perinatal outcome of singleton and twin pregnancies after COH, with or without artificial insemination, compared to pregnancies after natural conception.[85] We used the data from the regional registry of 661,065 births in Flanders (Belgium) during the period 1993 to 2003. Control subjects were matched for maternal age, parity, fetal sex, and place and year of birth. We found a significantly higher incidence of extreme prematurity (<32 weeks), very low birth weight (<1500 grams), stillbirths, and perinatal death for COH/artificial insemination singletons compared to naturally conceived singletons. In a following study, we studied a population-based cohort study with three exposure groups: a study group of pregnancies (1) after ovarian stimulation, with or without artificial insemination, (2) after IFV or ICSI, and (3) a naturally conceived comparison group. Data from the regional registry of all hospital deliveries in the Dutch-speaking part of Belgium during an 18-year period from January 1993 until December 2010 were used.[86] IVF/ICSI singletons had a significantly worse outcome when compared to ovarian stimulation and natural conception for almost all investigated perinatal parameters. Non-IVF/ovarian stimulation singletons were also significantly disadvantaged for prematurity and low birthweight when compared to natural conception. It seemed that all ART pregnancies, whether due to IVF/ ICSI or non-IVF treatment, have to be considered as risk pregnancies. According to a Danish national cohort study (2007–2012 data), singletons born after IUI had higher risk of adverse perinatal outcomes compared with naturally conceived. Stimulation with CC was associated with a higher risk of small for gestational age infants compared with natural cycle IUI, but follicle-stimulating hormone treatment did not seem to be associated with adverse outcomes.[87]

COST EFFECTIVENESS OF INTRAUTERINE INSEMINATION

The goal of research on cost effectiveness is to maximize health outcomes with a minimum use of resources. As costs linked to fertility care in many countries are not covered by government or insurance companies, the relative cost effectiveness of fertility treatments is a very important consideration.[88] Previous large cohort or randomized studies from individual centers have found IUI alone or IUI-COH to be the most cost-effective first-line therapy for heterosexual couples with infertility related to cervical factor, endometriosis, unexplained infertility, and relatively mild male factor infertility,[89,90] but the retrospective designs make it difficult to draw firm conclusions. Moolenaar et al.[91] studied the cost effectiveness of interventions for male infertility according to the TMSC. A computer-simulated cohort of infertile females with a partner with a prewash TMSC of 0 to 10 million was investigated. They compared IUI with and without COH, conventional IVF, and IVF/ICSI. Live birth rate was the main outcome parameter. Study results showed that above a prewash TMSC of 3 million, IUI is less costly than conventional IVF, and below a prewash TMSC of 3 million, IVF/ICSI is less costly. Another multicenter RCT from Scotland compared the outcomes of 6 months of natural cycle IUI, CC stimulation followed by normal intercourse, and expectant management in couples with 2 years of unexplained infertility.[92] Live birth rates were not significantly different. The authors recommended that IUI-OS should be the subject of future trials for unexplained infertility.

Most of the large retrospective cohort studies on cost effectiveness tend to become "dated," as both costs and outcomes change over time. It is well known that IVF CPRs have increased steadily over time and high-order multiple births have declined as there has been increased emphasis on the value of transferring fewer embryos. These changes have made conventional IVF a more attractive option from a cost-effective point of view compared to IUI or IUI-COH. Reindollar et al.[93] addressed the important issue of time to pregnancy, both to alleviate the suffering and disappointment of infertile couples and to avoid the negative effects of aging on their reproductive potential. Only females with unexplained infertility and a normal ovarian reserve were included in the study. Cost effectiveness was calculated by summing all insurance charges divided by the number of females having at least one live birth. Out-of-pocket expenses (indirect costs) to the patient and the cost of multiple gestations as well as their associated increased hospital perinatal costs were included in the analysis. They concluded that CC-IUI seems to be the best first-line therapy for couples with unexplained infertility and, if not pregnant after three cycles, moving

directly to conventional IVF was the most cost-effective approach.[93] In a multicenter randomized noninferiority trial in the Netherlands, the effectiveness of IVF with single embryo transfer or IVF in a modified natural cycle was compared with the effectiveness of IUI-OS, with an outcome indicator of a healthy live birth.[9] They showed that IUI-COH was the most cost-effective strategy for heterosexual couples with mild male factor or unexplained infertility with a poor prognosis of becoming pregnant with expectant management. In another cost-effectiveness study on the same cohort of participants and investigating direct healthcare costs, it was concluded that both IVF strategies were significantly more expensive compared with IUI-COH, without being significantly more effective.[10] Therefore IUI-COH is recommended as the initial treatment for mild male factor and unexplained infertility. Unfortunately, there are no strict criteria for how to define mild male factor. Bensdorp et al.[9] used a TMSC of between 3 and 10 million, although Cohlen et al.[57] showed that OS was only effective in couples with a TMSC above 10 million, which they defined as mild male infertility. Clear definitions of mild or moderate male infertility should be established before randomized trials can be started to define lower threshold levels of sperm parameters below which IUI with or without COH is no longer cost effective and IVF or IVF/ICSI should be the first-line treatment option.

Bordewijk et al.[94] performed an economic evaluation of ovulation induction with gonadotrophins compared with CC with or without IUI in a two-by-two factorial multicenter RCT in normogonadotropic anovulatory females not pregnant after six ovulatory cycles with CC. Gonadotrophins are more effective but more expensive than CC; therefore the use of gonadotrophins depends on society's willingness to pay for an additional child.

Recommendations for the Future

In the selection of couples to be treated with IUI or IVF/ICSI, it would be interesting to establish cut-off values of semen parameters above which IUI is a real alternative for IVF/ICSI in male subfertility. According to the actual literature, IMC and sperm morphology are the most valuable sperm parameters to predict IUI outcome.[95] A trend towards increasing conception rates with increasing IMC was reported, but the cut-off value above which IUI seems to be successful varies between 0.3 and 20 million. In a large number of studies,

5% normal forms and 1 million motile spermatozoa after sperm preparation are believed to be potential cut-off values to select couples for IUI treatment. More well-organized prospective studies are needed to establish the best cut-off values of sperm parameters below which IUI is not the optimal first-line treatment.

A better patient selection and some changes in the techniques of IUI have to be implemented if we want to justify IUI, considering the increase of success rate observed with IVF and IVF-related techniques.

SUMMARY

IUI should be promoted as the best first-line treatment in most cases of subfertility, provided at least one tube is patent and an IMC after sperm preparation of more than 1 million can be obtained. In this select group of patients, it is unwise to start with ARTs such as IVF and ICSI since these techniques are more invasive and less cost effective. The future of IUI will depend on our ability to maintain the multiple pregnancy rates at an acceptable level, and this will undoubtedly be the most important challenge in the near future. If the multiple pregnancy rate after artificial insemination is comparable to or lower than the multiple pregnancy rate after IVF, IUI with or without ovarian hyperstimulation should be used for most subfertile heterosexual couples and not only for heterosexual couples on a waiting list for IVF. Promoting IVF and ICSI to result in pregnancy "as quick as possible" ignores the advantages of artificial insemination completely.

REFERENCES

1. Ombelet W, Van Robays J. Artificial insemination history: hurdles and milestones. *Facts Views Vis Obgyn.* 2015;7(2): 137-143.
2. Guttmacher AF. The role of artificial insemination in the treatment of human sterility. *Bull N Y Acad Med.* 1943;19: 573-591.
3. Kohlberg K. Artificial insemination and the physician. *Dtsch Med Wochenschr.* 1953;78:855-856.
4. Steptoe PC, Edwards RG. Birth after the reimplantation of a human embryo. *Lancet.* 1978;2(8085):366. doi:10.1016/s0140-6736(78)92957-4.
5. Kerin JF, Kirby C, Peek J, et al. Improved conception rate after intrauterine insemination of washed spermatozoa from men with poor quality semen. *Lancet.* 1984;1(8376):533-535. doi:10.1016/s0140-6736(84)90932-2.
6. Sunde A, Kahn JA, Molne K. Intrauterine insemination: a European collaborative report. *Hum Reprod.* 1988;3 suppl 2:69-73. doi:10.1093/humrep/3.suppl_2.69.
7. te Velde ER, van Kooy RJ, Waterreus JJ. Intrauterine insemination of washed husband's spermatozoa: a controlled study. *Fertil Steril.* 1989;51(1):182-185. doi:10.1016/s0015-0282(16)60453-3.
8. Cohlen BJ, Vandekerckhove P, te Velde ER, Habbema JD. Timed intercourse versus intra-uterine insemination with or without ovarian hyperstimulation for subfertility in men. *Cochrane Database Syst Rev.* 2000;(2):CD000360. doi:10.1002/14651858.CD000360.
9. Bensdorp AJ, Tjon-Kon-Fat RI, Bossuyt PM, et al. Prevention of multiple pregnancies in couples with unexplained or mild male subfertility: randomised controlled trial of in vitro fertilisation with single embryo transfer or in vitro fertilisation in modified natural cycle compared with intrauterine insemination with controlled ovarian hyperstimulation. *BMJ.* 2015;350:g7771.
10. Tjon-Kon-Fat RI, Bensdorp AJ, Bossuyt PM, et al. Is IVF-served two different ways-more cost-effective than IUI with controlled ovarian hyperstimulation? *Hum Reprod.* 2015;30(10):2331-2339. doi:10.1093/humrep/dev193.
11. Ombelet W, Cooke I, Dyer S, Serour G, Devroey P. Infertility and the provision of infertility medical services in developing countries. *Hum Reprod Update.* 2008;14(6):605-621. doi:10.1093/humupd/dmn042.
12. Ombelet W, van Eekelen R, McNally A, Ledger W, Doody K, Farquhar C. Should couples with unexplained infertility have three to six cycles of intrauterine insemination with ovarian stimulation or in vitro fertilization as first-line treatment? *Fertil Steril.* 2020;114(6):1141-1148. doi:10.1016/j.fertnstert.2020.10.029.
13. Pont JC, Patrat C, Fauque P, Camp ML, Gayet V, Wolf JP. Pre-washing catheter dramatically improves the post intrauterine insemination pregnancy rate. *Gynecol Obstet Fertil.* 2012;40(6):356-359. doi:10.1016/j.gyobfe.2012.02.002.
14. Marschalek J, Egarter C, Vytiska-Binsdorfer E, et al. Pregnancy rates after slow-release insemination (SRI) and standard bolus intrauterine insemination (IUI) - a multicentre randomised, controlled trial. *Sci Rep.* 2020;10:7719. doi:10.1038/s41598-020-64164-4.
15. Ombelet W, Van der Auwera I, Bijnens H, et al. Improving IUI success by performing modified slow-release insemination and a patient-centred approach in an insemination programme with partner semen: a prospective cohort study. *Facts Views Vis Obgyn.* 2021;13(4):359-367. doi:10.52054/FVVO.13.4.045.
16. Gordts S, Gordts S, Puttemans P, Segaert I, Valkenburg M, Campo R. Systematic use of transvaginal hydrolaparoscopy as a minimally invasive procedure in the

exploration of the infertile patient: results and reflections. *Facts Views Vis Obgyn.* 2021;13(2):131-140. doi:10.52054/FVVO.13.2.014.

17. Cooper TG, Noonan E, von Eckardstein S, et al. World Health Organization reference values for human semen characteristics. *Hum Reprod Update.* 2010;16:231-245. doi:10.1093/humupd/dmp048.

18. Esteves SC, Zini A, Aziz N, et al. Critical appraisal of World Health Organization's new reference values for human semen characteristics and effect on diagnosis and treatment of subfertile men. *Urology.* 2012;79(1):16-22. doi:10.1016/j.urology.2011.08.003.

19. Hamilton JA, Cissen M, Brandes M, et al. Total motile sperm count: a better indicator for the severity of male factor infertility than the WHO sperm classification system. *Hum Reprod.* 2015;30(5):1110-1121. doi:10.1093/humrep/dev058.

20. Ombelet W, Dhont N, Thijssen A, Bosmans E, Kruger T. Semen quality and prediction of IUI success in male subfertility: a systematic review. *Reprod Biomed Online.* 2014;28(3):300-309. doi:10.1016/j.rbmo.2013.10.023.

21. Zollner U, Zollner KP, Dietl J, Steck T. Semen sample collection in medium enhances the implantation rate following ICSI in patients with severe oligoasthenoteratozoospermia. *Hum Reprod.* 2001;16(6):1110-1114. doi:10.1093/humrep/16.6.1110.

22. Hunault CC, Habbema JD, Eijkemans MJ, Collins JA, Evers JL, te Velde ER. Two new prediction rules for spontaneous pregnancy leading to live birth among subfertile couples, based on the synthesis of three previous models. *Hum Reprod.* 2004;19(9):2019-2026. doi:10.1093/humrep/deh365.

23. Shangold GA, Cantor B, Schreiber JR. Treatment of infertility due to retrograde ejaculation: a simple, cost-effective method. *Fertil Steril.* 1990;54(1):175-177. doi:10.1016/s0015-0282(16)53660-7.

24. Jefferys A, Siassakos D, Wardle P. The management of retrograde ejaculation: a systematic review and update. *Fertil Steril.* 2012;97(2):306-312. doi:10.1016/j.fertnstert.2011.11.019.

25. Helmerhorst FM, Van Vliet HA, Gornas T, Finken MJ, Grimes DA. Intra-uterine insemination versus timed intercourse for cervical hostility in subfertile couples. *Cochrane Database Syst Rev.* 2005;2005(4):CD002809. doi:10.1002/14651858.CD002809.pub2.

26. Steures P, van der Steeg JW, Hompes PG, et al. Effectiveness of intrauterine insemination in subfertile couples with an isolated cervical factor: a randomized clinical trial. *Fertil Steril.* 2007;88(6):1692-1696. doi:10.1016/j.fertnstert.2007.01.124.

27. Bensdorp AJ, Cohlen BJ, Heineman MJ, Vandekerckhove P. Intra-uterine insemination for male subfertility.

Cochrane Database Syst Rev. 2007;(4):CD000360. doi:10.1002/14651858.CD000360.pub4.

28. Van Waart J, Kruger TF, Lombard CJ, Ombelet W. Predictive value of normal sperm morphology in intrauterine insemination (IUI): a structured literature review. *Hum Reprod Update.* 2001;7(5):495-500. doi:10.1093/humupd/7.5.495.

29. Gupta S, Sharma R, Agarwal A, et al. Antisperm antibody testing: a comprehensive review of its role in the management of immunological male infertility and results of a global survey of clinical practices. *World J Mens Health.* 2022;40(3):380-398. doi:10.5534/wjmh.210164.

30. Ombelet W, Vandeput H, Janssen M, et al. Treatment of male infertility due to sperm surface antibodies: IUI or IVF? *Hum Reprod.* 1997;12(6):1165-1170. doi:10.1093/humrep/12.6.1165.

31. Ayeleke RO, Asseler JD, Cohlen BJ, Veltman-Verhulst SM. Intra-uterine insemination for unexplained subfertility. *Cochrane Database Syst Rev.* 2020;3(3):CD001838. doi:10.1002/14651858.CD001838.pub6.

32. Wang R, Danhof NA, Tjon-Kon-Fat RI, et al. Interventions for unexplained infertility: a systematic review and network meta-analysis. *Cochrane Database Syst Rev.* 2019;9(9):CD012692. doi:10.1002/14651858.CD012692.pub2.

33. Danhof NA, Wang R, van Wely M, et al. IUI for unexplained infertility-a network meta-analysis. *Hum Reprod Update.* 2020;26(1):1-15. doi:10.1093/humupd/dmz035.

34. Dunselman GA, Vermeulen N, Becker C, et al. ESHRE guideline: management of women with endometriosis. *Hum Reprod.* 2014;29(3):400-412. doi:10.1093/humrep/det457.

35. Werbrouck E, Spiessens C, Meuleman C, D'Hooghe T. No difference in cycle pregnancy rate and in cumulative live-birth rate between women with surgically treated minimal to mild endometriosis and women with unexplained infertility after controlled ovarian hyperstimulation and intrauterine insemination. *Fertil Steril.* 2006;86(3):566-571. doi:10.1016/j.fertnstert.2006.01.044.

36. Marcoux S, Maheux R, Bérubé S. Laparoscopic surgery in infertile women with minimal or mild endometriosis. Canadian Collaborative Group on Endometriosis. *N Engl J Med.* 1997;337(4):217-222. doi:10.1056/NEJM199707243370401.

37. Cai H, Xie J, Shi J, Wang H. Efficacy of intrauterine insemination in women with endometrioma-associated subfertility: analysis using propensity score matching. *BMC Pregnancy Childbirth.* 2022;22(1):12. doi:10.1186/s12884-021-04342-y.

38. Joint United Nations Programme on HIV/AIDS (UNAIDS). *Fact Sheet; 2021 Statistics.* Available at: http://www.unaids.org/en/resources/campaigns/HowAIDSchangedeverything/factsheet.

39. Baeten JM, Overbaugh J. Measuring the infectiousness of persons with HIV-1: opportunities for preventing sexual HIV-1 transmission. *Curr HIV Res.* 2003;1:69-86. doi:10.2174/1570162033352110.

40. Semprini AE, Levi-Setti P, Bozzo M, et al. Insemination of HIV-negative women with processed semen of HIV-positive partners. *Lancet.* 1992;340:1317-1319. doi:10.1016/0140-6736(92)92495-2.

41. Englert Y, Lesage B, Van Vooren JP, et al. Medically assisted reproduction in the presence of chronic viral diseases. *Hum Reprod Update.* 2004;10(2):149-162. doi:10.1093/humupd/dmh013.

42. Zafer M, Horvath H, Mmeje O, et al. Effectiveness of semen washing to prevent human immunodeficiency virus (HIV) transmission and assist pregnancy in HIV-discordant couples: a systematic review and meta-analysis. *Fertil Steril.* 2016;105(3):645-655. doi:10.1016/j.fertnstert.2015.11.028.

43. Carvalho WAP, Catafesta E, Rodart IF, Takata S, Estevam DL, Barbosa CP. Prevention of HIV transmission with sperm washing within fertile serodiscordant couples undergoing non-stimulated intrauterine insemination. *AIDS Care.* 2021;33(4):478-485. doi:10.1080/09540121.2020.1739201.

44. Savasi V, Parrilla B, Ratti M, Oneta M, Clerici M, Ferrazzi E. Hepatitis C virus RNA detection in different semen fractions of HCV/HIV-1 co-infected men by nested PCR. *Eur J Obstet Gynecol Reprod Biol.* 2010;151(1):52-55. doi:10.1016/j.ejogrb.2010.03.011.

45. Jaffe SB, Jewelewicz R, Wahl E, Khatamee MA. A controlled study for gender selection. *Fertil Steril.* 1991;56(2):254-258. doi:10.1016/s0015-0282(16)54481-1.

46. Schulman D, Karabinus DS. Scientific aspects of preconception gender selection. *Reprod Biomed Online.* 2005;10 suppl 1:111-115. doi:10.1016/s1472-6483(10)62217-1.

47. Khatamee MA, Horn SR, Weseley A, Farooq T, Jaffe SB, Jewelewicz R. A controlled study for gender selection using swim-up separation. *Gynecol Obstet Invest.* 1999;48(1):7-13. doi:10.1159/000010125.

48. Tomlinson MJ, Amissah-Arthur JB, Thompson KA, Kasraie JL, Bentick B. Prognostic indicators for intrauterine insemination (IUI): statistical model for IUI success. *Hum Reprod.* 1996;11(9):1892-1896. doi:10.1093/oxfordjournals.humrep.a019513.

49. Kamath MS, Bhave P, Aleyamma T, et al. Predictive factors for pregnancy after intrauterine insemination: a prospective study of factors affecting outcome. *J Hum Reprod Sci.* 2010;3(3):129-134. doi:10.4103/0974-1208.74154.

50. Merviel P, Heraud MH, Grenier N, Lourdel E, Sanguinet P, Copin H. Predictive factors for pregnancy after intrauterine insemination (IUI): an analysis of 1038 cycles and a review of the literature. *Fertil Steril.* 2010;93(1):79-88. doi:10.1016/j.fertnstert.2008.09.058.

51. Immediata V, Patrizio P, Parisen Toldin MR, et al. Twenty-one year experience with intrauterine inseminations after controlled ovarian stimulation with gonadotropins: maternal age is the only prognostic factor for success. *J Assist Reprod Genet.* 2020;37(5):1195-1201. doi:10.1007/s10815-020-01752-3.

52. Broekmans FJ, Soules MR, Fauser BC. Ovarian aging: mechanisms and clinical consequences. *Endocr Rev.* 2009;30(5):465-493. doi:10.1210/er.2009-0006.

53. Akl LD, Oliveira JB, Petersen CG, et al. Efficacy of the motile sperm organelle morphology examination (MSOME) in predicting pregnancy after intrauterine insemination. *Reprod Biol Endocrinol.* 2011;9:120. doi:10.1186/1477-7827-9-120.

54. Agarwal A, Parekh N, Panner Selvam MK, et al. Male oxidative stress infertility (MOSI): proposed terminology and clinical practice guidelines for management of idiopathic male infertility. *World J Mens Health.* 2019;37(3):296-312. doi:10.5534/wjmh.190055.

55. Panner Selvam MK, Agarwal A, Henkel R, et al. The effect of oxidative and reductive stress on semen parameters and functions of physiologically normal human spermatozoa. *Free Radic Biol Med.* 2020;152:375-385. doi:10.1016/j.freeradbiomed.2020.03.008.

56. Boomsma CM, Cohlen BJ, Farquhar C. Semen preparation techniques for intrauterine insemination. *Cochrane Database Syst Rev.* 2019;10(10):CD004507. doi:10.1002/14651858.CD004507.pub4.

57. Cohlen BJ, te Velde ER, van Kooij RJ, Looman CW, Habbema JD. Controlled ovarian hyperstimulation and intrauterine insemination for treating male subfertility: a controlled study. *Hum Reprod.* 1998;13(6):1553-1558. doi:10.1093/humrep/13.6.1553.

58. Cohlen BJ, Bijkerk A, Van der Poel S, Ombelet W. IUI: review and systematic assessment of the evidence that supports global recommendations. *Hum Reprod Update.* 2018;24(3):300-319. doi:10.1093/humupd/dmx041.

59. Erdem A, Erdem M, Atmaca S, Guler I. Impact of luteal phase support on pregnancy rates in intrauterine insemination cycles: a prospective randomized study. *Fertil Steril.* 2009;91(6):2508-2513. doi:10.1016/j.fertnstert.2008.04.029.

60. Seckin B, Turkcapar F, Yildiz Y, Senturk B, Yilmaz N, Gulerman C. Effect of luteal phase support with vaginal progesterone in intrauterine insemination cycles with regard to follicular response: a prospective randomized study. *J Reprod Med.* 2014;59(5-6):260-266.

61. Kyrou D, Fatemi HM, Tournaye H, Devroey P. Luteal phase support in normo-ovulatory women stimulated with clomiphene citrate for intrauterine insemination:

need or habit? *Hum Reprod.* 2010;25(10):2501-2506. doi:10.1093/humrep/deq223.

62. Huyghe S, Verest A, Thijssen A, Ombelet W. Influence of BMI and smoking on IUI outcome with partner and donor sperm. *Facts Views Vis Obgyn.* 2017;9(2):93-100.

63. Harlev A, Agarwal A, Ozgur Gunes S, et al. Smoking and male infertility: an evidence-based review. *World J Mens Health.* 2015;33:143-160. doi:10.5534/wjmh.2015.33.3.143.

64. Guzick DS, Carson SA, Coutifaris C, et al. Efficacy of superovulation and intrauterine insemination in the treatment of infertility. National Cooperative Reproductive Medicine Network. *N Engl J Med.* 1999;340(3):177-183. doi:10.1056/NEJM199901213400302.

65. Zavos A, Daponte A, Garas A, et al. Double versus single homologous intrauterine insemination for male factor infertility: a systematic review and meta-analysis. *Asian J Androl.* 2013;15(4):533-538. doi:10.1038/aja.2013.4.

66. Polyzos NP, Tzioras S, Mauri D, Tatsioni A. Double versus single intrauterine insemination for unexplained infertility: a meta-analysis of randomized trials. *Fertil Steril.* 2010;94(4):1261-1266. doi:10.1016/j.fertnstert.2009.06.052.

67. Rakic L, Kostova E, Cohlen BJ, Cantineau AE. Double versus single intrauterine insemination (IUI) in stimulated cycles for subfertile couples. *Cochrane Database Syst Rev.* 2021;7(7):CD003854. doi:10.1002/14651858.CD003854.pub2.

68. Suarez SS, Pacey AA. Sperm transport in the female reproductive tract. *Hum Reprod Update.* 2006;12(1):23-37. doi:10.1093/humupd/dmi047.

69. Saleh A, Tan SL, Biljan MM, Tulandi T. A randomized study of the effect of 10 minutes of bed rest after intrauterine insemination. *Fertil Steril.* 2000;74(3):509-511. doi:10.1016/s0015-0282(00)00702-0.

70. Custers IM, Flierman PA, Maas P, et al. Immobilisation versus immediate mobilisation after intrauterine insemination: randomised controlled trial. *BMJ.* 2009;339:b4080. doi:10.1136/bmj.b4080.

71. Scholten I, Custers IM, Moolenaar LM, et al. Long-term follow up of couples initially randomized between immobilization and immediate mobilization subsequent to IUI. *Reprod Biomed Online.* 2014;29(1):125-130. doi:10.1016/j.rbmo.2014.03.012.

72. De Jonge C, LaFromboise M, Bosmans E, Ombelet W, Cox A, Nijs M. Influence of the abstinence period on human sperm quality. *Fertil Steril.* 2004;82(1):57-65. doi:10.1016/j.fertnstert.2004.03.014.

73. Depuydt CE, Verstraete L, Berth M, et al. Human papillomavirus positivity in women undergoing intrauterine insemination has a negative effect on pregnancy rates. *Gynecol Obstet Invest.* 2016;81(1):41-46. doi:10.1159/000434749.

74. Depuydt CE, Donders GGG, Verstraete L, et al. Infectious human papillomavirus virions in semen reduce clinical pregnancy rates in women undergoing intrauterine insemination. *Fertil Steril.* 2019;111(6):1135-1144. doi:10.1016/j.fertnstert.2019.02.002.

75. Garolla A, Pizzol D, Bertoldo A, De Toni L, Barzon L, Foresta C. Association, prevalence, and clearance of human papillomavirus and antisperm antibodies in infected semen samples from infertile patients. *Fertil Steril.* 2013;99(1):125-131.e2. doi:10.1016/j.fertnstert.2012.09.006.

76. Lavie O, Margalioth EJ, Geva-Eldar T, Ben-Chetrit A. Ultrasonographic endometrial changes after intrauterine insemination: a comparison of two catheters. *Fertil Steril.* 1997;68(4):731-714. doi:10.1016/s0015-0282(97)00281-1.

77. Miller PB, Acres ML, Proctor JG, Higdon HL III, Boone WR. Flexible versus rigid intrauterine insemination catheters: a prospective, randomized, controlled study. *Fertil Steril.* 2005;83(5):1544-1546. doi:10.1016/j.fertnstert.2004.11.069.

78. Muharib NS, Abdel Gadir A, Shaw RW. Slow release intrauterine insemination versus the bolus technique in the treatment of women with cervical mucus hostility. *Hum Reprod.* 1992;7(2):227-229. doi:10.1093/oxfordjournals.humrep.a137622.

79. Marschalek J, Franz M, Gonen Y, et al. The effect of slow release insemination on pregnancy rates: report of two randomized controlled pilot studies and meta-analysis. *Arch Gynecol Obstet.* 2017;295(4):1025-1032. doi:10.1007/s00404-017-4290-3.

80. Marschalek J, Egarter C, Vytiska-Binsdorfer E, et al. Pregnancy rates after slow-release insemination (SRI) and standard bolus intrauterine insemination (IUI) - A multicentre randomised, controlled trial. *Sci Rep.* 2020;10(1):7719. doi:10.1038/s41598-020-64164-4.

81. Ombelet W, Van der Auwera I, Bijnens H, et al. Improving IUI success by performing modified slow-release insemination and a patient-centred approach in an insemination programme with partner semen: a prospective cohort study. *Facts Views Vis Obgyn.* 2021;13(4):359-367. doi:10.52054/FVVO.13.4.045.

82. Nuojua-Huttunen S, Gissler M, Martikainen H, Tuomivaara L. Obstetric and perinatal outcome of pregnancies after intrauterine insemination. *Hum Reprod.* 1999;14(8):2110-2115. doi:10.1093/humrep/14.8.2110.

83. Wang JX, Norman RJ, Kristiansson P. The effect of various infertility treatments on the risk of preterm birth. *Hum Reprod.* 2002;17(4):945-949. doi:10.1093/humrep/17.4.945.

84. Gaudoin M, Dobbie R, Finlayson A, Chalmers J, Cameron IT, Fleming R. Ovulation induction/intrauterine insemination in infertile couples is associated with low-birth-weight infants. *Am J Obstet Gynecol.* 2003;188(3):611-616. doi:10.1067/mob.2003.5.

85. Ombelet W, Martens G, De Sutter P, et al. Perinatal outcome of 12,021 singleton and 3108 twin births after non-IVF-assisted reproduction: a cohort study. *Hum Reprod.* 2006;21(4):1025-1032. doi:10.1093/humrep/dei419.

86. Ombelet W, Martens G, Bruckers L. Pregnant after assisted reproduction: a risk pregnancy is born! 18-years perinatal outcome results from a population-based registry in Flanders, Belgium. *Facts Views Vis Obgyn.* 2016; 8(4):193-204.

87. Malchau SS, Loft A, Henningsen AK, Nyboe Andersen A, Pinborg A. Perinatal outcomes in 6,338 singletons born after intrauterine insemination in Denmark, 2007 to 2012: the influence of ovarian stimulation. *Fertil Steril.* 2014;102(4):1110-1116.e2. doi:10.1016/j.fertnstert.2014. 06.034.

88. Moolenaar LM, Nahuis MJ, Hompes PG, van der Veen F, Mol BW. Cost-effectiveness of treatment strategies in women with PCOS who do not conceive after six cycles of clomiphene citrate. *Reprod Biomed Online.* 2014;28(5):606-613. doi:10.1016/j.rbmo.2014.01.014.

89. Guzick DS, Sullivan MW, Adamson GD, et al. Efficacy of treatment for unexplained infertility. *Fertil Steril.* 1998;70(2):207-213. doi:10.1016/s0015-0282(98)00177-0.

90. Goverde AJ, McDonnell J, Vermeiden JP, Schats R, Rutten FF, Schoemaker J. Intrauterine insemination or in-vitro fertilisation in idiopathic subfertility and male subfertility: a randomised trial and cost-effectiveness analysis. *Lancet.* 2000;355(9197):13-18. doi:10.1016/S0140-6736(99)04002-7.

91. Moolenaar LM, Cissen M, de Bruin JP, et al. Cost-effectiveness of assisted conception for male subfertility. *Reprod Biomed Online.* 2015;30(6):659-666. doi:10.1016/j.rbmo.2015.02.006.

92. Bhattacharya S, Harrild K, Mollison J, et al. Clomifene citrate or unstimulated intrauterine insemination compared with expectant management for unexplained infertility: pragmatic randomised controlled trial. *BMJ.* 2008;337:a716. doi:10.1136/bmj.a716.

93. Reindollar RH, Regan MM, Neumann PJ, et al. A randomized clinical trial to evaluate optimal treatment for unexplained infertility: the fast track and standard treatment (FASTT) trial. *Fertil Steril.* 2010;94(3):888-899. doi:10.1016/j.fertnstert.2009.04.022.

94. Bordewijk EM, Weiss NS, Nahuis MJ, et al. Gonadotrophins versus clomiphene citrate with or without IUI in women with normogonadotropic anovulation and clomiphene failure: a cost-effectiveness analysis. *Hum Reprod.* 2019;34(2):276-284. doi:10.1093/humrep/dey359.

95. Sallam HN, Ezzeldin F, Sallam A, Agameya AF, Farrag A. Sperm velocity and morphology, female characteristics, and the hypo-osmotic swelling test as predictors of fertilization potential: experience from the IVF model. *Int J Fertil Womens Med.* 2003;48(2):88-95.

23

In Vitro Fertilization/Intracytoplasmic Sperm Injection

Melissa A. Mathes, Achilleas Papatheodorou, Chara Oraiopoulou, Erlisa Bardhi, Samantha B. Schon, and Panagiotis Drakopoulos

KEY POINTS

- In vitro fertilization (IVF) was initially developed for patients with fallopian tube disease.
- Louise Brown is the first live child from an IVF pregnancy and was delivered in England in 1978.
- It is estimated that almost 2% of all infants born in the United States are a result of assisted reproductive technology interventions.
- Intracytoplasmic sperm injection (ICSI) technique was initially developed for patients with male factor infertility.

- Nowadays, ICSI accounts for around 70% of all treatments worldwide.
- Advances in ICSI technique involve new methods for sperm selection.
- Success rates of IVF/ICSI in terms of live births have steadily increased since Louise Brown. However, the safety of these techniques in terms of perinatal outcomes is still under scrutiny.

INTRODUCTION

Assisted reproductive technology (ART) involves the manipulation of gametes outside of the human body. This encompasses many techniques but the most utilized and arguably the most effective remains in vitro fertilization (IVF). IVF involves a sequence of highly coordinated events involving removal of oocytes from the ovaries followed by fertilization in vitro and return of the subsequent embryo to the uterus, all with the end goal of helping females achieve pregnancy. Since the emergence of IVF in 1976, significant improvements have been made to each step of the process, including ovarian stimulation, follicular monitoring, oocyte retrieval, micromanipulation of gametes, genetic testing of embryos, and transfer of embryos into the uterus. Each small advancement has resulted in incremental improvements to the process, ultimately increasing the chance of successful pregnancy and live birth.

The aim of this chapter is to review the history and indications for IVF and to describe improvements in methodology over the past 30 years.

History of In Vitro Fertilization

IVF was introduced in the 1970s as a method to treat tubal factor infertility. The fallopian tubes are critical for normal transport of the oocyte, sperm, and embryo; thus patients with blockage of the fallopian tubes were unable to naturally achieve pregnancy at that time. The first clinical pregnancy as a result of IVF was in 1976; however, it resulted in an ectopic pregnancy. With continued persistence, Louise Brown, the first live child from an IVF pregnancy, was delivered in England in 1978.[1]

Over the years, the use of IVF has become increasingly common. With higher success rates and increased insurance coverage, many females now utilize IVF to help build their family. In 2019, there were a reported 209,687 ART cycles in the United States resulting in 83,946 live births.[2] An additional 121,086 cycles were initiated for banking purposes (oocyte or embryo cryo-preservation).

It was recently estimated that almost 2% of all infants born in the United States are a result of ART interventions.[3] Globally, it is estimated that more than 8 million babies have been born from IVF since the birth of Louise Brown.[4] There have been significant advancements in the IVF process over the last 40-plus years that have resulted in continued improvement in success rates. In this chapter we will describe these major discoveries, as well as the current state of IVF.

INDICATIONS FOR IN VITRO FERTILIZATION

While egg and embryo banking are currently the most common indication for IVF, there are a variety of conditions, both male- and female-related, that ultimately require the utilization of IVF (Fig. 23.1).

Tubal Disease

As mentioned above, IVF was initially developed for patients with fallopian tube disease. The procurement of a mature oocyte during a natural menstrual cycle, embryo creation in vitro, and transfer of the resulting embryo into the uterus was used to bypass the diseased

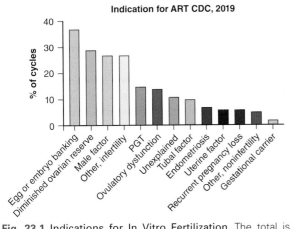

Fig. 23.1 Indications for In Vitro Fertilization. The total is greater than 100%, as more than one diagnosis can be listed for each cycle. *ART,* Assisted reproductive technology; *CDC,* Centers for Disease Control and Prevention; *PGT,* preimplantation genetic testing. (Adapted from 2019 Assisted Reproductive Technology Fertility Clinic and National Summary Report. Centers for Disease Control and Prevention. https://www.cdc.gov/art/reports/2019/fertility-clinic.htmlwebsite.)

fallopian tubes. Tubal disease remains an important reason for IVF, and in 2019 it was the indication for 10% of ART cycles in the United States (see Fig. 23.1). The pathophysiology of tubal disease includes inflammation secondary to ascending bacterial infection, adhesions caused from surgery, endometriosis, previous ectopic pregnancies, and previous tubal sterilization.[5] There are also a significant number of females who undergo tubal sterilization and decide later to further grow their families via IVF. Approximately 600,000 tubal sterilizations are performed each year in the United States. Regret of sterilization is estimated at 10% to 13% of cases and is secondary to a variety of circumstances. Factors contributing to regret include young age at time of sterilization and new partner or marriage.[6,7] Tubal factor infertility can be treated with microsurgical reconstruction of the diseased fallopian tube or with IVF. Both the severity and location of tubal disease are considered when recommending therapy. Mild distal tubal disease can be treated with laparoscopic revision. Reported success rates vary from about 20% to 33% and are similar to microsurgical techniques.[8–10] The risk of ectopic pregnancy after tubal disease revision remains higher than with IVF, and IVF remains the treatment of choice in cases of severe distal tubal disease. Additionally, the success of IVF is typically much higher than tubal reconstruction. Other factors considered include female age, number of desired children, any male factor infertility, type of previous sterilization procedure, and cost.

In addition to tubal obstruction, females diagnosed with hydrosalpinges are generally counseled towards surgical removal of the abnormal tube prior to proceeding with IVF. This recommendation comes from substantial evidence of improved pregnancy rates and decreased miscarriage rates with removal of hydrosalpinges.[11–14] Aspiration of hydrosalpinges may provide some brief benefit but due to the rapid reaccumulation of fluid, is not recommended.[14]

Ovulatory Dysfunction

Ovulatory dysfunction includes diseases that result in infrequent or lack of ovulation. This may be due to thyroid disorders, hyperprolactinemia, hypothalamic hypogonadism, and polycystic ovary syndrome (PCOS). While thyroid dysfunction and hyperprolactinemia may be treated medically, ovulatory dysfunction secondary to PCOS and hypothalamic hypogonadism require fertility interventions. PCOS is one of the most common causes of infertility and affects between 4% to 18% of reproductive-age females.[15] While oral ovulation induction can often result in pregnancy, many females still require more aggressive interventions such as IVF. Similarly, females with hypothalamic hypogonadism require treatment with gonadotropins for ovarian stimulation. While pregnancy can be achieved with timed intercourse or intrauterine insemination (IUI), females may eventually require IVF. Patients with PCOS and hypothalamic hypogonadism can have a profound response to exogenous gonadotropins. IVF allows ovarian stimulation to occur while balancing the risks of ovarian hyperstimulation syndrome (OHSS) and multiple gestations compared to other management strategies.

Male Factor

Male factor infertility was a subsequent and significant indication for IVF. Male factor infertility is diagnosed when any parameter falls outside of the "normal" range of the semen analysis.[16] Compared to timed intercourse and intrauterine insemination, IVF allows for fertilization when sperm parameters are well below the normal limits for natural fertilization.[5] The introduction of intracytoplasmic sperm injection (ICSI; described in detail later) revolutionized pregnancy outcomes for couples with severe male factor infertility. A male factor is the sole cause of infertility in about 20% to 30% of infertile couples but may contribute to approximately 50% of all cases of infertility.[17] Male factor was listed in about 27% of ART cycles in 2019 (see Fig. 23.1).

Endometriosis

Endometriosis is frequently identified in patients with infertility. While the exact pathophysiology of endometriosis is unclear, it is evident that endometriosis can result in damage to the reproductive tract and ovary. Endometriosis may result in pelvic adhesions, thereby distorting the normal reproductive anatomy. There are also known changes to the peritoneal fluid that may alter the normal functioning of the oocyte, sperm, and fallopian tube. Furthermore, there is evidence of endometrial dysfunction that may alter fecundity in females with endometriosis.[18] Prior studies estimate that 25% to 50% of females with infertility have endometriosis;[18] however, endometriosis was listed as the indication for only 7% of ART cycles in 2019 (see Fig. 23.1).

Many females with endometriosis may at some point undergo surgical management of their disease. At the time of surgery, endometriosis should be staged to allow clear communication between providers. Notably, stage severity does not correlate with dysmenorrhea and infertility. Prior surgery for endometriosis and endometriomas may impact ovarian reserve via direct insult to the ovarian cortex, which may result in a decreased number of oocytes retrieved in subsequent IVF cycles.[19] In addition to the known decrease in ovarian reserve with surgical management of endometriosis, there seems to be a direct impact of endometriosis on the oocyte itself, with decreased fertilization and implantation rates noted in females with endometriosis.[18,20]

There is evidence to support surgical treatment of stage III and IV endometriosis prior to infertility treatment, especially in patients with significant symptoms due to their disease. However, surgical intervention is often not recommended in asymptomatic patients or patients with mild disease.[18] Care must be taken to preserve ovarian tissue and to avoid any damage to ovarian blood supply. A previous study documented cumulative fecundity rates in the first 6 months following laparoscopic surgery for all stages of endometriosis to be 25%. This dropped to 10% in the following 6 months. After 1 year, pregnancy rates were less than 8%.[21] Pregnancy attempts following laparoscopic surgery should be purposeful and calculated.

Despite attempts to return pelvic structures to their anatomic locations and downregulation of worsening disease, females with endometriosis often require additional treatment for pregnancy. Thus many females will seek IVF as a treatment option. Endometriosis is associated with need for higher gonadotropin dose, lower oocyte yield, and lower pregnancy rates compared with tubal disease.[22] A gonadotropin-releasing hormone (GnRH) agonist is often utilized prior to IVF as some studies suggest increased pregnancy rates in females with endometriosis.[23]

Unexplained Infertility

Ten to thirty percent of couples who present for infertility care are diagnosed with unexplained infertility. That is, there is no identifiable cause to their infertility after full evaluation of ovarian, tubal, and sperm factors.[24] Females with unexplained infertility have several treatment options, including expectant management, superovulation with or without IUI, or IVF. It is generally recommended that females with unexplained infertility first undergo a trial of superovulation with oral medication combined with IUI. If not pregnant after three to four cycles, IVF is the next recommended treatment.[25] Unexplained infertility is the indication for 11% of ART cycles (see Fig. 23.1). Within the unexplained infertility population, those who choose to undergo IVF may have an increased risk of fertilization failure in IVF cycles. Some recommend use of ICSI in these patients as additional therapy.[26,27] While the use of ICSI may be associated with decreased rates of failed fertilization, it has not been shown to improve live birth outcomes in this population.[28]

Fertility Preservation

Initially, oocyte cryopreservation was introduced for patients with cancer or medical conditions necessitating gonadotoxic therapy. Today, many seek fertility preservation when diagnosed with a malignant disease, particularly breast cancer and hematologic malignancies. Fertility preservation should be offered prior to induction of cytotoxic chemotherapy, radiotherapy, and/or surgery that can induce premature ovarian insufficiency.[1] Other indications for fertility preservation include conditions that carry risk of premature ovarian insufficiency, such as bilateral ovarian tumors, endometriosis and endometriomas, and recurrent ovarian torsion. Currently, the majority of females seeking fertility preservation do so for "social" or personal reasons where, for a variety of indications, females choose to postpone childbearing. Reasons often cited include career aspirations, financial concerns, or current lack of a partner. In 2019, 37% of ART cycles were for egg or embryo banking indications (see Fig. 23.1). With the advent of vitrification, oocyte cryopreservation is the preferred option to allow females the chance to conceive with their own genetic offspring at a later time. In 2016, Cobo et al. released a multicenter retrospective observational study of a total of 1468 females undergoing elective fertility preservation in Spain. In total, 9.3% returned to use their oocytes, with overall survival rate of 85.2%. Improved live birth rate was noted in those less than 35 years at time of cryopreservation, with significantly increased live birth rates with eight oocytes versus five oocytes cryopreserved.[29] With increased utilization of oocyte cryopreservation for nonmedical indications, additional counseling tools have been developed to help patients understand their chance of future live birth, based on their current age and number of oocytes cryopreserved.[30]

For those patients who are prepubertal or if therapy cannot be postponed to allow for ovarian stimulation and retrieval of oocytes, another option is cryopreservation of ovarian tissue, although this remains experimental. Most often, a slow freezing technique is utilized.[31] Ovarian tissue can then be reimplanted into the pelvic cavity, and reportedly more than 95% of cases may have ovarian activity restored.[31] After this, ovarian function typically lasts 4 to 5 years but is dependent on the follicular density of the ovarian tissue originally preserved.[31] Pregnancy rates have been documented up to 53%, and live birth rates have been documented up to 42%.[32–34] There are many conceptions that are documented as spontaneous conceptions, but some required IVF.

Oocyte and Sperm Donation

The utilization of donor oocytes has become increasingly more common. Initially, due to need for laparoscopy under general anesthesia for oocyte retrieval, there was resistance to using donor oocytes given surgical and anesthetic risks. The advent of transvaginal ultrasound allowed oocyte retrieval to be completed in an office setting using conscious sedation and has revolutionized the concept of donated oocytes.[1] It is now a viable option to use donor oocytes for advanced maternal age, poor ovarian reserve, or same-sex male couples.

Gestational Surrogates

Indications for gestational surrogates include absent or compromised uterus, medical disease that would worsen with pregnancy, failed IVF, recurrent pregnancy loss, poor obstetric outcomes, same-sex male couples, or single males.[1] Gestational carrier cycles accounted for 2% of all ART cycles performed in 2019 (see Fig. 23.1). The use of a gestational carrier is complex, and there are published recommendations from the American Society of Reproductive Medicine. This guide was created to reduce complications of gestational carriers as well as to provide guidance to the complex medical, psychological, and legal obstacles that the gestational carrier, intended parents, and children may face.[35]

CURRENT TECHNIQUE OF IN VITRO FERTILIZATION

The IVF process requires a coordinated sequence of events involving ovarian stimulation, with the goal of multifollicular development, induction of oocyte maturity, oocyte retrieval and fertilization, and ultimately embryo transfer. Recombinant and purified gonadotropins (follicle-stimulating hormone [FSH] and luteinizing hormone [LH]) are initiated to stimulate multifollicular growth in the ovary. During this time, GnRH analogs (agonist or antagonist) are also utilized to suppress the endogenous LH surge, thereby preventing premature ovulation. Serum estradiol and ultrasounds are obtained every 1 to 3 days during the stimulation process to evaluate ovarian response and the need for medication adjustments.[36] Most often, females require 8 to 12 days of stimulation.[37–40] When multiple dominant follicles are visible (follicles measuring 18–20 mm), oocyte maturation is achieved through subcutaneous or intramuscular administration of human chorionic gonadotropin or a GnRH agonist. This is known as ovulation triggering.[41–43] Various ovarian stimulation protocols exist and are beyond the scope of this chapter. Approximately 36 hours following ovulation trigger, oocyte collection takes place. In most cases, this is completed via a transvaginal approach while the patient is under intravenous sedation. Using a 16- to 17-gauge needle and transvaginal ultrasound guidance, each follicle is drained, causing the follicle walls to collapse.[44,45] Semen is collected, most commonly by masturbation, at the time of the oocyte retrieval. In conventional IVF, oocytes and sperm are placed in same dish for about 12 to 18 hours. Alternatively, ICSI can be utilized for fertilization (see later). Once fertilized, the embryo is cultured in a dish an additional 3 to 7 days. Embryos cultured in the dish may remain in a single medium throughout development (single step) or may undergo a two-step formulation with different media designed for different developmental needs (sequential media).[46] If proceeding with a fresh embryo transfer in the same cycle, an embryo(s) is typically transferred on either day 3 or 5 of development under ultrasound guidance. The remaining embryos are then frozen using vitrification technique. With a planned frozen embryo cycle, all of the embryos are frozen at the day 5 and 6 blastocyst stage (although occasionally, embryos may be vitrified at an alternative stage such as day 1 when they are the two pronuclei stage or on day 7). Some IVF centers recommend all frozen embryo transfers, while others will do a fresh transfer with vitrification of any remaining embryos. A freeze-all approach may also be employed when there is concern about the development of OHSS or for patients undergoing preimplantation genetic testing (PGT) to allow for the results of genetic testing. Estrogen and progesterone supplementation are also utilized in patients undergoing a fresh or frozen transfer to support an early pregnancy (the protocol varies by institution and indication).[47,48] Pregnancy supplementation is continued until 8 to 10 weeks, when the placenta is producing enough progesterone to support the pregnancy.

Current Success Rates of In Vitro Fertilization

There are many prognostic factors of an IVF cycle. Factors include age, ovarian reserve, prior reproductive success, and infertility diagnosis. It is well known that as a female ages, her reproductive capacity declines, likely related to a decline in oocyte number and increasing rates of meiotic aneuploidy with age. As of 2019, the national reported live birth rates for females using autologous oocytes in the United States were 49.7% per embryo transfer in females ages less than 35 years, 44.8% per transfer in females ages 35 to 37 years, 39.6% per transfer in females ages 38 to 40 years, and 22.6% in females over the age of 40 years.[2]

IMPROVEMENTS IN IN VITRO FERTILIZATION TECHNIQUES OVER THE PAST 30 YEARS

Stimulation Protocols

The first IVF cycles utilized the natural menstrual cycle with the goal of obtaining a single mature oocyte.[1] Given the inefficiency of this process, ovarian stimulation was introduced to increase the oocyte yield of each cycle. Because embryo freezing was not available, all embryos created with each cycle were transferred, significantly increasing the rates of multiple gestations.[1] The selective estrogen receptor modulator clomiphene citrate was first utilized in the process of controlled ovarian hyperstimulation.[49] The discovery of human menopausal gonadotropins, a combination of both FSH and LH obtained from the urine of postmenopausal females, allowed for more aggressive ovarian stimulation.[49–52] Today, gonadotropins are created both recombinantly and through purification and are used in various combinations. Importantly, downregulation of endogenous gonadotropins with GnRH agonists and antagonists was introduced to decrease the rate of premature ovulation by inhibiting the endogenous LH surge.[52–54] Today, a number of different protocols are available for ovarian stimulation depending on the underlying diagnosis (i.e. patients with diminished ovarian reserve, those with a history of endometriosis, patients at high risk of OHSS). The method of oocyte trigger also varies widely depending on the particular protocol employed.

Oocyte Retrievals

Laparoscopy was initially used for oocyte retrievals and remained the standard of care for about 5 years.[1] This technique required the patient to undergo general anesthesia and risks of the surgical procedure.[44] The first proposed alternative to laparoscopic oocyte retrieval was reported out of Denmark in 1982 and involved percutaneous transabdominal-transvesical aspiration with ultrasound guidance under local anesthesia.[55] Due to pain related to the transvesical portion, this approach was not widely accepted. Given the requirement for laparoscopy and the improvements in IVF outlined later, these invasive procedures are rarely performed today.

In 1983, the first vaginal directed oocyte retrievals using abdominal ultrasound guidance were reported.[44,56] The following year, the first pregnancies as a result of transvaginal oocyte retrieval and IVF were reported.[44] With results of the vaginal approach as effective as laparoscopy, by the late 1980s, many centers were performing most of their oocyte retrievals by vaginal route.[57] In 1984, transvaginal ultrasound was introduced as a method to monitor ovarian follicles in patients with difficult visualization from an abdominal approach secondary to obesity or adhesive disease.[58,59] With the introduction of transvaginal ultrasonography, there was a major push to use this method to allow for closer monitoring of follicles but also allow for less invasive methods of oocyte retrieval. In 1986, transvaginal ultrasound with transvaginal oocyte retrieval was reported, with a high recovery rate.[60,61] Now, transvaginal ultrasound-guided oocyte retrieval is the standard of care.[1,62] Abdominal retrievals may still be necessary; however, this is still performed via ultrasound guidance rather than laparoscopy.

Assisted Hatching

Hatching of the blastocyst describes the embryo expansion before implantation, leaving behind the zona pellucida (ZP). With assisted hatching, a defect is created in the zona to thin or open the zona. Prior studies suggest that assisted hatching does not increase live birth rates compared to no assistance with hatching; thus this technique is not routinely utilized in the United States except for patients undergoing PGT.[63]

Preimplantation Genetic Testing–A and Preimplantation Genetic Testing–M

Decisions regarding the best embryo to transfer have traditionally relied on morphologic assessment of the embryo. Significant effort has been placed into advanced methodologies for assessing embryo quality. Initially, enzymatic activity was measured in the four-cell stage embryo to detect inborn errors of metabolism. Later, polar body biopsy was introduced to evaluate oocyte genetic material. Next, biopsy of cleavage-stage embryo was completed followed by development of blastocyst biopsy. Today, five to ten cells are commonly removed from the trophectoderm of the blastocyst as to limit the damage to the embryo.[1]

PGT is frequently used for whole chromosomal complement evaluation. It can also evaluate for monogenetic defects (PGT-M). Typically, the blastocyst trophectoderm is biopsied on day 5 or 6 of development, and then the embryo is vitrified. The tissue is sent for chromosome assessment (frequently via next-generation sequencing [NGS]) to determine whether an embryo has an overall normal number of chromosomes (euploid) or abnormal number of chromosomes (aneuploid). Results may also reveal mosaicism, indicating both euploid and aneuploid cells. Testing can also be performed simultaneously to assess for pathogenic single-gene mutations resulting in diseases such as cystic fibrosis and spinal muscular atrophy. Transfer of a euploid (or unaffected) embryo is then completed in a frozen/thaw cycle.[64]

Implementation of PGT varies widely both nationally and internationally. It has been suggested that females aged 38 years or older should consider PGT to evaluate for aneuploid embryos. The transfer of known euploid embryos increases implantation and pregnancy rates while decreasing rate of miscarriage.[65] However, in patients under the age of 35 years, it is controversial whether or not PGT-A provides an increase in live births.[66] In addition, the national ART surveillance systems found no improved pregnancy and live birth rates in those cycles that used PGT in females less than or equal to 37 years.[67] It is unlikely there is a benefit of using PGT-A in donor oocyte cycles, with the exception of paternal age greater than 50 years.[67] In patients with recurrent pregnancy loss, PGT-A does not appear to improve pregnancy or miscarriage rates and does not decrease time to pregnancy.[68]

Methodology for chromosome assessment has also significantly changed over the years.

Initially, fluorescence in situ hybridization (FISH) was used to evaluate a subset of chromosomes. At its advent, only five to nine chromosomes were evaluated. Later, all chromosomes were able to be assessed.[1] The first studies of FISH did not prove beneficial in improving pregnancy rates, and this is rarely used today.[67] With the development of polymerase chain reaction (PCR) in the mid 1980s, researchers were able to amplify specific short fragments of DNA. Later researchers were able to apply this to test for single-gene mutations (PGT-M). Array comparative genetic hybridization (aCGH) allows for 3000 fragments of DNA with accurate copy number analysis. The DNA in question is amplified and labeled green. This is then cohybridized with a control that is labeled red. The red and green signals are subsequently measured. In euploid samples, there are equal amounts of red and green. If monosomy is present, there is more red than green, whereas if a trisomy is present, there is more green than red.[1] A randomized controlled trial in females aged less than 35 years undergoing IVF for the first time with embryo selection based on morphology alone versus day 5 trophectoderm biopsy with aCGH found that clinical pregnancy rates were higher in the aCGH group versus morphology alone.[69] Real-time quantitative PCR and aCGH reportedly have similar sensitivities.[67] Another technology, single nucleotide polymorphism (SNP) microarray technology, allows for marking of biallelic SNPs to detect deletions and duplications of small regions as well as whole chromosomes. SNP microarray is most commonly used for identifying monogenic diseases. NGS utilizes whole-genome amplification technology. Once amplified, the DNA is chopped into small pieces and mixed with linker oligonucleotides. The intensity of these linker oligonucleotides is measured and compared to reference DNA. With increasing utilization and technology development, NGS has allowed for decrease in price and is used most often for PGT-A.[1]

There are several limitations to PGT-A. First, it is important to highlight that the chromosomal status of the embryo is inferred from biopsy of the trophectoderm.

This is especially relevant when considering mosaic results. As mentioned above, instead of simply euploid or aneuploid, biopsy results may also report mosaicism, indicating intermediate chromosome copy number. With the increasing utilization of NGS and its improved sensitivity, this has become a more common phenomenon, estimated at 3% to 20%.[70,71] The counseling regarding utilization of mosaic embryos and which mosaicism to prioritize is complicated and requires a multidisciplinary approach, including thorough genetic counseling. There is also concern that this technology increases the rate of embryo discard that may have resulted in a healthy pregnancy. Additionally, as mentioned above, there is still controversy regarding the best population to utilize PGT-A.

Laboratory Equipment, Culture Media, and Environment

The in vivo environments of the oviduct and uterus vary to align with the needs of the oocyte, sperm, or embryo. For example, the fallopian tubes have low levels of glucose and higher levels of pyruvate and lactate. The opposite is true of the uterus. Initial culture media was very basic in formulation and included simple salt solutions. Subsequent alterations in media attempted to mimic the female reproductive tract. Early embryos are fairly quiescent and are cultured in pyruvate and nonessential amino acids. Morula- and blastocyst-stage embryos are much more active and are cultured in glucose and essential amino acids. Previously used media was unable to support the rapid development of the blastocyst, which was initially the reason for transfer of pronuclear- and cleavage-stage embryos. Later developments involved sequential media, which accounts for the changing embryonic needs after the compaction stage. Single-step media contains all necessary nutrients for the various stages of embryo development. Both media are currently used, with studies demonstrating conflicting results regarding blastocyst rates; however, both media appear to have equivalent pregnancy rates.[46,72] The improvement of media to support a postcompaction embryo has resulted in the ability to transfer day 5 and 6 embryos.

In addition to the metabolic needs of the embryo, oxygen concentration is also critical. Culture media with low oxygen concentrations ($\sim$5%) increases live birth rates compared to culture media with oxygen concentrations near atmosphere levels ($\sim$20%). Higher than physiologic concentrations of oxygen negatively impact gene expression, metabolism, and the epigenome.[1] There is also an important buffering system within culture media to maintain the desired pH.[73] This maintains the appropriate bicarbonate and carbon dioxide concentrations. Beyond the media, temperature regulation of the culture remains important. Temperature aberrations from 37°C have been shown to impact the meiotic spindle of the oocyte and result in decreased fertilization, embryo development, and pregnancy rates.[73] An oil overlay is used to maintain the delicate balance of all components of media and to prevent evaporation and concentration of media.[73]

Initially, IVF labs utilized equipment designed for nonhuman gametes and somatic cell tissue.[1] Some of the first IVF-specific instruments developed were oocyte collection kits and pumps that provided gentle aspiration of oocytes follicular fluid.[1] The improvement of incubators allowed for a more stable environment for cellular culture. The advent of time-lapse microscopy allows for successive image extraction of the embryo during development and has been postulated for use in embryo selection. A single morphologic parameter or algorithm including multiple morphologic criteria has not been clinically proven to select the best embryo.[1]

Cryopreservation and Vitrification

Cryopreservation was first introduced in 1983.[74] The goal of cryopreservation is to preserve the human embryo while avoiding crystal formation of intracellular water content. During cryopreservation, cellular water is replaced by cryopreservative via osmosis. Initially, a process called slow freezing was utilized for embryo cryopreservation. In this methodology, embryos are placed in sealed containers and cooled in liquid nitrogen in a two-step process. Once the patient has decided to undergo embryo transfer, the reverse process is performed to expose the embryo to decreasing concentrations of cryopreservative. Vitrification was introduced in the 1990s, with the first live birth following oocyte vitrification reported in 1999.[75] With this process, embryos are rapidly frozen by immersing the embryo into liquid nitrogen. Vitrification has significantly improved the success of frozen embryo transfers. Prior to vitrification, survival rates remained less than 80%. Now, with vitrification, survival rates near 100%.[1]

Single Embryo Transfer Versus Double Embryo Transfer

As the rate of twins, triplets, and higher-order multiples increased with the advent of ART, there has been a public health initiative to decrease the number of multiple pregnancies. Multiple-gestation pregnancies place the mother at risk for poor obstetrical outcomes, including hypertensive disorders of pregnancy, gestational diabetes, and increased need for cesarean delivery, among other complications. Multiple pregnancies also increase the rates of neonatal morbidity and mortality, with increasing rates of preterm delivery and low birth weights. In 1992, congress passed the Fertility Clinical Success Rate and Certification Act, which requires all U.S. clinics performing ART procedures to report procedures, transfers, multiple pregnancy rates, and live-birth deliveries.[3] The rate of single embryo transfer in 2019 was 77.3%.[2] Over the last 10 years, the rate of singleton deliveries of ART-conceived infants has increased dramatically, and was 92.5% in 2019.[2]

Endometrium

Another area of interest lies within the endometrium. The classic "apposition, adhesion, invasion" process describes the very basics of embryo implantation. However, there are a number of evolving mechanisms critical for successful implantation. Initial disruption in the cytoskeleton allows adhesion of the blastocyst to the uterine epithelium.[1] Driven by progesterone, the decidualization process then begins and transforms the endometrial cells to a round and enlarged conformation via a complex rearrangement of intracellular cytoskeleton.[1] This is followed by trophoblast invasion and placentation, with subsequent covering of the implantation site by the uterine epithelium.[1]

The concept of endometrial receptivity in IVF began in the 1990s with histologic assessment.[76] Receptivity has been defined as the "period of endometrial maturation during which the trophectoderm of the blastocyst can attach to the endometrial epithelial cells and subsequently proceed to invade the endometrial stroma and vasculature."[77] In 2011, the transcriptomic signature of the receptive human endometrium was described.[78] Currently, NGS is combined with an algorithm to identify the window of implantation (WOI) specific to a particular patient. This testing, commonly known as endometrial receptivity array, was initially studied in patients with repeated implantation failure. Utilizing an array of 238 genes expressed at various stages of the endometrial cycle, it has been reported that there are higher rates of "nonreceptive" results in patients with repeated implantation failure.[79] A recent prospective cohort study documents no improvement in the general infertility population of using a personalized WOI compared to standard transfer timing.[80] While this technique remains controversial, it certainly provides space for additional investigation.

Embryo Transfer

The final step of an IVF cycle is the embryo transfer. It is the culmination of several weeks, and sometimes months or years, of work. Prior to the IVF cycle, a mock embryo transfer is performed to measure the cavity length and also to assess for possible technical difficulties prior to embryo transfer. At the time of the embryo transfer, a transabdominal ultrasound is used for guidance. Notably, the addition of ultrasound significantly improves pregnancy rates.[81] The provider performs handwashing and dons latex-free sterile gloves. A speculum is placed to visualize the cervix, and the cervix is cleansed with either gauze or a cotton swab with media or saline. A soft embryo transfer catheter is used and placed no closer than 1 cm to the fundus, which is also found to improve success rates. Current embryo transfer catheters consist of an outer and inner sheath. The embryo is expelled and the catheter is immediately removed. The catheter is evaluated to ensure there is no retained embryo. If a retained embryo is identified, the embryo is loaded into the catheter and transferred. No outcome differences have been seen when an embryo is retained and a second attempt is made at transfer. There is no recommended bed rest following the procedure.[81] There is known variance of clinical pregnancy rate following embryo transfer depending on the provider.[82,83] One study in particular calculates a 37% difference in clinical pregnancy rate when looking at different providers[83] (Fig. 23.2).

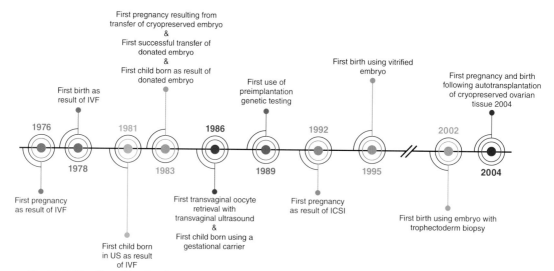

Fig. 23.2 Timeline of landmark events with in vitro fertilization (IVF). *ICSI*, Intracytoplasmic sperm injection; *US*, ultrasound. (From Niederberger C, Pellicer A, Cohen J, et al. Forty years of IVF. *Fertil Steril.* 2018;110(2):185-324; Donnez J, Dolmans MM. Fertility preservation in females. *N Engl J Med.* 2017;377(17):1657-1665; Trounson A, Mohr L. Human pregnancy following cryopreservation, thawing and transfer of an eight-cell embryo. *Nature.* 1983;305(5936):707-709; Kuleshova L, Gianaroli L, Magli C, Ferraretti A, Trounson A. Birth following vitrification of a small number of human oocytes: case report. *Hum Reprod.* 1999;14(12):3077-3079; Lutjen P, Trounson A, Leeton J, Findlay J, Wood C, Renou P. The establishment and maintenance of pregnancy using in vitro fertilization and embryo donation in a patient with primary ovarian failure. *Nature.* 1984;307(5947):174-175; Kemeter P, Feichtinger W. Trans-vaginal oocyte retrieval using a trans-vaginal sector scan probe combined with an automated puncture device. *Hum Reprod* 1986;1(1):21-24; Utian WH, Sheean L, Goldfarb JM, Kiwi R. Successful pregnancy after in vitro fertilization and embryo transfer from an infertile female to a surrogate. *N Engl J Med.* 1985;313(21):1351-1352; Donnez J, Silber S, Andersen CY, et al. Children born after autotransplantation of cryopreserved ovarian tissue. a review of 13 live births. *Ann Med.* 2011;43(6):437-450; de Boer KA, Catt JW, Jansen RP, Leigh D, McArthur S. Moving to blastocyst biopsy for preimplantation genetic diagnosis and single embryo transfer at Sydney IVF. *Fertil Steril.* 2004;82(2):295-298.)

ADVANCES OF INTRACYTOPLASMIC SPERM INJECTION—IMPROVEMENTS OVER THE LAST 30 YEARS

The Development of Intracytoplasmic Sperm Injection

The human IVF field was established with the birth of Louise Brown in 1978 after the pioneering work of Steptoe and Edwards.[89] It became obvious that many couples with infertility problems would benefit from this medical approach. However, the first decade (1980s) of the IVF era became notable in that a significant proportion of the infertility population would not find the solution to their problem using the conventional IVF method. Heterosexual couples with male factor infertility were still struggling to achieve proper fertilization rates, and although plenty of modifications to conventional IVF method were tested, like zona softening[90] or zona breaching,[91] successful fertilization was a rare, exceptional event.[92] It was apparent that a more manipulative technique would be the solution to the male origin infertility, and the subzonal insemination (SUZI) method was developed. In the SUZI technique, the ZP of the oocyte was breached with a needle, and plenty of spermatozoa were injected into the perivitelline space between the ZP and the oocyte.[93,94] Although this technique improved fertilization rates (from 5% to 40%)[95] and was proven to be successful for some cases, it did not serve the needs of heterosexual couples with severe male infertility. In 1992, a pioneer scientist, Gianluigi Palermo, who was working on gamete manipulation methods for fertilization at Brussels Free University, realized that when he was performing SUZI and accidently breaching the oolemma of the oocytes, the fertilization rate of these oocytes was relatively high. Palermo started performing ICSI in some oocytes and compared them with the SUZI oocytes from the same patients and realized that fertilization after ICSI was more consistent than after SUZI.[4] These findings were followed by the first report on pregnancies after intracytoplasmic injection of single spermatozoon into an oocyte.[96] Soon, ICSI was found to be more efficient that SUZI and become the dominant fertilization method.[97] Palermo continued to evolve the ICSI technique and proposed the immobilization of the selected spermatozoon before the insemination[98] and the apposition of the male gamete to a specific area of the oolemma.[99] These modifications, which are still being used today, increased the efficiency of the ICSI technique and led to fertilization rates up to a global average close to 76%.[100]

ICSI proved to be a big revolution in the IVF field. It began as a technique for treating male factor infertility but ended up as the preferable method for fertilization.[101] According to the International Committee for Monitoring Assisted Reproductive Technology, over 60 countries utilize ICSI as the preferred method of fertilization, ranging from 55% of oocyte retrieval cycles in Asia to nearly 100% of cycles in the Middle East.[102] Accordingly in Europe, 70% of oocyte pick up cycles are treated with ICSI and 30% with conventional IVF.[103]

Intracytoplasmic Sperm Injection for Male Factor Infertility

Nowadays, ICSI is used to treat effectively both male- and non male-factor conditions.[28] However, microinjection was first used to deal with male factor infertility since the direct injection of a spermatozoon into the oocyte can bypass several male-origin obstacles. Although low number of spermatozoa, impaired motility, or abnormal morphology were initially the main indications of ICSI,[104] the list of male factors leading to ICSI treatment is expanding.[105]

- Ejaculated spermatozoa
  - Oligozoospermia. There are cases, including cryptozoospermia, where ICSI is the only way of achieving pregnancy since as many normal spermatozoa can be recovered as there are mature oocytes to be inseminated.[106]
  - Asthenozoospermia. Although reduced motility of spermatozoa can result in male infertility,[107] the detection of motile spermatozoa in such samples and their subsequent microinjection can lead to successful fertilization.
  - Teratozoospermia. ICSI can bypass sperm defects in morphology that influence spermatozoa's ability to fertilize.[108] Cases of globozoospermia are included as well.
  - Immunological factors. Antisperm antibodies (ASAs) affect male fertility through reduction of sperm motility, impairment of the ability of spermatozoa to penetrate cervical mucus, and disablement of spermatozoon-oocyte interaction.[109] Direct injection of the spermatozoon into the oocyte can overcome these barriers.

- Ejaculatory dysfunction. In cases of retrograde ejaculation, urine can be used to recover a limited number of spermatozoa for microinjection.[106]
- Fertility preservation. Cryopreserved sperm samples of patients who underwent fertility preservation, for instance before starting chemotherapy, can be used for microinjection. ICSI usually requires the use of a part of the cryopreserved sperm sample—depending on the sperm parameters—so it is not necessary to warm the entirety of a possibly irreplaceable sample. Thus both high fertilization rates[110] and avoidance of the sample's wastage can be achieved.
- Previous total fertilization failure (TFF). The principal cause of TFF is oocyte activation deficiency, which is often caused by PLCζ abnormalities in spermatozoa.[111] Such deficient spermatozoa are unable to initialize oocyte activation through Ca^{2+} oscillations. Reports have shown that the levels of PLCζ are strongly associated to male subfertility.[112] The preferred method in these cases is ICSI treatment, followed by artificial oocyte activation (AOA).[113]
- Frozen oocytes. In cases of oocyte cryopreservation, either for fertility preservation or for oocyte pooling, the oocytes are completely denuded of surrounding cells prior to vitrification. Thus ICSI is the recommended fertilization method post oocyte warming, since conventional IVF requires insemination of the whole cumulus-oocyte complex.[114]
- Testicular or epididimal spermatozoa
  - Obstructive azoospermia (OA). OA can be successfully managed by sperm retrieval from testis or epididymis, as sperm recovery rate is close to 100%.[115] The combination of ICSI with the fact that the retrieved spermatozoa are usually motile leads to high pregnancy rates.
  - Nonobstructive azoospermia (NOA). In the majority of NOA patients, spermatogenesis cannot be restored.[116] Thus testicular biopsy followed by ICSI is the only available option.
  - Vasectomy. A significant number of patients who voluntarily proceeded to vasectomy wish to restore their fertility.[117] In cases where vasectomy reversal is not successful, the use of testicular spermatozoa in ICSI cycles does not negatively affect the clinical outcome.[118]
- Genetic conditions. Azoospermia could be a consequence of various genetic disorders.[119] Some of the most common conditions are listed below (Table 23.1).

Factors Affecting Intracytoplasmic Sperm Injection Outcomes

Even in heterosexual couples affected by male infertility, both male and female factors (e.g., the type of ovarian stimulation) can determine the ICSI outcome.[120] Although ICSI is a highly predictable method in terms of fertilization, clinical outcomes can be influenced by the type and severity of infertility. Several male factors can affect ICSI outcomes, while their impact ranges in a wide spectrum depending on the male condition's stringency.

FSH orchestrates cell–cell interactions and gene expression during spermatogenesis, along with LH.[121] High serum FSH concentration in males correlate to decreased blastocyst formation rate post ICSI. Particularly, if FSH concentration is higher than 10 IU/L, the probability of obtaining a blastocyst is four times lower than in males with normal FSH levels.[120]

According to the majority of published data, sperm motility plays a key role in the ICSI outcome as motility of ejaculated spermatozoa is an indicator of sperm integrity and DNA fragmentation.[122] In testicular samples, motile spermatozoa strongly influence the blastocyst formation in a positive way compared to the use of immotile spermatozoa.[120] However, motility is not a key factor for testicular spermatozoa's fertilization ability since they can be physiologically immotile in the testis.

TABLE 23.1   Genetic Conditions Linked to Azoospermia

Genetic Condition	Type of Azoospermia
Cystic fibrosis	Obstructive
Congenital bilateral absence of the vas deferens	Obstructive
Congenital unilateral absence of the vas deferens	Obstructive
Young syndrome	Obstructive
Klinefelter syndrome (47,XXY)	Nonobstructive
Y-chromosome microdeletions	Nonobstructive
Sertoli cell–only syndrome	Nonobstructive

Thus although the absence of motile testicular spermatozoa does not affect fertilization and pregnancy rates, it has an adverse effect on the available good quality day 3 embryos.[123]

The morphology of injected spermatozoa is a factor that was not thoroughly investigated in terms of its impact on the clinical outcome. There are studies indicating that the use of morphologically abnormal spermatozoa affects fertilization rate and implantation but not embryo formation.[124] On the other hand, the morphology of testicular spermatozoa has been correlated to reduced number of good quality day 3 embryos, but not to impaired fertilization or pregnancy rates.[123]

Sperm cryopreservation is widely applied in IVF treatments, especially in couples with mild male factor infertility, offering a back up plan in case of failure of sperm collection on the day of oocyte retrieval. Hence cryopreservation of sperm is an additional factor that could affect ICSI outcome, mainly in low-parameter sperm samples. Although cryopreserved sperm performs equally, in terms of fertilization and pregnancy rates, data suggest the use of fresh spermatozoa for patients with low sperm parameters, in both ejaculate[125] and testicular[123] samples, as rare cryopreserved spermatozoa do not maintain all properties postwarming.[126]

It is yet unclear whether ASAs have an adverse effect on ICSI outcome, while IVF is clearly affected.[109] However, ICSI is the proposed method to achieve the highest possible percentages in couples with ASA infertility[127] since microinjection of compromised sperm into the cytoplasm can minimize the inhibitory effects of ASAs.

Intracytoplasmic Sperm Injection: Recent Advances

The ICSI technique, in terms of manipulation maneuvers, has not changed a lot since 1996.[92] What is different nowadays is the effort that we make in order to select the best sperm possible. Therefore a list of sorting methods has been proposed in order to help embryologists select the male gamete that will contribute to a viable pregnancy. These methods are not in the category "one size fits all" but are alternatives approaches to different types of male factor infertility and are applied when strong evidence dictates their use.

Sperm Sorting Methods

- **Intracytoplasmic morphologically selected sperm injection (IMSI):** IMSI is an advanced ICSI approach.

During ICSI, the selection of spermatozoa to inject is being done under $200\times$ magnification. Teratozoospermia can affect the fertilization outcome and clinical rates, as it is associated with aneuploidies.[128] The need for a more detailed morphologically based selection led to the use of higher magnification lenses ($6000\times$) gave birth to the IMSI procedure[41] and gave the possibility to better evaluate the sperm morphology and to visualize the acrosome region and the presence of vacuoles in the sperm head. The clinical use of IMSI is controversial. The most recent Cochrane review reports that IMSI has no clinical significance compared to ICSI and does not affect clinical pregnancy rates and miscarriage rate.[129] However, the latest metaanalysis on IMSI shows that this technique can benefit cases with severe male factor infertility by increasing the odds of implantation by 50% and the odds for pregnancy by 60%.[130]

- **Binding Test with Hyaluronic Acid (HA):** The human oocyte is surrounded by HA, which acts as a natural selector. Only mature spermatozoa that express receptors specific to HA can reach the oocyte and fertilize it. It has been reported that sperm that bind to HA are more likely to be of normal morphology, have lower levels of DNA fragmentation, and have lower rates of chromosomal aneuploidy.[131] There are a variety of products (e.g., PISCI dish, Sperm Slow, Sperm Catch) that have been developed as HA tests that are used mainly when it is suspected that the sperm chromatin integrity has been compromised.

- **Magnetic activated cell sorting (MACS):** This sorting technique uses MACS with colloidal superparamagnetic microbeads conjugated with annexin V. The sample is passed through a column containing annexin V microbeads, and sperm expressing externalized phosphatidylserine are deselected. Using this technique, sperm remaining after deselection have been shown to be of higher quality, based on nuclear DNA integrity and a number of other markers.[132]

- **Microfluidic chambers:** Microfluidics involves the study and control of fluids, ranging from picoliters to microliters, inside micrometer-sized channels. It is ideally suited to sperm as it can be used to simulate the geometry of microconfined regions within the female reproductive tract, thereby allowing for biomimicry-based selection approaches that are more representative of the in vivo selection environment, as long as other characteristics, such as temperature and fluid composition, also reflect the in vivo environment.[133] It has been reported that the use of microfluidic chambers for sperm sorting before ICSI improves the clinical outcome in cases with increased DNA fragmentation and repetitive IVF failures.[134,135]

Intracytoplasmic Sperm Injection and Perinatal Outcomes

As of 2022, over 10 million babies have been born worldwide due to ART.[136] This branch of medicine has been subject to escalating progress in the last decades, and its objective has expanded in order to include not only the live birth of a healthy singleton baby but also reduced economic input, reduced time to pregnancy, increased patient safety, and favorable perinatal outcomes.[137,138] While success rates of IVF/ICSI in terms of live births have steadily increased since Louise Brown, the safety of these techniques in terms of perinatal outcomes is still under scrutiny. It has been noticed that, compared to naturally conceived ones, ART pregnancies present with higher risks of maternal-fetal complications, even in singleton gestations, including but not limited to low birthweight (LBW), fetal growth restriction, perinatal mortality and morbidity, placental anomalies (placenta previa or placental abruption), hypertensive disorders, antepartum hemorrhage, and preterm births (PTB).[138–149] Plausible reasons for these findings include parental age, infertility itself, the asynchrony between the embryo development and endometrial receptivity due to the altered endocrine milieu following ovarian stimulation, embryo-specific epigenetic modifications due to the IVF techniques, or even vascular endothelial dysfunction due to sex steroid depletion related with ovarian aging.[138,139,150–154]

ICSI was initially introduced in 1992 for the treatment of severe male infertility. However, its use has expanded over the years, and nowadays it accounts for around 70% of all treatments worldwide.[136,155] This procedure raises concerns over the health of its resulting children given its invasive nature, the arbitrary selection of the spermatozoa, and the epigenetic parental factors.

In 2012, a metaanalysis was published highlighting differences over the obstetric and neonatal outcomes of singleton pregnancies following IVF/ICSI compared to spontaneous ones.[145] Indeed, it was found that ART singleton gestations presented higher risks of antepartum hemorrhage (2.49, 95% confidence interval [CI]: 2.30,

2.69), congenital anomalies (1.67, 95% CI: 1.33, 2.09), hypertensive disorders of pregnancy (1.49, 1.39 −1.59), preterm rupture of membranes (1.16, 95% CI: 1.07, 1.26), cesarean section (1.56, 95% CI: 1.51, 1.60), LBW (1.65, 95% CI: 1.56, 1.75), perinatal mortality (1.87, 95% CI: 1.48, 2.37), PTB (1.54, 95% CI: 1.47, 1.62), gestational diabetes (1.48, 95% CI: 1.33, 1.66), induction of labor (1.18, 95% CI: 1.10, 1.28), and small for gestational age (1.39, 95% CI: 1.27, 1.53).[145]

However, within the ART pregnancies, most large studies have found similar or lower risks of PTB, LBW, and peri-neonatal mortality in singletons born after ICSI compared to those born after IVF.[138] In 2013, Pinborg et al. reported on singletons born after ICSI (fresh or frozen/thawed cycles) versus singletons born after IVF (fresh or frozen/thawed cycles), including 10 studies in the analysis.[139] ICSI singleton gestations presented with lower risk of PTB compared to IVF ones (adjusted odds ratio 0.80, 95% CI: 0.69, 0.93).[139]

A national population-based cohort study in Norway including 5824 singleton pregnancies after IVF and ICSI treatment found no differences in maternal complications such as preeclampsia, hypertension, and diabetes between the two groups. However, IVF pregnancies had a 60% increased risk PTB compared to ICSI pregnancies.[156] Another study that included 80 children conceived via ICSI and 450 children conceived via IVF found the mean Apgar values after 1 minute and after 10 minutes were lower in the ICSI group compared to that of the IVF group.[157] Moreover, ICSI-conceived children had to be hospitalized more often at a neonatal intensive care unit. However, no differences were seen in pH of the umbilical artery or in major congenital malformations between the two groups.[157] On the other hand, the authors observed higher need for hospitalization and more maternal obstetric complications (i.e., premature rupture of membranes, cervical insufficiency, and premature uterine contractions) after IVF rather than ICSI, so they concluded that the course of pregnancies is more complicated after conventional IVF, whereas ICSI pregnancies encompass worse fetal outcomes.[157] Observational studies have reported mostly an increased risk for congenital malformation; the risk of congenital malformations is 7.1% in ICSI and 4.0% in the general population (odds ratio 1.99, 95% CI: 1.87, 2.11).[158] However, infertility treatment by ICSI does not adversely affect growth during childhood, and the children's general health seems satisfactory.[159] Nonetheless, semen parameters of young adult males conceived by ICSI for male infertility were found to be significantly lower than spontaneously conceived peers.[160]

As a procedure, ICSI is based on either ejaculated or surgically acquired sperm; the surgical methods for acquiring sperm include percutaneous epididymal sperm aspiration, testicular sperm aspiration, and microdissection testicular sperm extraction (micro-TESE). A recently published retrospective study analyzed live birth and neonatal outcomes discriminating between the different methods of obtaining sperm.[161] While live birth rates were higher in the surgically acquired sperm group, no significant difference was found in terms of neonatal outcomes of the two groups.[161]

Nonetheless, the results of these studies need to be cautiously interpreted, given the small numbers and at times skewed population.

In this unclear scenario, given the fast expansion of ART use in order to overcome shortcomings in fertility, it becomes of paramount importance for future research, to shed light over the perinatal outcomes of ART babies, particularly of the more invasive procedures such as ICSI. Necessary steps need to be undertaken towards the exploration of what is expected to ultimately define IVF/ART success: the health outcomes of the IVF offspring.

CLINICAL CASE SCENARIOS

CASE 1

The patient was a 35-year-old male who visited an IVF clinic along with his 32-year-old spouse to investigate the fact that they could not achieve pregnancy during the last 1.5 year. Investigation revealed male factor infertility. Specifically, two different semen analyses confirmed azoospermia, with FSH 12.1 IU/L and LH 8.1 IU/L. Consequently, he underwent a TESE procedure, during which a very limited number of motile spermatozoa was found. The testicular sample was cryopreserved for future use. After 2 months, the ovarian stimulation of his partner resulted in the retrieval of seven mature oocytes, which were injected with three motile and four nonmotile frozen-thawed testicular spermatozoa. The viability of nonmotile spermatozoa was confirmed by hypoosmotic swelling test.[162] Upon day 5, one blastocyst of average morphology (2BB, according to Gardner grading system) was produced by an oocyte injected with a motile spermatozoon. The

embryo was vitrified and transferred on a next cycle, with no pregnancy.

The couple decided to proceed to a second IVF treatment. At that time, it was decided to tailor treatment according to patient's clinical history and synchronize the oocyte retrieval with the testicular biopsy, so as fresh testicular motile-only spermatozoa could be used for ICSI. In that way, a possible detrimental effect of cryopreservation on the scarce motile testicular spermatozoa would be avoided. Indeed, the ovarian stimulation produced eight mature oocytes that were injected with motile fresh testicular spermatozoa obtained on the same morning. On day 5, two blastocysts of very good quality (3AB and 4BA) were produced. Both embryos were vitrified and transferred on a following cycle and led to a live birth of one healthy baby.

CASE 2

A couple consisting of a 36-year-old female and a 31-year-old male visited an IVF clinic after three failed attempts of IUI and a diagnosis of unexplained infertility. The selected treatment was to proceed to ovarian stimulation, after which nine mature oocytes were collected. Embryologists decided that the sperm sample's parameters were not suitable for IVF (1.2 mL, 12.5 × 10^6/mL, 20% motility), so they proceeded to ICSI. On day 1, all oocytes failed to fertilize.

Three months later, the couple started a second treatment cycle. That time, seven mature oocytes were collected. Due to the previous TFF, the it was decided to follow ICSI protocol and AOA. Following microinjection, oocyte activation medium was used for all seven oocytes. On day 1, there were three pronucleate zygotes, which were evaluated on day 5 as one good-quality blastocyst (3AB), one average-quality blastocyst (3BB), and one arrested embryo. Both blastocysts were transferred and led to an ongoing pregnancy.

SUMMARY

In vitro fertilization (IVF), which has given hope to so many infertile couples, changed the field of reproductive medicine. The details of the two primary IVF procedures applied in human reproduction—traditional IVF and intracytoplasmic sperm injection (ICSI)—are reviewed in this chapter. This chapter aims to give doctors, researchers, and everyone interested in assisted reproductive technologies a comprehensive understanding of various techniques. The conventional IVF technique, in which a female's eggs are removed and mixed with sperm in a culture dish so as to allow fertilization to occur spontaneously, is explained in the chapter's opening paragraphs. Controlled ovarian stimulation, egg harvesting, sperm preparation, fertilization, and embryo transfer are some of the crucial procedures that are explained. The success rates and potential hazards of traditional IVF are reviewed, along with the indications for the procedure, such as female factor infertility, unexplained infertility, and tubal factor infertility. The breakthrough ICSI procedure, which has transformed the management of male factor infertility, is also explored in this chapter. In ICSI, a single sperm is injected directly into an egg, bypassing any potential barriers to fertilization. The process and complexities of sperm selection are thoroughly discussed, as are the criteria for ICSI, which include severe male factor infertility, prior IVF failure, and genetic abnormalities. The efficacy and safety issues related to ICSI are also covered, including the effects on embryonic development and perinatal outcomes. This chapter provides readers the required knowledge for selecting assisted reproductive technologies carefully by providing a thorough examination of traditional IVF and ICSI. In order to improve the success rates and general patient satisfaction in the field of human IVF, it emphasizes the significance of tailored treatment techniques based on patient-specific criteria.

REFERENCES

1. Niederberger C, Pellicer A, Cohen J, et al. Forty years of IVF. *Fertil Steril.* 2018;110(2):185-324.e5. doi:10.1016/j.fertnstert.2018.06.005.
2. Centers for Disease Control and Prevention. *2019 Assisted Reproductive Technology Fertility Clinic and National Summary Report.* U.S. Dept of Health and Human Services. Available at: https://www.cdc.gov/art/reports/2019/fertility-clinic.html.
3. Sunderam S, Kissin DM, Zhang Y, et al. Assisted reproductive technology surveillance - United States, 2017. *MMWR Surveill Summ.* 2020;69(9):1-20. doi:10.15585/mmwr.ss6909a1.
4. *More Than 8 Million Babies Born from IVF Since the World's First in 1978.* European Society of Human Reproduction and Embryology website. Available at: https://www.eshre.eu/Annual-Meeting/Barcelona-2018/ESHRE-2018-Press-releases/De-Geyter. Accessed.
5. Diedrich K, al-Hasani S, van der Ven H, Bauer O, Werner A, Krebs D. Indications for in-vitro fertilization and results. *Hum Reprod.* 1992;7 suppl 1:115-121. doi:10.1093/humrep/7.suppl_1.115.
6. American College of Obstetricians and Gynecologists' Committee on Practice Bulletins-Gynecology. ACOG Practice Bulletin No. 208: benefits and risks of sterilization. *Obstet Gynecol.* 2019;133(3):e194-e207. doi:10.1097/AOG.0000000000003111.
7. Danvers AA, Evans TA. Risk of sterilization regret and age: an analysis of the national survey of family growth, 2015-2019. *Obstet Gynecol.* 2022;139(3):433-439. doi:10.1097/AOG.0000000000004692.
8. Dubuisson JB, Bouquet de Joliniere J, Aubriot FX, Darai E, Foulot H, Mandelbrot L. Terminal tuboplasties by laparoscopy: 65 consecutive cases. *Fertil Steril.* 1990;54(3):401-403. doi:10.1016/s0015-0282(16)53751-0.
9. Canis M, Mage G, Pouly JL, Manhes H, Wattiez A, Bruhat MA. Laparoscopic distal tuboplasty: report of 87 cases and a 4-year experience. *Fertil Steril.* 1991;56(4):616-621. doi:10.1016/s0015-0282(16)54589-0.
10. Dlugi AM, Reddy S, Saleh WA, Mersol-Barg MS, Jacobsen G. Pregnancy rates after operative endoscopic treatment of total (neosalpingostomy) or near total (salpingostomy) distal tubal occlusion. *Fertil Steril.* 1994;62(5):913-920. doi:10.1016/s0015-0282(16)57050-2.
11. Meyer WR, Castelbaum AJ, Somkuti S, et al. Hydrosalpinges adversely affect markers of endometrial receptivity. *Hum Reprod.* 1997;12(7):1393-1398. doi:10.1093/humrep/12.7.1393.
12. Cohen MA, Lindheim SR, Sauer MV. Hydrosalpinges adversely affect implantation in donor oocyte cycles. *Hum Reprod.* 1999;14(4):1087-1089. doi:10.1093/humrep/14.4.1087.
13. Strandell A, Lindhard A. Why does hydrosalpinx reduce fertility? The importance of hydrosalpinx fluid. *Hum Reprod.* 2002;17(5):1141-1145. doi:10.1093/humrep/17.5.1141.
14. Farquhar C, Marjoribanks J. Assisted reproductive technology: an overview of Cochrane Reviews. *Cochrane Database Syst Rev.* 2018;8:CD010537. doi:10.1002/14651858.CD010537.pub5.
15. Dennett CC, Simon J. The role of polycystic ovary syndrome in reproductive and metabolic health: overview and approaches for treatment. *Diabetes Spectr.* 2015;28(2):116-120. doi:10.2337/diaspect.28.2.116.
16. Schlegel PN, Sigman M, Collura B, et al. Diagnosis and treatment of infertility in men: AUA/ASRM guideline part I. *Fertil Steril.* 2021;115(1):54-61. doi:10.1016/j.fertnstert.2020.11.015.
17. Vander Borght M, Wyns C. Fertility and infertility: definition and epidemiology. *Clin Biochem.* 2018;62:2-10. doi:10.1016/j.clinbiochem.2018.03.012.

18. Practice Committee of the American Society for Reproductive Medicine. Endometriosis and infertility: a committee opinion. *Fertil Steril.* 2012;98(3):591-598. doi:10.1016/j.fertnstert.2012.05.031.

19. Ho HY, Lee RK, Hwu YM, Lin MH, Su JT, Tsai YC. Poor response of ovaries with endometrioma previously treated with cystectomy to controlled ovarian hyperstimulation. *J Assist Reprod Genet.* 2002;19(11):507-511. doi:10.1023/a:1020970417778.

20. Barnhart K, Dunsmoor-Su R, Coutifaris C. Effect of endometriosis on in vitro fertilization. *Fertil Steril.* 2002;77(6):1148-1155.

21. Coccia ME, Rizzello F, Cammilli F, Bracco GL, Scarselli G. Endometriosis and infertility surgery and ART: an integrated approach for successful management. *Eur J Obstet Gynecol Reprod Biol.* 2008;138(1):54-59. doi:10.1016/j.ejogrb.2007.11.010.

22. Coccia ME, Rizzello F, Mariani G, Bulletti C, Palagiano A, Scarselli G. Impact of endometriosis on in vitro fertilization and embryo transfer cycles in young women: a stage-dependent interference. *Acta Obstet Gynecol Scand.* 2011;90(11):1232-1238. doi:10.1111/j.1600-0412.2011.01247.x.

23. Cao X, Chang HY, Xu JY, et al. The effectiveness of different down-regulating protocols on in vitro fertilization-embryo transfer in endometriosis: a meta-analysis. *Reprod Biol Endocrinol.* 2020;18(1):16. doi:10.1186/s12958-020-00571-6.

24. Gunn DD, Bates GW. Evidence-based approach to unexplained infertility: a systematic review. *Fertil Steril.* 2016;105(6):1566-1574.e1. doi:10.1016/j.fertnstert.2016.02.001.

25. Practice Committee of the American Society for Reproductive Medicine. Electronic address asrm@asrm.org; Practice Committee of the American Society for Reproductive Medicine. Evidence-based treatments for couples with unexplained infertility: a guideline. *Fertil Steril.* 2020;113(2):305-322. doi:10.1016/j.fertnstert.2019.10.014.

26. Takeuchi S, Minoura H, Shibahara T, Shen X, Futamura N, Toyoda N. In vitro fertilization and intracytoplasmic sperm injection for couples with unexplained infertility after failed direct intraperitoneal insemination. *J Assist Reprod Genet.* 2000;17(9):515-520. doi:10.1023/a:1009445909023.

27. Ruiz A, Remohi J, Minguez Y, Guanes PP, Simon C, Pellicer A. The role of in vitro fertilization and intracytoplasmic sperm injection in couples with unexplained infertility after failed intrauterine insemination. *Fertil Steril.* 1997;68(1):171-173. doi:10.1016/s0015-0282(97)81497-5.

28. Practice Committees of the American Society for Reproductive Medicine, The Society for Assisted Reproductive Technology. Electronic address: asrm@asrm.org. Intracytoplasmic sperm injection (ICSI) for non-male factor indications: a committee opinion. *Fertil Steril.* 2020;114(2):239-245. doi:10.1016/j.fertnstert.2020.05.032.

29. Cobo A, Garcia-Velasco JA, Coello A, Domingo J, Pellicer A, Remohi J. Oocyte vitrification as an efficient option for elective fertility preservation. *Fertil Steril.* 2016;105(3):755-764.e8. doi:10.1016/j.fertnstert.2015.11.027.

30. Goldman RH, Racowsky C, Farland LV, Munne S, Ribustello L, Fox JH. Predicting the likelihood of live birth for elective oocyte cryopreservation: a counseling tool for physicians and patients. *Hum Reprod.* 2017;32(4):853-859. doi:10.1093/humrep/dex008.

31. Donnez J, Dolmans MM. Fertility preservation in women. *N Engl J Med.* 2017;377(17):1657-1665. doi:10.1056/NEJMra1614676.

32. Donnez J, Dolmans MM. Ovarian cortex transplantation: 60 reported live births brings the success and worldwide expansion of the technique towards routine clinical practice. *J Assist Reprod Genet.* 2015;32(8):1167-1170. doi:10.1007/s10815-015-0544-9.

33. Meirow D, Ra'anani H, Shapira M, et al. Transplantations of frozen-thawed ovarian tissue demonstrate high reproductive performance and the need to revise restrictive criteria. *Fertil Steril.* 2016;106(2):467-474. doi:10.1016/j.fertnstert.2016.04.031.

34. Donnez J, Dolmans MM, Diaz C, Pellicer A. Ovarian cortex transplantation: time to move on from experimental studies to open clinical application. *Fertil Steril.* 2015;104(5):1097-1098. doi:10.1016/j.fertnstert.2015.08.005.

35. Practice Committee of the American Society for Reproductive Medicine, Practice Committee of the Society for Assisted Reproductive Technology. Electronic address: ASRM@asrm.org; Practice Committee of the American Society for Reproductive Medicine, Practice Committee of the Society for Assisted Reproductive Technology. Recommendations for practices utilizing gestational carriers: a committee opinion. *Fertil Steril.* 2017;107(2):e3-e10. doi:10.1016/j.fertnstert.2016.11.007.

36. Kwan I, Bhattacharya S, Kang A, Woolner A. Monitoring of stimulated cycles in assisted reproduction (IVF and ICSI). *Cochrane Database Syst Rev.* 2014;(8):CD005289. doi:10.1002/14651858.CD005289.pub3.

37. Alport B, Case A, Lim H, Baerwald A. Does the ovarian stimulation phase length predict in vitro fertilization outcomes? *Int J Fertil Steril.* 2011;5(3):134-141.

38. Macklon NS, Stouffer RL, Giudice LC, Fauser BC. The science behind 25 years of ovarian stimulation for in vitro fertilization. *Endocr Rev.* 2006;27(2):170-207. doi:10.1210/er.2005-0015.

39. Sarkar P, Ying L, Plosker S, Mayer J, Ying Y, Imudia AN. Duration of ovarian stimulation is predictive of in-vitro

fertilization outcomes. *Minerva Ginecol.* 2019;71(6):419-426. doi:10.23736/S0026-4784.19.04455-1.

40. Chuang M, Zapantis A, Taylor M, et al. Prolonged gonadotropin stimulation is associated with decreased ART success. *J Assist Reprod Genet.* 2010;27(12):711-717. doi:10.1007/s10815-010-9476-6.

41. Casper RF. Introduction: Gonadotropin-releasing hormone agonist triggering of final follicular maturation for in vitro fertilization. *Fertil Steril.* 2015;103(4):865-866. doi:10.1016/j.fertnstert.2015.01.012.

42. Jones BP, Al-Chami A, Gonzalez X, et al. Is oocyte maturity influenced by ovulation trigger type in oocyte donation cycles? *Hum Fertil (Camb).* 2021;24(5):360-366. doi:10.1080/14647273.2019.1671614.

43. Segal S, Casper RF. Gonadotropin-releasing hormone agonist versus human chorionic gonadotropin for triggering follicular maturation in in vitro fertilization. *Fertil Steril.* 1992;57(6):1254-1258.

44. Dellenbach P, Nisand I, Moreau L, Feger B, Plumere C, Gerlinger P. Transvaginal sonographically controlled follicle puncture for oocyte retrieval. *Fertil Steril.* 1985;44(5):656-662. doi:10.1016/s0015-0282(16)48983-1.

45. Seyhan A, Ata B, Son WY, Dahan MH, Tan SL. Comparison of complication rates and pain scores after transvaginal ultrasound-guided oocyte pickup procedures for in vitro maturation and in vitro fertilization cycles. *Fertil Steril.* 2014;101(3):705-709. doi:10.1016/j.fertnstert.2013.12.011.

46. Sfontouris IA, Martins WP, Nastri CO, et al. Blastocyst culture using single versus sequential media in clinical IVF: a systematic review and meta-analysis of randomized controlled trials. *J Assist Reprod Genet.* 2016;33(10):1261-1272. doi:10.1007/s10815-016-0774-5.

47. Zhang XM, Lv F, Wang P, et al. Estrogen supplementation to progesterone as luteal phase support in patients undergoing in vitro fertilization: systematic review and meta-analysis. *Medicine (Baltimore).* 2015;94(8):e459. doi:10.1097/MD.0000000000000459.

48. Wu H, Zhang S, Lin X, Wang S, Zhou P. Luteal phase support for in vitro fertilization/intracytoplasmic sperm injection fresh cycles: a systematic review and network meta-analysis. *Reprod Biol Endocrinol.* 2021;19(1):103. doi:10.1186/s12958-021-00782-5.

49. Garcia JE, Jones GS, Acosta AA, Wright Jr G. Human menopausal gonadotropin/human chorionic gonadotropin follicular maturation for oocyte aspiration: phase I, 1981. *Fertil Steril.* 1983;39(2):167-173. doi:10.1016/s0015-0282(16)46814-7.

50. Garcia JE, Jones GS, Acosta AA, Wright Jr G. Human menopausal gonadotropin/human chorionic gonadotropin follicular maturation for oocyte aspiration: phase II,

1981. *Fertil Steril.* 1983;39(2):174-179. doi:10.1016/s0015-0282(16)46815-9.

51. Laufer N, DeCherney AH, Haseltine FP, et al. The use of high-dose human menopausal gonadotropin in an in vitro fertilization program. *Fertil Steril.* 1983;40(6):734-741. doi:10.1016/s0015-0282(16)47472-8.

52. Neveu S, Hedon B, Bringer J, et al. Ovarian stimulation by a combination of a gonadotropin-releasing hormone agonist and gonadotropins for in vitro fertilization. *Fertil Steril.* 1987;47(4):639-643. doi:10.1016/s0015-0282(16)59115-8.

53. Wildt L, Diedrich K, van der Ven H, al Hasani S, Hubner H, Klasen R. Ovarian hyperstimulation for in-vitro fertilization controlled by GnRH agonist administered in combination with human menopausal gonadotrophins. *Hum Reprod.* 1986;1(1):15-19. doi:10.1093/oxfordjournals.humrep.a136334.

54. Smitz J, Devroey P, Braeckmans P, et al. Management of failed cycles in an IVF/GIFT programme with the combination of a GnRH analogue and HMG. *Hum Reprod.* 1987;2(4):309-314. doi:10.1093/oxfordjournals.humrep.a136540.

55. Lenz S, Lauritsen JG. Ultrasonically guided percutaneous aspiration of human follicles under local anesthesia: a new method of collecting oocytes for in vitro fertilization. *Fertil Steril.* 1982;38(6):673-677. doi:10.1016/s0015-0282(16)46692-6.

56. Gleicher N, Friberg J, Fullan N, et al. EGG retrieval for in vitro fertilisation by sonographically controlled vaginal culdocentesis. *Lancet.* 1983;2(8348):508-509. doi:10.1016/s0140-6736(83)90530-5.

57. Dellenbach P, Nisand I, Moreau L, et al. The transvaginal method for oocyte retrieval. An update on our experience (1984-1987). *Ann N Y Acad Sci.* 1988;541:111-124. doi:10.1111/j.1749-6632.1988.tb22247.x.

58. Meldrum DR, Chetkowski RJ, Steingold KA, Randle D. Transvaginal ultrasound scanning of ovarian follicles. *Fertil Steril.* 1984;42(5):803-805. doi:10.1016/s0015-0282(16)48212-9.

59. Schwimer SR, Lebovic J. Transvaginal pelvic ultrasonography. *J Ultrasound Med.* 1984;3(8):381-383. doi:10.7863/jum.1984.3.8.381.

60. Feichtinger W, Kemeter P. Transvaginal sector scan sonography for needle guided transvaginal follicle aspiration and other applications in gynecologic routine and research. *Fertil Steril.* 1986;45(5):722-725. doi:10.1016/s0015-0282(16)49349-0.

61. Wikland M, Enk L, Hammarberg K, Nilsson L. Use of a vaginal transducer for oocyte retrieval in an IVF/ET program. *J Clin Ultrasound.* 1987;15(4):245-251. doi:10.1002/jcu.1870150405.

62. Yuzpe AA, Brown SE, Casper RF, Nisker J, Graves G, Shatford L. Transvaginal, ultrasound-guided oocyte

retrieval for in vitro fertilization. *J Reprod Med.* 1989; 34(12):937-942.

63. Carney SK, Das S, Blake D, Farquhar C, Seif MM, Nelson L. Assisted hatching on assisted conception (in vitro fertilisation (IVF) and intracytoplasmic sperm injection (ICSI). *Cochrane Database Syst Rev.* 2012;12:CD001894. doi:10.1002/14651858.CD001894.pub5.

64. Wells D, Kaur K, Grifo J, et al. Clinical utilisation of a rapid low-pass whole genome sequencing technique for the diagnosis of aneuploidy in human embryos prior to implantation. *J Med Genet.* 2014;51(8):553-562. doi:10.1136/jmedgenet-2014-102497.

65. Scott Jr RT, Upham KM, Forman EJ, et al. Blastocyst biopsy with comprehensive chromosome screening and fresh embryo transfer significantly increases in vitro fertilization implantation and delivery rates: a randomized controlled trial. *Fertil Steril.* 2013;100(3):697-703. doi:10.1016/j.fertnstert.2013.04.035.

66. Yan J, Qin Y, Zhao H, et al. Live birth with or without preimplantation genetic testing for aneuploidy. *N Engl J Med.* 2021;385(22):2047-2058. doi:10.1056/NEJMoa2103613.

67. Practice Committees of the American Society for Reproductive Medicine, The Society for Assisted Reproductive Technology. Electronic address: ASRM@asrm.org; Practice Committees of the American Society for Reproductive Medicine, The Society for Assisted Reproductive Technology. The use of preimplantation genetic testing for aneuploidy (PGT-A): a committee opinion. *Fertil Steril.* 2018;109(3):429-436. doi:10.1016/j.fertnstert.2018.01.002.

68. Murugappan G, Shahine LK, Perfetto CO, Hickok LR, Lathi RB. Intent to treat analysis of in vitro fertilization and preimplantation genetic screening versus expectant management in patients with recurrent pregnancy loss. *Hum Reprod.* 2016;31(8):1668-1674. doi:10.1093/humrep/dew135.

69. Yang Z, Liu J, Collins GS, et al. Selection of single blastocysts for fresh transfer via standard morphology assessment alone and with array CGH for good prognosis IVF patients: results from a randomized pilot study. *Mol Cytogenet.* 2012;5(1):24. doi:10.1186/1755-8166-5-24.

70. Scott Jr RT, Galliano D. The challenge of embryonic mosaicism in preimplantation genetic screening. *Fertil Steril.* 2016;105(5):1150-1152. doi:10.1016/j.fertnstert.2016.01.007.

71. Practice Committee and Genetic Counseling Professional Group of the American Society for Reproductive Medicine. Electronic address: asrm@asrm.org. Clinical management of mosaic results from preimplantation genetic testing for aneuploidy (PGT-A) of blastocysts: a committee opinion. *Fertil Steril.* 2020;114(2):246-254. doi:10.1016/j.fertnstert.2020.05.014.

72. Werner MD, Hong KH, Franasiak JM, et al. Sequential versus Monophasic Media Impact Trial (SuMMIT): a paired randomized controlled trial comparing a sequential media system to a monophasic medium. *Fertil Steril.* 2016;105(5):1215-1221. doi:10.1016/j.fertnstert.2016.01.005.

73. Wale PL, Gardner DK. The effects of chemical and physical factors on mammalian embryo culture and their importance for the practice of assisted human reproduction. *Hum Reprod Update.* 2016;22(1):2-22. doi:10.1093/humupd/dmv034.

74. Trounson A, Mohr L. Human pregnancy following cryopreservation, thawing and transfer of an eight-cell embryo. *Nature.* 1983;305(5936):707-709. doi:10.1038/305707a0.

75. Kuleshova L, Gianaroli L, Magli C, Ferraretti A, Trounson A. Birth following vitrification of a small number of human oocytes: case report. *Hum Reprod.* 1999;14(12):3077-3079. doi:10.1093/humrep/14.12.3077.

76. Navot D, Scott RT, Droesch K, Veeck LL, Liu HC, Rosenwaks Z. The window of embryo transfer and the efficiency of human conception in vitro. *Fertil Steril.* 1991;55(1):114-118. doi:10.1016/s0015-0282(16)54069-2.

77. Lessey BA, Young SL. What exactly is endometrial receptivity? *Fertil Steril.* 2019;111(4):611-617. doi:10.1016/j.fertnstert.2019.02.009.

78. Diaz-Gimeno P, Horcajadas JA, Martinez-Conejero JA, et al. A genomic diagnostic tool for human endometrial receptivity based on the transcriptomic signature. *Fertil Steril.* 2011;95(1):50-60, 60.e1-e15. doi:10.1016/j.fertnstert.2010.04.063.

79. Ruiz-Alonso M, Blesa D, Diaz-Gimeno P, et al. The endometrial receptivity array for diagnosis and personalized embryo transfer as a treatment for patients with repeated implantation failure. *Fertil Steril.* 2013;100(3):818-824. doi:10.1016/j.fertnstert.2013.05.004.

80. Riestenberg C, Kroener L, Quinn M, Ching K, Ambartsumyan G. Routine endometrial receptivity array in first embryo transfer cycles does not improve live birth rate. *Fertil Steril.* 2021;115(4):1001-1006. doi:10.1016/j.fertnstert.2020.09.140.

81. Practice Committee of the American Society for Reproductive Medicine. Electronic address: ASRM@asrm.org, Penzias A, Bendikson K, et al. ASRM standard embryo transfer protocol template: a committee opinion. *Fertil Steril.* 2017;107(4):897-900. doi:10.1016/j.fertnstert.2017.02.108.

82. Angelini A, Brusco GF, Barnocchi N, El-Danasouri I, Pacchiarotti A, Selman HA. Impact of physician performing embryo transfer on pregnancy rates in an assisted reproductive program. *J Assist Reprod Genet.* 2006;23(7-8):329-332. doi:10.1007/s10815-006-9032-6.

83. Hearns-Stokes RM, Miller BT, Scott L, Creuss D, Chakraborty PK, Segars JH. Pregnancy rates after embryo transfer depend on the provider at embryo transfer. *Fertil Steril.* 2000;74(1):80-86. doi:10.1016/s0015-0282(00)00582-3.

84. Lutjen P, Trounson A, Leeton J, Findlay J, Wood C, Renou P. The establishment and maintenance of pregnancy using in vitro fertilization and embryo donation in a patient with primary ovarian failure. *Nature.* 1984;307(5947):174-175. doi:10.1038/307174a0.

85. Kemeter P, Feichtinger W. Trans-vaginal oocyte retrieval using a trans-vaginal sector scan probe combined with an automated puncture device. *Hum Reprod.* 1986;1(1):21-24. doi:10.1093/oxfordjournals.humrep.a136335.

86. Utian WH, Sheean L, Goldfarb JM, Kiwi R. Successful pregnancy after in vitro fertilization and embryo transfer from an infertile woman to a surrogate. *N Engl J Med.* 1985;313(21):1351-1352. doi:10.1056/nejm198511213132112.

87. Donnez J, Silber S, Andersen CY, et al. Children born after autotransplantation of cryopreserved ovarian tissue. a review of 13 live births. *Ann Med.* 2011;43(6):437-450. doi:10.3109/07853890.2010.546807.

88. de Boer KA, Catt JW, Jansen RP, Leigh D, McArthur S. Moving to blastocyst biopsy for preimplantation genetic diagnosis and single embryo transfer at Sydney IVF. *Fertil Steril.* 2004;82(2):295-298. doi:10.1016/j.fertnstert.2003.11.064.

89. Steptoe PC, Edwards RG. Birth after the reimplantation of a human embryo. *Lancet.* 1978;2(8085):366. doi:10.1016/s0140-6736(78)92957-4.

90. Kiessling AA, Loutradis D, McShane PM, Jackson KV. Fertilization in trypsin–treated oocytes. *Ann N Y Acad Sci.* 1988;541(1):614-620. doi:10.1111/j.1749-6632.1988.tb22298.x.

91. Gordon JW, Grunfeld L, Garrisi GJ, Talansky BE, Richards C, Laufer N. Fertilization of human oocytes by sperm from infertile males after zona pellucida drilling. *Fertil Steril.* 1988;50(1):68-73. doi:10.1016/S0015-0282(16)60010-9.

92. O'Neill CL, Chow S, Rosenwaks Z, Palermo GD. Development of ICSI. *Reproduction.* 2018;156(1):F51-F58. doi:10.1530/REP-18-0011.

93. Fishel S, Antinori S, Jackson P, et al. Twin birth after subzonal insemination. *Lancet.* 1990;335(8691):722-723. doi:10.1016/0140-6736(90)90834-R.

94. Palermo G, Joris H, Devroey P, Van Steirteghem AC. Induction of acrosome reaction in human spermatozoa used for subzonal insemination. *Hum Reprod.* 1992;7(2):248-254. doi:10.1093/oxfordjournals.humrep.a137626.

95. Fishel S, Timson J, Lisi F, Rinaldi L. Evaluation of 225 patients undergoing subzonal insemination for the procurement of fertilization in vitro. *Fertil Steril.* 1992;57(4):840-849. doi:10.1016/S0015-0282(16)54968-1.

96. Palermo G, Joris H, Devroey P, Steirteghem ACV. Pregnancies after intracytoplasmic injection of single spermatozoon into an oocyte. *Lancet.* 1992;340(8810):17-18. doi:10.1016/0140-6736(92)92425-F.

97. Palermo G, Joris H, Derde MP, Camus M, Devroey P, Van Steirteghem A. Sperm characteristics and outcome of human assisted fertilization by subzonal insemination and intracytoplasmic sperm injection. *Fertil Steril.* 1993;59(4):826-835. doi:10.1016/S0015-0282(16)55867-1.

98. Palermo GD, Schlegel PN, Colombero LT, Zaninovic N, Moy F, Rosenwaks Z. Aggressive sperm immobilization prior to intracytoplasmic sperm injection with immature spermatozoa improves fertilization and pregnancy rates. *Hum Reprod.* 1996;11(5):1023-1029. doi:10.1093/oxfordjournals.humrep.a019290.

99. Palermo GD, Alikani M, Bertoli M, et al. Oolemma characteristics in relation to survival and fertilization patterns of oocytes treated by intracytoplasmic sperm injection. *Hum Reprod.* 1996;11(1):172-176. doi:10.1093/oxfordjournals.humrep.a019012.

100. Palermo GD, Neri QV, Rosenwaks Z. To ICSI or Not to ICSI. *Semin Reprod Med.* 2015;33(2):92-102. doi:10.1055/s-0035-1546825.

101. Fishel S, Aslam I, Lisi F, et al. Should ICSI be the treatment of choice for all cases of in-vitro conception? *Hum Reprod.* 2000;15(6):1278-1283. doi:10.1093/humrep/15.6.1278.

102. Dyer S, Chambers GM, de Mouzon J, et al. International Committee for Monitoring Assisted Reproductive Technologies world report: Assisted Reproductive Technology 2008, 2009 and 2010. *Hum Reprod.* 2016;31(7):1588-1609. doi:10.1093/humrep/dew082.

103. European IVF-Monitoring Consortium (EIM) for the European Society of Human Reproduction and Embryology (ESHRE), Wyns C, Geyter CD, et al. ART in Europe, 2017: results generated from European registries by ESHRE. *Hum Reprod Open.* 2021;2021(3):hoab026. doi:10.1093/hropen/hoab026.

104. O'Neill CL, Chow S, Rosenwaks Z, Palermo GD. Development of ICSI. *Reproduction.* 2018;156(1):F51-F58. doi:10.1530/REP-18-0011.

105. Pereira N, Palermo GD. Intracytoplasmic Sperm injection: history, indications, technique, and safety. In: Palermo G, Sills E, eds. *Intracytoplasmic Sperm Injection.* Springer, Cham; 2018. https://doi.org/10.1007/978-3-319-70497-5_2.

106. Elder K, Dale B. Micromanipulation techniques. In: *In-Vitro Fertilization.* Cambridge: Cambridge University Press; 2020:284-310. doi:10.1017/9781108611633.014.

107. Vogiatzi P, Pouliakis A, Sakellariou M, et al. Male age and progressive sperm motility are critical factors af-

fecting embryological and clinical outcomes in oocyte donor ICSI cycles. *Reprod Sci.* 2021;29(3):883-895. doi:10.1007/S43032-021-00801-1.

108. Palermo GD, Kocent J, Monahan D, Neri VQ, Rosenwaks Z. Treatment of male infertility. *Methods Mol Biol.* 2014;1154:385-405. doi:10.1007/978-1-4939-0659-8_18.

109. Lu SM, Li X, Wang SL, et al. Success rates of in vitro fertilization versus intracytoplasmic sperm injection in men with serum anti-sperm antibodies: a consecutive cohort study. *Asian J Androl.* 2019;21(5):473. doi:10.4103/AJA.AJA_124_18.

110. Aggarwal B, Evans AL, Ryan H, Martins da Silva SJ. IVF or ICSI for fertility preservation? *Reprod Fertil.* 2021;2(1):L1-L3. doi:10.1530/RAF-20-0059.

111. Parrington J, Arnoult C, Fissore RA. The eggstraordinary story of how life begins. Molecular reproduction and development. *Mol Reprod Dev.* 2019;86(1):4-19. doi:10.1002/MRD.23083.

112. Kashir J, Mistry VB, BuSaleh L, et al. Phospholipase C zeta profiles are indicative of optimal sperm parameters and fertilisation success in patients undergoing fertility treatment. *Andrology.* 2020;8(5):1143-1159. doi:10.1111/ANDR.12796.

113. Lv M, Zhang D, He X, et al. Artificial oocyte activation to improve reproductive outcomes in couples with various causes of infertility: a retrospective cohort study. *Reprod Biomed Online.* 2020;40(4):501-509. doi:10.1016/J.RBMO.2020.01.001.

114. Takeshige Y, Takahashi M, Hashimoto T, Kyono K. Six-year follow-up of children born from vitrified oocytes. *Reprod Biomed Online.* 2021;42(3):564-571. doi:10.1016/j.rbmo.2020.11.005.

115. Medhavi S, Stephen WL. Azoospermia. 2022:74-76.

116. Chiba K, Enatsu N, Fujisawa M. Management of non-obstructive azoospermia. *Reprod Med Biol.* 2016;15(3):165-173.

117. Hervás I, Valls L, Rivera-Egea R, et al. TESE-ICSI outcomes per couple in vasectomized males are negatively affected by time since the intervention, but not other comorbidities. *Reprod Biomed Online.* 2021;43(4):708-717. doi:10.1016/j.rbmo.2021.05.013.

118. Esteves SC, Agarwal A. Reproductive outcomes, including neonatal data, following sperm injection in men with obstructive and nonobstructive azoospermia: Case series and systematic review. *Clinics.* 2013;68(suppl 1):141-149. doi:10.6061/clinics/2013(Sup01)16.

119. Hamada AJ, Esteves SC, Agarwal A. A comprehensive review of genetics and genetic testing in azoospermia. *Clinics.* 2013;68(suppl 1):39-60. doi:10.6061/clinics/2013(Sup01)06.

120. Zorn B, Virant-Klun I, Drobni S, Šinkovec J, Meden-Vrtovec H. Male and female factors that influence ICSI

outcome in azoospermia or aspermia. *Reprod Biomed Online.* 2009;18(2):168-176. doi:10.1016/S1472-6483(10)60252-0.

121. Oduwole OO, Huhtaniemi IT, Misrahi M. The roles of luteinizing hormone, follicle-stimulating hormone and testosterone in spermatogenesis and folliculogenesis revisited. *Int J Mol Sci.* 2021;22(23):12735. doi:10.3390/ijms222312735.

122. Meijerink AM, Cissen M, Mochtar MH, et al. Prediction model for live birth in ICSI using testicular extracted sperm. *Hum Reprod.* 2016;31(9):1942-1951. doi:10.1093/humrep/dew146.

123. Oraiopoulou C, Vorniotaki A, Taki E, Papatheodorou A, Christoforidis N, Chatziparasidou A. The impact of fresh and frozen testicular tissue quality on embryological and clinical outcomes. *Andrologia.* 2021;53(5):1-8. doi:10.1111/and.14040.

124. De Vos A, Van de Velde H, Joris H, Verheyen G, Devroey P, Van Steirteghem A. Influence of individual sperm morphology on fertilization, embryo morphology, and pregnancy outcome of intracytoplasmic sperm injection. *Fertil Steril.* 2003;79(1):42-48. doi:10.1016/S0015-0282(02)04571-5.

125. Miller CM, Duong S, Weaver AL, Zhao Y, Shenoy CC. Outcomes of frozen oocyte donor in vitro fertilization (IVF) cycles using fresh versus frozen sperm. *Reprod Sci.* 2022;29(4):1226-1231. doi:10.1007/S43032-021-00796-9.

126. Madureira C, Cunha M, Sousa M, et al. Treatment by testicular sperm extraction and intracytoplasmic sperm injection of 65 azoospermic patients with non-mosaic Klinefelter syndrome with birth of 17 healthy children. *Andrology.* 2014;2(4):623-631. doi:10.1111/j.2047-2927.2014.00231.x.

127. Chiu WWC, Chamley LW. Clinical associations and mechanisms of action of antisperm antibodies. *Fertil Steril.* 2004;82(3):529-535. doi:10.1016/j.fertnstert.2003.09.084.

128. De Vos A, Van de Velde H, Bocken G, et al. Does intracytoplasmic morphologically selected sperm injection improve embryo development? A randomized sibling-oocyte study. *Hum Reprod.* 2013;28(3):617-626. doi:10.1093/humrep/des435.

129. Teixeira DM, Barbosa MA, Ferriani RA, et al. Regular (ICSI) versus ultra-high magnification (IMSI) sperm selection for assisted reproduction. *Cochrane Database Syst Rev.* 2013;(7):CD010167. doi:10.1002/14651858.CD010167.pub2.

130. Setti AS, Braga DPAF, Figueira RCS, Iaconelli A, Borges E. Intracytoplasmic morphologically selected sperm injection results in improved clinical outcomes in couples with previous ICSI failures or male factor infertility: a meta-analysis. *Eur J Obstet Gynecol Reprod Biol.* 2014;183:96-103. doi:10.1016/j.ejogrb.2014.10.008.

131. Parmegiani L, Cognigni GE, Ciampaglia W, Pocognoli P, Marchi F, Filicori M. Efficiency of hyaluronic acid (HA) sperm selection. *J Assist Reprod Genet*. 2010;27(1):13-16. doi:10.1007/s10815-009-9380-0.

132. Nadalini M, Tarozzi N, Di Santo M, Borini A. Annexin V magnetic-activated cell sorting versus swim-up for the selection of human sperm in ART: is the new approach better then the traditional one? *J Assist Reprod Genet*. 2014;31(8):1045-1051. doi:10.1007/s10815-014-0267-3.

133. Smith G, Takayama S. Application of microfluidic technologies to human assisted reproduction. *Mol Hum Reprod*. 2017;23:gaw076. doi:10.1093/molehr/gaw076.

134. Quinn MM, Jalalian L, Ribeiro S, et al. Microfluidic sorting selects sperm for clinical use with reduced DNA damage compared to density gradient centrifugation with swim-up in split semen samples. *Hum Reprod*. 2018;33(8):1388-1393. doi:10.1093/humrep/dey239.

135. Parrella A, Keating D, Cheung S, et al. A treatment approach for couples with disrupted sperm DNA integrity and recurrent ART failure. *J Assist Reprod Genet*. 2019;36(10):2057-2066. doi:10.1007/s10815-019-01543-5.

136. *ESHRE Factsheet 2022*. European Society of Human Reproduction and Embryology. Available at: https://www.eshre.eu/Press-Room/Resources.

137. Bardhi E, Blockeel C, Cools W, et al. Is ovarian response associated with adverse perinatal outcomes in GnRH antagonist IVF/ICSI cycles? Reproductive biomedicine online 2020;41(2):263-270. doi:10.1016/j.rbmo.2020.03.010.

138. Berntsen S, Soderstrom-Anttila V, Wennerholm UB, et al. The health of children conceived by ART: 'the chicken or the egg?'. *Hum Reprod Update*. 2019;25(2):137-158. doi:10.1093/humupd/dmz001.

139. Pinborg A, Wennerholm UB, Romundstad LB, et al. Why do singletons conceived after assisted reproduction technology have adverse perinatal outcome? Systematic review and meta-analysis. *Hum Reprod Update*. 2013;19(2):87-104. doi:10.1093/humupd/dms044.

140. Romundstad LB, Romundstad PR, Sunde A, von During V, Skjaerven R, Vatten LJ. Increased risk of placenta previa in pregnancies following IVF/ICSI; a comparison of ART and non-ART pregnancies in the same mother. *Hum Reprod*. 2006;21(9):2353-2358. doi:10.1093/humrep/del153.

141. Romundstad LB, Romundstad PR, Sunde A, et al. Effects of technology or maternal factors on perinatal outcome after assisted fertilisation: a population-based cohort study. *Lancet*. 2008;372(9640):737-743. doi:10.1016/S0140-6736(08)61041-7.

142. Healy DL, Breheny S, Halliday J, et al. Prevalence and risk factors for obstetric haemorrhage in 6730 singleton births after assisted reproductive technology in Victoria Australia. *Hum Reprod*. 2010;25(1):265-274. doi:10.1093/humrep/dep376.

143. Calhoun KC, Barnhart KT, Elovitz MA, Srinivas SK. Evaluating the association between assisted conception and the severity of preeclampsia. *ISRN Obstet Gynecol*. 2011;2011:928592. doi:10.5402/2011/928592.

144. Esh-Broder E, Ariel I, Abas-Bashir N, Bdolah Y, Celnikier DH. Placenta accreta is associated with IVF pregnancies: a retrospective chart review. *BJOG*. 2011;118(9):1084-1089. doi:10.1111/j.1471-0528.2011.02976.x.

145. Pandey S, Shetty A, Hamilton M, Bhattacharya S, Maheshwari A. Obstetric and perinatal outcomes in singleton pregnancies resulting from IVF/ICSI: a systematic review and meta-analysis. *Hum Reprod Update*. 2012;18(5):485-503. doi:10.1093/humupd/dms018.

146. Maheshwari A, Pandey S, Shetty A, Hamilton M, Bhattacharya S. Obstetric and perinatal outcomes in singleton pregnancies resulting from the transfer of frozen thawed versus fresh embryos generated through in vitro fertilization treatment: a systematic review and meta-analysis. *Fertil Steril*. 2012;98(2):368-377.e1-9. doi:10.1016/j.fertnstert.2012.05.019.

147. Declercq E, Luke B, Belanoff C, et al. Perinatal outcomes associated with assisted reproductive technology: the Massachusetts Outcomes Study of Assisted Reproductive Technologies (MOSART). *Fertil Steril*. 2015;103(4):888-895. doi:10.1016/j.fertnstert.2014.12.119.

148. Tandberg A, Klungsoyr K, Romundstad LB, Skjaerven R. Pre-eclampsia and assisted reproductive technologies: consequences of advanced maternal age, interbirth intervals, new partner and smoking habits. *BJOG*. 2015;122(7):915-922. doi:10.1111/1471-0528.13051.

149. Qin J, Liu X, Sheng X, Wang H, Gao S. Assisted reproductive technology and the risk of pregnancy-related complications and adverse pregnancy outcomes in singleton pregnancies: a meta-analysis of cohort studies. *Fertil Steril*. 2016;105(1):73-85.e1-6. doi:10.1016/j.fertnstert.2015.09.007.

150. Herrington DM, Espeland MA, Crouse JR III, et al. Estrogen replacement and brachial artery flow-mediated vasodilation in older women. *Arterioscler Thromb Vasc Biol*. 2001;21(12):1955-1961. doi:10.1161/hq1201.100241.

151. Vita JA, Keaney Jr JF. Hormone replacement therapy and endothelial function: the exception that proves the rule? *Arterioscler Thromb Vasc Biol*. 2001;21(12):1867-1869.

152. Sunkara SK, La Marca A, Seed PT, Khalaf Y. Increased risk of preterm birth and low birthweight with very high number of oocytes following IVF: an analysis of 65 868 singleton live birth outcomes. *Hum Reprod*.

2015;30(6):1473-1480. doi:10.1093/humrep/dev076.

153. Pereira N, Elias RT, Christos PJ, et al. Supraphysiologic estradiol is an independent predictor of low birth weight in full-term singletons born after fresh embryo transfer. *Hum Reprod.* 2017;32(7):1410-1417. doi:10.1093/humrep/dex095.

154. Ribeiro VC, Santos-Ribeiro S, De Munck N, et al. Should we continue to measure endometrial thickness in modern-day medicine? The effect on live birth rates and birth weight. *Reprod Biomed Online.* 2018;36(4):416-426. doi:10.1016/j.rbmo.2017.12.016.

155. Palermo G, Joris H, Devroey P, Van Steirteghem AC. Pregnancies after intracytoplasmic injection of single spermatozoon into an oocyte. *Lancet.* 1992;340(8810): 17-18. doi:10.1016/0140-6736(92)92425-f.

156. Morken NH. Preterm delivery in IVF versus ICSI singleton pregnancies: a national population-based cohort. *Eur J Obstet Gynecol Reprod Biol.* 2011;154(1):62-66. doi:10.1016/j.ejogrb.2010.08.025.

157. Nouri K, Ott J, Stoegbauer L, Pietrowski D, Frantal S, Walch K. Obstetric and perinatal outcomes in IVF versus ICSI-conceived pregnancies at a tertiary care center—a pilot study. *Reprod Biol Endocrinol.* 2013;11:84. doi:10.1186/1477-7827-11-84.

158. Lacamara C, Ortega C, Villa S, Pommer R, Schwarze JE. Are children born from singleton pregnancies conceived by ICSI at increased risk for congenital malformations when compared to children conceived naturally? A systematic review and meta-analysis. *JBRA Assist Reprod.* 2017;21(3):251-259. doi:10.5935/1518-0557. 20170047.

159. Bonduelle M, Bergh C, Niklasson A, et al. Medical follow-up study of 5-year-old ICSI children. *Reprod Biomed Online.* 2004;9(1):91-101. doi:10.1016/s1472-6483(10)62116-5.

160. Belva F, Bonduelle M, Roelants M, et al. Semen quality of young adult ICSI offspring: the first results. *Hum Reprod.* 2016;31(12):2811-2820. doi:10.1093/humrep/dew245.

161. Du M, Zhang J, Li Z, Liu Y, Wang K, Guan Y. Clinical and neonatal outcomes of children born after ICSI with or without surgically acquired sperm: a retrospective cohort study. *Front Endocrinol (Lausanne).* 2021; 12:788050. doi:10.3389/fendo.2021.788050.

162. Rossato M, Galeazzi C, Ferigo M, Foresta C. Antisperm antibodies modify plasma membrane functional integrity and inhibit osmosensitive calcium influx in human sperm. *Hum Reprod.* 2004;19(8):1816-1820. doi:10.1093/humrep/deh317.

24

Techniques for Selection of Surgically Retrieved Sperm for Intracytoplasmic Sperm Injection

Rafael Favero Ambar, Filipe Tenorio Lira Neto, and Thais Serzedello de Paula

KEY POINTS

- The laboratory has a crucial role to facilitate sperm search, to select the best quality spermatozoa for intracytoplasmic sperm injection (ICSI), and to manage the sperm fertilizing competence.
- Several methods may be used for sperm searching in a surgically retrieved sample, such as mechanical dissection, erythrocyte lysis, and enzymatic digestion.

- Sperm motility stimulants may be a useful tool to improve sperm selection.
- In order to select a viable spermatozoon for ICSI, embryologists can make use of specific techniques such as hypoosmotic test, sperm tail flexibility test, laser-assisted immotile sperm selection, and intracytoplasmic morphologically selected sperm injection.

INTRODUCTION

The development of intracytoplasmic sperm injection (ICSI) has completely revolutionized the treatment of males with azoospermia.[1] According to the etiology of azoospermia and to anatomical factors, sperm can be surgically retrieved from the epididymis or the testis, by different techniques such as percutaneous epididymal sperm aspiration (PESA), microsurgical epididymal sperm aspirations (MESA), testicular sperm aspiration (TESA), testicular sperm extraction (TESE), and microsurgical testicular sperm extraction (micro- TESE).[1]

In cases of nonobstructive azoospermia (NOA), the histopathology of testis is compromised, resulting in severely impaired or nonexistent sperm production.[2] It accounts for about 5% of infertile males, and harvesting testicular sperm is the last chance of fatherhood for these patients.[3] Sperm recovery rate in NOA patients is approximately 50% and has not significantly changed in the last two decades, despite the efforts of clinicians and researchers.[4]

Handling testicular tissue provided by the surgeon is often challenging. The embryologists have the difficult mission of finding sperm suitable for ICSI in the surgically retrieved specimen.[5] Notwithstanding, testicular sperm is, frequently, fragile and nonmotile.[1] For this reason, a thorough and assertive management conducted in the andrology laboratory is crucial.[3] To achieve this objective three critical aspects must be accomplished: (1) good quality surgically retrieved specimen, (2) adequate tissue handling to improve sperm recovery, and (3) sperm potential enhancement with stimulant agents and appropriate selection of viable sperm in case of total immotile.[1] The techniques involved in this process are discussed in this chapter.

SURGICALLY RETRIEVED SPERM SELECTION

Dissection Methods

The most important outcome when assessing sperm extraction is the sperm retrieval rate (SRR). The SRR indicates the percentage of success in sperm recovery.[6,7] In males with obstructive azoospermia (OA), the SRR is usually almost 100%. Nonetheless, the SRR in NOA is about 50% due to the low sperm motility and the poor concentration resulting from partial and heterogeneous preserved focal spermatogenesis.[4,6] However, higher SRR does not indicate good outcomes, nor does a lower SRR indicate poor outcomes.[8]

Therefore greater attention should be paid during dissection methods. The laboratory has a crucial role to facilitate sperm search, to select the best quality spermatozoa for ICSI, and to manage the sperm fertilizing competence. In order to achieve these aims, the andrologists should reduce iatrogenic damage during sperm processing (centrifugation patterns, ultraviolet light exposure, temperature variation, laboratory air quality, dilution and washing steps, quality of reagents, culture media, and disposable materials) and improve sperm fertilizing potential.[7] A minimal search time in the laboratory is recommended to ensure adequate outcomes. By aligning effort with procedural complexity, laboratory staff are better prepared for the task at hand.[9]

In males with OA, sperm may be retrieved by PESA or by MESA. In any of these techniques, sperm retrieval is more easily found, and almost all the times assured.[10] These procedures need less laboratory manipulation since sperm is extracted directly from the epididymis, without dissection.[6]

The biggest challenge is sperm retrieval in males with NOA because just a few of them will have scarce sperm in the testis and the distribution of these sperm may be completely different.[10] In the TESA technique, the aspirate, consisting of fluid and tiny pieces of testicular tissue, is examined, looking for sperm. Although the procedure seems to be innocuous, it is essentially traumatic to the testis, as the multiple passages in different directions macerate the tissue and causes intratesticular bleeding.[10]

TESE or micro-TESE have higher SRR than epididymal recovery, whereas micro-TESE is the most effective and safe method to retrieve sperm from males with NOA but requires gentle manipulation and special expertise.[10,11] This technique allows magnification of the testis parenchyma under an operating microscope, allowing selection of the seminiferous tubules with active spermatogenesis, which appear larger and more opaque than those without active production.[4,9] Scissors cutting, scalpel tear, or a 26-G needle dissection are applied to the testicular tissue to release seminiferous tubule

content.[6] When a testis sperm extraction is performed 24 hours before oocyte retrieval, it is possible to incubate the sample on a supplemented culture medium in order to improve sperm motility.[6]

Erythrocyte Lysis

Surgically retrieved sperm samples usually have red blood cells, which may preclude sperm identification, especially if they are immotile.[6] In order to achieve their goals, laboratory staff should receive the best quality surgically retrieved specimen, with minimal or no red blood cells.[7,12] The laboratory team must dominate processing techniques to minimize iatrogenic cellular damage during sperm preparation.[12]

In such cases, the use of an erythrocyte lysis buffer (ELB) solution, which does not affect sperm viability, is a possible alternative. After tissue cutting, the sample is centrifuged at $750 \times$ g for 5 min. The supernatant is aspirated and discarded, and the pellet is resuspended in 1 to 2 mL of ELB (155 mM NH_4Cl, 10 mM $KHCO_3$, and 2 mM ethylenediaminetetracetic acid; pH 7.2). The mixture is incubated at room temperature for 5 minutes, followed by filling up the tube with buffered medium to dilute the ELB, and centrifuged at $750 \times$ g for 5 min. The supernatant is completely aspirated and discarded, and pellet is resuspended in 0.5 to 1 mL buffered medium. From this fraction, a dish with 10-μL droplets under oil is prepared to perform ICSI.[12] This procedure enhances the efficiency of sperm collection, reducing time of sperm searching and improving the sperm selection process without affecting sperm fertilization potential after ICSI.[6,13]

Enzymatic Digestion

When sperm is not easily found in surgical samples, an enzyme digestion is an alternative to improve sperm recovery, especially in males with NOA, where most of the spermatozoa are adhered to testicular tissue.[6] The use of the enzymatic approach might improve sperm retrieval in subjects where no spermatozoa were detected after the mechanical approach.[4]

Mechanical disruption of the tubules is typically achieved by vigorous tissue shredding or squeezing using needled-tuberculin syringes or undergoing the suspensions through a 24-gauge angiocatheter.[11] Despite solving the testicular adherence, mechanical technique is unproductive and, when improperly performed, might damage sperm.[6] By contrast, enzymatic digestion is carried out by incubation of testicular suspensions with collagenase, combined or not with DNAse and ELB.[11] Both collagenase type IA and collagenase type IV have been used successfully to digest collagen as component of the basement membrane and extracellular matrix. Enzyme solution consists of buffered medium with 1000 IU/mL collagenase IV, 25 μg/mL DNase, and 1.6 mM $CaCl_2$. After exposure of the tissue pellet at 37°C for 1 hour to 1 to 2 mL collagenase solution and meanwhile regularly shaking the tubes, the reaction is stopped by adding 10 mL buffered medium. The digested tissue solution is gently centrifuged at 50 × g for 5 minutes in order to remove residual nondigested pieces or debris. The supernatant cell suspension is washed twice with buffered medium, and the resuspended pellet is used to prepare droplets under oil. In case of high numbers of red blood cells, ELB treatment is preceding the double-washing step.[13]

The enzymes digest the extracellular matrix and facilitate spermatozoa to release from the seminiferous tubules without affecting sperm motility.[11] Consequently, performing enzymatic digestion of testicular tissue is an efficient tool to improve sperm recovery.[6,13] Nevertheless, the procedure may still require several hours, depending on the number of sperm found and the number of oocytes to be injected.[13] In addition, embryologists' experience has a significant effect. However, a recent review and metaanalysis showed no consensus regarding SRR comparing mechanical only or mixed mechanical–enzymatic sperm separation.[4]

Primordial Cell Identification

Nuclear fast/picroindigocarmine staining (NF-PICS) is a rapid and noninvasive tool that may be used in the clinical management of azoospermic patients. The aim of this technique is to identify primordial germ cells in ejaculate or testicular tissue, indicating a possible spermatogenesis focus.[14,15]

Azoospermia is defined as the complete absence of sperm from the ejaculate. For a precise diagnosis, it is necessary to centrifuge the entire semen sample and search for sperm in the pellet to make sure it is completely absent.[16] However, the observer may have difficulty in applying this technique due to an extremely low sperm count not to mention its altered morphology, which hinders its identification.

NF-PICS stains sperm head red and sperm tails green. The same staining pattern may be observed in primordial cells (spermatids and spermatogonia) (Fig. 24.1).

In the case of testis sperm extraction, primordial cells, identification may be of great value because this finding indicates a possible focus of spermatogenesis. Occasionally, the morphology of these cells may be altered due to the extraction method of microtubules; hence applying a differential and specific staining may help identifying these cells.

NF-PICS stain is obtained by dissolving 5 g of aluminum sulfate in 200 mL of hot distilled water and adding 0.1 g of nuclear fast red before stirring with a glass rod.[17] To obtain picroindigocarmine stain, add 150 mL of saturated picric acid solution to a glass beaker, dissolve 0.5 g of indigocarmine dye in the solution, filter, and store in a brown bottle (light sensitive).[17]

In 1998, a study was carried out to compare histological findings of prognostic testicular biopsy and NF-PICS staining in centrifuged ejaculates. A positive correlation was observed between both analyses, concluding that the use of staining may avoid a surgical testicular biopsy procedure.[15] Recently, the benefit of this technique in identifying spermatozoa in samples of males previously considered as azoospermic was confirmed again.[17] NF-PICS can be easily included in andrology laboratory routines in order to achieve a better evaluation of males with azoospermia.[15]

SPERM SELECTION METHODS

Pentoxifylline

Pentoxifylline is a phosphodiesterase enzyme inhibitor derived from methylxanthine. It inhibits the cyclic adenosine monophosphate (cAMP) phosphodiesterase, increasing intracellular cAMP concentration and tyrosine phosphorylation at the sperm tail level.[18] It has been suggested that cAMP is the primary signal for the onset of progressive motility under proper conditions.[19]

A 5 mM pentoxifylline solution can be obtained by dissolving 1.391 mg pentoxifylline in 1 mL of HEPES-buffered culture medium.[1] After that, an aliquot of testicular sperm suspension is loaded into a solution microdroplet and incubated for 20 minutes.[1] In cases of success, a motility pattern will be noticed.

Pentoxifylline has become a tool to increase sperm motility and fertilization capacity in asthenozoospermic samples or in selecting immotile testicular sperm, however, still with controversial results.[20,21]

Some studies reported an improvement in fertilization rate and consequently in the number of available

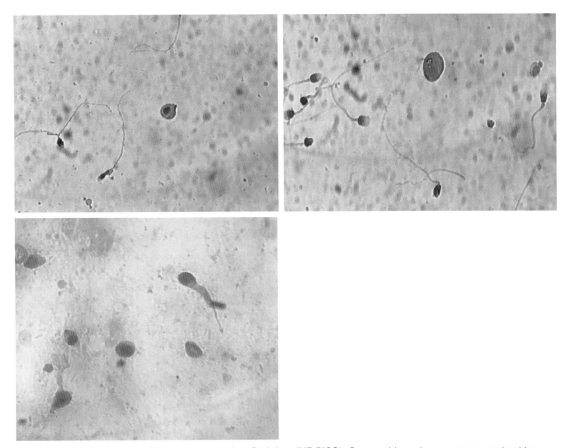

Fig. 24.1 Nuclear Fast/Picroindigocarmine Staining (NF-PICS). Spermatids and spermatozoa stained by the NF-PICS method, where the head stains red and the tail stains green.

embryos, but no benefit in clinical results was found.[22,23] Other authors have shown no difference in any of the evaluated parameters.[24]

An important highlight is that pentoxifylline concentration in adopted protocol may affect laboratory results. In animal models, concentrations in micromolar ranges did not have a negative influence on embryo development, but in millimolar, however, it demonstrated deleterious effects, leading to developmental embryo block in early stages.[25]

Theophylline

The rationale involved in the use of this technique is similar to pentoxifylline, increasing intracellular cAMP.

The evidence on theophylline benefit is scarce. There is a single, well-structured study with 65 patients submitted to TESE by various causes. The samples were frozen to perform ICSI in the near future. After thawing, samples were divided into two groups: in one, theophylline was added to sample, and in the other, not. The results showed that 98.5% of the samples with theophylline had improved seminal motility as well as oocyte fertilization and pregnancy rates.[26]

Although there is concern regarding the toxic effects of motility-enhancing chemicals on embryo development, no evidence of anomalies in offspring has been shown.[27,28]

Calcium Ionophore

Intracytoplasmic injection was developed to overcome infertility due to severe male factor. There is a 60% to 70% fertilization rate in ICSI, but total fertilization failure occurs in 2% to 3% of ICSI cycles.[29] Among many other factors, fertilization failure after ICSI might be explained by inability of sperm to activate oocytes despite proper injection of spermatozoa.[30]

Sperm with lack of motility, commonly found in testicular samples, are associated with fertilization failure in assisted reproductive technology (ART).[29]

The calcium oscillation during oocyte activation may influence the fertilization rates, as well as embryo development. Calcium ionophore has been the most frequently used method for artificial oocyte activation.[31]

A study evaluating the impact of incubation of post-ICSI oocytes (injected with immotile testicular sperm) in culture medium containing 10 μM calcium ionophore for 5 minutes concluded that oocyte activation is a useful method to ensure fertilization in TESE-ICSI cycles in cases of unsuccessful motility improvement with pentoxifylline and after a previous ICSI cycle with low fertilization rate.[29]

Unfortunately, these results are not demonstrated by all researchers, and there is still controversy about the use of calcium ionophore.[32]

Hypoosmotic Swelling Test

The hypoosmotic swelling test (HOS) is a vitality test used for selecting immotile sperm when performing ICSI once this technique does not damage the sperm.

This test is based on the integrity of the cell membrane in viable sperm. It is performed by placing 100 μL of liquefied semen or any sperm-containing media, such as samples from testicular and epididymal sperm extraction procedures, in 1 mL of hypoosmotic solution (i.e., medium diluted 1:1 in embryo toxicity–tested distilled water) and incubating for 5 minutes.[33] Droplets of 20 μL are placed in a petri dish and covered with mineral oil. After 20 minutes, the drops are observed under an inverted microscope. Live spermatozoa become hyperosmotic with respect to the medium, which causes an influx of water to the intracellular compartment; therefore their tails become swollen, while dead spermatozoa with damage to the cell membrane do not change due to the free flow of solutes between the intracellular compartment and the medium, as shown in Fig. 24.2. An important highlight is that live swollen sperm are very fragile and may be damaged by ICSI because injecting pipettes have an internal diameter of 4 to 5 mm. Instead, these sperm should be handled with specially prepared fine glass needles with an inner diameter of 7 to 9 mm and an angle of 35 degrees. The sperm should also be

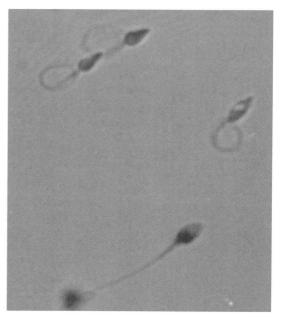

Fig. 24.2 Hypoosmotic Swelling Test. Live cells are distinguished by evidence of swelling of the sperm tail, and dead cells by the absence of swelling.

washed thoroughly in normosmolar sperm preparation medium and stored in a 10-μL droplet before ICSI.[34]

To avoid damage to swollen sperm, an alternative technique of HOS is to aspirate a single immotile spermatozoon with normal morphology by the head with a pipette and moving only the sperm tail out into the hypoosmotic solution. After 5 to 10 seconds, it is observed if a tail tip swelling occurs.[1,35] If swelling or curling is visible, the sperm is taken quickly and completely into the needle and washed in another droplet of normal medium until it regains its normal shape before being stored in a polyvinylpyrrolidone (PVP) droplet.[36]

There is a well-established correlation between the HOS test and eosin test in fresh semen samples, and the HOS test is a good sperm selection technique when motility is low. Furthermore, the HOS test has been shown to select sperm with higher DNA integrity and fewer chromosomal abnormalities.[37,38] However, it should not be used to assess vitality in cryopreserved samples because of spontaneous tail curling after thawing.[39]

Sperm Tail Flexibility Test

Another option for testing individual sperm vitality during sperm selection for ICSI is the sperm tail flexibility test. This test is simple to perform but requires embryologists with extensive experience. Using a microinjection pipette, immotile sperm with normal morphology are aspirated from the culture medium and transferred to a microdroplet of PVP. The sperm tail is manually moved up and down using the micropipette tip and if the tail is flexible, moving independently of the head, the sperm is considered viable. If the tail remains rigid and moves in a single block with the head, the sperm is considered unviable.[40,41] Like the HOS test, the sperm tail flexibility test might be suboptimal for cryopreserved samples.[36]

Laser-Assisted Immotile Sperm Selection

Recently, laser has been used in ART, with different objectives such as assisted hatching, embryo biopsies, and sperm immobilization.[42] In 2004, Aktan et al. used laser to identify viable spermatozoa for the first time.[43] Laser-assisted immotile sperm selection (LAISS) is performed by a single laser shot of 129 μJ for approximately 1.2 milliseconds directed to the tips of the tails of immotile sperm. If the spermatozoon is viable, the tail will coil or curl after the shot. The ability of LAISS to detect live immotile sperm is comparable to that of the HOS test. In addition, when LAISS is used to select sperm for ICS, there is a significant increase in the fertilization and live birth rates in comparison with randomly selected sperm.[36] A retrospective study reported no negative effects on perinatal and neonatal outcome when LAISS was used to select testicular sperm compared with traditional motility-based sperm selection.[42] This method is easily reproducible and does not use any additional chemical reagent, decreasing the possibility of adverse effects. Conversely, LAISS has a high cost, since it requires expensive equipment and an embryologist well trained in the use of the laser. Furthermore, despite exciting preliminary evidence, more robust data from clinical trials are necessary to establish LAISS as an effective and safe method of sperm selection.

INTRACYTOPLASMIC MORPHOLOGICALLY SELECTED SPERM INJECTION

Intracytoplasmic morphologically selected sperm injection (IMSI) employs high sperm magnification to select live sperm for ICSI based on several morphological features such as the head shape, the presence of a vacuole in the nucleus, and the head base. In fact, IMSI is the application of motile sperm organelle morphology examination (MSOME) during ICSI.[44] The most important aspects evaluated by MSOME are the presence, location, and number of vacuoles in the sperm head due to their association with DNA damage, chromosomal alterations, and decreased pregnancy rate (Fig. 24.3).[45–48]

IMSI is carried out by loading spermatozoa in a PVP droplet in a glass-bottomed culture dish. A preliminary selection of motile spermatozoa in the PVP drop is performed at 630× to 1000× magnification under a Nomarski interferential inverted microscope. In this step, spermatozoa with normal oval head shape as well as absence of both cytoplasmic extrusions and tail defects are selected. Then selected spermatozoa are immobilized and their morphology reevaluated under magnifications ranging between 6600× and 12,000× using a variable zoom lens and a digital camera.[49] A scoring scale based on the normalcy of the head (2 points if normal), the symmetry of the base (1 point if normal), and the absence of vacuole (3 points if absent) is used, and the spermatozoa are classified into three grades: high-quality spermatozoa (score 4–6), medium-quality spermatozoa (score 1–3), and low-quality spermatozoa (score 0).[50] The primary goal is to choose spermatozoa without vacuoles for injection into the oocytes. However, if this is not possible, spermatozoa with the least number of vacuoles and/or other abnormalities are selected for injection. The entire procedure can be time-consuming, especially in cases of a very low percentage of morphological normal sperm and large number of oocytes.

Despite the promising results of several studies, a recent Cochrane metaanalysis of 13 randomized controlled trials (RCTs) reported that IMSI use did not improve live birth and miscarriage rates, with only marginal improvement in clinical pregnancy rate compared with traditional sperm selection techniques.[51] These results were confirmed by a different metaanalysis that found improvement in the reproductive outcomes only when observational studies were included.[52] Conversely, IMSI decreased the risk of congenital malformations, as demonstrated by another metaanalysis.[53] In clinical practice, IMSI may be useful in heterosexual couples with severe male factor and repetitive in vitro fertilization/ICSI failure.[54]

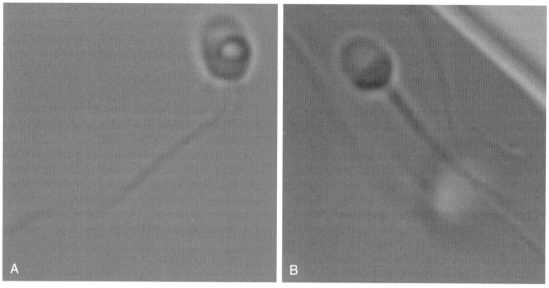

Fig. 24.3 Classification of spermatozoa analyzed at high magnification (6600×) into two different categories: morphologically normal sperm (A) and sperm with large nuclear vacuoles (B).

Magnetic-Activated Cell Sorting

During spermatogenesis, apoptosis serves to control the number and quality of germ cells. In fact, around 50% to 70% of developing germ cells are discarded.[55] Apoptotic sperm cells express apoptotic marker residues in their outer plasma membrane, such as phosphatidylserine, that are recognized by Sertoli cells, leading to the elimination of these cells.[56] However, under certain pathological conditions, some sperm cells that initiated apoptosis may escape detection and elimination by Sertoli cells.[57] The DNA of apoptotic spermatozoa is usually damaged due to the action of nuclear endonucleases that induce double-strand breaks. The sperm DNA breaks are commonly referred to as sperm DNA fragmentation (SDF) and are typically found in the ejaculates of infertile males.[58,59] While elevated SDF is mainly observed in males with abnormal semen parameters, namely count, motility, and morphology, it can also coexist with normozoospermia.[60] Elevated levels of SDF are associated with infertility and decreased pregnancy rates, even with medically assisted reproduction.

Magnetic-activated cell sorting (MACS) is a technique employed to identify and eliminate apoptotic sperm cells from the ejaculate. Briefly, the method works by mixing sperm cells with annexin V conjugated with a magnetic microbead. Annexin has a high affinity for phosphatidylserine, binding to this marker on the membrane of apoptotic sperm cells. Then, the sperm/microbead suspension is loaded into a separation column with a MACS magnet that retains the apoptotic spermatozoa attached to the microbead, allowing only the nonapoptotic ones to pass through.[61]

Concerning the ability of selecting sperm with less DNA damage, MACS has been shown to greatly decrease SDF levels, especially in males with baseline SDF greater than 30%.[61–63] In addition, the use of MACS has been shown to improve implantation rates, pregnancy rates, and live birth rates in most retrospective[56,64] and prospective[65–67] studies. However, most studies included males with abnormal semen analysis (SA) parameters or high SDF levels.[56,65–68]

A retrospective study including 305 males with SDF greater than 30% and nonsevere male factor (volume >1.5 mL, sperm concentration $\geq 5 \times 10^6$/mL, progressive motility >15%, and normal sperm morphology ≥ 1%) revealed that albeit effective in selecting sperm with less DNA damage, the use addition of MACS to density gradient centrifugation (DGC) did not increase the live birth rate compared with density gradient alone.[69]

In contrast, an RCT comparing DGC plus MACS with DGC alone in males with SDF levels greater than 20% and at least 1×10^6 progressive motile sperm also showed increased clinical pregnancy rate when MACS was used.[66] Moreover, another RCT including 80 males with abnormal SA parameters demonstrated significant increase in pregnancy rate (54.54% vs. 24.25%, p = 0.01), implantation rate (36.3% vs. 15.7%, p = 0.02), and live birth rate (45% vs. 15%, p value not reported) when DGC plus MACS was compared with DCG.[65] A similar RCT including males with abnormal SA parameters revealed higher implantation rate (61.4% vs. 45.9%, p < 0.05) with MACS.[70] Similarly, a retrospective analysis of 724 cycles including only males with SDF levels greater than 20% demonstrated increased pregnancy rate (60.7% vs. 51.5%, p = 0.01) and live birth rate (47.4 vs. 31.2%, p = 0.001) when MACS was used.[56] The technique was also effective in improving the cumulative live birth rates as reported by Mei and colleagues in an RCT including 80 males with SDF levels greater than 30%,[67] as well as by Julia and colleagues in a retrospective study including more than 49,000 cycles in unselected couples.[64]

A Cochrane metaanalysis reported no benefit of MACS in improving live birth rate (risk ratio [RR] 1.95; 95% confidence interval [CI]: 0.89, 4.29; one RCT, 62 females), clinical pregnancy rate (RR 1.05; 95% CI: 0.84, 1.31; three RCTs, 413 females; $I^2 = 81\%$), or miscarriage rate (RR 0.95; 95% CI: 0.16, 5.63; two RCTs, 150 females; $I^2 = 0\%$) compared with standard sperm selection techniques.[71] However, the low number of included studies limited the level of evidence.

Regarding the safety of MACS, no differences in obstetric and perinatal outcomes were observed in a post hoc analysis of data from an RCT comparing MACS with swim-up.[72] This technique is better used in males with persistently high SDF levels and normal or moderately reduced sperm count, allowing the selection of sperm with less DNA damage, and is thus more suitable for ICSI.

MICROFLUIDICS-BASED SPERM SELECTION TECHNIQUES

Microfluidics is the science of manipulating small amounts of fluids with volumes ranging from microliters to picoliters at the submillimeter scale.[73] Microfluidics can be used to simulate the geometry of natural routes that are navigated by spermatozoa. Most microfluidic devices contain microchannels that resemble the tubal channels, leading to the selection of progressive motile spermatozoa that reach to the end of such structures.[74] In addition, other microfluidic approaches such as active flow, rheotaxis, and chemical-based sorting have been used to efficiently isolate good quality sperm.[75,76] These techniques mimic the in vivo sperm selection process that takes place while the male gametes are traveling from the cervix to the ovarian tube. Studies have described a positive correlation between motility characteristics and DNA quality;[77,78] thus selecting highly motile sperm improves the chances that spermatozoa with lower SDF are selected.[79]

Usually, microfluidic devices are easy to use, but the process varies with the selection techniques employed by each device. The most frequently used technique is the passive flow. Microchips that use this approach are first primed with some sort of sperm incubation medium, then raw semen is placed into an inlet chamber of the microchip. After some time, usually 10 to 30 minutes, the sorted sperm are collected from an outlet chamber.

Some authors have demonstrated that elevated gravitational forces used in traditional sperm selection techniques may induce the production reactive oxygen species.[80,81] In addition, these techniques require up to 3 hours of processing, another factor that could induce SDF.[82] Therefore another advantage of microfluidic sperm selection (MSS) is that by bypassing centrifugation and shortening the time of processing, it reduces SDF during sperm selection. In fact, MSS has consistently been shown to select sperm not only with higher motility but also with decreased SDF levels compared with swim-up or DCG, both in the general male population[79,83–85] and in males with high baseline sperm DNA damage.[79,86,87] This technique is also able to select sperm with lower oxidative reduction potential, a marker of oxidative stress.[88]

The ZyMoT-Multi and ZyMoT-ICSI (formerly known as Fertile and Fertile Plus; DxNow, Inc.) devices are the most-studied MSS tools to date. Reports employing these devices have shown increased fertilization rate, total number of blastocysts, and number of top-quality blastocysts compared with DGC.[89–93] However, improved pregnancy and live birth rates were demonstrated only when the devices were used in couples with male factor infertility.[91,94]

Despite selecting sperm with better motility and lower DNA damage, the devices used for MSS are yet to be definitively proven useful in increasing pregnancy rates and live birth rates. This selection technique is best used in males with high SDF levels and with sperm concentration of at least 1×10^6 sperm/mL.

CLINICAL CASE SCENARIOS

CASE 1

A 44-year-old male presented to the fertility clinic requesting a male fertility factor evaluation. He had a previous vasectomy 10 years ago and wanted to have a new conception with his new 29-year-old wife. At that time, his wife had a simultaneously fertility evaluation and no abnormalities were found. Two options were offered to the couple: vasectomy reversal or ICSI, and they chose the second one. At the same time, a percutaneous epididymal sperm extraction was performed, and an adequate amount of sperm for fresh use and cryopreservation was harvested. After using DGC to process the sample, spermatozoa were selected for injection by the traditional method. The fertilization rate was 45%, and no embryo survived to day 5.

Soon after the failed ICSI, the couple decided to undergo a second ICSI cycle. The same antagonist protocol was used, 12 mature oocytes were retrieved, and cryopreserved spermatozoa were used. However, fertilization rate was 40%, and only one low-quality embryo reached day 5. A fresh embryo transfer was performed, but the embryo failed to implant.

After the second ICSI, the wife was again thoroughly reevaluated, but no additional findings or conditions were found. After discussion of the case during grand rounds, IMSI technique was offered to the couple, which was accepted. For the third ICSI cycle, the same ovarian stimulation protocol was used and 13 mature oocytes were retrieved, but MSOME was applied to select thawed spermatozoa. During sperm selection, it was revealed that most spermatozoa, including the ones with motility, contained vacuoles in their heads. The embryologist was able to select 10 high-quality and three medium-quality spermatozoa for injection. The fertilization rate was 82%, and five embryos reached the blastocyst stage at day 5. A fresh single embryo transfer was performed, resulting in an ongoing singleton pregnancy.

CASE 2

A 35-year-old male was admitted for fertility evaluation, reporting primary infertility for 5 years. He had an unremarkable past medical and surgical history. On physical examination, both testes were normally descended, with decreased size and consistency. No other abnormalities were identified. His spouse was 29 years old and had no gynecological problems. Two semen analyses confirmed azoospermia after centrifugation. Laboratory work up showed no abnormalities, except for karyotype 47,XXY.

The patient was counseled about treatment alternatives and decided to proceed with diagnostic TESA before ART. After TESA sample processing, no sperm were identified; however, when NF-PICS was applied, primordial germ cells were stained. Despite the previous diagnosis of azoospermia, in light of the NF-PICS finding, it was decided to proceed with an attempt at sperm retrieval by micro-TESE along with ovarian stimulation for ICSI on the day before oocyte aspiration. Concerning the micro-TESE sample, immotile sperm were identified after careful shredding and mincing of the tissue. Due to immobility, pentoxifylline was used to increase motility, ensuring the use of viable motile sperm for ICSI.

SUMMARY

Tissue and sperm handling prior to assisted reproductive technology is often challenging. The embryologists have the difficult mission of finding sperm suitable for intracytoplasmic sperm injection (ICSI) in the surgically retrieved specimen, in patients with nonobstructive azoospermia. Notwithstanding, testicular sperm is, frequently, fragile and nonmotile. For this reason, a thorough and assertive management conducted in the andrology laboratory is crucial. This chapter explores widely used techniques to improve sperm search and selection for ICSI.

REFERENCES

1. Esteves SC, Varghese AC. Laboratory handling of epididymal and testicular spermatozoa: What can be done to improve sperm injections outcome. *J Hum Reprod Sci.* 2012;5(3):233-243.
2. Popal W, Nagy ZP. Laboratory processing and intracytoplasmic sperm injection using epididymal and testicular spermatozoa: what can be done to improve outcomes? *Clinics (Sao Paulo).* 2013;68 Suppl 1(suppl 1):125-130.

3. Pan MM, Hockenberry MS, Kirby EW, Lipshultz LI. Male infertility diagnosis and treatment in the era of in vitro fertilization and intracytoplasmic sperm injection. *Med Clin North Am.* 2018;102(2):337-347.

4. Corona G, Minhas S, Giwercman A, et al. Sperm recovery and ICSI outcomes in men with non-obstructive azoospermia: a systematic review and meta-analysis. *Hum Reprod Update.* 2019;25(6):733-757.

5. Verheyen G, Popovic-Todorovic B, Tournaye H. Processing and selection of surgically-retrieved sperm for ICSI: a review. *Basic Clin Androl.* 2017;27:6.

6. Ambar RF, Gava MM, Ghirelli-Filho M, Yoshida IH, De Paula TS, Glina S. Tissue and sperm handling before assisted reproductive technology (ART): a systematic review. *Arab J Urol.* 2021;19(3):238-246.

7. Esteves SC, Miyaoka R, Agarwal A. Sperm retrieval techniques for assisted reproduction. *Int Braz J Urol.* 2011;37(5):570-583.

8. Zhang HLL, Zhao LMM, Mao JMM, et al. Sperm retrieval rates and clinical outcomes for patients with different causes of azoospermia who undergo microdissection testicular sperm extraction-intracytoplasmic sperm injection. *Asian J Androl.* 2021;23(1):59-63.

9. Shin DH, Turek PJ. Sperm retrieval techniques. *Nat Rev Urol.* 2013;10(12):723-730.

10. Shah R, Gupta C. Advances in sperm retrieval techniques in azoospermic men: a systematic review. *Arab J Urol.* 2018;16(1):125-131.

11. Achermann APP, Pereira TA, Esteves SC. Microdissection testicular sperm extraction (micro-TESE) in men with infertility due to nonobstructive azoospermia: summary of current literature. *Int Urol Nephrol.* 2021;53(11):2193-2210.

12. Miyaoka R, Orosz JE, Achermann AP, Esteves SC. Methods of surgical sperm extraction and implications for assisted reproductive technology success. *Panminerva Med.* 2019;61(2):164-177.

13. Verheyen G, Popovic-Todorovic B, Tournaye H. Processing and selection of surgically-retrieved sperm for ICSI: a review. *Basic Clin Androl.* 2017;27:6.

14. Hallak J, Cocuzza M, Sarkis AS, Athayde KS, Cerri GG, Srougi M. Organ-sparing microsurgical resection of incidental testicular tumors plus microdissection for sperm extraction and cryopreservation in azoospermic patients: surgical aspects and technical refinements. *Urology.* 2009;73(4):887-892.

15. Hendin BN, Patel B, Levin HS, Thomas AJJ, Agarwal A. Identification of spermatozoa and round spermatids in the ejaculates of men with spermatogenic failure. *Urology.* 1998;51(5):816-819.

16. WHO. *Examination and Processing of Human Semen.* 5th ed. World Health Organization; 2010:286.

17. Sharma RK, Gupta S, Agarwal A, et al. Role of cytocentrifugation combined with nuclear fast picroindigocarmine staining in detecting cryptozoospermia in men diagnosed with azoospermia. *World J Mens Health.* 2022;40(4):627-635.

18. Tournaye H, Wieme P, Janssens R, Verheyen G, Devroey P, Van Steirteghem A. Incubation of spermatozoa from asthenozoospermic semen samples with pentoxifylline and 2-deoxyadenosine: variability in hyperactivation and acrosome reaction rates. *Hum Reprod.* 1994;9(11):2038-2043.

19. Morisawa M, Okuno M. Cyclic AMP induces maturation of trout sperm axoneme to initiate motility. *Nature.* 1982;295(5851):703-704.

20. Fountain S, Rizk B, Avery SP, et al. An evaluation of the effect of pentoxifylline on sperm function and treatment outcome of male-factor infertility: a preliminary study. *J Assist Reprod Genet.* 1995;12(10):704-709.

21. Laokirkkiat P, Kunathikom S, Choavaratana R, Petyim S, Prechapanich J. Comparison between sperm treated with pentoxifylline and 2-deoxyadenosine using hypo-osmotic swelling test. *J Med Assoc Thai.* 2007;90(2):211-215.

22. Kovačič B, Vlaisavljević V, Reljič M. Clinical use of pentoxifylline for activation of immotile testicular sperm before ICSI in patients with azoospermia. *J Androl.* 2006;27(1):45-52.

23. Griveau JF, Lobel B, Laurent MC, Michardière L, Le Lannou D. Interest of pentoxifylline in ICSI with frozen-thawed testicular spermatozoa from patients with non-obstructive azoospermia. *Reprod Biomed Online.* 2006;12(1):14-18.

24. Terriou P, Hans E, Giorgetti C, et al. Pentoxifylline initiates motility in spontaneously immotile epididymal and testicular spermatozoa and allows normal fertilization, pregnancy, and birth after intracytoplasmic sperm injection. *J Assist Reprod Genet.* 2000;17(4):194-199.

25. Tournaye H, Van der Linden M, Van den Abbeel E, Devroey P, Van Steirteghem A. Effect of pentoxifylline on implantation and post-implantation development of mouse embryos in vitro. *Hum Reprod.* 1993;8(11):1948-1954.

26. Ebner T, Tews G, Mayer RB, et al. Pharmacological stimulation of sperm motility in frozen and thawed testicular sperm using the dimethylxanthine theophylline. *Fertil Steril.* 2011;96(6):1331-1336.

27. Aydos K, Aydos OS. Sperm selection procedures for optimizing the outcome of ICSI in patients with NOA. *J Clin Med.* 2021;10(12):2687.

28. Ebner T, Shebl O, Mayer RB, Moser M, Costamoling W, Oppelt P. Healthy live birth using theophylline in a case of retrograde ejaculation and absolute asthenozoospermia. *Fertil Steril.* 2014;101(2):340-343.

29. Kang HJ, Lee SH, Park YS, et al. Artificial oocyte activation in intracytoplasmic sperm injection cycles using testicular sperm in human in vitro fertilization. *Clin Exp Reprod Med.* 2015;42(2):45-50.

30. Nasr-Esfahani MH, Deemeh MR, Tavalaee M. Artificial oocyte activation and intracytoplasmic sperm injection. *Fertil Steril.* 2010;94(2):520-526.

31. Ozil JP, Banrezes B, Tóth S, Pan H, Schultz RM. Ca2+ oscillatory pattern in fertilized mouse eggs affects gene expression and development to term. *Dev Biol.* 2006;300(2):534-544.

32. Borges E, de Almeida Ferreira Braga DP, de Sousa Bonetti TC, Iaconelli A, Franco JG. Artificial oocyte activation using calcium ionophore in ICSI cycles with spermatozoa from different sources. *Reprod Biomed Online.* 2009;18(1):45-52.

33. Verheyen G, Joris H, Crits K, Nagy Z, Tournaye H, Van Steirteghem A. Comparison of different hypo-osmotic swelling solutions to select viable immotile spermatozoa for potential use in intracytoplasmic sperm injection. *Hum Reprod Update.* 1997;3(3):195-203.

34. Mangoli V, Mangoli R, Dandekar S, Suri K, Desai S. Selection of viable spermatozoa from testicular biopsies: a comparative study between pentoxifylline and hypoosmotic swelling test. *Fertil Steril.* 2011;95(2):631-634.

35. Sallam HN, Farrag A, Agameya AF, El-Garem Y, Ezzeldin F. The use of the modified hypo-osmotic swelling test for the selection of immotile testicular spermatozoa in patients treated with ICSI: a randomized controlled study. *Hum Reprod.* 2005;20(12):3435-3440.

36. Nordhoff V. How to select immotile but viable spermatozoa on the day of intracytoplasmic sperm injection? An embryologist's view. *Andrology.* 2015;3(2):156-162.

37. Bloch A, Rogers EJ, Nicolas C, et al. Detailed cell-level analysis of sperm nuclear quality among the different hypo-osmotic swelling test (HOST) classes. *J Assist Reprod Genet.* 2021;38(9):2491-2499.

38. Rouen A, Carlier L, Heide S, et al. Potential selection of genetically balanced spermatozoa based on the hypo-osmotic swelling test in chromosomal rearrangement carriers. *Reprod Biomed Online.* 2017;35(4):372-378.

39. Hossain A, Osuamkpe C, Hossain S, Phelps JY. Spontaneously developed tail swellings (SDTS) influence the accuracy of the hypo-osmotic swelling test (HOS-test) in determining membrane integrity and viability of human spermatozoa. *J Assist Reprod Genet.* 2010 ;27(2-3):83-86.

40. Oliveira NM, Vaca Sánchez R, Rodriguez Fiesta S, et al. Pregnancy with frozen-thawed and fresh testicular biopsy after motile and immotile sperm microinjection, using the mechanical touch technique to assess viability. *Hum Reprod.* 2004;19(2):262-265.

41. Soares JB, Glina S, Antunes NJ, Wonchockier R, Galuppo AG, Mizrahi FE. Sperm tail flexibility test: a simple test for selecting viable spermatozoa for intracytoplasmic sperm injection from semen samples without motile spermatozoa. *Rev Hosp Clin Fac Med Sao Paulo.* 2003;58(5):250-253.

42. Chen H, Wang C, Zhou H, et al. Laser-assisted selection of immotile spermatozoa has no effect on obstetric and neonatal outcomes of TESA-ICSI pregnancies. *Reprod Biol Endocrinol.* 2021;19(1):159.

43. Aktan TM, Montag M, Duman S, Gorkemli H, Rink K, Yurdakul T. Use of a laser to detect viable but immotile spermatozoa. *Andrologia.* 2004;36(6):366-369.

44. Bartoov B, Berkovitz A, Eltes F. Selection of spermatozoa with normal nuclei to improve the pregnancy rate with intracytoplasmic sperm injection. *N Engl J Med.* 2001;345(14):1067-1068.

45. Mangoli E, Khalili MA, Talebi AR, et al. Association between early embryo morphokinetics plus transcript levels of sperm apoptotic genes and clinical outcomes in IMSI and ICSI cycles of male factor patients. *J Assist Reprod Genet.* 2020;37(10):2555-2567.

46. Cassuto NG, Hazout A, Hammoud I, et al. Correlation between DNA defect and sperm-head morphology. *Reprod Biomed Online.* 2012;24(2):211-218.

47. Perdrix A, Travers A, Chelli MH, et al. Assessment of acrosome and nuclear abnormalities in human spermatozoa with large vacuoles. *Hum Reprod.* 2011;26(1):47-58.

48. Berkovitz A, Eltes F, Ellenbogen A, Peer S, Feldberg D, Bartoov B. Does the presence of nuclear vacuoles in human sperm selected for ICSI affect pregnancy outcome? *Hum Reprod.* 2006;21(7):1787-1790.

49. Vanderzwalmen P, Hiemer A, Rubner P, et al. Blastocyst development after sperm selection at high magnification is associated with size and number of nuclear vacuoles. *Reprod Biomed Online.* 2008;17(5):617-627.

50. Cassuto NG, Bouret D, Plouchart JM, et al. A new real-time morphology classification for human spermatozoa: a link for fertilization and improved embryo quality. *Fertil Steril.* 2009;92(5):1616-1625.

51. Teixeira DM, Hadyme Miyague A, Barbosa MA, Navarro PA, Raine-Fenning N, Nastri CO, et al. Regular (ICSI) versus ultra-high magnification (IMSI) sperm selection for assisted reproduction. *Cochrane Database Syst Rev.* 2020;2:CD010167.

52. Duran-Retamal M, Morris G, Achilli C, et al. Live birth and miscarriage rate following intracytoplasmic morphologically selected sperm injection vs intracytoplasmic sperm injection: an updated systematic review and meta-analysis. *Acta Obstet Gynecol Scand.* 2020;99(1):24-33.

53. Dieamant F, Petersen CG, Vagnini LD, et al. Impact of intracytoplasmic morphologically selected sperm injection (IMSI) on birth defects: a systematic review and meta-analysis. *JBRA Assist Reprod.* 2021;25(3):466-472.

54. Karabulut S, Aksunger O, Korkmaz O, Eren Gozel H, Keskin I. Intracytoplasmic morphologically selected sperm injection, but for whom? *Zygote.* 2019;27(5):299-304.

55. Neto FT, Bach PV, Najari BB, Li PS, Goldstein M. Spermatogenesis in humans and its affecting factors. *Semin Cell Dev Biol*. 2016;59:10-26.

56. Pacheco A, Blanco A, Bronet F, Cruz M, García-Fernández J, García-Velasco JA. Magnetic-activated cell sorting (MACS): a useful sperm-selection technique in cases of high levels of sperm DNA fragmentation. *J Clin Med*. 2020;9(12):3976.

57. Sakkas D, Seli E, Bizzaro D, Tarozzi N, Manicardi GC. Abnormal spermatozoa in the ejaculate: abortive apoptosis and faulty nuclear remodelling during spermatogenesis. *Reprod Biomed Online*. 2003;7:428-432.

58. Blumer CG, Fariello RM, Restelli AE, Spaine DM, Bertolla RP, Cedenho AP. Sperm nuclear DNA fragmentation and mitochondrial activity in men with varicocele. *Fertil Steril*. 2008;90:1716-1722.

59. Esteves SC, Zini A, Coward RM, et al. Sperm DNA fragmentation testing: Summary evidence and clinical practice recommendations. *Andrologia*. 2021;53:e13874.

60. Jeremias JT, Belardin LB, Okada FK, et al. Oxidative origin of sperm DNA fragmentation in the adult varicocele. *Int Braz J Urol*. 2021;47:275-283.

61. Said TM, Agarwal A, Grunewald S, Rasch M, Glander HJ, Paasch U. Evaluation of sperm recovery following annexin V magnetic-activated cell sorting separation. *Reprod Biomed Online*. 2006;13:336-369.

62. Martínez MG, Sánchez-Martín P, Dorado-Silva M, et al. Magnetic-activated cell sorting is not completely effective at reducing sperm DNA fragmentation. *J Assist Reprod Genet*. 2018;35:2215-2221.

63. Degheidy T, Abdelfattah H, Seif A, Albuz FK, Gazi S, Abbas S. Magnetic activated cell sorting: an effective method for reduction of sperm DNA fragmentation in varicocele men prior to assisted reproductive techniques. *Andrologia*. 2015;47:892-896.

64. Gil Juliá M, Hervás I, Navarro-Gómez Lechón A, et al. Sperm Selection by magnetic-activated cell sorting before microinjection of autologous oocytes increases cumulative live birth rates with limited clinical impact: a retrospective study in unselected males. *Biology (Basel)*. 2021;10(5):430.

65. Ziarati N, Tavalaee M, Bahadorani M, Nasr Esfahani MH. Clinical outcomes of magnetic activated sperm sorting in infertile men candidate for ICSI. *Hum Fertil (Cambridge, England)*. 2019;22:118-125.

66. Hozyen M, Hasanen E, Elqusi K, et al. Reproductive outcomes of different sperm selection techniques for ICSI patients with abnormal sperm DNA fragmentation: a randomized controlled trial. *Reprod Sci*. 2022;29:220-228.

67. Mei J, Chen LJ, Zhu XX, et al. Magnetic-activated cell sorting of nonapoptotic spermatozoa with a high DNA fragmentation index improves the live birth rate and decreases transfer cycles of IVF/ICSI. *Asian J Androl*. 2022;24:367-372.

68. Norozi-Hafshejani M, Tavalaee M, Najafi MH, Shapour F, Arbabian M, Nasr-Esfahani MH. MACS-DGC versus DGC sperm wash procedure: comparing clinical outcomes in couples with male factor infertility undergoing ICSI: a clinical trial study. *Int J Fertil Steril*. 2022;16:17-22.

69. Sánchez-Martín P, Dorado-Silva M, Sánchez-Martín F, González Martínez M, Johnston SD, Gosálvez J. Magnetic cell sorting of semen containing spermatozoa with high DNA fragmentation in ICSI cycles decreases miscarriage rate. *Reprod Biomed Online*. 2017;34:506-512.

70. Dirican EK, Ozgün OD, Akarsu S, et al. Clinical outcome of magnetic activated cell sorting of non-apoptotic spermatozoa before density gradient centrifugation for assisted reproduction. *J Assist Reprod Genet*. 2008;25:375-381.

71. Lepine S, McDowell S, Searle LM, Kroon B, Glujovsky D, Yazdani A. Advanced sperm selection techniques for assisted reproduction. *Cochrane Database Syst Rev*. 2019;7:Cd010461.

72. Romany L, Garrido N, Cobo A, Aparicio-Ruiz B, Serra V, Meseguer M. Obstetric and perinatal outcome of babies born from sperm selected by MACS from a randomized controlled trial. *J Assist Reprod Genet*. 2017;34:201-207.

73. Sackmann EK, Fulton AL, Beebe DJ. The present and future role of microfluidics in biomedical research. *Nature*. 2014;507:181-189.

74. Nosrati R, Graham PJ, Zhang B, et al. Microfluidics for sperm analysis and selection. *Nat Rev Urol*. 2017;14:707-730.

75. Vasilescu SA, Khorsandi S, Ding L, et al. A microfluidic approach to rapid sperm recovery from heterogeneous cell suspensions. *Sci Rep*. 2021;11:7917.

76. Romero-Aguirregomezcorta J, Laguna-Barraza R, Fernández-González R, et al. Sperm selection by rheotaxis improves sperm quality and early embryo development. *Reproduction*. 2021;161:343-352.

77. Velez de la Calle JF, Muller A, Walschaerts M, et al. Sperm deoxyribonucleic acid fragmentation as assessed by the sperm chromatin dispersion test in assisted reproductive technology programs: results of a large prospective multicenter study. *Fertil Steril*. 2008;90:1792-1799.

78. Elbashir S, Magdi Y, Rashed A, Ibrahim MA, Edris Y, Abdelaziz AM. Relationship between sperm progressive motility and DNA integrity in fertile and infertile men. *Middle East Fertil Soc J*. 2018;23:195-198.

79. Riordon J, Tarlan F, You JB, et al. Two-dimensional planar swimming selects for high DNA integrity sperm. *Lab Chip*. 2019;19:2161-2167.

80. Zalata A, Hafez T, Comhaire F. Evaluation of the role of reactive oxygen species in male infertility. *Hum Reprod (Oxford, England)*. 1995;10:1444-1451.

81. Zini A, Finelli A, Phang D, Jarvi K. Influence of semen processing technique on human sperm DNA integrity. *Urology*. 2000;56:1081-1084.

82. Zhang XD, Chen MY, Gao Y, Han W, Liu DY, Huang GN. The effects of different sperm preparation methods and incubation time on the sperm DNA fragmentation. *Hum Fertil (Cambridge, England)*. 2011;14:187-191.

83. Quinn MM, Jalalian L, Ribeiro S, et al. Microfluidic sorting selects sperm for clinical use with reduced DNA damage compared to density gradient centrifugation with swim-up in split semen samples. *Hum Reprod (Oxford, England)*. 2018;33:1388-1393.

84. Nosrati R, Vollmer M, Eamer L, et al. Rapid selection of sperm with high DNA integrity. *Lab Chip*. 2014;14:1142-1150.

85. Kishi K, Ogata H, Ogata S, et al. Frequency of sperm DNA fragmentation according to selection method: comparison and relevance of a microfluidic device and a swim-up procedure. *J Clin Diagn Res*. 2015;9:QC14-QC16.

86. Parrella A, Keating D, Cheung S, et al. A treatment approach for couples with disrupted sperm DNA integrity and recurrent ART failure. *J Assist Reprod Genet*. 2019;36:2057-2066.

87. Pujol A, García-Peiró A, Ribas-Maynou J, Lafuente R, Mataró D, Vassena R. A microfluidic sperm-sorting device reduces the proportion of sperm with double-stranded DNA fragmentation. *Zygote*. 2022;30:200-205.

88. Gode F, Gürbüz AS, Tamer B, Pala I, Isik AZ. The effects of microfluidic sperm sorting, density gradient and swim-up methods on semen oxidation reduction potential. *Urol J*. 2020;17:397-401.

89. Keskin M, Pabuçcu EG, Arslanca T, Demirkıran Ö D, Pabuçcu R. Does microfluidic sperm sorting affect embryo euploidy rates in couples with high sperm DNA fragmentation? *Reprod Sci*. 2022;29:1801-1808.

90. Mirsanei JS, Sheibak N, Zandieh Z, et al. Microfluidic chips as a method for sperm selection improve fertilization rate in couples with fertilization failure. *Arch Gynecol Obstet*. 2022;306:901-910.

91. Yildiz K, Yuksel S. Use of microfluidic sperm extraction chips as an alternative method in patients with recurrent in vitro fertilisation failure. *J Assist Reprod Genet*. 2019;36:1423-1429.

92. Yetkinel S, Kilicdag EB, Aytac PC, Haydardedeoglu B, Simsek E, Cok T. Effects of the microfluidic chip technique in sperm selection for intracytoplasmic sperm injection for unexplained infertility: a prospective, randomized controlled trial. *J Assist Reprod Genet*. 2019;36:403-409.

93. Guler C, Melil S, Ozekici U, Donmez Cakil Y, Selam B, Cincik M. Sperm selection and embryo development: a comparison of the density gradient centrifugation and microfluidic chip sperm preparation methods in patients with astheno-teratozoospermia. *Life (Basel)*. 2021;11(9):933.

94. Ozcan P, Takmaz T, Yazici MGK, et al. Does the use of microfluidic sperm sorting for the sperm selection improve in vitro fertilization success rates in male factor infertility? *J Obstet Gynaecol Res*. 2021;47:382-388.

25

Sperm Banking

Israel Maldonado-Rosas, Liliana Ramirez-Dominguez,
Christina Anagnostopoulou, and Ashok Agarwal

KEY POINTS

- The laboratory has a crucial role to facilitate sperm search, to select the best quality spermatozoa for intracytoplasmic sperm injection (ICSI), and to manage the sperm fertilizing competence.
- Several methods may be used for sperm searching in a surgically retrieved sample, such as mechanical dissection, erythrocyte lysis, and enzymatic digestion.

- Sperm motility stimulants may be a useful tool to improve sperm selection.
- In order to select a viable spermatozoon for ICSI, embryologists can make use of specific techniques such as the hypoosmotic test, the sperm tail flexibility test, laser-assisted immotile sperm selection, and intracytoplasmic morphologically selected sperm injection.

INTRODUCTION

Sperm banking is defined as the practice of freezing sperm at low temperatures of around −80°C to −196°C. The frozen sperm are stored long-term for use in assisted conception. Initially, this process was done for improving cattle breeding by use of bull sperm that had been frozen. The first reported use of banked sperm for human assisted conception utilizing the artificial insemination technique resulted in three successful pregnancies with viable embryonic development.[1] In 1954, the first live birth was reported with the use of frozen sperm. In these initial studies sperm was frozen in glycerol 10% and then thawed for use.[1,2]

Sperm cryopreservation is a highly complex procedure and needs to be performed by technically skilled personnel.[3–6] The semen sample can be obtained either by masturbation or with invasive surgical retrieval methods such as testicular aspiration or biopsy techniques. It is highly important to preserve the cell membrane integrity and minimize damage during freezing

and thawing.[7] There is a body of literature regarding sperm cryopreservation and its significance in the assisted reproductive technique (ART) field.[8–10]

INDICATIONS OF SPERM CRYOPRESERVATION

Reproduction is central to human experience, and there is a growing list of indications for fertility preservation, including both pediatric or adult cancer patients.[11,12] Quality of life of the cancer survivors is compromised, and sperm banking is good insurance to enhance quality of life.[13,14] The current recommendation from multiple professional societies is that sperm cryopreservation is standard of care for cancer patients.[13,15] In 2013, there were 854,790 new cases of cancer reported in males, and 47% occurred in males less than 45 years of age. Postcancer quality-of-life studies revealed that male factor infertility is a devastating side effect of cancer treatment. The advances in cancer therapeutics have led to high cancer survival rates. Usage rates of banked sperm are increasing by up to 10% to 15%, and use of cryopreserved sperm may lead to pregnancies in more than half of these couples.[13]

Currently, there are diverse indications for sperm banking, including fertility preservation in males with cancer, prior to gonadotoxic therapies for medical conditions, emergency cryopreservation for testicular injury, or testicular torsion and other indications.[16]

Urgent need for cryopreservation includes scrotal trauma in a patient with or without a history of previous contralateral cryptorchidism, bilateral scrotal trauma, testicular torsion in a solitary testis, and bilateral synchronous testicular torsion. Scrotal trauma can lead to severe consequences: testicular fracture, hematoma, avulsion, or damage to the epididymis.[16] Hence scrotal exploration is recommended, but there is the potential limitation of an emergency testicular sperm extraction and need for immediate access to an andrology laboratory.

An emerging important indication for sperm cryopreservation is fertility preservation in transwomen.[17] A transwoman is a person who was assigned male at birth and suffers distress brought upon by the discrepancy between their gender identity and the sex assigned at birth. Fertility preservation before cross-gender hormonal treatment is increasingly being used. Sexual orientation will determine how the sperm is used. The World Professional Association for Transgender Health Standards of Care (American Psychiatric Association) has recommended discussing fertility issues with transgender patients.[18] In a study conducted in Europe, only 15% of transwomen patients chose to freeze their sperm. The prefreeze semen parameter data in transwomen showed a high incidence of oligozoospermia (27.5%), asthenozoospermia (31%), and teratozoospermia (31%). The mean sperm concentration was 46.9×10^6 mL, mean percent motility was 42.9%, and mean percent normal sperm morphology (Kruger's) was 7.98%.[17]

Other indications include inability of the male to produce a semen sample on the day of intrauterine insemination (IUI) or ART due to a psychological block or freezing the sperm for future use in ART when the male cannot be present on the day of oocyte retrieval. Cryopreservation of the sperm is also necessary in sperm donation programs.

Cryopreservation Media

Cryopreservation allows patients likely to have impaired fertility potential to be able to have a biological child in the future and meet individual family goals. Cryopreservation can greatly reduce sperm parameters and increase sperm DNA damage; the addition of cryopreservation media allows improved cryosurvival.[12,19–21] Optimum combinations of glycerol, animal versus human protein, antioxidants, and other additives remains highly debated and researched.[2,22,23] Cryopreservation can induce damage to the sperm due to pH variations, glycerol toxicity, and induction of osmotic shock. HEPES and MOPS are better zwitterion buffering agents to maintain a pH of 7.2 and preserve sperm membrane integrity. Media needs to obey the recommended 6% to 7% glycerol concentration for adequate sperm survival.[2]

Cryoprotectants are highly soluble molecules that diminish cell cryodamage, reducing osmotic stress and helping to reach optimal cooling and thawing rates. The cryoprotective agents can be permeating; examples of these are glycerol, ethylene glycol, dimethyl sulfoxide, propylene glycol, and methyl formamide. On the other hand, nonpermeating cryoprotective chemicals that are included in media are sugar compounds such as sucrose or trehalose. The sperm plasma membrane stabilizing agents added include egg yolk, milk, and albumin. The other components of cryopreservation media are chelating agents, pH buffers such as glycine and TRIS, or zwitterionic buffers such as HEPES and antibiotics. Antioxidants such as glutathione and dithiothreitol have been reported to provide protection against lipid peroxidation during cryopreservation.[24]

Calcium lactate, also known as a gelling activator, helps to form a thin film in the presence of Ca^{2+} when added to the freezing media. Kolliphore P is a surfactant added to the medium to help mediate separation/interface between protein contents from liquefied semen and sperm for higher sperm survival rates. Inositol, an alcohol-based sugar, helps sustain sperm motility and the number of spermatozoa retrieved.[25,26]

SPERM CRYOPRESERVATION

Cryopreservation of ejaculated sperm is standard of care for patients with cancer.[14] There is an array of methods available to freeze sperm, including slow cryopreservation, rapid cryopreservation with or without programmable freezing, sperm vitrification, and single-sperm vitrification using special cell devices.

Slow Cryopreservation

Slow cryopreservation is a systematic procedure with slow addition of the cryoprotectant mixture in equal aliquots. The regulated addition helps the cryoprotectants to equilibrate well across the sperm cell membrane and results in stabilization of the cells. Sperm cryopreservation is a controlled procedure. If not done properly, it can damage the sample, leaving it unusable for subsequent ART procedures post thaw. The main factors that result in cellular cryodamage are intracellular ice formation, osmotic stress, and oxidative stress induced as a result of rapid changes in temperature.

The most common cryoprotectants for sperm freezing include mixtures of egg yolk and pH buffer systems such as TEST with zwitterions. TEST buffer is a combination of TES [*N*Tris (hydroxymethyl) methyl2aminoethanesulfonic acid, pH 7.5] and Tris [(hydroxymethyl) aminomethane]. The fresh egg yolk, dextrose, and antibiotics are additives to form the cryobuffer known as TEST (TES and Tris) yolk buffer (TYB).[27,28] TYB is used and favored for sperm cryopreservation. It preserves sperm motility with higher post thaw recovery compared with other cryoprotectant methods such as Sperm Freezing Medium (Cooper Surgical, Trumbull, CT) and Enhance Sperm Freeze (Conception Technologies, San Diego, CA).[27–29]

A graduated, piecemeal addition of equal aliquots of the cryoprotectant is performed. Once the cryoprotective agent has been added in a ratio of 1:1 to the semen sample, the sample is transferred to cryovials or straws for storage. They are then placed in a freezer at a temperature of −20°C for 8 minutes and next at −96°C in liquid nitrogen vapor for another 2 hours. Finally, they are immersed in liquid nitrogen at −196°C for long-term storage.

There are other available cryoprotectants such as Sperm Freeze Medium from Origio, which is used at a dilution of 1:1 with semen, as well as Arctic Sperm Cryopreservation Medium, where the dilution is 1:2 (medium:semen). The protocol involves determining the volume of media, and the total volume is divided by 10 for the volume of each media aliquot to be added per minute. The initial aliquot is added and the 10-minute dilution begun. Every minute, an aliquot of the cryopreservation medium is added until the final total volume of cryomedium is achieved. In between medium aliquots, semen is mixed utilizing the Vari Mix Test Tube Rocker (Thermo-Scientific). After 10 minutes, dilution is completed. Postmix parameters are obtained. After addition of the cryopreservation media, samples are immediately placed in cryovials in a refrigerator at 4°C for 10 minutes. Samples are next placed into liquid nitrogen vapor for 60 minutes and then submerged in liquid nitrogen for 24 hours.

Sperm Vitrification

Sperm vitrification is a technique that entails precipitous reduction in temperatures at the rate of greater than 1000°C per minute.[30] The process involves creation of a solid glasslike state with increase in viscosity and prevents intracellular ice formation.[31] Sperm vitrification is reported to be safer and induces less damage on sperm vitality, DNA fragmentation, and sperm motility.[32] In a study comparing epigenetic changes in slow cryopreservation versus vitrification, it was proven that cryopreservation of spermatozoa is an epigenetically safe process and does not impact the genes related to fertilization.[32] Isachenko et al.[33] introduced the technique of cryopreservation-free vitrification by utilizing sucrose compound. Cryoprotectant-free vitrification is an innocuous method and still needs more research for clinical applicability.[33]

Options for Sperm Storage Following Cryopreservation

Plastic straws and cryovials are available and have been traditionally used for semen storage. Cryovials are easy to use for storage and then for thawing the semen sample. They have a disadvantage in that they cannot be sealed and thus have a higher risk of contamination.[34] If the cryocap seal is not secure and leaks, then the liquid nitrogen can seep into the sample and could cause an explosion. Small-width tubes such as straws provide efficient heat exchange and seal well, thus preventing mishaps. Straws are manufactured with polyvinyl chloride (PVC) or polyethylene terephthalate glycol (PETG). However, only PETG is used currently. PVC is no longer used as it disintegrates with radiation sterilization. The straws have a storage capacity from 25 μL to 500 μL of sample.

Thawing and Preparation of Cryopreserved Sperm

Thawing of sperm is a process with maximum probability of inducing sperm damage. Initially, the cryovial or straw is withdrawn from the liquid nitrogen tank and then kept at room temperature for 5 minutes. Following this, it is immersed under water in a water bath at 37°C for 20 minutes. The semen sample is then processed to remove the cryoprotectants and the buffers by addition of a sperm-washing medium such as modified human tubular fluid in a ratio of 1:2. The semen–wash medium mixture is next subjected to centrifugation at 350 g for 5 to 10 minutes. Following centrifugation the pellet is aspirated and suspended in nutrient-rich medium for use in IUI/in vitro fertilization (IVF).

Assisted Reproductive Outcomes of Male Cancer Survivors

Fertility preservation in males with cancer is yielding fair reproductive outcomes and helps improve quality of life in survivors. A retrospective review has reported a usage rate for banked sperm in IVF as 10.7%.[35] The authors of the latter study reported high effectiveness, with 77% of patients achieving parenthood with ART. The live birth rate per IVF cycle was 29% versus an average of less than or equal to 20% in earlier studies. A major limitation of this study was that a large proportion of patients using their semen for ART went to other fertility clinics (18/96 patients: 19%). The recent studies also report that little is known about the mutation load of the semen of cancer patients after chemotherapy and/or radiotherapy.[35]

In a prospective review of assisted reproductive outcomes with banked semen specimens, a total of 87 ART cycles were performed, and 18.3% resulted in pregnancy (7% IUI, 23% IVF, and 37% ICSI), and 75% of the pregnancies resulted in a live birth (100% IUI, 83% IVF, and 57% ICSI).[14] There was no significant difference in the outcomes when the results were stratified by type of ART and malignancy.

In a medical records review for 682 patients, 70 patients withdrew their frozen sperm for fertility treatments over a 20-year period.[36] Conception was achieved in 46/184 ART cycles (25%), and this resulted in 36 deliveries. The pregnancy rate was 37.4% with ICSI and 11.5% with IUI, similar to other groups of infertile couples.

There are a variety of newer innovative techniques such as single-sperm vitrification that are emerging with good outcomes, even for a small numbers of sperm.[37] Cryobank facilities should be geared up to store the samples in a low-risk manner, with continuous monitoring for long periods of time. Cryopreserved gametes are the only chance for some patients to father a biological child in the future.

ASSISTED REPRODUCTIVE TECHNIQUE OUTCOMES WITH FROZEN DONOR SPERM

Donor sperm use in ART is reported to be increasing in the United States.[38] Reported data in the literature can support the provider to counsel patients regarding probable cycle success rates and possible pregnancy complications. In a large study conducted in China, the four major reasons for donor rejection were suboptimal semen quality (90.27%), sexually transmitted diseases (STDs) (6.26%), dropping out (2.65%), and chromosomal abnormalities (0.35%). The most common reason for the rejection of donors with an STD was a positive test for mycoplasmas (49.05%), followed by hepatitis B virus (27.56%).[39] Appropriate donor screening is important as demand for donor sperm use is rising.

As statistically significant higher odds ratio for live birth was reported in females greater than 40 years of age undergoing IVF with donor sperm versus partner sperm after removing the effect of the confounding factors.[40] Several studies have demonstrated similar or even higher live birth rates in IVF cycles with donor sperm.[41] However, there are several limitations associated with the design of these studies.

EMERGENCE OF FIELD OF ONCOFERTILITY AND ITS IMPORTANCE IN ASSISTED REPRODUCTIVE TECHNIQUE

Oncofertility is an emerging field and is being developed as a consortium with collaborative efforts of oncologists, reproductive urologists, and male infertility specialists. Cancer therapies are being fine tuned by oncologists to have less impact on fertility. There has been a huge headway made in the technologies of assisted reproduction, cryopreservation procedures, and cancer research, but still more research is needed in these fields. Baseline semen quality is reported to be poor in patients with cancer, and the cancer itself negatively impacts the hypothalamic pituitary axis as well as spermatogenesis. Ultimately, it is crucial to develop cancer therapies that are less harmful to fertility. This includes developing new therapies and ensuring that new chemotherapeutics are tested for gonadotoxicity prior to administration. There is also increasing research being conducted on gonadoprotective agents and therapeutics such as gonadotropin-releasing hormone analogs.[42] Collaborative efforts from the oncofertility consortiums also strive to decrease the incidence of disease-related fertility loss by finding noninterventional or medical ways to eliminate a young person's risk of losing his fertility due to cancer treatment.[42]

Procedures like testicular tissue surgical retrieval and freezing for prepubertal cancer patients are done under the ambit of experimental research protocols with institutional review board guidelines; however, there are several challenges with these experimental procedures regarding their translation application in clinical practice. There is a significant need for raising the awareness of the gonadotoxic effects of oncological treatments on future fertility. This will help to increase the referrals for sperm banking. As the side effects of cancer therapy receive more attention, oncofertility will emerge as a growing field, with more research and translational applications.

MANAGEMENT OF CRYOBANKING SERVICES AND FACILITIES

The guidelines from the American Society for Reproductive Medicine (ASRM) emphasize the importance of availability of cryopreservation facilities and quick accessibility for patients with cancer or other indications.[43] The ASRM recommends that ART programs should have a full-service associated cryopreservation program capable of offering both ejaculated and testicular tissue cryopreservation.

GENERAL REQUIREMENTS FOR SPERM BANKING

The management of a sperm bank must be led by qualified staff who are able to perform an efficient quality control and supervision. Proper standard operating procedures for sperm cryopreservation and storage include the correct sample labeling of analytical, processing, and preparation samples.

All the required equipment, including Class 2 biological safety hoods, liquid nitrogen storage tanks with continuous monitoring alarm systems, protective cryogloves, and face shields, needs to be available in the facility. The staff need to be trained in safety issues related to liquid nitrogen use. There are strict guidelines by the College of American Pathologists regarding monitoring

of cryobanking facilities. The technologists must measure both the liquid nitrogen and temperature levels for the cryotanks at defined intervals. Round-the-clock monitoring of the two parameters can be done with remote monitoring systems installed by various vendors.

Screening and testing guidelines for patients and donors for sperm cryopreservation have been established by several associations:

- Testing for serologic testing for human immunodeficiency virus (HIV) type 1 antibody (AB) and nucleic acid testing (NAT); HIV-2 AB and NAT, and the HIV group 0 AB; hepatitis C AB and NAT; hepatitis B surface antigen; hepatitis B core antibody (IgG and IgM); serology for syphilis, human T-lymphotropic virus types 1 and 2; and *Neisseria gonorrhea* and *Chlamydia trachomatis*. Testing for HIV 1 and 2 and for hepatitis B and C is recommended to diminish the risk of transmission to partners and offspring. In 2013, the Practice Committee of the ASRM released actual hands-on recommendations for andrology and IVF labs for autologous gamete handling and cryopreservation.[43]

Some countries like the United Kingdom have recently stated 55 years of maximum storage in IVF facilities for human gametes,[44] with consent renewal every 10 years. Patients should sign an informed consent form for cryopreservation and storage. However, currently few countries have specific regulations for gamete preservation and fate; therefore, patient counseling is important for them to decide the future of the cryopreserved sperm.

CONCLUSIONS

Besides other indications, sperm banking is now playing a pivotal role in fertility preservation. Reproductive specialists, endocrinologists, and oncologists need to ensure that males receive counseling regarding sperm banking preceding their undergoing gonadotoxic treatment or surgical removal of gonads. Reproductive-age males can be engaged in discussions about their future fertility and benefit from these counseling sessions. Many males in various stages such as prepubertal, pubertal, or adult stages could benefit from utilizing sperm cryopreservation. The different disease conditions can impact their future fertility directly or indirectly such as cancer, hematologic conditions, renal disorders of glomerulonephritis, gender reassignment hormone therapy, infertility related to varicocele, or other infertility associated with oligospermia. Clear communication with patients helps remove the barriers to sperm cryopreservation and helps them make informed decisions for preventing future fertility loss along with their caregivers. It is the physician's duty to ensure that they do not preclude the patient's options of having a biological child of his own and help him achieve his parenthood goals in future and prior to undergoing cancer treatment, gonadotoxic exposure, or conditions like varicocele that are detrimental to future fertility.

SUMMARY

Sperm cryopreservation is an important component of the range of services offered at an ART facility. The indications for sperm banking can be either for autologous or homologous use. Evidence suggests that there is no difference in ART outcomes with use of cryopreserved sperm compared to fresh sperm. This chapter discusses the materials, methods, and organization of sperm banking services in ART laboratories. The chapter also provides updated information regarding sperm freezing, its indications, and the latest techniques for cryopreservation. In addition, the chapter provides comprehensive information to the clinicians about fertility preservation options and new innovative methods. Oncologists can utilize comprehensive information to counsel their patients regarding sperm banking and the importance and indications of fertility preservation. Furthermore, the chapter will help understand the impact of different types of cancer on fertility, outcomes of the use of cryopreserved sperm, the need for development of better cryoprotective media, and sperm banking in transwomen and emergency sperm banking.

REFERENCES

1. Bunge RG, Sherman JK. Fertilizing capacity of frozen human spermatozoa. *Nature.* 1953;172:767-768. doi:10.1038/172767b0.
2. Bunge RG, Keettel WC, Sherman JK. Clinical use of frozen semen: report of four cases. *Fertil Steril.* 1954;5:520-529. doi:10.1016/s0015-0282(16)31802-7.
3. Tomlinson M. Therapeutic sperm cryopreservation. In: Björndahl L, Giwercman A, Tournaye H, Weidner W, eds. *Clinical Andrology EAU/ESAU Course Guidelines.* London: Informa Healthcare; 2010:124-133.
4. Ping P, Zhu WB, Zhang XZ, et al. Sperm banking for male reproductive preservation: a 6-year retrospective multicentre study in China. *Asian J Androl.* 2010;12:356-362. doi:10.1038/aja.2010.12.
5. Gupta S, Sekhon LH, Agarwal A. Sperm banking: when, why, and how? In: Sabanegh ES, ed. *Male Infertility: Problems and Solutions.* Totowa, NJ: Humana Press; 2011:107-108.
6. Hu H, Shi X, Ji G, et al. Studies on the basic issues relevant to sperm cryopreservation in humans. *Ther Adv Reprod Health.* 2020;14:263349412090937. doi:10.1177/2633494120909375.
7. Mazur P. Kinetics of water loss from cells at subzero temperatures and the likelihood of intracellular freezing. *J Gen Physiol.* 1963;47:347-369. doi:10.1085/jgp.47.2.347.
8. Wolf DP, Patton PE. Sperm cryopreservation: state of the art. *J In Vitro Fertil Embryo Transfer.* 1989;6:325-327.
9. Hourvitz A, Goldschlag DE, Davis OK, Gosden LV, Palermo GD, Rosenwaks Z. Intracytoplasmic sperm injection (ICSI) using cryopreserved sperm from men with malignant neoplasm yields high pregnancy rates. *Fertil Steril.* 2008;90:557-563. doi:10.1016/j.fertnstert.2007.03.002.
10. Freour T, Mirallie S, Jean M, Barriere P. Sperm banking and assisted reproductive outcome in men with cancer: a 10 years' experience. *Int J Clin Oncol.* 2012;17:598-603. doi:10.1007/s10147-011-0330-3.
11. Ragheb AM, Jones SJ, Sabanegh Jr ES. Invited review implications of cancer on male fertility. *Arch Med Sci Spec Issues.* 2008;2009:69.
12. Agarwal A, Ranganathan P, Kattal N, et al. Fertility after cancer: a prospective review of assisted reproductive outcome with banked semen specimens. *Fertil Steril.* 2004;81:342-348. doi:10.1016/j.fertnstert.2003.
13. American Cancer Society. *Cancer Facts & Figures 2013.* Atlanta: American Cancer Society; 2013.
14. Agarwal A, Allamaneni SSR. Disruption of spermatogenesis by the cancer disease process. *JNCI Monographs.* 2005;(34):9-12. doi:10.1093/JNCIMONOGRAPHS/LGI005.
15. Practice Committee of the American Society for Reproductive Medicine Fertility Preservation in Patients Undergoing Gonadotoxic Therapy or Gonadectomy: a Committee Opinion. *Fertil Steril.* 2019;112:1022-1033. doi:10.1016/j.fertnstert.2019.09.013.
16. Gadda F, Spinelli MG, Cozzi G, Paffoni A, Carmignani L, Rocco F. Emergency testicular sperm extraction after scrotal trauma in a patient with a history of contralateral orchiopexy for cryptorchidism: case report and review of the literature. *Fertil Steril.* 2012;97:1074-1077. doi:10.1016/j.fertnstert.2012.02.017.
17. Hamada A, Kingsberg S, Wierckx K, et al. Semen characteristics of transwomen referred for sperm banking before sex transition: a case series. *Andrologia.* 2015;47:832-838. doi:10.1111/and.12330.
18. Meyer W, Bockting WO, Cohen-Kettenis P, et al. The Harry Benjamin International Gender Dysphoria Association's standards of care for gender identity disorders, sixth version. *J Psychol Human Sex.* 2002;13:1-30. doi:10.1300/J056v13n01_01.

19. Donnelly ET, McClure N, Lewis SEM. Cryopreservation of human semen and prepared sperm: effects on motility parameters and DNA integrity. *Fertil Steril.* 2001;76: 892-900.

20. Bahadur G, Ozturk O, Muneer A, et al. Semen quality before and after gonadotoxic treatment. *Hum Reprod.* 2005;20:774-781. doi:10.1093/humrep/deh671.

21. Edelstein A, Yavetz H, Kleiman SE, et al. Effect of long-term storage on deoxyribonucleic acid damage and motility of sperm bank donor specimens. *Fertil Steril.* 2008;90:1327-1330. doi:10.1016/j.fertnstert.2007.07.1343.

22. Kaden R, Klippel FF, Katzorke T, Propping D, Schone D. A new instant cryoprotectant for human sperm. *Syst Biol Reprod Med.* 1985;14:133-137. doi:10.3109/ 01485018508988288.

23. Owen DH, Katz DF. A review of the physical and chemical properties of human semen and the formulation of a semen simulant. *J Androl.* 2005;26:459-469.

24. Björndahl L, Mortimer D, Barratt CLR, et al. Sperm Cryobanking. In: *A Practical Guide to Basic Laboratory Andrology.* Cambridge: Cambridge University Press; 2010:189-218.

25. Foskett JK, White C, Cheung KH, Mak DOD. Inositol trisphosphate receptor Ca2+ release channels. *Physiol Rev.* 2007;87:593-658. doi:10.1152/PHYSREV.00035.2006.

26. Condorelli RA, la Vignera S, Bellanca S, Vicari E, Calogero AE. Myoinositol: does it improve sperm mitochondrial function and sperm motility? *Urology.* 2012; 79:1290-1295. doi:10.1016/j.urology.2012.03.005.

27. Hallak J, Rakesh K, Sharma MD, Wellstead C, Agarwal M. Cryopreservation of human spermatozoa: comparison of TEST-yolk buffer and glycerol. *Int J Fertil Womens Med.* 2000;45(1):38-42.

28. Kobayashi H, Ranganathan P, Mahran R, Sharma R, Thomas AJ, Agarwal A. Comparison of two cryopreservation protocols for freezing human spermatozoa. *Fertil Steril.* 2001;76:S229-S230. Available at: https://doi. org/10.1016/S0015-0282(01)02684-X.

29. Glander HJ, Schaller J. Binding of annexin V to plasma membranes of human spermatozoa: a rapid assay for detection of membrane changes after cryostorage. *Mol Human Rep.* 1999;5(2):109-115.

30. Tao Y, Sanger E, Saewu A, Leveille MC. Human sperm vitrification: the state of the art. *Reprod Biol Endocrinol.* 2020;18(1):17.

31. Shah, D, Rasappan, Shila, et al. A simple method of human sperm vitrification. *MethodsX.* 2019;6:2198-2204. doi:10.1016/j.mex.2019.09.022.

32. Wang M, Todorov P, Wang W, et al. Cryoprotectants-free vitrification and conventional freezing of human spermatozoa: a comparative transcript profiling. *Int J Mol Sci.* 2022;23(6):3047. doi:10.3390/ijms23063047.

33. Isachenko V, Maettner R, Petrunkina AM, et al. Vitrification of Human ICSI/IVF spermatozoa without cryoprotectants: new capillary technology. *J Androl.* 2012;33: 462-468. doi:10.2164/jandrol.111.013789.

34. Clarke GN. Sperm cryopreservation: is there a significant risk of cross-contamination? *Human Rep.* 1999;14: 2941-2943.

35. Muller I, Oude Ophuis RJA, Broekmans FJM, Lock TMTW. Semen cryopreservation and usage rate for assisted reproductive technology in 898 men with cancer. *Reprod Biomed Online.* 2016;32:147-153. doi:10.1016/j. rbmo.2015.11.005.

36. Botchan A, Karpol S, Lehavi O, et al. Preservation of sperm of cancer patients: extent of use and pregnancy outcome in a tertiary infertility center. *Asian J Androl.* 2013;15:382-386. doi:10.1038/aja.2013.3.

37. Cohen J, Garrisi GJ, Congedo-Ferrara TA, Kieck KA, Schimmel TW, Scott RT. Cryopreservation of single human spermatozoa. *Hum Reprod.* 1997;12:994-1001.

38. Diego D, Medline A, Shandley LM, Kawwass JF, Hipp HS. Donor sperm recipients: fertility treatments, trends, and pregnancy outcomes. *J Assist Reprod Genet.* 2022;39:2303-2310. doi:10.1007/S10815-022-02616-8/TABLES/4.

39. Liu S, Li F. Cryopreservation of single-sperm: where are we today? *Reprod Biol Endocrinol.* 2020;18(1):41. doi: 10.1186/S12958-020-00607-X.

40. Bortoletto P, Willson S, Romanski PA, Davis OK, Rosenwaks Z. Reproductive outcomes of women aged 40 and older undergoing IVF with donor sperm. *Hum Reprod.* 2021;36:229-235. doi:10.1093/HUMREP/DEAA286.

41. Lansac J, Thepot F, Mayaux MJ, et al. Pregnancy outcome after artificial insemination or IVF with frozen semen donor: a collaborative study of the French CECOS federation on 21 597 pregnancies. *Eur J Obstet Gynecol Reprod Biol.* 1997;74(2):223-228. doi:10.1016/S0301-2115(97) 00102-4.

42. Achille MA, Rosberger Z, Robitaille R, et al. Facilitators and obstacles to sperm banking in young men receiving gonadotoxic chemotherapy for cancer: the perspective of survivors and health care professionals. *Hum Reprod.* 2006;21(12):3206-3216. doi:10.1093/humrep/del307.

43. Practice Committee of American Society for Reproductive Medicine recommendations for reducing the risk of viral transmission during fertility treatment with the use of autologous gametes: a committee opinion. *Fertil Steril.* 2013;99:340-346. doi:10.1016/j.fertnstert.2012.08.028.

44. Human Fertilisation & Embryology Authority. *New Law Comes into Force Giving Greater Flexibility for Fertility Patients.* Human Fertilisation & Embryology Authority. Available at: https://www.hfea.gov.uk/about-us/news-and-press-releases/2022-news-and-press-releases/new-law-comes-into-force-giving-greater-flexibility-for-fertility-patients/#:~:text=From%201%20July%20 2022%2C%20all,their%20sperm%2C%20eggs%20 or%20embryos. Accessed: January 22, 2023.

SECTION 7

Clinical Practice Guidelines for Male Infertility

26

Guidelines of the American Society for Reproductive Medicine, American Urological Association, and European Association of Urology

Kadir Bocu and Murat Gül

KEY POINTS

- Infertility is a global health problem, and 8% to 12% of couples who want to have children worldwide suffer from this condition.
- The American Urological Association/American Society for Reproductive Medicine guidelines and the 2 provide a concise and clear summary of the literature on male infertility for all reproductive health professionals.
- Although the result of semen analysis is not a definitive predictor of male infertility except for

azoospermia, it is the first test to be requested to guide male infertility management.
- The development of in vitro fertilization techniques and the introduction of intracytoplasmic sperm injection may offer a chance to males with nonobstructive azoospermia to become fathers.
- Treatment may be scheduled with or without assisted reproductive techniques for infertile heterosexual couples with a male factor, depending on the underlying etiology.

INTRODUCTION

The World Health Organization (WHO) considers infertility a global health problem and defines it as the inability to achieve pregnancy despite regular, unprotected sexual intercourse for at least 12 months.[1] According to available data, more than 186 million people currently have infertility, and 8% to 12% of couples are not able to conceive despite 1 year of consecutive unprotected intercourse worldwide.[2] Also, male infertility is responsible for 20% and general male factor–related infertility is responsible for approximately 50% of infertile heterosexual couples. However, determining the true unbiased prevalence of global male infertility remains a challenge due to the lack of a commonly defined population, variances in the definition of infertility, and inconsistency in current study outcomes.[3]

Studies on male infertility have shown that sperm concentration, total sperm count, and semen quality have decreased in the last few decades.[4–6] Furthermore, male infertility has become a health issue related to the deterioration of males's overall health and systemic comorbidities beyond the desire to have a child.[7] On the economic side, reproductive health care for infertile males includes assisted reproductive technologies (ARTs) and couples treatment, representing a significant financial burden to the health system and couples.[8] Pregnancy could be achieved even in couples with highly poor semen quality by in vitro fertilization (IVF) or intracytoplasmic sperm injection (ICSI). Especially, the clinical practice of ICSI has gained worldwide popularity, with the simultaneous revolutionary development of surgical sperm retrieval methods in the management of male infertility.[9] However, some azoospermic males still cannot provide a single spermatozoon, even with testicular sperm extraction procedure (TESE). Studies are ongoing on some experimental treatment modalities such as stem cell transplantation, testicular tissue grafting, xenograft, and in vitro spermatogenesis.[10,11]

Today, there are still many controversial issues regarding male infertility, and clinicians' approaches to male infertility–related problems differ in their clinical practices. For this reason, standardization in the evaluation and management of males suffering from infertility is of significant importance. This chapter presents the all-around clinical approach to male infertility for all reproductive medicine professionals, according to the latest European Association of Urology (EAU) and American Urological Association/American Society for Reproductive Medicine (AUA/ASRM) guidelines.

CAUSES AND RISK FACTORS OF MALE INFERTILITY

Spermatogenesis is a process that requires the proper functioning of many factors. Hormonal, neuronal, and immunological systems, as well as gene expression sequences, chromosomal structure formations, intact genital anatomical structures, and appropriate genetic and epigenetic environments play interwoven roles.[12,13] Any factor affecting the complex pathways of spermatogenesis can lead to male infertility. According to the latest EAU and AUA/ASRM guidelines, the male factor is involved in 50% of the infertile heterosexual couple's etiology. Unexplained infertility is also common: EAU and AUA/ASRM guidelines report a rate of 20% to 30%. Idiopathic male infertility is defined as the absence of any pathological finding for etiology in males with abnormal semen parameters. It has been reported that it constitutes 30% of all infertile males.[14,15] Recently, environmental factors, reactive oxygen species, sperm DNA damage, genetic factors, and epigenetic factors have been thought to cause idiopathic male infertility.[16]

Considering the identifiable causes and risk factors in male infertility, EUA Sexual and Reproductive Health guidelines have classified male infertility under subheadings such as infertility of known (possible) cause, hypogonadism, general systemic diseases, cryopreservation due to malignant disease, and erection/ejaculation disorder (Fig. 26.1).[17] Although the AUA/ASRM guidelines state that data on specific causes of male infertility are limited, they have mentioned that demographics, lifestyle, medical treatments, and environmental exposures

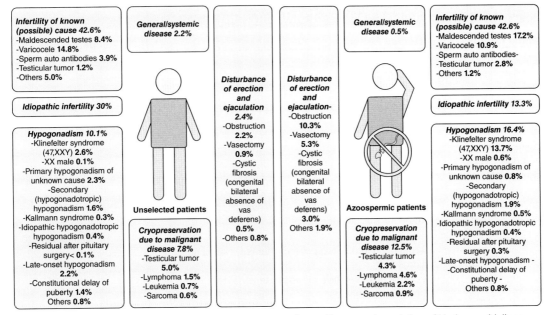

Fig. 26.1 Causes and distribution of male infertility according to European Association of Urology guidelines. *NP,* Nonprogressive; *PR,* progressive (a+b motility).

play a role in male infertility.[18] The comorbidities associated with male infertility, cancer, the general health of infertile males, and mortality rates relative to fertile males are discussed in more detail in this guideline.[14] A few of the important points addressed in both of these most recent guidelines are that maternal age is the strongest predictive factor for couples seeking fertility treatment, and advancing paternal age is one of the main risk factors associated with the progressive increase in the prevalence of male factor infertility.[19,20] Risk factors and causes of male infertility can be classified more systematically as congenital, acquired, and idiopathic (Table 26.1).[21]

DIAGNOSIS OF MALE INFERTILITY

History of Male Partners for Initial Infertility Evaluation

EAU and AUA/ASRM guidelines recommend that couples seeking medical care for infertility should be evaluated simultaneously. In both guidelines, infertility evaluation is recommended after having the inability to achieve pregnancy in 12 months despite regular unprotected intercourse in couples. However, these guidelines recommend starting research on infertility at six months for couples with female partners over the age

of 35 due to diminished fertility potential with increasing maternal age.[22,23] The AUA/ASRM guideline indicates that reproductive history should be included in the initial male infertility assessment under the clinical principles category. In addition, this guideline presents a solid recommendation to perform one or more semen analyses (SA) for initial evaluation.[22] The latest EAU guideline also states at a strong recommendation level that a comprehensive medical history, physical examination, and SA are the keystones of male infertility assessment.[23]

The medical history of the male partner is essential to reveal the potential causes of male infertility and comorbidities associated with male infertility. A medical history, including information on the duration of infertility, previous pregnancy and miscarriages, lifestyle factors, sexual history, surgical history, gonadotoxic exposure, and family history, provides significant findings and can guide the clinician (Fig. 26.2).[21]

Physical Examination

Male infertility evaluation should start with a systematic assessment. The characteristic features of faces of male and female phenotypes may guide the clinician about sexual dysmorphism.[24] Secondary sexual characteristics

TABLE 26.1   Causes and Risk Factors of Male Infertility

Congenital Factors	Acquired Factors	Idiopathic Risk Factors
Anorchia	Varicocele	Smoking
Congenital absence of vas deferens	Testicular trauma	Alcohol
Cryptorchidism	Testicular torsion	Recreational drugs
Y chromosome micro-deletions	Germ cell tumors	Obesity
Chromosomal or genetic abnormalities	Acquired hypogonadotrophic hypogonadism	Psychological stress
Genetic endocrinopathy	Recurrent urogenital infection (prostatitis, prostatovesciculitis)	Advanced paternal age
Congenital obstruction	Postinflammatory conditions (epididymitis, mumps orchitis)	Dietary factors
	Urogenital tract obstruction	Environmental or occupational exposure to toxins
	Exogenous factors (e.g., chemotherapy, medications, radiation, heat)	
	Systemic diseases (live cirrhosis, renal failure)	
	Antisperm antibodies	
	Surgeries that can comprise vascularization of the testis	
	Sexual dysfunction (erectile or ejaculatory dysfunction)	

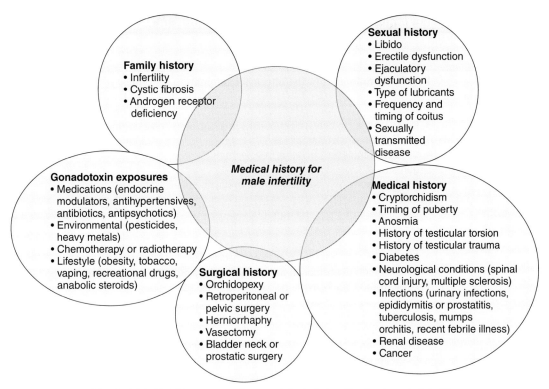

Family history
• Infertility
• Cystic fibrosis
• Androgen receptor deficiency

Sexual history
• Libido
• Erectile dysfunction
• Ejaculatory dysfunction
• Type of lubricants
• Frequency and timing of coitus
• Sexually transmitted disease

Gonadotoxin exposures
• Medications (endocrine modulators, antihypertensives, antibiotics, antipsychotics)
• Environmental (pesticides, heavy metals)
• Chemotherapy or radiotherapy
• Lifestyle (obesity, tobacco, vaping, recreational drugs, anabolic steroids)

Medical history for male infertility

Medical history
• Cryptorchidism
• Timing of puberty
• Anosmia
• History of testicular torsion
• History of testicular trauma
• Diabetes
• Neurological conditions (spinal cord injury, multiple sclerosis)
• Infections (urinary infections, epididymitis or prostatitis, tuberculosis, mumps orchitis, recent febrile illness)
• Renal disease
• Cancer

Surgical history
• Orchidopexy
• Retroperitoneal or pelvic surgery
• Herniorrhaphy
• Vasectomy
• Bladder neck or prostatic surgery

Fig. 26.2 Medical history according to etiological classification in male infertility.

such as the face, trunk, axillary, and pubic hair should be evaluated to assess androgenization.[25] Eunuchoid body structure, reduced body hair, and gynecomastia may indicate Klinefelter syndrome, increased estradiol levels, or hyperprolactinemia.[26] Obesity, a significant component of metabolic syndrome, must also be noted. Many mechanisms such as low testosterone levels in obese males, increased aromatase activity, transformations in the hypothalamic-pituitary axis, increased leptin, and insulin resistance have been shown to affect male fertility negatively.[27]

Male genital examination must follow the systemic assessment. Scrotum, phallus, testes and epididymis, spermatic cord, penis, prostate, and seminal vesicles should be evaluated during the examination. Visual observation of the scrotum should be performed. The hypoplastic side may be the sign of cryptorchidism. Additionally, hydrocele, infectious diseases, and clinical varicocele (grade 3) can be identified. Testicular size and consistency should be checked with palpation, and potential testicular masses should not be overlooked. The epididymis and the presence of spermatic cords should

be palpated. Penile abnormalities such as hypospadias, epispadias, fibrous plaque, curvature, and phimosis should be revealed. Although a digital rectal examination is not indicated for every patient, it should be performed in patients with low semen volume. The consistency of the prostate size should be checked, and midline cysts or possible dilated seminal vesicles should raise the suspicion of obstruction of ductal ejaculators.[28] The steps for the physical examination of male infertility are listed in the AUA/ASRM guidelines, and the typical outcomes of testicular insufficiency are specified in the EAU guidelines (Table 26.2).[22,23]

Semen Analysis

Semen analysis (SA) is essential for the clinical evaluation of the male partner, especially in infertile heterosexual couples, and it can guide the management of male infertility. An appropriate SA should include total sperm count, sperm concentration, sperm pH, agglutination, sperm motility, the viability of the spermatozoa, and the concentration of positive peroxide cells.[29] The current AUA/ASRM guidelines recommend performing

TABLE 26.2   Physical Examination Steps and Typical Findings in Male Infertility

AUA/ASRM Guidelines		EAU Guideline
Sections of the physical examination	Potential findings from the physical examination	Typical results suggesting testicular insufficiency, based on EAU guideline
General	• Body habitus, as overweight/obesity is associated with impaired spermatogenesis. • Virilization to assess pubertal development/androgen status. • Gynecomastia may be a marker for endocrine disorders.	Abnormal secondary sexual characteristics
Abdominal exam	• Examination of any scars from prior surgical procedures that may involve the pelvis or impact the urogenital system.	Abnormal testicular volume and/or consistency
Phallus	• Meatal location, as hypospadias/epispadias may make semen deposition in the vagina challenging. • Penile plaque, as Peyronie disease may make vaginal intercourse difficult. • Penile lesions/ulcers/discharge may be a sign of sexually transmitted infection.	Testicular masses (potentially suggestive of cancer)
Scrotum/Testes	• Examination for prior scars suggesting prior scrotal surgery/trauma. • Location, as scrotal position of the testes is important for normal function. • Size/consistency/contours, as a majority of the testis is devoted to spermatogenesis. The exam may also reveal masses consistent with a testicular cancer.	Absence of testes (uni- or bilaterally)
Epididymides	• Shape/consistency, as normal development should be identified to determine atresia that could be identified by the presence of a *CFTR* mutation. • Induration/dilation could suggest obstruction. Epididymal cysts or spermatoceles may also lead to obstruction.	Gynecomastia
Vas deferens	• Shape/consistency, as normal development and contour should be confirmed to rule out agenesis, as may be seen in the presence of a *CFTR* mutation or aberrant Wolffian duct embryogenesis. • The presence/location of any vasectomy defect or granuloma should also be assessed.	Varicocele
Digital rectal examination	• Midline prostatic cysts or dilated seminal vesicles may assist in the diagnosis of EDO.	

AUA/ASRM, American Urological Association/American Society for Reproductive Medicine; *CFTR,* cystic fibrosis transmembrane conductance regulator; *EAU,* European Association of Urology; *EDO,* ejaculatory duct obstruction.

at least two SAs a month apart, particularly if the first result of SA is not typical.[14] The EAU guidelines stated that, if there is a normal SA result, a single test is sufficient, according to the WHO criteria. Still, at least two abnormal SA results are required for further evaluation.[23]

The WHO has recently published the sixth edition of the laboratory manual for the examination and processing of human semen. In a previous edition of the WHO manual, the lower fifth percentile of SA results from 1800 males who contributed to achieving pregnancy within one year was specified as definitive reference values for normal SA. However, these reference values have been removed in the most recent edition.[29] SA is never predictive of fertility for an individual patient, so reference intervals for commonly measured sperm parameter variables cannot be a clear indicator of male infertility.[30] SA distinguishes between fertile and infertile males only when there is azoospermia (complete absence of spermatozoa in the semen).

However, the AUA/ASRM guidelines use reference limits for SA from the fifth edition of the WHO manual to decide how to manage infertile or subfertile males in clinical practice.[31] On the other hand, the EAU guidelines reported both lower reference limits that were similar to each other as determined in the fifth and sixth editions of the WHO manual.[29,31] Although individual semen parameters alone are not diagnostic for male infertility, it is important in the clinical approach to identify pathological findings such as oligozoospermia: less than 15 million spermatozoa/mL; asthenozoospermia: less than 32%

progressive motile spermatozoa; and teratozoospermia: less than 4% normal forms (Table 26.3).

Hormonal Evaluation of the Male Partner

Hormone assessment is critical because spermatogenesis is strongly dependent on intratesticular testosterone synthesis. Although many clinics perform routine hormonal evaluation in the clinical approach to male infertility, current guidelines do not recommend it as an initial test for every patient.[32] The AUA/ASRM guidelines recommend hormonal evaluation for male infertility, including follicle-stimulating hormone (FSH) and testosterone, as an expert opinion when decreased libido, erectile dysfunction, oligozoospermia or azoospermia, atrophic testes, or findings suggestive of endocrinological pathology are found during on physical examination.[22] The EAU guideline recommends a weak strength rating for a hormonal assessment, including total serum testosterone and FSH/luteinizing hormone (LH) in cases of oligospermia and azoospermia.[23]

The serum testosterone level should be measured between 7:00 and 11:00 in the morning while fasting because it shows a circadian rhythm and is affected by food intake.[33,34] Different threshold values have been adopted for testosterone levels in diagnosing hypogonadism in both guidelines. The AUA/ASRM guidelines accepted the 300 ng/dL threshold, and the EAU acknowledged the 345 ng/dL threshold.[35,36] In cases where the total testosterone level is low, repeat measurement of total and free testosterone (or bioactive testosterone)

TABLE 26.3 World Health Organization Lower Reference Limits for Semen Characteristics		
Parameter	The 5th Edition of the WHO Manual for Human Semen Analysis Lower reference limit[a] (range)	The 6th Edition of the WHO Manual for Human Semen Analysis Lower reference limit[a] (range)
Semen volume (mL)	1.5 (1.4–1.7)	1.4 (1.3–1.5)
Total sperm number (10^6/ejaculate)	39 (33–46)	39 (35–40)
Sperm concentration (10^6/mL)	15 (12–16)	16 (15–18)
Total motility (progressive + nonprogressive)	40 (38–42)	42 (40–43)
Progressive motility (%)	32 (31–34)	30 (29–31)
Vitality (live spermatozoa, %)	58 (55–63)	54 (50–56)
Sperm morphology (normal forms, %)	4 (3.0–4.0)	4 (3.9–4.0)
pH	>7.2	>7.2
Peroxidase-positive leukocytes (10^6/mL)	<1.0	<1.0

[a]5th percentiles and 95% confidence intervals.
WHO, World Health Organization.

and determination of serum LH, estradiol, and prolactin levels are required. These results can help clinicians differentiate between possible pathologies such as primary hypogonadism, secondary hypogonadism, or hyperprolactinemia (Fig. 26.3).[37] Testosterone levels are typically decreased or normal in patients with primary hypogonadism (testicular deficiency), whereas FSH and LH levels are increased.[38] Clinicians may consequently measure plasma FSH to indicate spermatogenesis.[39] In addition, a retrospective study showed that 96% of males with obstructive azoospermia (OA) had an FSH test value of 7.6 IU/L or less and a long testicular axis greater than 4.6 cm. This study stated that 89% of males with azoospermia due to spermatogenic dysfunction had FSH values above 7.6 IU/L, and the long axis of the testis was less than 4.6 cm.[40] However, in males with normal spermatogonia counts, if there is a maturation arrest at the spermatocyte or spermatid level, the FSH

level is usually within the normal range. FSH level is not precise in predicting foci of spermatogenesis in patients scheduled for TESE.[41]

Genetic Assessment

Genetic factors are responsible for at least 15% of male infertility.[42] Azoospermic males have a 25% possibility of harboring and being carriers of genetic anomalies. The detection rates of genetic abnormalities increase as sperm counts decrease.[43] Although many genetic factors cause male infertility, they may be discussed under three practical headings in the clinical approach.

Chromosomal Abnormalities

The first test in the genetic assessment of male infertility is karyotype analysis because 15% of patients with NOA and 4% of patients with moderate oligospermia (<10 million spermatozoa per mL) have harbored

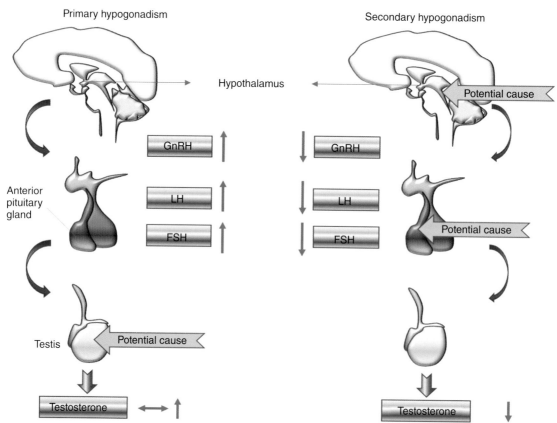

Fig. 26.3 Hormonal evaluation of male infertility. *FSH*, Follicle-stimulating hormone; *GnRH*, gonadotropin-releasing hormone; *LH*, luteinizing hormone.

chromosomal abnormalities.[44] Chromosomal abnormalities can be detected as structural and numerical chromosome defects. The most common chromosomal anomaly in NOA is Klinefelter syndrome and its variants (47,XXY and mosaics 46,XY/47,XXY). In these patients, spermatogenesis is adversely affected and semen phenotype is compatible with azoospermia in at least 90% of the patients, while in the rest, it is compatible with cryptozoospermia or severe oligozoospermia.

The sperm retrieval rate (SRR) is approximately 50% with the microdissection TESE (micro-TESE) in infertile males with Klinefelter syndrome.[45] These patients, including those with different types of mosaicism, have a risk of sex chromosome aneuploidy in their offspring, so patients should be informed about the preimplantation genetic diagnosis (PGD).[46]

Structural abnormalities in the chromosome are ten times more common in males with oligospermia than in normozoospermic males.[44] The most common structural chromosomal defects include Robertsonian translocations, inversions, and reciprocal translocations. Genetic counseling regarding PGD and the necessity of ART should be provided in infertile couples due to these aberrations and the possible risk of aneuploidy in offspring.[47]

Y Chromosome Microdeletions

Y chromosome microdeletions occur in regions that contain genes required for spermatogenesis and are defined as azoospermia factor (AZF). These deletions are the second most common cause of male infertility and are detected in 8% to 12% of azoospermic males and 3% to 7% of oligozoospermic males.[48] Complete or partial deletions in the AZFa, AZFb, and AZFc regions are important for managing male infertility from a clinical perspective. Complete deletions involving the AZFa region are associated with Sertoli cell–only syndrome, and complete AZFb deletions are associated with the spermatogenic arrest.[49] Carriers of complete AZFa and AZFb deletion have a poor prognosis, and sperm retrieval fails with TESE.[50] AZFc microdeletions are the most common deletions, with a 65% to 70% rate among Y chromosome microdeletions. In these latter microdeletion carriers, the success of SRR with TESE varies between 50% and 75%.[51]

Cystic Fibrosis Gene Mutations

Mutations in the cystic fibrosis transmembrane conductance regulator (CFTR) gene located on chromosome 7p affect membrane protein, which functions as an ion channel in the ejaculatory duct, seminal vesicle, vas deferens, and distal two-thirds of the epididymis.[52] It is stated that approximately 80% of patients with congenital bilateral absence of vas deferens (CBAVD) and 20% of males with congenital unilateral absence of vas deferens have CFTR gene mutations.[53] Both partners should be tested for CFTR gene mutations containing the 5-thymidine (5T) allele for males with congenital vas deferens structural abnormalities.[54]

The recommendations and statements of the EAU and AUA/ASRM guidelines that will facilitate the approach for clinicians regarding the genetic evaluation in male infertility, which was mentioned earlier, are indicated in Table 26.4.

Imaging

Imaging techniques may be necessary for specific situations in the diagnostic evaluation of male infertility. Mainly, scrotal ultrasonography (US) is widely used by clinicians in daily practice in patients with oligozoospermia or azoospermia.[55] The scrotal US contributes to the physical examination in detecting testicular volume, testicular anatomy, testicular parenchyma homogeneity, possible testicular masses associated with testicular dysgenesis, signs of OA (rete testis dilatation, enlarged epididymis with cystic lesions, or absence of vas deferens), and varicocele suspected on palpation.[56]

However, the current AUA/ASRM guidelines state that the scrotal US should not be routinely performed in the initial evaluation of an infertile male (expert opinion).[22] The EAU guidelines, on the other hand, recommend performing the scrotal US in patients with infertility, as there is a risk of testis cancer (weak strength rating).[23]

The transrectal US, another imaging modality, describes the anatomy of primary organs/structures related to ejaculation, including the prostate, seminal vesicles, vasal ampulla, and ejaculatory ducts.[57] The current guidelines (EAU and AUA/ASRM) do not recommend transrectal US in the initial evaluation of infertile males. However, both guidelines recommend transrectal US for patients with low seminal volume (<1.5 mL), acidic pH (pH<7.0), and suspected obstruction with severe oligozoospermia or azoospermia.[22,23]

TABLE 26.4 Genetic Diagnostic Work-Up According to Current Guidelines

AUA/ASRM Guidelines (2020) (Statements)	EAU Guideline (2022) (Recommendations)
Karyotype and Y-chromosome microdeletion analysis should be recommended for males with primary infertility and azoospermia or severe oligozoospermia (<5 million sperm/mL) with elevated FSH or testicular atrophy or a presumed diagnosis of impaired sperm production as the cause of azoospermia. (**Expert Opinion**)	Offer standard karyotype analysis and genetic counseling to all males with azoospermia and oligozoospermia (spermatozoa <10 million/mL) for diagnostic purposes. (**Strong**)
Clinicians should recommend cystic fibrosis transmembrane conductance regulator (*CFTR*) gene mutation carrier testing (including assessment of the 5T allele) in males with vasal agenesis or idiopathic obstructive azoospermia. (**Expert Opinion**)	Do not test for Y-chromosome microdeletions in males with pure obstructive azoospermia, as spermatogenesis will be normal. (**Strong**)
For males who harbor a *CFTR* mutation, genetic evaluation of the female partner should be recommended. (**Expert Opinion**)	Y chromosome microdeletion testing may be offered in males with sperm concentrations of <5 million sperm/mL but must be mandatory in males with sperm concentrations of <1 million sperm/mL. (**Strong**)
Sperm DNA fragmentation analysis is not recommended in the initial evaluation of the infertile couple. (**Moderate Recommendation; Evidence Level: Grade C**)	Inform males with Yq microdeletion and their partners who wish to proceed with intracytoplasmic sperm injection that microdeletions will be passed to their sons but not to their daughters. (**Strong**)
For couples with recurrent pregnancy loss (RPL), males should be evaluated with karyotype (**Expert Opinion**) and sperm DNA fragmentation. (**Moderate Recommendation; Evidence Level Grade: C**)	In males with structural abnormalities of the vas deferens (unilateral or bilateral absence with no renal agenesis), test the male and his partner for *CFTR* gene mutations, which should include common point mutations and the 5T allele. (**Strong**)
	Provide genetic counseling in all couples with a genetic abnormality found on clinical or genetic investigations and in patients who carry a (potential) inheritable disease. (**Strong**)
	Sperm DNA fragmentation testing should be performed in the assessment of couples with recurrent pregnancy loss from natural conception and assisted reproductive technology or males with unexplained infertility. (**Strong**)

MANAGEMENT OF MALE INFERTILITY BEFORE THE ASSISTED REPRODUCTIVE TECHNOLOGY STAGE

The use of ARTs in infertile couples, and especially the increasing role of ICSI in clinical practice, has brought about a revolution in the management of male infertility.[58] In the ICSI era, the female partners of heterosexual couples maintain their importance, especially in carrying the embryo and fetus; however, there is no absolute necessity to reveal the male factor to achieve live birth with ARTs.[59] This condition may result in ignoring appropriate male partner evaluation and treatment. Therefore it is

crucial in clinical practice to approach correctable male infertility pathologies to contribute to the success of ARTs and achieve pregnancy without ART.[60]

Noninvasive Treatment Modalities for Male Infertility
Empirical Treatments for Idiopathic Male Infertility and Oligoasthenoteratozoospermia

Idiopathic oligoasthenoteratozoospermia (OAT) is characterized by decreased sperm count, motile sperm, and sperm morphology percentage.[61] Despite performing all diagnostic procedures, in 30% of males with abnormal semen parameters, the etiology is undetectable and is defined as idiopathic male infertility.[42]

The AUA/ASRM guidelines recommend that clinicians discuss risk factors associated with male infertility, such as lifestyle, drug use, and environmental exposures. They advise patients that available data on most of the risk factors is limited (conditional recommendation; Evidence Level Grade: C).[22] The EAU guidelines also stated that lifestyle changes such as losing weight, increasing physical activity, quitting smoking, and reducing alcohol intake in males with idiopathic OAT can improve sperm quality and the chance of conception, with a weak strength rating recommendation.[23]

It has been shown that oxidative stress and its end products, reactive oxygen species, can impair sperm function by various mechanisms and play an essential role in the pathogenesis of idiopathic male infertility.[62] However, there are conflicting studies such as that antioxidant therapy has positive effects on improving semen parameters and reducing oxidative stress in males with infertility, or there is no significant difference with placebo. Furthermore, it is still challenging to obtain a clear image of antioxidant therapy due to certain limitations in these studies.[63,64] Consequently, the AUA/ASRM guidelines recommend that clinicians inform patients that the clinical benefit of supplements (e.g., antioxidants, vitamins) in treating male infertility is questionable. In addition, they indicated that the available data were insufficient to provide recommendations on specific agents to use for this purpose (conditional recommendation; level of evidence rating: B).[22] The EAU guidelines also state that although the use of antioxidants can improve semen parameters, no clear recommendation can be made for the treatment of patients with idiopathic infertility with antioxidants.[23]

Other approaches to the empirical treatment of idiopathic male infertility include selective estrogen receptor modulators (SERMs) and aromatase inhibitors (AIs) that inhibit the cytochrome p450 aromatase enzyme. While these agents work through different pathways, their primary goal is to increase endogenous testosterone production and stimulate spermatogenesis.[65,66] Although studies confirmed spermatogenesis and positive hormonal effects of both treatment molecules, definite recommendations could not be present due to the insufficient quality of the studies and the necessity of prospective randomized controlled studies.[32] The AUA/ASRM guidelines recommend that clinicians inform males suffering from idiopathic infertility that the use of SERMs has limited advantages over the results of ART (expert opinion). For infertile males with low serum testosterone, this guideline states that AIs, human chorionic gonadotropin (hCG), SERMs, or a combination of these can be used (conditional recommendation; Evidence Level Grade: C).[22] Definite recommendations cannot be made regarding the use of SERMs in males with idiopathic infertility or the use of steroidal (testolactone) or nonsteroidal (anastrozole and letrozole) AIs in the EAU guidelines (weak strength rating).[23]

Hormonal Therapy

Treatment with gonadotropins and gonadotropin-releasing hormone (GnRH) analogs to improve semen parameters in infertile males dates back half a century.[67] Treatment of gonadotropin is the reference treatment for infertile males with hypogonadotropic hypogonadism (secondary hypogonadism). A positive natural or assisted pregnancy result can often be achieved in this group of patients.[68] In males with prepubertal-onset congenital hypogonadotropic hypogonadism, combined therapy with hCG and FSH by subcutaneous administration may be considered, or GnRH therapy by pulsed administration using a subcutaneous pump is also optional.[69] However, the need for special devices for intravenous or subcutaneous pulsatile release of GnRH therapy and patient incompatibility limit the use of GnRH.[70]

In patients with prepubertal-onset secondary hypogonadism, hCG is started at 1000 IU twice a week and can be increased to 5000 IU two or three times a week until normal testosterone levels are achieved.[71] When testosterone reaches normal levels, subcutaneous FSH 75 to 150 IU should be started three times weekly.[72] In postpubertal-onset secondary hypogonadism, an initial dose of 250 IU twice weekly is recommended, and hCG doses can be increased up to 2000 IU twice weekly until normal testosterone levels are achieved. Afterwards, 75 IU of FSH three times a week and 150 IU of FSH three times a week can be added as required.[73]

Gonadotropins may be suppressed as a result of hyperprolactinemia. In this case, the treatment should be planned according to the etiology. Dopamine agonists may be started as pharmacological and first-line therapy, or surgery for pituitary adenoma may be considered. If the underlying cause is not pituitary adenoma, other causes that may increase the prolactin level should be focused on.[74]

Evidence for the effectiveness of gonadotropin therapy in the presence of testicular failure (primary hypogonadism) is insufficient and contradictory.[75] It has been shown that FSH treatment affects sperm parameters positively in idiopathic infertile males with normal FSH levels. A metaanalysis of 15 controlled studies found that idiopathic infertile males in the FSH treatment arm had higher pregnancy rates. However, this study was limited due to the heterogeneity of the included studies and the high risk of bias.[76] No statistically significant positive effect of hCG treatment could be demonstrated in terms of SRR, pregnancy rate, or live birth rate in the study on empirical hormonal therapy in the case of NOA.[77] Another nonrandomized comparative study in 108 males with NOA compared FSH treatment before TESE with nondrug treatment. While there was no sperm recovery in the ejaculate in both groups, FSH treatment showed a statistically significant positive effect in terms of surgical SRR.[78] As briefly mentioned above, the findings concerning empirical hormone treatment regimens in idiopathic male infertility, primary hypogonadism, and NOA are not satisfactory. Recommendations and statements of current guidelines for the practical clinical approach are given in Table 26.5.

Surgical Treatment Modalities for Male Infertility

Varicocelectomy

Varicocele is the enlargement of the pampiniform plexus vessels that provide venous return from the testicles. The incidence of varicocele in males with primary infertility is 35% to 44%, and the incidence in males with secondary infertility may increase up to 45% to 81%.[79] There are radiological procedures such as sclerotherapy and embolization in varicocele treatment, but surgical repair is the primary approach in treatment.[80] Although varicocele repair can be performed with different surgical treatment methods from past to present, the microsurgical inguinal or subinguinal approach has the lowest recurrence and hydrocele rates.[23]

Current guidelines on the management of varicocele have presented similar recommendations. The EAU guidelines strongly recommend varicocele treatment for clinical varicocele, abnormal semen parameters, and unexplained infertile couples with female partners with good ovarian reserve.[23] The AUA/ASRM guidelines also recommend that surgical varicocelectomy is considered in males attempting to conceive who have a palpable varicocele, infertility, and abnormal semen parameters, except for azoospermic males (moderate recommendation; Evidence Level Grade: B).[22] Both the EAU and AUA/ASRM guidelines do not recommend varicocele repair in males with subclinical varicocele and normal semen parameters.[22,23]

The EAU guidelines for males with NOA and clinical varicoceles provided a summary of evidence that showed although there are no prospective randomized trials, the available metaanalyses suggest that varicocele repair results in the appearance of sperm in the ejaculate of males with NOA. The AUA/ASRM guidelines also state that couples should be informed before ART that there is no conclusive evidence to support varicocele repair for males with clinical varicocele and NOA (expert opinion).[22,23]

In adolescents with clinical varicocele, prophylactic varicocele repair is recommended only when there is a decrease in ipsilateral testicular volume or deterioration in semen parameters in serial US and physical examination.[81] Although there are no precise results in the patient group with clinical varicocele and some specific accompanying conditions (high DNA fragmentation, unexplained infertility, recurrent pregnancy loss, embryogenesis, implantation failure, and ART failure), varicocele treatment can be planned.[82]

Sperm Retrieval Methods

Sperm retrieval techniques have been developed especially for azoospermic males who want to achieve pregnancy with ART. Microsurgical epididymal sperm aspiration (MESA) was first described in 1985, and live birth was reported with the help of this technique.[83] Subsequently, percutaneous epididymal sperm aspiration (PESA), which is another sperm collection method from the epididymis, and testicular sperm aspiration (TESA), conventional TESE (cTESE), and micro-TESE, which are testicular sperm retrieval methods, have been described (Fig. 26.4).[84]

Management of Obstructive Azoospermia

In patients with azoospermia, OA and NOA should be differentiated, with the help of some diagnostic tests at the first stage. OA is less common in etiology than NOA in azoospermic males and is generally characterized by normal FSH, testicular volume, and enlargement of the epididymis.[85] Males with OA may have options in disease

TABLE 26.5   Hormonal Therapy in Specific Cases of Male Infertility According to Current Guidelines

AUA/ASRM Guidelines (2020) (Statements)	EAU Guideline (2022) (Recommendations)
The patient presenting with hypogonadotropic hypogonadism should be evaluated to determine the etiology of the disorder and treated based on diagnosis. **(Clinical Principle)**	Hypogonadotropic hypogonadism (secondary hypogonadism), including congenital causes, should be treated with combined human chorionic gonadotropin (hCG) and follicle-stimulating hormone (FSH) (recombinant FSH; highly purified FSH) or pulsed gonadotropin-releasing hormone (GnRH) via pump therapy to stimulate spermatogenesis. **(Strong)**
Clinicians may use aromatase inhibitors (AIs), hCG, selective estrogen receptor modulators (SERMs), or a combination thereof for infertile males with low serum testosterone. **(Conditional Recommendation; Evidence Level Grade: C)**	In males with hypogonadotropic hypogonadism, induce spermatogenesis by an effective drug therapy (hCG; human menopausal gonadotropins; recombinant FSH; highly purified FSH). **(Strong)**
For the male interested in current or future fertility, testosterone monotherapy should not be prescribed. **(Clinical Principle)**	Do not use testosterone therapy for the treatment of male infertility. **(Strong)**
The infertile male with hyperprolactinemia should be evaluated for the etiology and treated accordingly. **(Expert Opinion)**	Provide testosterone therapy for symptomatic patients with primary and secondary hypogonadism who are not considering parenthood. **(Strong)**
Clinicians should inform the male with idiopathic infertility that the use of SERMs has limited benefits relative to results of assisted reproductive technology. **(Expert Opinion)**	The use of GnRH therapy is more expensive and does not offer any advantages compared to gonadotropins for the treatment of hypogonadotropic hypogonadism. **(Strong)**
For males with idiopathic infertility, a clinician may consider treatment using an FSH analog with the aim of improving sperm concentration, pregnancy rate, and live birth rate. **(Conditional Recommendation; Evidence Level Grade: B)**	In males with idiopathic oligozoospermia and FSH values within the normal range, FSH treatment may ameliorate spermatogenesis outcomes. **(Weak)**
Patients with nonobstructive azoospermia (NOA) should be informed of the limited data supporting pharmacologic manipulation with SERMs, AIs, and gonadotropins prior to surgical intervention. **(Conditional Recommendation; Evidence Level Grade: C)**	No conclusive recommendations can be given on the use of high-dose FSH in males with idiopathic infertility and prior microdissection testicular sperm extraction (TESE) and therefore cannot be routinely advocated. **(Weak)**
	In the presence of hyperprolactinemia, dopamine agonist therapy may improve spermatogenesis. **(Weak)**
	No conclusive recommendations on the routine use of medical therapy (e.g., recombinant FSH; highly purified FSH; hCG; AIs or selective SERMs) in patients with NOA can be drawn and are not therefore currently recommended routinely before TESE. **(Weak)**

management according to the level of obstruction. Congenital or intratesticular obstruction can be detected in 15% of OA patients. In these patients, sperm can be obtained for ICSI only with cTESE and micro-TESE.[86] Epididymal obstruction is the most common cause among males with OA. Epididymal obstruction may be congenital or acquired secondary to infections, trauma, and surgical procedures.[87] Epididymal sperm retrieval techniques such as MESA and PESA are indicated for males with CBAVD. In addition, in cases where sperm cannot be obtained in the epididymis, testicular sperm retrieval techniques such as TESA, cTESE, and micro-TESE

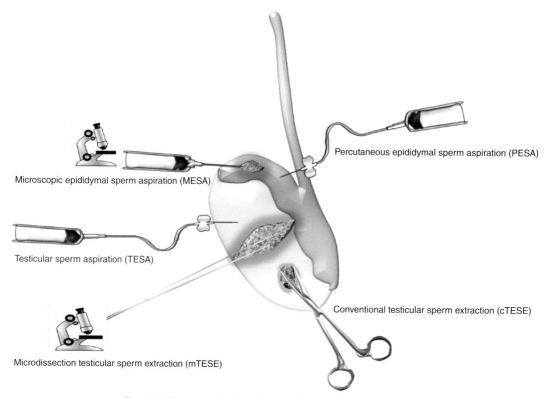

Percutaneous epididymal sperm aspiration (PESA)

Microscopic epididymal sperm aspiration (MESA)

Testicular sperm aspiration (TESA)

Conventional testicular sperm extraction (cTESE)

Microdissection testicular sperm extraction (mTESE)

Fig. 26.4 Sperm retrieval techniques from epididymis and testis.

can be used.[88] In cases of acquired epididymal obstruction, microsurgical epididymovasostomy (EV) is recommended if the partner has a good ovarian reserve. Obstruction may also occur in the vas deferens associated with vasectomy, inguinal hernia repair, or CBAVD accompanied by cystic fibrosis. In this group of patients, sperm can be retrieved for ICSI and cryopreservation with microscopic procedures such as EV and vasovasostomy.[23] Ejaculatory duct obstruction (EDO) is rare in OA cases. Detection of some findings in clinical diagnostic tests (anteroposterior diameter of seminal vesicle >15 mm, ejaculatory duct diameter >2.3 mm, dilated vasal ampulla >6 mm, prostate cysts in transrectal ultrasound, and presence of sperm in seminal vesicle aspiration) suggest EDO.[89] Transurethral resection of the ejaculatory ducts in males with EDO has been shown to improve semen parameters in 63% to 83% of these males.[22]

Management of Nonobstructive Azoospermia

Infertile males with NOA usually have primary testicular dysfunction and impaired spermatogenesis. The probability of successful testicular sperm retrieval in NOA is significantly lower than in males with OA.[21] Surgical techniques for sperm retrieval in males with NOA include TESA, cTESE, and micro-TESE, and SRRs are up to 50% in different techniques. Moreover, it was observed that micro-TESE in NOA resulted in 1.5 times more successful extraction than cTESE, and testicular sperm extraction was two times more successful compared to TESA.[90] Therefore both the EAU and AUA/ASRM guidelines recommend using micro-TESE for sperm retrieval in males with NOA.[22,23]

Many factors such as testicular histology, hormone profile, testicular volume, diagnostic biopsy, fine-needle aspiration, and fine-needle mapping have been defined to predict surgical sperm retrieval in patients with NOA. Although there are significant positive results that some of these are predictive of sperm retrieval, current guidelines do not recommend their routine clinical use for any of these factors. The only situation clearly stated in both guidelines is that it is not possible with surgical sperm retrieval techniques in patients with complete AZFa and AZFb deletions.[22,23]

MALE INFERTILITY MANAGEMENT WITH ASSISTED REPRODUCTIVE TECHNIQUES

ART has provided a treatment option for couples who cannot conceive naturally and various ART techniques have been described from the past to the present. The first randomized controlled study on the use of IUI, one of the relatively older techniques in male infertility, was published in 1984 and reported that IUI had a positive outcome compared to natural sexual intercourse.[91] This procedure is an infertility treatment based on the rationale of placing the prepared sperm into the uterine cavity, with or without ovarian stimulation, and increasing the maximum number of healthy sperm reaching the fertilization site. Although IUI with ovarian stimulation is a safer and cheaper alternative to IVF in managing couples with unexplained and mild male factor infertility, it is contraindicated in males with severe oligospermia due to the lower success of IUI cycles in infertile couples with male factor.[92]

IVF is a technique developed primarily for the treatment of female infertility. Following controlled ovarian hyperstimulation for the cycle in conventional IVF, oocytes are collected by aspiration and mixed with semen in a petri dish, and sperm fertilize the oocyte naturally. After culture incubation, the formed embryos are placed in the transcervical uterus as frozen-thawed or fresh embryos.[93] IVF in infertile couples with male factors like oligozoospermia and oligoasthenozoospermia have a 40-year history.[94] In the following years, conventional IVF was enhanced with various techniques such as high insemination concentration IVF and microscopic IVF to achieve pregnancy at lower motile sperm or lower sperm concentrations.[95] A review that evaluated studies comparing IVF and ICSI results showed that IVF and ICSI provide equal efficacy in cases of male infertility factors caused by moderate OAT, isolated teratozoospermia, and antisperm antibodies.[60]

The ICSI technique was defined for infertile couples with severe male factor infertility or failed cycles of non–male factor IVF in 1992. This technique allows fertilizing the oocyte regardless of the morphology and/or motility of the injected sperm.[96] The ICSI represents the majority of ART cycles conducted and is the most commonly used ART method today. In the United States, ICSI utilization for all indications increased from 36.4% to 76.2% from 1996 to 2012.[97] After ICSI interventions were performed with different age groups and all different types of spermatozoa, it was found that fertilization was about 70% to 80%, and clinical pregnancy rates were 45%. Although available evidence suggests that ICSI is associated with better fertilization rates in couples with unexplained infertility, it does not definitively support ICSI as a replacement for IVF with nonmale factor infertile heterosexual couples undergoing ART.[60]

Considering the results of ICSI in azoospermic patients, classification as NOA and OA have been shown to impact the success of ICSI. Live birth rates with the ICSI procedure have been reported as 21.4% for males with NOA, 37.5% for males with OA, and 32.3% for the general male infertility population using ejaculate sperm.[98] In addition, it has been shown that there is no statistical difference between the use of fresh or frozen-thawed spermatozoa in terms of ICSI pregnancy outcomes for both OA and NOA patients.[99,100] The AUA/ASRM guidelines state that fresh or cryopreserved sperm can be used for ICSI (moderate recommendation; Evidence Level Grade: C).[22] Although the current guidelines cannot provide clear recommendations about which ART method clinicians should use in male infertility, the summary of the methods to be used in the possible causes that will guide the clinical decision in male factor infertility or nonmale factor infertility is given in Table 26.6.[60]

TABLE 26.6 Fertilization Methods for Male Factor and Nonmale Factor Infertility

Type of Infertility	Fertilization Method
Male factor infertility	
Azoospermia	ICSI mandatory
Severe OAT	ICSI highly recommended
Moderate OAT	IVF and ICSI equally effective
Isolated teratozoospermia	IVF and ICSI equally effective
Absolute asthenozoospermia	ICSI mandatory

Continued

TABLE 26.6 Fertilization Methods for Male Factor and Nonmale Factor Infertility—cont'd

Type of Infertility	Fertilization Method
Globozoospermia	ICSI mandatory
Antisperm antibodies	IVF and ICSI equally effective
Sperm DNA fragmentation	ICSI recommended
Nonmale factor infertility	
General nonmale factor population	Equally effective, slightly in favor of IVF
Unexplained infertility	Equally effective, but sibling oocyte studies suggest that ICSI is superior to IVF for fertilization, whereas the reproductive outcome is not significantly different
Poor-quality oocytes and advanced maternal age	Equally effective, slightly in favor of IVF
Poor responders	Equally effective, slightly in favor of IVF
Preimplantation genetic testing	ICSI highly recommended
Tubal ligation	IVF preferable
Serodiscordant couples	Equally effective

ICSI, Intracytoplasmic sperm injection; *IVF*, in vitro fertilization; *OAT*, oligoasthenoteratozoospermia.
From Esteves SC, Roque M, Bedoschi G, Haahr T, Humaidan P. Intracytoplasmic sperm injection for male infertility and consequences for offspring. *Nat Rev Urol.* 2018;15(9):535-562.

CLINICAL/LABORATORY CASE SCENARIO

CASE 1

A 31-year-old male patient has a history of unprotected intercourse for 4 years and seeks medical care for primary infertility. General physical examination and the secondary sex characteristics revealed no pathology. In the urogenital examination, both testicles were normal, and both testicular volumes were found to be above 20 mL, according to the Prader orchidometer measurement. There is a grade 3 varicocele on the left side (Fig. 26.5). His partner's age is 28 years and gynecological evaluation and laboratory findings were unremarkable.

Semen Analysis Parameters	First Semen Analysis Results	Second Semen Analysis Results
Sperm volume (mL)	2	3
Semen pH	7.5	7.5
Sperm concentration (10^6/mL)	7.3	8.5
Total sperm count (10^6/ejaculate)	14.6	25.5
Total motility (progressive + nonprogressive, %)	40	35
Progressive motility (%)	0	0
Sperm morphology (normal forms, %)	1	1

What would be the best approach based on the available evidence?

Microscopic approach (inguinal/subinguinal) varicocelectomy

EAU: Treat infertile males with a clinical varicocele, abnormal semen parameters, and otherwise unexplained infertility in a heterosexual couple where the female partner has a good ovarian reserve to improve fertility rates (strong).

AUA/ASRM: Surgical varicocelectomy should be considered in males attempting to conceive who have palpable varicocele(s), infertility, and abnormal semen parameters except for azoospermic males (moderate recommendation; evidence level grade: B).

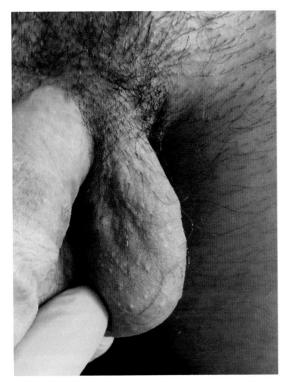

Fig. 26.5 Grade 3 varicocele image on examination.

SUMMARY

Infertility is a global health problem, and 8% to 12% of couples worldwide who want to have children suffer from this condition. The AUA/ASRM guideline and the EAU guideline provide a concise and clear summary of the literature on male infertility for all reproductive health professionals. Although the result of SA is not a definitive predictor of male infertility except for azoospermia, it is the first test to be requested to guide male infertility management. The development of IVF techniques and the introduction of ICSI may offer a chance to males with NOA to become fathers. Treatment may be scheduled with or without ART for infertile heterosexual couples with a male factor, depending on the underlying etiology. In this chapter, we strove to gather the evidence around elements of male infertility from its diagnosis to its management in the direction of the most recent AUA/ASRM and EAU guidelines.

The current guidelines provide evidence-based statements and recommendations that maintain a balance between overtreatment and undertreatment concerning the clinical assessment, diagnosis, and disease management of male infertility. These guidelines for male infertility are constantly being updated and are leading in this field. Each guideline uses an evidence-based system (a level of evidence or strength rating system) according to their consensus. This condition provides more objective and scientific guidance for clinicians to decide on male infertility management. Although there are minor nuances regarding male infertility, both guidelines contain similar assessments.

REFERENCES

1. Zegers-Hochschild F, Adamson GD, Dyer S, et al. The international glossary on infertility and fertility care, 2017. *Fertil Steril.* 2017;108(3):393-406.
2. Vander Borght M, Wyns C. Fertility and infertility: definition and epidemiology. *Clin Biochem.* 2018;62:2-10.
3. Barratt CLR, Björndahl L, De Jonge CJ, et al. The diagnosis of male infertility: an analysis of the evidence to support the development of global WHO guidance-challenges and future research opportunities. *Hum Reprod Update.* 2017;23(6):660-680.
4. Geoffroy-Siraudin C, Loundou AD, Romain F, et al. Decline of semen quality among 10 932 males consulting for couple infertility over a 20-year period in Marseille, France. *Asian J Androl.* 2012;14(4):584-590.
5. Romero-Otero J, Medina-Polo J, García-Gómez B, et al. Semen quality assessment in fertile men in Madrid during the last 3 decades. *Urology.* 2015;85(6):1333-1338.
6. Wang L, Zhang L, Song XH, Zhang HB, Xu CY, Chen ZJ. Decline of semen quality among Chinese sperm bank donors within 7 years (2008-2014). *Asian J Androl.* 2017;19(5):521-525.
7. Choy JT, Eisenberg ML. Male infertility as a window to health. *Fertil Steril.* 2018;110(5):810-814.
8. Meacham RB, Joyce GF, Wise M, Kparker A, Niederberger C. Male infertility. *J Urol.* 2007;177(6):2058-2066.
9. Zheng D, Nguyen QN, Li R, Dang VQ. Is intracytoplasmic sperm injection the solution for all in unexplained infertility? *Semin Reprod Med.* 2020;38(1):36-47.
10. Gul M, Hildorf S, Dong L, et al. Review of injection techniques for spermatogonial stem cell transplantation. *Hum Reprod Update.* 2020;26(3):368-391.
11. Jensen CFS, Dong L, Gul M, et al. Fertility preservation in boys facing gonadotoxic cancer therapy. *Nat Rev Urol.* 2022;19(2):71-83.
12. Rajender S, Avery K, Agarwal A. Epigenetics, spermatogenesis and male infertility. *Mutat Res.* 2011;727(3):62-71.

13. Neto FTL, Bach PV, Najari BB, Li PS, Goldstein M. Spermatogenesis in humans and its affecting factors. *Semin Cell Dev Biol.* 2016;59:10-26.

14. Schlegel PN, Sigman M, Collura B, et al. Diagnosis and treatment of infertility in men: AUA/ASRM guideline part I. *Fertil Steril.* 2021;115(1):54-61.

15. Jungwirth A, Giwercman A, Tournaye H, et al. European Association of Urology guidelines on male infertility: the 2012 update. *Eur Urol.* 2012;62(2):324-332.

16. Agarwal A, Parekh N, Panner Selvam MK, et al. Male oxidative stress infertility (MOSI): proposed terminology and clinical practice guidelines for management of idiopathic male infertility. *World J Mens Health.* 2019;37(3):296-312.

17. Salonia A, Bettocchi C, Boeri L, et al. European Association of Urology guidelines on sexual and reproductive health—2021 update: male sexual dysfunction. *Eur Urol.* 2021;80(3):333-357.

18. Schlegel PN, Sigman M, Collura B, et al. Diagnosis and treatment of infertility in men: AUA/ASRM Guideline part I. *J Urol.* 2021;205(1):36-43.

19. Dunson DB, Baird DD, Colombo B. Increased infertility with age in men and women. *Obstet Gynecol.* 2004;103(1):51-56.

20. Brandt JS, Cruz Ithier MA, Rosen T, Ashkinadze E. Advanced paternal age, infertility, and reproductive risks: a review of the literature. *Prenat Diagn.* 2019;39(2):81-87.

21. Agarwal A, Baskaran S, Parekh N, et al. Male infertility. *Lancet (London, England).* 2021;397(10271):319-333.

22. Schlegel PN, Sigman M, Collura B, et al. Diagnosis and treatment of infertility in men: AUA/ASRM guideline part I. *Fertil Steril.* 2021;115(1):54-61.

23. Minhas S, Bettocchi C, Boeri L, et al. European Association of Urology Guidelines on Male Sexual and Reproductive Health: 2021 Update on Male Infertility. *Eur Urol.* 2021;80(5):603-620.

24. Velemínská J, Bigoni L, Krajíček V, et al. Surface facial modelling and allometry in relation to sexual dimorphism. *Homo.* 2012;63(2):81-93.

25. Sigman M, Lipshultz LI, Howard SS. Office evaluation of the subfertile male. In: Lipshultz LI, Howards SS, Niederberger CS, eds. *Infertility in the Male.* 4th ed. Cambridge: Cambridge University Press; 2009:153-176.

26. Sigman M. Klinefelter syndrome: how, what, and why? *Fertil Steril.* 2012;98(2):251-252.

27. Leisegang K, Sengupta P, Agarwal A, Henkel R. Obesity and male infertility: mechanisms and management. *Andrologia.* 2021;53(1):e13617.

28. Witthaus MW, O'Brien J. Assessment of the male partner. In: Allahbadia GN, Ata B, Lindheim SR, Woodward BJ, Bhagavath B, eds. *Textbook of Assisted Reproduction.* Singapore: Springer Singapore; 2020:37-42.

29. WHO. *WHO Laboratory Manual for the Examination and Processing of Human Semen.* 6th ed. WHO. Available at: https://www.who.int/publications/i/item/9789240030787. Accessed December 3, 2021.

30. Björndahl LJHF. What is normal semen quality? On the use and abuse of reference limits for the interpretation of semen analysis results. *Hum Fertil (Camb).* 2011;14(3):179-186.

31. World Health Organization. *WHO Laboratory Manual for the Examination and Processing of Human Semen.* 6th ed. WHO Press: Geneva, Switzerland; 2021. Available on: https://www.who.int/publications/i/item/9789240030787. Accessed: December 3, 2021.

32. Ring JD, Lwin AA, Köhler TS. Current medical management of endocrine-related male infertility. *Asian J Androl.* 2016;18(3):357-363.

33. Guay A, Miller MG, McWhirter CL. Does early morning versus late morning draw time influence apparent testosterone concentration in men aged > or =45 years? Data from the Hypogonadism In Males study. *Int J Impot Res.* 2008;20(2):162-167.

34. Gagliano-Jucá T, Li Z, Pencina KM, et al. Oral glucose load and mixed meal feeding lowers testosterone levels in healthy eugonadal men. *Endocrine.* 2019;63(1):149-156.

35. Hackett G, Kirby M, Edwards D, et al. British Society for Sexual Medicine guidelines on adult testosterone deficiency, with statements for UK practice. *J Sex Med.* 2017;14(12):1504-1523.

36. Wang C, Nieschlag E, Swerdloff RS, et al. ISA, ISSAM, EAU, EAA and ASA recommendations: investigation, treatment and monitoring of late-onset hypogonadism in males. *Aging Male.* 2009;12(1):5-12.

37. Practice Committee of the American Society for Reproductive Medicine. Diagnostic evaluation of the infertile male: a committee opinion. *Fertil Steril.* 2015;103(3):e18-e25.

38. Martin-du-Pan RC, Bischof P. Increased follicle stimulating hormone in infertile men. Is increased plasma FSH always due to damaged germinal epithelium? *Hum Reprod.* 1995;10(8):1940-1945.

39. Hauser R, Temple-Smith PD, Southwick GJ, de Kretser D. Fertility in cases of hypergonadotropic azoospermia. *Fertil Steril.* 1995;63(3):631-636.

40. Schoor RA, Elhanbly S, Niederberger CS, Ross LS. The role of testicular biopsy in the modern management of male infertility. *J Urol.* 2002;167(1):197-200.

41. Ramasamy R, Lin K, Gosden LV, Rosenwaks Z, Palermo GD, Schlegel PN. High serum FSH levels in men with non-obstructive azoospermia does not affect success of microdissection testicular sperm extraction. *Fertil Steril.* 2009;92(2):590-593.

42. Tournaye H, Krausz C, Oates RD. Novel concepts in the aetiology of male reproductive impairment. *Lancet Diabetes Endocrinol.* 2017;5(7):544-553.

43. Krausz C, Riera-Escamilla A. Genetics of male infertility. *Nat Rev Urol.* 2018;15(6):369-384.

44. Vincent MC, Daudin M, De MP, et al. Cytogenetic investigations of infertile men with low sperm counts: a 25-year experience. *J Androl.* 2002;23(1):18-45.

45. Corona G, Pizzocaro A, Lanfranco F, et al. Sperm recovery and ICSI outcomes in Klinefelter syndrome: a systematic review and meta-analysis. *Hum Reprod Update.* 2017;23(3):265-275.

46. Staessen C, Tournaye H, Van Assche E, et al. PGD in 47,XXY Klinefelter's syndrome patients. *Hum Reprod Update.* 2003;9(4):319-330.

47. Nguyen MH, Morel F, Pennamen P, et al. Balanced complex chromosome rearrangement in male infertility: case report and literature review. *Andrologia.* 2015;47(2):178-185.

48. Colaco S, Modi D. Genetics of the human Y chromosome and its association with male infertility. *Reprod Biol Endocrinol.* 2018;16(1):14.

49. Hopps CV, Mielnik A, Goldstein M, Palermo GD, Rosenwaks Z, Schlegel PN. Detection of sperm in men with Y chromosome microdeletions of the AZFa, AZFb and AZFc regions. *Hum Reprod (Oxford, England).* 2003;18(8):1660-1665.

50. Park SH, Lee HS, Choe JH, Lee JS, Seo JT. Success rate of microsurgical multiple testicular sperm extraction and sperm presence in the ejaculate in Korean men with Y chromosome microdeletions. *Korean J Urol.* 2013;54(8):536-540.

51. Abur U, Gunes S, Ascı R, et al. Chromosomal and Y-chromosome microdeletion analysis in 1,300 infertile males and the fertility outcome of patients with AZFc microdeletions. *Andrologia.* 2019;51(11):e13402.

52. De Boeck K. Cystic fibrosis in the year 2020: a disease with a new face. *Acta Paediatr (Oslo, Norway: 1992).* 2020;109(5):893-899.

53. Chillon M, Casals T, Mercier B, et al. Mutations in the cystic fibrosis gene in patients with congenital absence of the vas deferens. *N Engl J Med.* 1995;332(22):1475-1480.

54. Gul M, Carvajal A, Serefoglu EC, Minhas S, Salonia A. European Association of Urology guidelines for sexual and reproductive health 2020: What is new? *Int J Impot Res.* 2020;32(5):477-479.

55. Armstrong JM, Keihani S, Hotaling JM. Use of ultrasound in male infertility: appropriate selection of men for scrotal ultrasound. *Curr Urol Rep.* 2018;19(8):58.

56. Lotti F, Maggi M. Ultrasound of the male genital tract in relation to male reproductive health. *Hum Reprod Update.* 2015;21(1):56-83.

57. Jurewicz M, Gilbert BR. Imaging and angiography in male factor infertility. *Fertil Steril.* 2016;105(6):1432-1442.

58. Esteves SC, Miyaoka R, Agarwal A. Surgical treatment of male infertility in the era of intracytoplasmic sperm injection - new insights. *Clinics (Sao Paulo, Brazil).* 2011;66(8):1463-1478.

59. Agarwal A, Cho CL. Clinical andrology: the missing jigsaw pieces. *Indian J Urol.* 2017;33(3):186-187.

60. Esteves SC, Roque M, Bedoschi G, Haahr T, Humaidan P. Intracytoplasmic sperm injection for male infertility and consequences for offspring. *Nat Rev Urol.* 2018;15(9):535-562.

61. Majzoub A, Agarwal A. Antioxidant therapy in idiopathic oligoasthenoteratozoospermia. *Indian J Urol.* 2017;33(3):207-214.

62. Sidorkiewicz I, Zaręba K, Wołczyński S, Czerniecki J. Endocrine-disrupting chemicals-Mechanisms of action on male reproductive system. *Toxicol Ind Health.* 2017;33(7):601-609.

63. Smits RM, Mackenzie-Proctor R, Yazdani A, Stankiewicz MT, Jordan V, Showell MG. Antioxidants for male subfertility. *Cochrane Database Syst Rev.* 2019;3(3):CD007411.

64. Steiner AZ, Hansen KR, Barnhart KT, et al. The effect of antioxidants on male factor infertility: the Males, Antioxidants, and Infertility (MOXI) randomized clinical trial. *Fertil Steril.* 2020;113(3):552-560.e3.

65. Cannarella R, Condorelli RA, Mongioì LM, Barbagallo F, Calogero AE, La Vignera S. Effects of the selective estrogen receptor modulators for the treatment of male infertility: a systematic review and meta-analysis. *Expert Opin Pharmacother.* 2019;20(12):1517-1525.

66. Del Giudice F, Busetto GM, De Berardinis E, et al. A systematic review and meta-analysis of clinical trials implementing aromatase inhibitors to treat male infertility. *Asian J Androl.* 2020;22(4):360-367.

67. Gemzell C, Kjessler B. Treatment of infertility after partial hypophysectomy with human pituitary gonadotrophins. *Lancet (London, England).* 1964;1(7334):644.

68. Fraietta R, Zylberstejn DS, Esteves SC. Hypogonadotropic hypogonadism revisited. *Clinics (Sao Paulo, Brazil).* 2013;68 Suppl 1(suppl 1):81-88.

69. El Meliegy A, Motawi A, El Salam MAA. Systematic review of hormone replacement therapy in the infertile man. *Arab J Urol.* 2018;16(1):140-147.

70. Salonia A, Rastrelli G, Hackett G, et al. Paediatric and adult-onset male hypogonadism. *Nat Rev Dis Primers.* 2019;5(1):38.

71. Bouloux P, Warne DW, Loumaye E. Efficacy and safety of recombinant human follicle-stimulating hormone in men with isolated hypogonadotropic hypogonadism. *Fertil Steril.* 2002;77(2):270-273.

72. Warne DW, Decosterd G, Okada H, Yano Y, Koide N, Howles CM. A combined analysis of data to identify predictive factors for spermatogenesis in men with

hypogonadotropic hypogonadism treated with recombinant human follicle-stimulating hormone and human
chorionic gonadotropin. *Fertil Steril.* 2009;92(2):
594-604.

73. Rastrelli G, Corona G, Mannucci E, Maggi M. Factors
affecting spermatogenesis upon gonadotropin-
replacement therapy: a meta-analytic study. *Andrology.*
2014;2(6):794-808.

74. Melmed S, Casanueva FF, Hoffman AR, et al. Diagnosis
and treatment of hyperprolactinemia: an Endocrine Society clinical practice guideline. *J Clin Endocrinol Metab.*
2011;96(2):273-288.

75. Corona G, Rastrelli G, Maggi M. The pharmacotherapy
of male hypogonadism besides androgens. *Expert Opin
Pharmacother.* 2015;16(3):369-387.

76. Santi D, Granata AR, Simoni M. FSH treatment of male
idiopathic infertility improves pregnancy rate: a meta-
analysis. *Endocr Connect.* 2015;4(3):R46-R58.

77. Gul Ü. The effect of human chorionic gonadotropin
treatment before testicular sperm extraction in non-
obstructive azoospermia. *J Clin Anal Med.* 2014;7.
doi:10.4328/JCAM.3332

78. Aydos K, Ünlü C, Demirel LC, et al. The effect of pure
FSH administration in non-obstructive azoospermic
men on testicular sperm retrieval. *Eur J Obstet Gynecol
Reprod Biol.* 2003;108(1):54-58.

79. Jensen CFS, Østergren P, Dupree JM, Ohl DA, Sønksen J,
Fode M. Varicocele and male infertility. *Nat Rev Urol.*
2017;14(9):523-533.

80. Shridharani A, Owen RC, Elkelany OO, Kim ED. The significance of clinical practice guidelines on adult varicocele detection and management. *Asian J Androl.*
2016;18(2):269-275.

81. Silay MS, Hoen L, Quadackaers J, et al. Treatment of varicocele in children and adolescents: a systematic review
and meta-analysis from the European Association of
Urology/European Society for Paediatric Urology Guidelines panel. *Eur Urol.* 2019;75(3):448-461.

82. Machen GL, Sandlow JI. Extended indications for
varicocelectomy. *F1000Research* 2019;8:F1000 Faculty
Rev-1579.

83. Temple-Smith PD, Southwick GJ, Yates CA, Trounson
AO, de Kretser DM. Human pregnancy by in vitro fertil-
ization (IVF) using sperm aspirated from the epididymis.
J In Vitro Fert Embryo Transf. 1985;2(3):119-122.

84. Shin DH, Turek PJ. Sperm retrieval techniques. *Nat Rev
Urol.* 2013;10(12):723-730.

85. Wosnitzer MS, Goldstein M. Obstructive azoospermia.
Urol Clin North Am. 2014;41(1):83-95.

86. Hendry WF. Azoospermia and Surgery for Testicular Obstruction. In: Hargreave TB, ed. *Male Infertility.* London:
Springer London; 1994:337-363. doi:10.1007/978-1-
4471-1029-3_17

87. Han H, Liu S, Zhou XG, Tian L, Zhang XD. Aetiology
of obstructive azoospermia in Chinese infertility
patients. *Andrologia.* 2016;48(7):761-764.

88. Esteves SC, Miyaoka R, Agarwal A. Sperm retrieval
techniques for assisted reproduction. *Int Braz J Urol.*
2011;37(5):570-583.

89. Meacham RB, Hellerstein DK, Lipshultz LI. Evaluation
and treatment of ejaculatory duct obstruction in the
infertile male. *Fertil Steril.* 1993;59(2):393-397.

90. Bernie AM, Mata DA, Ramasamy R, Schlegel PN. Comparison of microdissection testicular sperm extraction,
conventional testicular sperm extraction, and testicular
sperm aspiration for non-obstructive azoospermia: a
systematic review and meta-analysis. *Fertil Steril.*
2015;104(5):1099-1103.e1-e3.

91. Kerin JF, Kirby C, Peek J, et al. Improved conception
rate after intrauterine insemination of washed spermatozoa from men with poor quality semen. *Lancet
(London, England).* 1984;1(8376):533-535.

92. Group ECW. Intrauterine insemination. *Hum Reprod
Update.* 2009;15(3):265-277.

93. Merchant R, Gandhi G, Allahbadia GN. In vitro fertil-
ization/intracytoplasmic sperm injection for male infertility. *Indian J Urol.* 2011;27(1):121-132.

94. Cohen J, Edwards R, Fehilly C, et al. In vitro fertilization: a treatment for male infertility. *Fertil Steril.* 1985;
43(3):422-432.

95. Hall J, Fishel S. In vitro fertilization for male infertility:
when and how? *Baillieres Clin Obstet Gynaecol.* 1997;
11(4):711-724.

96. Palermo G, Joris H, Devroey P, Van Steirteghem AC.
Pregnancies after intracytoplasmic injection of single
spermatozoon into an oocyte. *Lancet (London, England).*
1992;340(8810):17-18.

97. Boulet SL, Mehta A, Kissin DM, Warner L, Kawwass JF,
Jamieson DJ. Trends in use of and reproductive outcomes associated with intracytoplasmic sperm injection. *JAMA.* 2015;313(3):255-263.

98. Esteves SC, Agarwal A. Reproductive outcomes, including neonatal data, following sperm injection in men
with obstructive and non-obstructive azoospermia: case
series and systematic review. *Clinics (Sao Paulo, Brazil).*
2013;68 Suppl 1(suppl 1):141-150.

99. Van Peperstraten A, Proctor ML, Johnson NP, Philipson
G. Techniques for surgical retrieval of sperm prior to in-
tra-cytoplasmic sperm injection (ICSI) for azoospermia.
Cochrane Database Syst Rev. 2008;2008(2):CD002807.

100. Ohlander S, Hotaling J, Kirshenbaum E, Niederberger
C, Eisenberg ML. Impact of fresh versus cryopreserved
testicular sperm upon intracytoplasmic sperm injection
pregnancy outcomes in men with azoospermia due to
spermatogenic dysfunction: a meta-analysis. *Fertil Steril.*
2014;101(2):344-349.

27

Expert Opinion: Management of Male Infertility in the Postintracytoplasmic Sperm Injection Era

Rupin Shah and Armand Zini

KEY POINTS

- Though intracytoplasmic sperm injection (ICSI) has shifted the focus from the infertile male to a single sperm, it is still vital to evaluate and treat an infertile male to improve the success of ICSI by improving sperm quality and for psychosocial, medical, and financial reasons.
- While semen analysis is no longer considered a reliable discriminator between fertile and infertile males,

it does provides valuable information for deciding further evaluation and therapy prior to considering ICSI, and the results of special tests like sperm DNA fragmentation are relevant to the outcome of ICSI.
- Detailed genetic testing of the infertile male will be used far more extensively in the future and will impact decision making in couples planned for ICSI.

INTRODUCTION

The advent of intracytoplasmic sperm injection (ICSI) has changed the way in which male infertility can be managed. Even males with very low sperm counts or motility can father a child without any intervention to improve semen quality. Hence assisted reproductive technology (ART) specialists tend to focus on the sperm and not concern themselves with evaluation or treatment of the infertile male.[1]

However, there are numerous reasons why it is important to evaluate and treat a male with infertility, even though ICSI may offer a shortcut. Various chapters in this book have already discussed in great detail all aspects of investigation and management of male infertility and have provided clear clinical guidelines. The preceding chapter has summarized the management recommendations from international professional societies. Hence in this chapter, we will focus on discussing why it is important to evaluate and treat infertile males despite the availability of ICSI, and also highlight

key recommendations that are relevant in the ICSI era from the previous chapters.

THE IMPORTANCE OF EVALUATING AND TREATING MALE INFERTILITY

Fertility treatment is much more than just getting a sperm and egg together. It has social, psychological, and health-related implications. Any male whose fertility history or semen analysis reveal him to be subfertile deserves to be evaluated for the following reasons.
- *Joy of natural conception:* every couple would like to conceive naturally, if possible. ICSI is a compromise, not a preference. Also, since the genetic consequences of ICSI are still uncertain,[2] heterosexual couples would prefer a natural conception, if that is feasible, by improving the male's fertility.
- *Self-image:* being infertile can be a huge blow to a male's self-image and his ego[3-5] and may also affect his sex life.[6] It is common to see males in the clinic who agonize: "Doc, my health is fine, my sex life is

great, I have a healthy lifestyle—how can I have such a low sperm count?" Improvement of semen parameter can increase a male's self-esteem, especially if it leads to a natural pregnancy, while the need for ART may be associated with depression.[7]

- *Financial:* the cost of therapies (medical, surgical, or lifestyle) to improve semen quality are much lower than the costs of ART.[8] Hence treatment of the male factor, when possible, is economically beneficial.
- *Marker for other illnesses:* male infertility may be the consequence of or associated with other illnesses. It is associated with a greater risk of malignancy,[9] and evaluation of an infertile male may also help uncover other significant medical conditions.[10]
- *Motivation for lifestyle changes:* since lifestyle changes may improve a male's fertility in some cases,[11] the treatment of an infertile male provides the opportunity to improve his overall health since the prospect of improving his semen quality can be a strong motivator for a male to improve his lifestyle.
- *Paternal health affects health of offspring:* evidence suggests that paternal health at the time of conception can impact the health of the offspring through epigenetic changes in the sperm.[12] Understanding this will also motivate infertile males to work towards optimal health.
- *Sperm quality may affect ICSI outcome:* many events related to fertilization and early implantation can be affected by sperm quality,[13,14] and hence it is important to improve sperm quality and minimize iatrogenic damage to sperm as much as possible prior to ICSI.

CONTROVERSIES IN EVALUATION OF AN INFERTILE MALE

In this section, we comment on some of the controversial areas related to male infertility in the context of ICSI.

Interpretation of Semen Analysis

The sixth edition of the World Health Organization (WHO) manual on examination and processing of semen[15] presents data on the distribution of sperm parameters in heterosexual couples with a time to pregnancy of 1 year or less, much like the fifth edition of the WHO manual. The data presented in the sixth edition have been further expanded (relative to the fifth edition) and complemented with data from around 3500 males in 12 countries.

As such, the distribution results in the sixth edition are more robust and globally representative than those in the fifth edition manual but interestingly, the distributions do not differ much from the fifth edition manual. As in the fifth edition, the authors of the sixth edition suggest that the lower fifth percentile can be used to interpret results from an individual patient. However, they caution that overinterpretation of the fifth percentile values should be avoided as these values do not represent a limit between fertile and infertile males.[16] Moreover, they caution that there is significant overlap of semen results between fertile and infertile males.

What is new in the sixth edition[15] on the interpretation of semen analysis is the suggestion that other methods for evaluating semen examination results be used. The authors propose that a multiparametric approach (with combined reference limits) may be useful, although they acknowledge that this has not yet been developed. The authors also consider using decision limits to help identify infertile males but do not provide further details on this approach. As such, it is implied that there is no ideal interpretation of the semen analysis. Combining semen parameters with duration of infertility can give a more accurate prediction of a male's fertility potential[17] and thus help decide when ICSI is needed. Further, the clinician should not label a male fertile and withhold treatment just because his semen parameters are above the fifth percentile (as per norms of the fifth edition). Offering therapy to improve semen parameters to a higher percentile may increase the probability of and reduce the time to pregnancy.[18,19]

Testing for Sperm DNA Fragmentation

Despite many studies and systematic reviews,[20] there is still controversy about the utility of sperm DNA fragmentation (SDF) testing,[21] about which test and threshold to use,[22] and about when and how to manage males with raised SDF.[23] To date, the level of evidence supporting the use of SDF testing in the management of heterosexual couple infertility and as a predictor of reproductive outcomes remains modest.[24] It is advisable for clinicians to work with one standardized test and evaluate it in fertile males to establish their own norms and to periodically review the utility (discriminatory and predictive) of SDF testing in their populations of infertile males. This will enable clinicians to make their own informed decisions until further research provides greater clarity.

Genetic Testing

Male infertility can be due to a variety of genetic causes.[25] With the widespread availability and greater affordability of genomic testing together with artificial intelligence-based algorithms to analyze the data, a significant proportion of males with azoospermia, severe oligozoospermia, or monomorphic sperm defects will be found to have a genetic basis for their problem. Finding of a genetic defect would have major impact on the subsequent ICSI procedure. Thus clinicians can expect genetic testing to assume a major role in future evaluation of male infertility,[26] especially when ICSI is planned.[27]

Varicocele

There will continue to be a role for varicocele repair (VR) in the ICSI era.[28] Cost analysis has shown that VR is significantly more cost effective than intrauterine insemination or ICSI in achieving a live birth.[29] VR for an infertile male targets the problem (the male) instead of shifting the burden of therapy on to the healthy person (the female partner). Even when ICSI is contemplated, correcting the varicocele prior to ICSI appears to result in a higher live birth rate.[30] When ICSI is planned with surgical sperm retrieval, then prior VR may increase the likelihood of finding sperm in the ejaculate[31] or the testis.[32]

Azoospermia

A thorough andrological evaluation is needed before a male can be scheduled for sperm retrieval with ICSI. In some cases, the problem may turn out to be obstructive, and a permanent cure may be possible by microsurgical bypass of an epididymal obstruction[33] or by transurethral resection of an ejaculatory duct block.[34] If the obstructive azoospermia is due to vas aplasia, then genetic testing is needed.[35] If the azoospermia is due to testicular failure, then genetic testing, screening for malignancy, and planning the surgical sperm retrieval would be needed. Occasionally, the problem may be due to hypogonadotropic hypogonadism. This would need a detailed medical evaluation, followed by a long course of hormone therapy.

CONCLUSION

Though ICSI has made it possible to achieve a pregnancy even when only very few sperm are present, this does not mean that the infertile male should not be treated. As discussed in this chapter, there are numerous reasons why it is vital to evaluate and treat an infertile male despite the availability of ICSI. It is very important to remember this fact when ART procedures grow more sophisticated and automated and tend to ignore the vital human element in all infertility-related issues.

SUMMARY

The advent of intracytoplasmic sperm injection (ICSI) has made it possible to achieve pregnancy with very low numbers of sperm retrieved from the ejaculate or the testes. However, it is still very important to evaluate the infertile male for a variety of reasons. Improving a male's fertility may result in a natural pregnancy, which would avoid a large financial expense and a major medical intervention on a healthy female partner, while improving the male's self-esteem and psychological well-being. Even if ICSI is eventually required, improving sperm quality may increase chances of a live birth. Treatment of male infertility involves lifestyle changes to improve paternal health and this may, in turn, improve the health of the offspring through epigenetic modifications. Finally, male infertility is linked with greater health problems, which could be uncovered during an infertility evaluation. As assisted reproductive techniques become more widespread, it is important not to focus just on the sperm and forget the male behind it.

REFERENCES

1. Wong MY, Ledger WL. Is ICSI risky? *Obstet Gynecol Int.* 2013;2013:473289. doi:10.1155/2013/473289.
2. Georgiou I, Syrrou M, Pardalidis N, et al. Genetic and epigenetic risks of intracytoplasmic sperm injection method. *Asian J Androl.* 2006;8(6):643-673.
3. Swierkowski-Blanchard N, Alter L, Salama S, et al. To be or not to be [fertile], that is the question. *Basic Clin Androl.* 2016;26:12. doi: 10.1186/s12610-016-0040-9.
4. Peronace LA, Boivin J, Schmidt L. Patterns of suffering and social interactions in infertile men: 12 months after unsuccessful treatment. *J Psychosom Obstet Gynaecol.* 2007;28(2):105-114.
5. Throsby K, Gill R. "It's different for men": masculinity and IVF. *Men Masculinities.* 2004;6(4):330-348.
6. Smith JF, Walsh TJ, Shindel AW, et al; Infertility Outcomes Program Project Group. Sexual, marital, and social impact of a man's perceived infertility diagnosis. *J Sex Med.* 2009;6(9):2505–2515.

7. Samorinha C, Tendais I, Silva S, Figueiredo B. Antenatal paternal adjustment and paternal attitudes after infertility treatment. *Hum Reprod.* 2018;33(1):109-115.

8. Meng MV, Greene KL, Turek PJ. Surgery or assisted reproduction? A decision analysis of treatment costs in male infertility. *J Urol.* 2005;174(5):1926-1931.

9. Hotaling JM, Walsh TJ. Male infertility: a risk factor for testicular cancer. *Nat Rev Urol.* 2009;6(10):550-556.

10. Minhas S, Bettocchi C, Boeri L, et al. European Association of Urology guidelines on male sexual and reproductive health: 2021 update on male infertility. *Eur Urol.* 2021;80(5):603-620.

11. Zampieri N, Zamboni C, Ottolenghi A, Camoglio FS. The role of lifestyle changing to improve the semen quality in patients with varicocele. *Minerva Urol Nefrol.* 2008;60(4):199-204.

12. Craig JR, Jenkins TG, Carrell DT, Hotaling JM. Obesity, male infertility, and the sperm epigenome. *Fertil Steril.* 2017;107(4):848-859.

13. McQueen DB, Zhang J, Robins JC. Sperm DNA fragmentation and recurrent pregnancy loss: a systematic review and meta-analysis. *Fertil Steril.* 2019;112(1):54-60.

14. Colaco S, Sakkas D. Paternal factors contributing to embryo quality. *J Assist Reprod Genet.* 2018;35(11): 1953-1968.

15. World Health Organization. *WHO Laboratory Manual for the Examination and Processing of Human Semen.* 6th ed. Geneva: World Health Organization; 2021.

16. Boitrelle F, Shah R, Saleh R, et al. The sixth edition of the WHO manual for human semen analysis: a critical review and SWOT analysis. *Life (Basel).* 2021;11(12):1368. doi:10.3390/life11121368.

17. Hargreave TB, Elton RA. Is conventional sperm analysis of any use? *Br J Urol.* 1983;55(6):774-749.

18. Keihani S, Verrilli LE, Zhang C, et al. Semen parameter thresholds and time-to-conception in subfertile couples: how high is high enough? *Hum Reprod.* 2021;36(8): 2121-2133.

19. Romero Herrera JA, Bang AK, Priskorn L, Izarzugaza JMG, Brunak S, Jørgensen N. Semen quality and waiting time to pregnancy explored using association mining. *Andrology.* 2021;9(2):577-587.

20. Agarwal A, Majzoub A, Baskaran S, et al. Sperm DNA fragmentation: a new guideline for clinicians. *World J Mens Health.* 2020;38(4):412-471.

21. Ten J, Guerrero J, Linares Á, et al. Sperm DNA fragmentation on the day of fertilisation is not associated with assisted reproductive technique outcome independently of gamete quality. *Hum Fertil (Camb).* 2022;25(4):706-715.

22. Javed A, Talkad MS, Ramaiah MK. Evaluation of sperm DNA fragmentation using multiple methods: a comparison of their predictive power for male infertility. *Clin Exp Reprod Med.* 2019;46(1):14-21.

23. Esteves SC, Zini A, Coward RM, et al. Sperm DNA fragmentation testing: summary evidence and clinical practice recommendations. *Andrologia.* 2021;53(2):e13874. doi:10.1111/and.13874.

24. Agarwal A, Majzoub A, Esteves SC, Ko E, Ramasamy R, Zini A. Clinical utility of sperm DNA fragmentation testing: practice recommendations based on clinical scenarios. *Transl Androl Urol.* 2016;5(6):935-950.

25. Cioppi F, Rosta V, Krausz C. Genetics of azoospermia. *Int J Mol Sci.* 2021;22(6):3264. doi:10.3390/ijms22063264.

26. Fakhro KA, Elbardisi H, Arafa M, et al. Point-of-care whole-exome sequencing of idiopathic male infertility. *Genet Med.* 2018;20(11):1365-1373.

27. Kherraf ZE, Cazin C, Bouker A, et al. Whole-exome sequencing improves the diagnosis and care of men with non-obstructive azoospermia. *Am J Hum Genet.* 2022;109(3):508-517.

28. Sönmez MG, Haliloğlu AH. Role of varicocele treatment in assisted reproductive technologies. *Arab J Urol.* 2018;16(1):188-196.

29. Masson P, Brannigan RE. The varicocele. *Urol Clin North Am.* 2014;41(1):129-144.

30. Esteves SC, Roque M, Agarwal A. Outcome of assisted reproductive technology in men with treated and untreated varicocele: systematic review and meta-analysis. *Asian J Androl.* 2016;18(2):254-258.

31. Weedin JW, Khera M, Lipshultz LI. Varicocele repair in patients with nonobstructive azoospermia: a meta-analysis. *J Urol.* 2010;183(6):2309-2315.

32. Haydardedeoglu B, Turunc T, Kilicdag EB, et al. The effect of prior varicocelectomy in patients with nonobstructive azoospermia on intracytoplasmic sperm injection outcomes: a retrospective pilot study. *Urology.* 2010;75(1):83-86.

33. Chan PT. The evolution and refinement of vasoepididymostomy techniques. *Asian J Androl.* 2013;15(1):49-55.

34. Fisch H, Lambert SM, Goluboff ET. Management of ejaculatory duct obstruction: etiology, diagnosis, and treatment. *World J Urol.* 2006;24(6):604-610.

35. Bieth E, Hamdi SM, Mieusset R. Genetics of the congenital absence of the vas deferens. *Hum Genet.* 2021;140(1):59-76.

Insights Into the Future of Male Infertility

28

Clinical Perspective in the Postintracyoplasmic Sperm Injection Era

Hussein Kandil and Ramadan Saleh

KEY POINTS

The main issues highlighted in the current review include:

- Relationship between epigenetic disorders and male infertility and the potential role of epigenetics in the management of infertile males.
- Impact of proteomics on sperm biology and functional state and the clinical implications of proteomic alterations in male infertility.
- Advances in the management of infertile males with nonobstructive azoospermia, with focus on

molecular markers of future modalities of sperm retrieval in this selected category.

- Advances in sperm selection methods for intracytoplasmic sperm injection, highlighting their advantages, disadvantages, and clinical outcomes.
- The potential of stem cell therapy in the treatment of male infertility.
- Advances in fertility preservation of cancer patients.
- The role of artificial intelligence in the management of male infertility.

INTRODUCTION

Male factor solely accounts for 20% to 30% of cases of infertility, and a male cause contributes in additional 20% of heterosexual couples' infertility.[1] The etiological and risk factors of male infertility are wide ranging and are generally categorized into congenital or acquired causes.[2] However, the etiology is not clear in up to 50% of male infertility cases and no identifiable female factor is detected; hence a diagnosis of idiopathic infertility is given.[3] Despite the presence of several tests for evaluation of male infertility, they are limited by low diagnostic and prognostic capabilities,[4] and failure to explain the underlying mechanisms at a molecular level of spermatozoa.[5] The introduction of intracytoplasmic sperm injection (ICSI) has revolutionized the treatment of infertility and enabled couples with severe male factor to initiate pregnancy, e.g., following surgical sperm retrieval in cases of nonobstructive azoospermia (NOA).[6] Despite great advances in assisted reproductive

techniques (ARTs) in the last two decades, the outcome of ICSI for severe male factor remains unsatisfactory.

In this review, we highlight the potential role of epigenetics and proteomics in the management of male infertility. We also discuss the molecular markers that may help predict sperm retrieval in patients with NOA and future modalities of sperm retrieval for this category. In addition, we summarize the methods of optimizing sperm selection for ICSI. Furthermore, we discuss fertility preservation (FP) in cancer patients. Finally, we provide future insights on the role of artificial intelligence (AI) and stem cells in the management of male infertility.

ROLE OF EPIGENETICS IN THE MANAGEMENT OF MALE INFERTILITY

There is mounting evidence supporting a relationship between male infertility and epigenetic disorders.[7] Epigenetics involves the heritable alteration in genetic expression and gene activities without alteration in the DNA sequence.[8] Male germ cells have a distinctive epigenetic pattern compared to somatic cells. Many epigenetic steps take place during the different phases of spermatogenesis; this includes DNA methylation and chromatic remodeling during chromatin compaction, which is the transition from histones to protamines.[9] Subsequently, aberration in the epigenetic regulator genes is believed to attribute to spermatogenic failure.[9]

Methylation

This involves methyl group transfer to the DNA cytosine ring in a step that is catalyzed by DNA methyl transferases.[10] Methylation is a crucial epigenetic process that is regulated by many mediators and is important in many reactions involving the DNA and RNA. Methylene-tetrahydrofolate reductase (MTHFR) is a regulatory enzyme that is involved in the methylation process by generating methyl donors[11] and is more prominent in the testes compared to other human tissues.[12] MTHFR-altered genetic expression is associated with alteration in spermatogenesis.[12] The transcriptional process is repressed when cytosine methylation occurs at the CpG level.[13] In a study evaluating the differences in DNA methylation profiles between NOA and obstructive azoospermia (OA), DNA hypomethylation was demonstrated in 78 of 212 CpG sites compared to 134 DNA hypermethylation patterns in the NOA group compared to the OA counterparts.[14]

Acetylation

Acetylation is an epigenetic step that affects gene expression by allowing access to transcription factors.[15] Chromatin remodeling taking place during spermiogenesis that is consistent with histone-protamine transition appears to be linked to histone H4 hyperacetylation.[16] Faure et al. demonstrated that in specimens from testes with absence of germ cells (as in Sertoli cell–only syndrome) or absence of spermatocytes and spermatids, an increased state of hyperacetylation of H4 in the Sertoli cells nuclei was observed when compared to specimens with normal spermatogenesis, where Sertoli cell chromatin hypoacetylation prevails.[17] It was also shown that spermatids in patients with maturation arrest at the round spermatid level demonstrated reduced histone(H4) acetylation.[18]

Phosphorylation

Phosphorylation is governed by kinases and is associated with reduced activity when the epigenetic modifier proteins are phosphorylated, which subsequently alters the interactions between proteins.[19] Calmodulin-dependent protein kinase is essential for protamine 2 phosphorylation, and mutations involving it can result in male infertility.[20] Alterations in genetic expression resulting from aberrant DNA protamine packaging are expected to result in spermatogenesis failure.[21]

Ubiquitination (Ubiquitylation)

Ubiquitination of the mitochondria is considered an important step during spermatogenesis and is involved in the paternal mitochondrial degeneration following fertilization, which is believed to permit the inheritance of the maternal mitochondrial DNA.[22] Ubiquitination enzymes are highly expressed in the testis, reflecting the importance of the ubiquitin system for spermatogenesis, being partially involved in histone degradation process taking place during the histone to protamine transition.[23]

Epigenetics and Male Infertility-Associated Conditions

It has been found that NOA patients have 1.8 times more identified rare, nonsilent variants (22.5% carrier frequency) compared to controls (13.7% carrier frequency), suggesting that defects in the key epigenetic regulators may alter spermatogenesis, hence explaining their role in NOA.[9] In a study investigating the epigenetic status of the extraembryonic spermatogenesis homeobox 1 gene (*ESX1*), it was demonstrated that 81.3% of subjects lacked *ESX1* expression when their histologic examination showed absence of spermatogenesis. Furthermore, transcriptional analysis demonstrated that *ESX1* gene expression reached 95.4% and 18.7% in patients with and without proven spermatogenesis, respectively, and hence could be used as a marker for spermatogenesis and sperm retrieval.[24] In a study of the transcriptional and posttranscriptional gene expression regulated by microRNA (miRNA) and noncoding RNA, it was found that the expression profile differed according to the different testicular histologic patterns. Moreover, the presence of miR-34 and miR-449 in the testicular tissues was different between patients presenting with azoospermia and counterparts with intact spermatogenesis.[25] Enzymatic knockout to the germ cell specific enzymes involved in the formation of mature miRNA can result in alteration in spermatogenesis.[26] Additionally, it is believed that DNA methylation of the tissue-specific differentially methylated region (TDMR) is associated with transcriptional suppression, further justifying the epigenetic role in the pathogenesis of male infertility. This was further demonstrated in a study on patients with NOA, which revealed that subjects with hypospermatogenesis (HS) had higher levels of DNA methylation at TDMR of the *GTF2A1L* gene promoter compared to healthy controls, highlighting the impact of abnormal methylation to various testis-specific gene promoters, which is believed to induce postmeiotic failure in patients with HS.[7] In a study assessing the DNA methylation state in patients with NOA, testicular DNA hypermethylation was observed in 53% of patients with NOA compared to none in the control group. Furthermore, when the peripheral blood was assessed, no difference was observed in the methylation profiles between both groups, suggesting a distinct testicular DNA hypermethylation occurring in NOA patients.[11]

ROLE OF PROTEOMICS IN THE MANAGEMENT OF MALE INFERTILITY

Over the last decade, there has been a tremendous increase in human sperm proteomics research to investigate the role of key proteins in the pathophysiology of male infertility.[27] Proteomic analysis of spermatozoa and seminal plasma provides invaluable information on the molecular pathways involved in sperm function and fertilizing potential.[28] In addition, sperm proteomics helps in understanding the mechanisms of posttranslational modifications and protein–protein interactions associated with normal gametogenesis.[27] It has been shown that the proteome of ejaculate sperm can impact the fertilization process.[29] The proteomic approach in sperm cells has been used in recent studies to explain the molecular mechanisms underlying male infertility in different clinical scenarios.[28,30–32]

Techniques of Sperm Proteomics

The techniques used for proteomic analysis include two-dimensional (2D) gel electrophoresis based on the isoelectric focusing property and molecular weight of peptides, a modified version known as difference gel electrophoresis that is used to identify differentially expressed proteins (DEPs) with a minimum error of less than 10%,[33] and 2D gel electrophoresis coupled with matrix-assisted laser

desorption/ionization time-of-flight.[34] An algorithm for assessment of sperm proteomics is shown in Fig. 28.1.

Spermatozoa are excellent target for proteomic research, as they can be easily purified and separated from seminal plasma. In addition, spermatozoa are transcriptionally and translationally quiescent and do not generate new proteins, thus reducing the complexity of sperm proteomic profiling.[35] Therefore more studies on sperm proteomics are expected in near future that can help the development of biomarker panels for the management of infertile males. However, identification of an ideal biomarker sperm protein for prognosis or diagnosis of a specific male infertility condition remains a major challenge.[27] In addition, the use of sperm proteomics in clinical setup for fertility management is still limited. This is mainly due to the involvement of very expensive and sophisticated instruments that require a great deal of training and skills.

Diagnostic and Prognostic Potentials of Sperm Proteomics in Male Infertility

An in-depth proteomic analysis of sperm may help identify the mechanisms underlying different abnormalities of male infertility. Recent clinical studies on the topic have paved the way for identifying DEPs related to various clinical scenarios associated with male infertility.[27] Altered protein expression has been associated with axoneme activation and cellular response to stress and nucleosome assembly.[36] In addition, asthenozoospermic samples revealed differential expression of some components of the proteasome complex, indicating a possible role of this complex in sperm motility abnormalities.[37] The DEPs found in asthenozoospermic samples have been correlated with sperm mitochondrial dysfunction and oxidative stress.[38] This latter finding led to the speculation that oxidative stress may play a role in impairment of mitochondrial energy metabolism resulting in mitochondrial dysfunction and reduction of sperm motility. In addition, mitochondrial structure proteins were under expressed in infertile patients with the diagnosis of varicocele.[32] Furthermore, varicocele patients demonstrated increased generation of reactive oxygen species and prooxidant-associated proteins, resulting in an altered seminal plasma proteomic profile.[28,39] Infertile males with globozoospermia were found to have significantly decreased expression of perinuclear theca proteins, which play a role in acrosome development.[40]

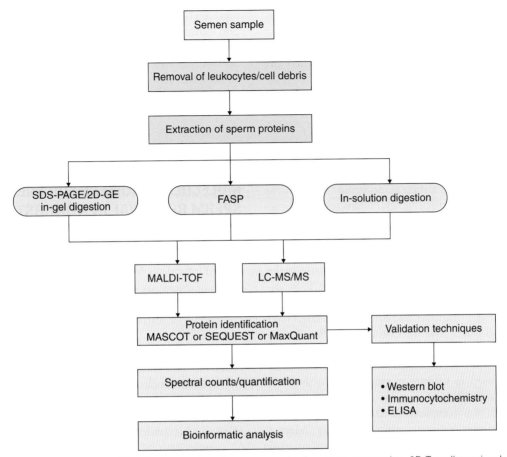

Fig. 28.1 Workflow involving the processing of semen samples for sperm proteomics. *2D*, Two-dimensional; *DEPs*, differentially expressed proteins; *ELISA*, enzyme-linked immunosorbent assay; *FASP*, filter-aided sample preparation; *LC*, liquid chromatography; *MALDI-TOF*, matrix-assisted laser desorption/ionization time-of-flight; *MS*, mass spectrometry; *PBS*, phosphate-buffered saline; *RIPA*, radioimmunoprecipitation assay; *SDS-PAGE*, sodium dodecyl sulfate–polyacrylamide gel electrophoresis. (From Agarwal A, Panner Selvam MK, Baskaran S. Proteomic analyses of human sperm cells: understanding the role of proteins and molecular pathways affecting male reproductive health. *Int J Mol Sci.* 2020;21(5):1621.)

In the context of ART, altered expression of the proteins involved in chromatin assembly have been found in spermatozoa from normozoospermic infertile males with in vitro fertilization (IVF) failure.[41] Similarly, an array of proteins involved in spermatogenesis, including NME5, TSSK2, MYCBP, MYCBPAP, NDRG3, ROPN1L, and SPATA24, were underexpressed in spermatozoa, leading to poor blastocyst formation and IVF failure.[42]

In conclusion, the sperm proteomics have a great potential not only to expand our understanding of sperm biology but also to enhance the clinical management of male infertility. The research focus should be directed towards identification of ideal set of proteins for clinical validation in specific male infertility conditions.

OPTIMIZING SPERM SELECTION TECHNIQUES FOR INTRACYTOPLASMIC SPERM INJECTION

Currently, ICSI is the standard treatment of males with severe oligozoospermia, OA, and NOA.[43] The direct injection of a sperm into an oocyte in ICSI allows the bypass of all natural selection barriers, thus increasing the risk of transferring paternal defects such as sperm DNA fragmentation (SDF) and genomic abnormalities to the offspring.[44] Conventional sperm processing methods, such as swim up and density gradient centrifugation, help select sperm based on their density and/or motility, characteristics that do not reflect their fertilizing potential. Hence these methods in ICSI may introduce a defective sperm into the oocyte, leading to undesirable reproductive outcomes. To overcome this limitation, other sperm-processing methods have been developed based on different selection mechanisms such as sperm apoptotic markers.[45] This includes magnetic-activated cell sorting (MACS), which uses annexin V beads to bind phosphatidylserine on the surface of apoptotic sperm and remove them, thereby lowering SDF.[46] In a recent retrospective study, infertile males with SDF greater than 20% who underwent ICSI following MACS had significantly higher clinical pregnancy and live birth rates and lower miscarriage rates compared to males who underwent ICSI after density gradient centrifugation alone.[47] Another technique is physiologic ICSI (P-ICSI), in which hyaluronic acid binding is used to capture mature sperm with lower SDF.[48] Outcomes of ICSI were not significantly different when P-ICSI was compared to MACS.[49] A third technique is intracytoplasmic morphologically selected sperm injection (IMSI), in which high-powered microscopy (magnification 6000–10,000×) is used to choose the highest quality sperm devoid of vacuoles in their heads that contain less SDF.[50] A metaanalysis indicates significantly higher implantation rates and pregnancy rates in IMSI as compared to conventional ICSI, while no difference was found in miscarriage rates.[51]

As for the use of testicular-derived sperm for ICSI in cases with persistently high SDF, a metaanalysis indicated significantly higher clinical pregnancy and live birth rates and lower miscarriage rates as compared to ICSI using ejaculate sperm.[52] However, the evidence for the use of testicular sperm for ICSI in males with high SDF is of poor quality.[53] Additionally, no SDF test is standardized for testicular sperm. The latest approach is to select sperm by their response to external cues in microfluidics.[54] Microfluidic sperm sorters allow the passage of sperm through microchannels using fluid dynamics to choose high quality sperm with least SDF.[55]

In conclusion, data are scarce regarding the benefit of the current sperm selection methods in improving reproductive outcomes in ICSI. An optimal sperm selection technique for ICSI should incorporate multiple tools that help identify sperm with high fertilization potential at molecular level and monitor their interactions to external environments that mimic the female reproductive tract in vitro such as microfluidic system.[44] New, well-designed studies are warranted to investigate the effect of various sperm selection methods for infertile males and to determine their impact on ART outcomes.

MOLECULAR MARKERS FOR PREDICTING SPERM RETRIEVAL IN NONOBSTRUCTIVE AZOOSPERMIA

NOA is a serious form of male infertility affecting nearly 10% of infertile male patients.[56] The sperm retrieval rate (SRR) of microsurgical testicular sperm extraction (micro-TESE) in NOA can reach 50% to 60%.[57] SRR is governed by a learning curve, which could significantly affect SRR.[58] Many believe microdissection can result in major parenchymal disruption, causing further deterioration of testicular function.[59] Hence the need for markers that can predict sperm recovery prior to testicular biopsy remains crucial to minimize the need for nonindicated surgeries. In a study investigating the use of *ESX1* as a marker for spermatogenesis in NOA patients, 62 samples (out of 65) demonstrated the presence of *ESX1* transcript in subjects proven to have spermatogenesis.[24] Another study analyzed the different gene expression in Y chromosome comparing the findings between patients with NOA and fertile counterparts and showed that 18 transcripts (out of 41) were downregulated in NOA, compared to normal counterparts. Moreover, it is believed that transcripts including *HSFY1-1*, *HSFY1-3*, *BPY2-1*, *KDM5C2*, *RBMX2*, and *DAZL1* showed significant expression differences among maturation arrest (MA) patients with and without successful sperm recovery, justifying their utility as markers in NOA management.[60] Round spermatid miRNA expression was compared between NOA patients and OA controls using RNA deep sequencing and demonstrated differential expression of 378 miRNAs between both groups.[26] Zinc-finger CCHC gene (*ZCCHC13*) had lower expression in patients with NOA compared to subjects with normal spermatogenesis, suggesting that *ZCCHC13* is a signaling molecular biomarker for spermatogenesis.[61] Recently, histone variant H3.5 was identified in human testicular tissue, being expressed in the spermatogonia and preleptotene/leptotene primary spermatocytes, and was found less expressed in NOA compared to OA testes.[62] Additionally, it was shown that 86 testicular miRNAs were absent in NOA patients with failed sperm retrieval compared to patients with successful sperm recovery.[63] Expression of the epigenetic regulator Jumonji domain-containing 1a (*JMJD1A*), which is involved in sperm maturation during spermatogenesis, was significantly higher in azoospermic patients with successful sperm retrieval (p < 0.001) compared to those with failed SRR.[64] Testicular stage-specific genes were assessed in the semen as a noninvasive approach to predict sperm retrieval outcome in 110 azoospermic males and found that *DAZ* and *PRM2* were significantly correlated with the presence of germ cells, including spermatogenoia, spermatids, and spermatozoa.[65] Agarwal et al. studied the seminal fluid for DEPs comparing between NOA patients with and without follicle-stimulating hormone (FSH) elevation and control group, and demonstrated 68 DEPs out of 448 proteins in the group with normal FSH and 15 DEPs out of 436 proteins in the group with elevated FSH, respectively.[66]

Future Modalities of Sperm Retrieval for Patients with Nonobstructive Azoospermia

The use of microsurgical magnification during micro-TESE enables for better assessment of the seminiferous tubules, with an associated 1.5 times increase in SRR compared to non micro-TESE and two times higher than testicular sperm aspiration.[67] Moreover, more options are warranted to improve SRR without an associated testicular parenchymal disruption. What follows will discuss a few of the most recent innovations that still await further studies to validate their efficacy and, most importantly, safety.

Multiphoton Microscopy

This optical technology includes the utilization of laser technology (80 femtosecond pulses at 780 nm) and low-energy photons, which induces autofluorescence after excitation of the intrinsic fluorophores in unstained tissues. Multiphoton microscopy (MPM) penetrative power can reach 400 μm, offering adequate assessment of the seminiferous tubules.[68] The principle used in MPM entails the state of autoexcitation in a molecule after absorbing two low-energy photons.[69] In a rodent study, MPM could differentiate between Sertoli cell–only tubules, which demonstrated autofluorescence in the wavelength ranges of 420 to 490 nm and 550 to 650 nm, and the sperm-harboring tubules, which had autofluorescence at the 420- to 490-nm range only.[68] An ex vivo study showed an 86% concordance rate between MPM and hematoxylin and eosin–stained samples.[70] Presently, the need to assess MPM's safety, including the thermal-induced DNA damage, remains crucial before its application in sperm retrieval.[69]

ORBEYE

Microsurgical visualization can be enhanced by the utilization of a high-resolution 4K 3D exoscope.[71] This technology has already been used in other microsurgical fields, including neurosurgery.[72] ORBEYE was compared to traditional microscopy in the vasectomy reversal setting and no difference was found regarding time and outcome.[73] However, a different study showed that using a 4K 3D video microscope offered more comfort to the operating surgeon compared to a conventional operating microscope.[71]

Raman Spectroscopy

Raman spectroscopy (RS) is another laser-based technology that converts biochemical data using tissue-based molecular fingerprints into a Raman spectrum and which can deliver ample cellular information without the need for a labeling process.[74] In a rat model, Osterberg et al. were able to identify spermatogenesis in the Sertoli cell–only tubules of an ex vivo rat model with a sensitivity of 96% and a specificity of 100% (receiver operating characteristic area under the curve = 0.98).[75]

Full-Field Optical Coherence Tomography

Unlike MPM and RS, full-field optical coherence tomography (FFOCT) has a higher safety profile while using traditional light (tungsten halogen) and not laser beams, and hence bypasses the hazardous impact of laser-induced thermal DNA damage. This technology offers high-resolution images and is capable of discerning between tubules harboring sperm from those that do not. In a rodent model study, sperm-containing tubules were identified using FFOCT and were shown to have a mean diameter of 328 μm compared to void tubules, which had a mean diameter of 178 μm. The limitations of FFOCT reside in its low depth of assessment and that it analyzes ex vivo samples.[76]

THE FUTURE OF STEM CELL THERAPY IN MALE INFERTILITY

Subgroups of infertile males with NOA due to genetic abnormalities or toxic exposure are unable to use ICSI and are referred to donor insemination, where permitted.[77] Advances in stem cell research indicate that stem cell therapies represent a future potential avenue for allowing these sterile patients to produce their own biological offspring.[78] Generally, embryonic stem cells (ESCs), induced pluripotent stem cells (iPSCs), spermatogonial stem cells (SSCs), and mesenchymal stem cells (MSCs) are the methods used to treat male infertility. Embryonic stem cell transplantation is limited by ethical concerns and immunologic problems, while iPSCs and MSCs have minimal to no ethical concerns, and their use in reproductive medicine become more popular.[79] Spermatogonial stem cells are specialized germ cells that undergo self-renewal and differentiation to produce sperm.[80] In addition, no morphological or genetic change was observed in the offspring resulting from SSC transplantation treatment.[81] In an in vitro study, SSC-derived cells were found to have differentiation potential similar to ESCs, with potential to differentiate into haploid male germ cells.[82] Further, transplantations of SSCs into the rhesus testes resulted in improvement of testicular function and restoration of spermatogenesis.[83] However, research on utility of SSCs for treatment of male infertility is limited due to their small number in the testis and difficulties in identification and evaluation of their biological activity.[84] Despite promising results of the in vitro and in vivo studies on stem cell therapy of male infertility, providing suitable conditions for stem cell isolation and differentiation remains a significant challenge before it can be applied in clinical practice.[78] In addition, the use of stem cell therapy to treat different types of male infertility requires further clinical research.

In conclusion, stem cell therapy holds promise for the treatment of severe cases of infertility wishing to have their own genetically related offspring. However, additional clinical trials are warranted to obtain evidence of the safety and efficacy of this modality of treatment in the field of reproductive medicine.

FERTILITY PRESERVATION IN CANCER PATIENTS

Cancer therapy can negatively impact male reproductive function through alteration in cellular cycle, which could alter the replication and transcription processes of the DNA, resulting in cell death. FP offers protection to future fertility to patients with cancer or chronic illnesses, by overcoming the detrimental effect of different gonadotoxic-related treatments.[85] Unfortunately, many are not aware of the availability of such services and suffer infertility following cancer treatment. Furthermore, 76% of individuals suffering from cancer express their desire to have children in the future.[86] In a study by Selter et al. on 3648 males in their reproductive age suffering from different types of cancer, only 7.8% had FP, which increased from 6.6% to 12.4% between 2008 and 2017.[87] Patient counseling and FP-related educational programs and quick referral remain crucial.[88] Factors limiting FP could be the pressing need of the patient to start his cancer-related therapy without any delay,[89] lack of awareness due to deficient counseling process,[90] and the associated financial burden.[88] A UK-based survey showed that 21% of the surveyed hematologists and oncologists (n = 499) were unaware of local sperm preservation policies.[91] The fertility impairment secondary to cancer therapy could range from temporary to persistent infertility, in addition to the associated ejaculatory and/or erectile dysfunction. Most chemotherapeutic agents are gonadotoxic, causing variable degrees of DNA aberrations, with high risk of developing serious seminal abnormalities.[85,92,93] Radiation therapy induces chromatid damage, as it occurs during the G2 cell cycle phase,[94] resulting in infertility secondary to azoospermia and irreversible testicular damage (above 3–4 Gy).[95] The efficacy of sperm cryopreservation has been examined and has proven to be an effective method of male FP.[95] Sperm could be cryopreserved either by slow freezing (conventional), which is commonly used in ART, or vitrification, which is a faster process entailing the plunging of the sperm sample into liquid nitrogen and is not associated with damage due to ice crystallization.[96] With regards to children and adolescent boys with cancers, FP can be challenging, and the need for parental guidance and consenting prior to FP is crucial.[97] For children prone for spermatogonial stem cell loss due to cancer-related therapies, testicular tissue cryopreservation for possible future use has emerged as an experimental modality. Peripubertal patients could be offered to deliver a semen sample by masturbation, and, if present, sperm could be cryopreserved. Since delivering a semen sample could be a challenging task for patients at such an age, testicular aspiration could be performed and retrieved sperm cryopreserved; yet if no sperm was found, then patients could undergo testicular sperm extraction and retrieve spermatogonial stem cells for cryopreservation.[98]

ROLE OF ARTIFICIAL INTELLIGENCE IN THE PRACTICE OF MALE INFERTILITY

AI involves a complex process of machine learning which entails the utilization of a dataset of information (input and output variables) to train the computer, offering it to deduct patterns that enable it to execute predictive computing based on this knowledge.[99] An AI study conducted to examine the relationship between lifestyle hazards and semen parameters succeeded in achieving 86% and 73% to 76% accuracy of prediction for sperm concentration and motility, respectively.[100] Another study tested an artificial neural network (ANN) prediction model on 177 patients with semen parameters as an input variable and demonstrated high predictive results obtained for seminal biochemical markers, including protein, fructose, glucosidase, and zinc.[101] ANN was used in assessing sperm morphology after training the model using 3500 sperm images, which resulted in an accuracy of 100% in assessing and discriminating between normal and abnormal sperm morphology on nine samples.[102] A validated ANN model was more predictive to the presence of sperm in NOA before testicular biopsy compared to standard logistic regression (SLR), with a predictive value of the outcomes of 80.8% (59/73) for ANN compared to 65.7% for SLR, with a higher sensitivity for ANN reaching 68% compared to 28% for SLR (p < 0.0001).[103]

SUMMARY

This chapter provides clinical perspectives on the current advances of male infertility research. The role of epigenetics and proteomics in the management of male infertility is highlighted. We also discussed molecular markers for predicting sperm retrieval in patients with NOA and future modalities of sperm retrieval for these patients. In addition, we summarized the methods of optimizing sperm selection techniques for ICSI. Furthermore, we discussed FP in cancer patients. Finally, we provided future insights on the role of AI and stem cell therapy in male infertility. This review helps better understanding of sperm biochemistry and physiology and provides information that aids in improving reproductive outcomes in infertility patients.

REFERENCES

1. Anderson JE, Farr SL, Jamieson DJ, Warner L, Macaluso M. Infertility services reported by men in the United States: national survey data. *Fertil Steril*. 2009;91(6):2466-2470. doi:10.1016/j.fertnstert.2008.03.022.
2. Agarwal A, Baskaran S, Parekh N, et al. Male infertility. *Lancet*. 2021;397(10271):319-333. doi:10.1016/S0140-6736(20)32667-2.
3. Tournaye H, Krausz C, Oates RD. Novel concepts in the aetiology of male reproductive impairment. *Lancet Diabetes Endocrinol*. 2017;5(7):544-553. doi:10.1016/S2213-8587(16)30040-7.
4. Esteves SC. Are specialized sperm function tests clinically useful in planning assisted reproductive technology? *Int Braz J Urol*. 2020;46(1):116-123. doi:10.1590/s1677-5538.ibju.2020.01.03.
5. Agarwal A, Majzoub A, Baskaran S, et al. Sperm DNA fragmentation: a new guideline for clinicians. *World J Mens Health*. 2020;38(4):412. doi:10.5534/wjmh.200128.
6. Ramasamy R, Lin K, Gosden LV, Rosenwaks Z, Palermo GD, Schlegel PN. High serum FSH levels in men with nonobstructive azoospermia does not affect success of microdissection testicular sperm extraction. *Fertil Steril*. 2009;92(2):590-593. doi:10.1016/j.fertnstert.2008.07.1703.
7. Sugimoto K, Koh E, Iijima M, Taya M, Maeda Y, Namiki M. Aberrant methylation of the TDMR of the GTF2A1L promoter does not affect fertilisation rates via TESE in patients with hypospermatogenesis. *Asian J Androl*. 2013;15(5):634-639. doi:10.1038/aja.2013.56.
8. Gunes S, Arslan MA, Hekim GNT, Asci R. The role of epigenetics in idiopathic male infertility. *J Assist Reprod Genet*. 2016;33(5):553-569. doi:10.1007/s10815-016-0682-8.
9. Li Z, Huang Y, Li H, et al. Excess of rare variants in genes that are key epigenetic regulators of spermatogenesis in the patients with non-obstructive azoospermia. *Sci Rep*. 2015;5:8785. doi:10.1038/srep08785.
10. Jin B, Li Y, Robertson KD. DNA methylation: superior or subordinate in the epigenetic hierarchy? *Genes Cancer*. 2011;2(6):607-617. doi:10.1177/1947601910393957.
11. Khazamipour N, Noruzinia M, Fatehmanesh P, Keyhanee M, Pujol P. MTHFR promoter hypermethylation in testicular biopsies of patients with non-obstructive azoospermia: the role of epigenetics in male infertility. *Hum Reprod*. 2009;24(9):2361-2364. doi:10.1093/humrep/dep194.
12. Rezaeian A, Karimian M, Hossienzadeh Colagar A. Methylation status of MTHFR promoter and oligozoospermia risk: an epigenetic study and in silico analysis. *Cell J*. 2021;22(4):482-490. doi:10.22074/cellj.2021.6498.
13. Watt F, Molloy PL. Cytosine methylation prevents binding to DNA of a HeLa cell transcription factor required for optimal expression of the adenovirus major late promoter. *Genes Dev*. 1988;2(9):1136-1143. doi:10.1101/gad.2.9.1136.

14. Ferfouri F, Boitrelle F, Ghout I, et al. A genome-wide DNA methylation study in azoospermia. *Andrology.* 2013;1(6):815-821. doi:10.1111/j.2047-2927.2013.00117.x.

15. Gujral P, Mahajan V, Lissaman AC, Ponnampalam AP. Histone acetylation and the role of histone deacetylases in normal cyclic endometrium. *Reprod Biol Endocrinol.* 2020;18(1):84. doi:10.1186/s12958-020-00637-5.

16. Lahn BT, Tang ZL, Zhou J, et al. Previously uncharacterized histone acetyltransferases implicated in mammalian spermatogenesis. *Proc Natl Acad Sci.* 2002;99(13):8707-8712. doi:10.1073/pnas.082248899.

17. Faure AK. Misregulation of histone acetylation in Sertoli cell-only syndrome and testicular cancer. *Mol Hum Reprod.* 2003;9(12):757-763. doi:10.1093/molehr/gag101.

18. Sonnack V, Failing K, Bergmann M, Steger K. Expression of hyperacetylated histone H4 during normal and impaired human spermatogenesis. *Andrologia.* 2002;34(6):384-390. doi:10.1046/j.1439-0272.2002.00524.x.

19. Treviño LS, Wang Q, Walker CL. Phosphorylation of epigenetic "readers, writers and erasers": Implications for developmental reprogramming and the epigenetic basis for health and disease. *Prog Biophys Mol Biol.* 2015;118(1-2):8-13. doi:10.1016/j.pbiomolbio.2015.02.013.

20. Dada R, Kumar M, Jesudasan R, Fernández JL, Gosálvez J, Agarwal A. Epigenetics and its role in male infertility. *J Assist Reprod Genet.* 2012;29(3):213-223. doi:10.1007/s10815-012-9715-0.

21. Shamsi M, Kumar K, Dada R. Genetic and epigenetic factors: role in male infertility. *Indian J Urol.* 2011;27(1):110. doi:10.4103/0970-1591.78436.

22. Thompson WE, Ramalho-Santos J, Sutovsky P. Ubiquitination of prohibitin in mammalian sperm mitochondria: possible roles in the regulation of mitochondrial inheritance and sperm quality control. *Biol Reprod.* 2003;69(1):254-260. doi:10.1095/biolreprod.102.010975.

23. Sheng K, Liang X, Huang S, Xu W. The role of histone ubiquitination during spermatogenesis. *Biomed Res Int.* 2014;2014:870695. doi:10.1155/2014/870695.

24. Bonaparte E, Moretti M, Colpi GM, et al. ESX1 gene expression as a robust marker of residual spermatogenesis in azoospermic men. *Hum Reprod.* 2010;25(6):1398-1403. doi:10.1093/humrep/deq074.

25. Wosnitzer MS. Genetic evaluation of male infertility. *Transl Androl Urol.* 2014;3(1):17-26. doi:10.3978/j.issn.2223-4683.2014.02.04.

26. Yao C, Yuan Q, Niu M, et al. Distinct expression profiles and novel targets of MicroRNAs in human spermatogonia, pachytene spermatocytes, and round spermatids between OA patients and NOA patients. *Mol Ther Nucleic Acids.* 2017;9:182-194. doi:10.1016/j.omtn.2017.09.007.

27. Agarwal A, Panner Selvam MK, Baskaran S. Proteomic analyses of human sperm cells: understanding the role of proteins and molecular pathways affecting male reproductive health. *Int J Mol Sci.* 2020;21(5):1621. doi:10.3390/ijms21051621.

28. Panner Selvam M, Agarwal A, Baskaran S. Proteomic analysis of seminal plasma from bilateral varicocele patients indicates an oxidative state and increased inflammatory response. *Asian J Androl.* 2019;21(6):544. doi:10.4103/aja.aja_121_18.

29. Agarwal A, Bertolla RP, Samanta L. Sperm proteomics: potential impact on male infertility treatment. *Expert Rev Proteomics.* 2016;13(3):285-296. doi:10.1586/14789450.2016.1151357.

30. Panner Selvam MK, Agarwal A, Pushparaj PN. A quantitative global proteomics approach to understanding the functional pathways dysregulated in the spermatozoa of asthenozoospermic testicular cancer patients. *Andrology.* 2019;7(4):454-462. doi:10.1111/andr.12620.

31. Panner Selvam MK, Agarwal A, Pushparaj PN. Altered molecular pathways in the proteome of cryopreserved sperm in testicular cancer patients before treatment. *Int J Mol Sci.* 2019;20(3):677. doi:10.3390/ijms20030677.

32. Samanta L, Agarwal A, Swain N, et al. Proteomic signatures of sperm mitochondria in varicocele: clinical use as biomarkers of varicocele associated infertility. *J Urol.* 2018;200(2):414-422. doi:10.1016/j.juro.2018.03.009.

33. Gupta S, Ghulmiyyah J, Sharma R, Halabi J, Agarwal A. Power of proteomics in linking oxidative stress and female infertility. *Biomed Res Int.* 2014;2014:1-26. doi:10.1155/2014/916212.

34. Martínez-Heredia J, Estanyol JM, Ballescà JL, Oliva R. Proteomic identification of human sperm proteins. *Proteomics.* 2006;6(15):4356-4369. doi:10.1002/pmic.200600094.

35. Jodar M, Selvaraju S, Sendler E, Diamond MP, Krawetz SA. The presence, role and clinical use of spermatozoal RNAs. *Hum Reprod Update.* 2013;19(6):604-624. doi:10.1093/humupd/dmt031.

36. Saraswat M, Joenväärä S, Jain T, et al. Human spermatozoa quantitative proteomic signature classifies normo- and asthenozoospermia. *Mol Cell Proteomics.* 2017;16(1):57-72. doi:10.1074/mcp.M116.061028.

37. Martinez-Heredia J, de Mateo S, Vidal-Taboada JM, Ballesca JL, Oliva R. Identification of proteomic differences in asthenozoospermic sperm samples. *Hum Reprod.* 2008;23(4):783-791. doi:10.1093/humrep/den024.

38. Nowicka-Bauer K, Lepczynski A, Ozgo M, et al. Sperm mitochondrial dysfunction and oxidative stress as possible reasons for isolated asthenozoospermia. *J Physiol Pharmacol.* 2018;69(3):403-417. doi:10.26402/jpp.2018.3.05.

39. Panner Selvam MK, Samanta L, Agarwal A. Functional analysis of differentially expressed acetylated spermatozoal proteins in infertile men with unilateral and bilateral varicocele. *Int J Mol Sci.* 2020;21(9):3155. doi:10.3390/ijms21093155.

40. Alvarez Sedo C, Rawe VY, Chemes HE. Acrosomal biogenesis in human globozoospermia: immunocytochemical, ultrastructural and proteomic studies. *Hum Reprod.* 2012;27(7):1912-1921. doi:10.1093/humrep/des126.

41. Azpiazu R, Amaral A, Castillo J, et al. High-throughput sperm differential proteomics suggests that epigenetic alterations contribute to failed assisted reproduction. *Hum Reprod.* 2014;29(6):1225-1237. doi:10.1093/humrep/deu073.

42. McReynolds S, Dzieciatkowska M, Stevens J, Hansen KC, Schoolcraft WB, Katz-Jaffe MG. Toward the identification of a subset of unexplained infertility: a sperm proteomic approach. *Fertil Steril.* 2014;102(3):692-699. doi:10.1016/j.fertnstert.2014.05.021.

43. Mazzilli R, Vaiarelli A, Dovere L, et al. Severe male factor in in vitro fertilization: definition, prevalence, and treatment. An update. *Asian J Androl.* 2022;24(2):125. doi:10.4103/aja.aja_53_21.

44. Leung ETY, Lee CL, Tian X, et al. Simulating nature in sperm selection for assisted reproduction. *Nat Rev Urol.* 2022;19(1):16-36. doi:10.1038/s41585-021-00530-9.

45. Grunewald S, Paasch U. Sperm selection for ICSI using annexin V. *Methods Mol Biol.* 2013;927:257-262. doi:10.1007/978-1-62703-038-0_23.

46. Troya J, Zorrilla I. Annexin V-MACS in infertile couples as method for separation of sperm without DNA fragmentation. *JBRA Assist Reprod.* 2015;19(2):66-69. doi:10.5935/1518-0557.20150015.

47. Pacheco A, Blanco A, Bronet F, Cruz M, García-Fernández J, García-Velasco JA. Magnetic-activated cell sorting (MACS): a useful sperm-selection technique in cases of high levels of sperm DNA fragmentation. *J Clin Med.* 2020;9(12):3976. doi:10.3390/jcm9123976.

48. Parmegiani L, Cognigni GE, Bernardi S, Troilo E, Ciampaglia W, Filicori M. "Physiologic ICSI": hyaluronic acid (HA) favors selection of spermatozoa without DNA fragmentation and with normal nucleus, resulting in improvement of embryo quality. *Fertil Steril.* 2010;93(2):598-604. doi:10.1016/j.fertnstert.2009.03.033.

49. Hasanen E, Elqusi K, ElTanbouly S, et al. PICSI vs. MACS for abnormal sperm DNA fragmentation ICSI cases: a prospective randomized trial. *J Assist Reprod Genet.* 2020;37(10):2605-2613. doi:10.1007/s10815-020-01913-4.

50. Hammoud I, Boitrelle F, Ferfouri F, et al. Selection of normal spermatozoa with a vacuole-free head (x6300) improves selection of spermatozoa with intact DNA in patients with high sperm DNA fragmentation rates. *Andrologia.* 2013;45(3):163-170. doi:10.1111/j.1439-0272.2012.01328.x.

51. Setti AS, Braga DPAF, Figueira RCS, Iaconelli A, Borges E. Intracytoplasmic morphologically selected sperm injection results in improved clinical outcomes in couples with previous ICSI failures or male factor infertility: a meta-analysis. *European Journal of Obstetrics & Gynecology and Reproductive Biology.* 2014;183:96-103. doi:10.1016/j.ejogrb.2014.10.008.

52. Esteves SC, Roque M, Bradley CK, Garrido N. Reproductive outcomes of testicular versus ejaculated sperm for intracytoplasmic sperm injection among men with high levels of DNA fragmentation in semen: systematic review and meta-analysis. *Fertil Steril.* 2017;108(3):456-467.e1. doi:10.1016/j.fertnstert.2017.06.018.

53. Ambar RF, Agarwal A, Majzoub A, et al. The use of testicular sperm for intracytoplasmic sperm injection in patients with high sperm DNA damage: a systematic review. *World J Mens Health.* 2021;39(3):391. doi:10.5534/wjmh.200084.

54. Albertini DF, Crosignani P, Dumoulin J, et al. IVF, from the past to the future: the inheritance of the Capri Workshop Group. *Hum Reprod Open.* 2020;2020(3):hoaa040. doi:10.1093/hropen/hoaa040.

55. Shirota K, Yotsumoto F, Itoh H, et al. Separation efficiency of a microfluidic sperm sorter to minimize sperm DNA damage. *Fertil Steril.* 2016;105(2):315-321.e1. doi:10.1016/j.fertnstert.2015.10.023.

56. Kumar R. Medical management of non-obstructive azoospermia. *Clinics (Sao Paulo).* 2013;68(suppl 1):75-79. doi:10.6061/clinics/2013(sup01)08.

57. Schlegel PN, Sigman M, Collura B, et al. Diagnosis and treatment of infertility in men: AUA/ASRM guideline part I. *Fertil Steril.* 2021;115(1):54-61. doi:10.1016/j.fertnstert.2020.11.015.

58. Dabaja AA, Schlegel PN. Microdissection testicular sperm extraction: an update. *Asian J Androl.* 2013;15(1):35-39. doi:10.1038/aja.2012.141.

59. Ramasamy R, Yagan N, Schlegel PN. Structural and functional changes to the testis after conventional versus microdissection testicular sperm extraction. *Urology.* 2005;65(6):1190-1194. doi:10.1016/j.urology.2004.12.059.

60. Ahmadi Rastegar D, Sharifi Tabar M, Alikhani M, et al. Isoform-level gene expression profiles of human Y chromosome azoospermia factor genes and their X chromosome paralogs in the testicular tissue of non-obstructive azoospermia patients. *J Proteome Res.* 2015;14(9):3595-3605. doi:10.1021/acs.jproteome.5b00520.

61. Li Z, Chen S, Yang Y, Zhuang X, Tzeng CM. Novel biomarker ZCCHC13 revealed by integrating DNA methylation and mRNA expression data in non-obstructive

azoospermia. *Cell Death Discov.* 2018;4(1):36. doi:10. 1038/s41420-018-0033-x.

62. Shiraishi K, Shindo A, Harada A, et al. Roles of histone H3.5 in human spermatogenesis and spermatogenic disorders. *Andrology.* 2018;6(1):158-165. doi:10.1111/andr. 12438.

63. Fang N, Cao C, Wen Y, Wang X, Yuan S, Huang X. MicroRNA profile comparison of testicular tissues derived from successful and unsuccessful microdissection testicular sperm extraction retrieval in non-obstructive azoospermia patients. *Reprod Fertil Dev.* 2019;31(4):671. doi:10.1071/RD17423.

64. Eelaminejad Z, Favaedi R, Modarresi T, Sabbaghian M, Sadighi Gilani MA, Shahhoseini M. Association between JMJD1A expression and sperm retrieval in non-obstructive azoospermic patients. *Cell J.* 2018;19(4):660-665. doi:10.22074/cellj.2018.4409.

65. Aslani F, Modarresi MH, Soltanghoraee H, et al. Seminal molecular markers as a non-invasive diagnostic tool for the evaluation of spermatogenesis in non-obstructive azoospermia. *Syst Biol Reprod Med.* 2011;57(4):190-196. doi:10.3109/19396368.2011.569906.

66. Agarwal A, Sharma R, Cui Z, Sabanegh ES. Identification of Sertoli cell markers in men with non-obstructive azoospermia. *Fertil Steril.* 2015;104(3):e289. doi:10.1016/j. fertnstert.2015.07.905.

67. Bernie AM, Mata DA, Ramasamy R, Schlegel PN. Comparison of microdissection testicular sperm extraction, conventional testicular sperm extraction, and testicular sperm aspiration for nonobstructive azoospermia: a systematic review and meta-analysis. *Fertil Steril.* 2015;104(5):1099-1103.e3. doi:10.1016/j.fertnstert.2015.07.1136.

68. Ramasamy R, Sterling J, Fisher ES, et al. Identification of spermatogenesis with multiphoton microscopy: an evaluation in a rodent model. *J Urol.* 2011;186(6):2487-2492. doi:10.1016/j.juro.2011.07.081.

69. Katz MJ, Huland DM, Ramasamy R. Multiphoton microscopy: applications in urology and andrology. *Transl Androl Urol.* 2014;3(1):77-83. doi:10.3978/j.issn.2223-4683.2014.01.01.

70. Najari BB, Ramasamy R, Sterling J, et al. Pilot study of the correlation of multiphoton tomography of ex vivo human testis with histology. *J Urol.* 2012;188(2):538-543. doi:10.1016/j.juro.2012.03.124.

71. Best JC, Gonzalez D, Alawamlh OAH, Li PS, Ramasamy R. Use of 4K3D video microscope in male infertility microsurgery. *Urol Video J.* 2020;7:100046. doi:10.1016/j. urolvj.2020.100046.

72. Takahashi S, Toda M, Nishimoto M, et al. Pros and cons of using ORBEYE™ for microneurosurgery. *Clin Neurol Neurosurg.* 2018;174:57-62. doi:10.1016/j.clineuro.2018. 09.010.

73. Hayden RP, Chen H, Goldstein M, Li PSS. A randomized controlled animal trial: efficacy of a 4K3D video microscope versus an optical operating microscope for urologic microsurgery. *Fertil Steril.* 2019;112(3):e93. doi:10. 1016/j.fertnstert.2019.07.364.

74. Huang WE, Li M, Jarvis RM, Goodacre R, Banwart SA. Shining light on the microbial world: the application of Raman microspectroscopy. *Adv Appl Microbiol.* 2010;70:153-186. doi:10.1016/S0065-2164(10)70005-8.

75. Osterberg EC, Laudano MA, Ramasamy R, et al. Identification of spermatogenesis in a rat sertoli-cell only model using Raman spectroscopy: a feasibility study. *J Urol.* 2014;192(2):607-612. doi:10.1016/j.juro.2014.01.106.

76. Ramasamy R, Sterling J, Manzoor M, et al. Full field optical coherence tomography can identify spermatogenesis in a rodent sertoli-cell only model. *J Pathol Inform.* 2012;3:4. doi:10.4103/2153-3539.93401.

77. Easley CA, Simerly CR, Schatten G. Stem cell therapeutic possibilities: future therapeutic options for male-factor and female-factor infertility? *Reprod Biomed Online.* 2013;27(1):75-80. doi:10.1016/j.rbmo.2013.03.003.

78. Hajiesmailpoor A, Emami P, Kondori BJ, Ghorbani M. Stem cell therapy as a recent advanced approach in male infertility. *Tissue Cell.* 2021;73:101634. doi:10.1016/j. tice.2021.101634.

79. Saha S, Roy P, Corbitt C, Kakar SS. Application of stem cell therapy for infertility. *Cells.* 2021;10(7):1613. doi:10.3390/cells10071613.

80. Sharma S, Wistuba J, Pock T, Schlatt S, Neuhaus N. Spermatogonial stem cells: updates from specification to clinical relevance. *Hum Reprod Update.* 2019;25(3):275-297. doi:10.1093/humupd/dmz006.

81. Wu X, Goodyear SM, Abramowitz LK, et al. Fertile offspring derived from mouse spermatogonial stem cells cryopreserved for more than 14 years. *Hum Reprod.* 2012;27(5):1249-1259. doi:10.1093/humrep/des077.

82. Nolte J, Michelmann HW, Wolf M, et al. PSCDGs of mouse multipotent adult germline stem cells can enter and progress through meiosis to form haploid male germ cells in vitro. *Differentiation.* 2010;80(4-5):184-194. doi:10.1016/j.diff.2010.08.001.

83. Hermann BP, Sukhwani M, Winkler F, et al. Spermatogonial stem cell transplantation into rhesus testes regenerates spermatogenesis producing functional sperm. *Cell Stem Cell.* 2012;11(5):715-726. doi:10.1016/j.stem. 2012.07.017.

84. McLean DJ. Spermatogonial stem cell transplantation and testicular function. *Cell Tissue Res.* 2005;322(1): 21-31. doi:10.1007/s00441-005-0009-z.

85. Jensen JR, Morbeck DE, Coddington CC. Fertility preservation. *Mayo Clin Proc.* 2011;86(1):45-49. doi:10.4065/ mcp.2010.0564.

86. Schover LR, Rybicki LA, Martin BA, Bringelsen KA. Having children after cancer. A pilot survey of survivors' attitudes and experiences. *Cancer*. 1999;86(4):697-709. doi:10.1002/(sici)1097-0142(19990815)86:4<697::aid-cncr20>3.0.co;2-j.

87. Selter J, Huang Y, Williams SZ, et al. Use of fertility preservation services in male reproductive-aged cancer patients. *Gynecol Oncol Rep*. 2021;36:100716. doi:10.1016/j.gore.2021.100716.

88. Dorfman CS, Stalls JM, Mills C, et al. Addressing barriers to fertility preservation for cancer patients: the role of oncofertility patient navigation. *J Oncol Navig Surviv*. 2021;12(10):332-348.

89. Peddie VL, Porter MA, Barbour R, et al. Factors affecting decision making about fertility preservation after cancer diagnosis: a qualitative study. *BJOG*. 2012;119(9):1049-1057. doi:10.1111/j.1471-0528.2012.03368.x.

90. Hohmann C, Borgmann-Staudt A, Rendtorff R, et al. Patient counselling on the risk of infertility and its impact on childhood cancer survivors: results from a national survey. *J Psychosoc Oncol*. 2011;29(3):274-285. doi:10.1080/07347332.2011.563344.

91. Gilbert E, Adams A, Mehanna H, Harrison B, Hartshorne GM. Who should be offered sperm banking for fertility preservation? A survey of UK oncologists and haematologists. *Ann Oncol*. 2011;22(5):1209-1214. doi:10.1093/annonc/mdq579.

92. Sapkota Y, Wilson CL, Zaidi AK, et al. A novel locus predicts spermatogenic recovery among childhood cancer survivors exposed to alkylating agents. *Cancer Res*. 2020;80(17):3755-3764. doi:10.1158/0008-5472.CAN-20-0093.

93. Morris ID. Sperm DNA damage and cancer treatment1. *Int J Androl*. 2002;25(5):255-261. doi:10.1046/j.1365-2605.2002.00372.x.

94. Terzoudi GI, Jung T, Hain J, et al. Increased G2 chromosomal radiosensitivity in cancer patients: the role of cdk1/cyclin-B activity level in the mechanisms involved. *Int J Radiat Biol*. 2000;76(5):607-615. doi:10.1080/095530000138268.

95. Sharma V. Sperm storage for cancer patients in the UK: a review of current practice. *Hum Reprod*. 2011;26(11):2935-2943. doi:10.1093/humrep/der281.

96. Tao Y, Sanger E, Saewu A, Leveille MC. Human sperm vitrification: the state of the art. *Reprod Biol Endocrinol*. 2020;18(1):17. doi:10.1186/s12958-020-00580-5.

97. Wyns C, Collienne C, Shenfield F, et al. Fertility preservation in the male pediatric population: factors influencing the decision of parents and children. *Hum Reprod*. 2015;30(9):2022-2030. doi:10.1093/humrep/dev161.

98. Goossens E, Jahnukainen K, Mitchell RT, et al. Fertility preservation in boys: recent developments and new insights. *Hum Reprod Open*. 2020;2020(3):hoaa016. doi:10.1093/hropen/hoaa016.

99. Chu KY, Nassau DE, Arora H, Lokeshwar SD, Madhusoodanan V, Ramasamy R. Artificial intelligence in reproductive urology. *Curr Urol Rep*. 2019;20(9):52. doi:10.1007/s11934-019-0914-4.

100. Gil D, Girela JL, de Juan J, Gomez-Torres MJ, Johnsson M. Predicting seminal quality with artificial intelligence methods. *Expert Syst Appl*. 2012;39(16):12564-12573. doi:10.1016/j.eswa.2012.05.028.

101. Vickram AS, Kamini AR, Das R, et al. Validation of artificial neural network models for predicting biochemical markers associated with male infertility. *Syst Biol Reprod Med*. 2016;62(4):258-265. doi:10.1080/19396368.2016.1185654.

102. Thirumalaraju P, Bormann CL, Kanakasabapathy M, et al. Automated sperm morphology testing using artificial intelligence. *Fertil Steril*. 2018;110(4):e432. doi:10.1016/j.fertnstert.2018.08.039.

103. Samli MM, Dogan I. An artificial neural network for predicting the presence of spermatozoa in the testes of men with nonobstructive azoospermia. *J Urol*. 2004;171(6 Pt 1):2354-2357. doi:10.1097/01.ju.0000125272.03182.c3.

29

Research Perspectives in the Postintracytoplasmic Sperm Injection Era

Mausumi Das, Suks Minhas, and Ralf Reinhold Henkel

INTRODUCTION

While more than 267,987 articles (as of August 18, 2023) have been published on spermatozoa since their discovery by Antonie van Leeuwenhoek in the year 1677, only 38,082 articles on "male infertility" could be found on Scopus, the first being published in 1941.[1] Since that time, a constant increase in the annual number of articles published on male infertility can be noticed, with some landmark papers highlighting the important contribution of the male germ cells to the fertilization process and reproductive medicine as a whole.[2-5] Nevertheless, across social and medical sciences, the importance of the male contribution to a successful reproductive outcome has long been underrecognized and reflects the fact that research into reproduction is mainly focused on females.[6] The reasons for this are manifold and may include knowledge gaps in males about reproduction,[7] the perception that reproduction is a "female issue,"[8] or male attitude and ignorance. This often leads to the fact that females are taking the blame for the childlessness and even protect their infertile husbands.[9]

Intracytoplasmic sperm injection (ICSI) seemed to be a solution not only to this problem but also to declining semen quality[10,11] and is therefore often employed as the method of choice. However, a number of studies reported possible associations of ICSI with an increased risk for chromosomal abnormalities, autism, intellectual disabilities, and congenital defects compared with conventional in vitro fertilization (IVF).[12-15] On the other hand, these increased risks may also be due to the effects of poor semen quality and subfertility. Consequently, the use of ICSI has constantly increased over the years. In the United States, the use of ICSI increased from 36.4% in 1996 to 76.2% in 2012.[16] In 2016, the US Centers for Disease Control and Prevention reported the use of ICSI in male factor patients between 87% and 94% and for nonmale factor patients between 68% and 72%,[17] and a critical review of the available literature concluded that ICSI is overwhelmingly overused.[18] This could possibly be explained by fears of higher failure rates in standard IVF. In addition, males's perception that reproduction is a female issue and therefore do not see or only see a specialist after failed assisted reproductive technology (ART) leads to the fact that males are often not properly diagnosed. On the other hand, a recent population-based cohort study analyzing the results from 14,693 couples concluded that ICSI is not superior to IVF with regard to cumulative live birth rate in nonmale factor patients.[19]

Despite these challenges, progress has been made not only in development of advanced techniques to manage couples infertility and the understanding of the male contribution to the fertilization process and the success of assisted reproduction but also in the diagnostic and therapeutic techniques for male infertility. Nevertheless, more work has to be done, scientifically, medically, educationally, socially, and politically, in order to manage infertility and thereby reduce the costs for the infertility treatment by increasing the success rates of the treatment through utilization of less invasive techniques. Moreover, an understanding has to be adopted that the 2 rather than his sperm has to be treated so that less invasive techniques can be employed. Ideally, heterosexual couple infertility treatment will result in the couple achieving their goal to conceive naturally. Hence there must be an understanding that reproduction is the unification of male and female gametes and that therefore

BOTH partners play an EQUAL role and should carry an EQUAL responsibility and burden for the creation of their offspring. Eventually, "Men's health is family health."[20] In this chapter, new methods to achieve this goal will be discussed.

NEW DEVELOPMENTS IN ANDROUROLOGICAL DIAGNOSTICS

Artificial Intelligence in Semen Analysis

Standard semen analysis performed according to the guidelines provided by the World Health Organization (WHO)[21] is, despite standardization efforts of the WHO, although not predicting male fertility potential, still regarded as the cornerstone of male fertility evaluation.[22,23] However, sperm concentration and motility are not only biologically highly variable parameters, but the very nature of the standard semen analysis being performed manually is a major cause of limitations and concern because the procedure is prone to evaluator subjectivity, as well as intra- and interoperator and interlaboratory variability, and can therefore have a significantly impact on clinical decision making.[24,25] Therefore it is recommended to perform two consecutive semen analyses,[21,26] a procedure that increases costs, trouble, and inconvenience for the patients.

In efforts to overcome the problems and variability of the manual analysis, various computer-aided sperm analysis systems (e.g., Sperm Class Analyzer, SCA, Microptics SL, Barcelona, Spain; SQA-V GOLD, Medical Electronic Systems, Los Angeles, USA; IVOS, Hamilton-Thorne, Beverly, USA) with different optical systems and sperm recognition/tracking algorithms were developed since the 1980s.[27] Since such systems have the capability to minimize errors and also to reduce the time of the analysis,[28] results will be more accurate and a larger number of patients can be evaluated.

Crucial for an automated approach is that the system accurately recognizes and differentiates sperm from other cells or debris, quantifies motility, and recognizes the quality of motility, a task that includes sperm motion parameters such as motility, progressive motility, and sperm kinematics (e.g., velocity average path, velocity straight line, beat cross frequency, hyperactivation, etc.). In addition, because of its association with sperm functionality, normal sperm morphology also needs to be evaluated. However, evaluation of normal sperm morphology is the most difficult because of the three dimensionality of the male germ cell. The fact that

sperm are moving in a three-dimensional manner makes the evaluation even more complicated. Therefore early automated systems used fixed and stained semen smears. However, the aim should be to obtain information about sperm concentration, motility, and normal morphology in one evaluation. Therefore recent studies used artificial intelligence (AI), machine learning, or deep learning neural network approaches.

Agarwal and coworkers[29,30] evaluated the LensHooke X1 PRO, a novel AI-based semen analyzer, against manual semen analysis by a trained lab technologist, and reported a concordance correlation coefficients of r > 0.96 for sperm concentration, r = 0.94 for total motility, and r > 0.86 for progressive motility. A recent analysis in the United Kingdom basically confirmed this positive association, but at a significantly lower level.[31] A comparison of the LensHooke X1 PRO with the Hamilton-Thorne IVOS showed similarly high associations.[30] A comparison of normal sperm morphology showed that the X1 PRO provided significantly lower results than the manual evaluation.[30] Although great progress in the development of AI and machine-learning algorithms was made in recent years, these results indicate that there is still a long way to go for the routine application of automated semen analysis systems in clinical practice.

Alameri et al.[32] optimized sperm motility tracking using a modified Gaussian Mixture Model for video analyses of semen samples and succeeded in 92.3%, 96.3%, and 72.4% accuracy, sensitivity, and specificity, respectively, for the improved method as compared to the standard method. For sperm morphology, Riordon et al.[33] used VGG16, a deep convolutional neural network (CNN), initially trained on ImageNet, to classify human sperm and obtained 94.0%, 94.1%, and 94.7% accuracy, true positive rate, and positive predictive value, respectively, in an accurate and reliable manner with improved throughput rate. However, it needs to be understood that these morphology results were obtained from fixed and semen smears.

Home Test Kits

While the aforementioned methods are laboratory based, more recent approaches for a more patient-friendly semen analysis are home test kits. These testing systems are based on different technologies such as immunological reactions and microfluidics.[34] Recent developments are smartphone based such as the

Bemaner test (Createcare, Shenzhen, China), the Ex-Seed (ExSeed Health, Copenhagen, Denmark), the YO Home Sperm Test (Medical Electronics Systems, Los Angeles, USA), or the SEEM kit (Recruit Lifestyle Co, Tokyo, Japan). At the moment, depending on the type of system the patient is using, the home test systems are rather limited in the kind of parameters analyzed and their accuracy. Ideally, such home test kits would analyze sperm concentration; motility, including various kinematic parameters; and normal sperm morphology. Further refinement by using machine learning and AI approaches will make these systems more accurate with lower variability. For other sperm functional parameters such as sperm DNA fragmentation, however, sperm would have to be processed in order to obtain relevant results. However, this is only possible in a specialized laboratory.

On the other hand, these systems have tremendous advantages as the patient does not have to come to a laboratory, with its often uncomfortable environment. The sample can be produced in the privacy of the home. Furthermore, the software for smartphone-based home test kits can not only be updated and improved automatically, but the data of the semen samples that are obtained can be fed into machine-learning AI systems of the developer and can then be used to refine the system.

Measurement of Seminal Redox Stress

Oxidative stress is caused by an excessive amount of reactive oxygen species (ROS) and involved in the pathogenesis of many diseases, including male infertility, for which it has been found to be a major cause.[35,36] ROS in varying amounts are produced by any aerobic living cell, including sperm.[2,37] Leukocytes are producing about 1000 times more ROS than sperm.[38] Due to the extraordinarily high amount of polyunsaturated fatty acids in sperm plasma membranes,[39] which are essential for normal sperm function, however, male germ cells are prone to oxidative damage,[40] including damage to the DNA.[41] On the other hand, a small amount of ROS is essential for normal cell functions, including sperm capacitation and acrosome reaction.[42,43] Therefore too little amounts of ROS, a condition caused by excessive amounts of antioxidants, are also detrimental to fertility.[44,45] Therefore it is crucial that the bodily redox balance is properly maintained.[46] These conditions are either called oxidative or reductive stress,[47,48] with

reductive stress and oxidative stress being equally harmful to cells and organisms.[49]

The usual methods to determine the redox state of sperm or semen are luminescence with luminol,[50] colorimetry to determine the total antioxidant capacity,[51] the nitroblue tetrazolium assay,[52] determination of the ROS-TAC score,[53] determination of lipid peroxidation,[54] or the measurement of malondialdehyde as end product of lipid peroxidation.[55] The most recent development is the introduction of the MiOXSYS system, a galvanometric technique that measures the transfer of electron from electron donors (antioxidants) to electron acceptors (oxidants) as so-called oxidation-reduction potential (ORP).[56] In contrast to the other methods, this system can determine oxidative and reductive stress and uses much less semen that the other methods.

While initial studies to validate this method differentiated between donors and patients attending to an andrology unit and obtained cut-off values between 1.42 mV/10^6 sperm/mL and 1.34 mV/10^6 sperm/mL,[57,58] a study determined a cut-off value of 0.51 mV/10^6 sperm/mL[59] in 144 patients attending an ICSI program. The reason for this lower cut-off value might be that these authors used blastocyst development, ongoing pregnancy, and live birth as reproductive endpoint parameters for the calculation. The use of ICSI might have also contributed to the fact that the predictive power of the ORP testing for fertilization was low. On the other hand, since sperm were selected for apparent good morphology and motility by a trained and experienced embryologist, the impact of seminal OS on the DNA might be more obvious as the integrity of the DNA is one of the last functional parameters determined by the spermatozoa. Therefore it could be that the predictive value of ORP, including the calculated cutoff point after IVF or intrauterine insemination (IUI), is different from the one that was calculated. If this is true, measurement of seminal ORP might be a method to possibly categorize patients suitable for IUI, IVF, or ICSI.

Considering the potential in improving andrological diagnostics and treatment, an integration of the measurement of seminal ORP with semen analysis seems plausible and achievable. Devices for semen analysis using AI are already commercially available (e.g., Lens-Hooke X1 PRO). If this approach could be combined with the measurement of ORP in a device that can perform the analysis in one sample, this approach would save time and money.

UTILITY OF ARTIFICIAL INTELLIGENCE IN REPRODUCTIVE MEDICINE

Sperm Separation for Assisted Reproductive Technology

Current Sperm Separation Methods

Separation and isolation of viable and, most importantly, functional sperm is essential for any technique of assisted reproduction. At the time when assisted reproduction started, motile sperm were selected and isolated by means of the swim-up technique.[60] Later, various filtration techniques (glass wool, Sephadex, etc.) and density gradient centrifugation were developed.[61-63] With the introduction of ICSI in 1992[64] and the understanding to isolate the most capable sperm from poor ejaculates, it was realized that the most functional sperm had to be selected to achieve ongoing pregnancies and the birth of a healthy baby (for review, see Henkel, 2003, 2012[65,66]).

As a result of these efforts, techniques such as magnetic-activated sperm sorting (MACS),[67] hyaluronan binding,[68] physiological ICSI (PICSI),[69] zeta potential,[70] or intracytoplasmic morphologically selected sperm injection (IMSI)[71] were developed. Specifically, the "physiological" and morphological approaches for sperm selection for ICSI with PICSI and IMSI, respectively, have initially been reported to result in higher pregnancy and miscarriage rates.[69,72-74] In a direct comparison of MACS, PICSI, and ICSI, Troya and Zorrilla[75] report higher clinical pregnancy rates for MACS and PICSI. Similarly, a recent study by Hozyen et al.[76] showed significantly higher clinical pregnancy rates after sperm preparation with MACS and PICSI as compared to the conventional density gradient centrifugation and testicular sperm. Hyaluronic acid-bound sperm also exhibit significantly lower DNA fragmentation rates and better normal sperm morphology as compared to other methods,[69,77,78] which is important for a positive reproductive outcome.[79,80] On the other hand, more recent studies, including several Cochrane reviews, concluded that there is insufficient evidence deriving from low quality trials supporting the assumption that MACS, PICSI, or IMSI results in improved live birth rates. However, IMSI may reduce the miscarriage rate.[81-86] Hence there is a need to follow new paths for the development of new sperm separation/selection methods able to identify and select the most functional

sperm. Ideally, such methods will mimic sperm selection processes in the female reproductive tract.[66]

Sperm Movement Through the Female Reproductive Tract

In recent years, our understanding of sperm movement in the female reproductive tract and its selection of the most capable sperm for fertilization has increased dramatically. While millions of sperm are ejaculated in the vagina and deposited in its anterior part close to the cervical os, only a few hundred will reach the fertilization site in the ampulla and only one spermatozoon will eventually fertilize the oocyte,[87,88] i.e., a few hundred sperm per oocyte. In contrast, in IVF, Tournaye et al.[89] showed that 5000 to 20,000 sperm are necessary for successful fertilization, with higher fertilization rates at a ratio of 20,000 sperm per oocyte. This difference in the ratio clearly indicates that the female reproductive tract has additional highly efficient sperm selection mechanisms[90] that are still not fully understood in their complexity.

Although the sperm cells' ability to move is a major aspect of sperm separation, it was revealed in recent years that aspects which also include physical and biochemical interactions of the sperm with the female genital tract play a major role in the natural selection of sperm. Therefore it is important to understand these interactions and mimic them in a laboratory set-up.

In the bovine female reproductive tract, longitudinal microgrooves were observed.[91,92] Sperm seem to swim in the corners of these microgrooves.[93,94] These microgrooves enable sperm not only to move faster but also against the natural flow of liquid;[95] thus sperm are showing a positive rheotactic behavior.[94,96] Further, the fact that sperm swim along the microgrooves leads to interactions between the sperm and the epithelial lining of the female reproductive tract. It has been found that due to the glycocalyx being rich in sialic acid,[97] the sperm plasma membrane surface is negatively charged.[98,99] Sialoglycoproteins are mainly acquired during sperm epididymal maturation and cause an increase in the negative surface charge[100] called the zeta potential. Sperm selection using the zeta potential method resulted in significantly better sperm DNA integrity as compared to hyaluronic acid binding[101] and improved pregnancy rates.[102] If the sperm surface charge plays a role for physiological sperm selection and guidance through the female reproductive tract, then it would assist that the sperm be in close contact with the epithelium in the microgrooves as sperm move along the surface topography in the female reproductive tract.[93,95] This process could be assisted by thermotaxis[103] and chemotaxis.[104]

In the rabbit, David et al.[105] observed a 2°C higher temperature at the fertilization site than at the isthmus. Boryshpolets et al.[106] showed that human sperm swim up a temperature gradient and that this gradient modulates speed and hyperactivation of the sperm. On the other hand, one should not neglect the impact of the biochemical interactions, chemotaxis, and direct interactions based on sperm surface characteristics between the female reproductive system and the sperm. In this regard, it has been shown that the oocyte and the surrounding cumulus cells secrete chemoattractants.[107] However, the chemical nature of the chemoattractants is still controversially discussed. While Teves et al.[108] propose that progesterone at picomolar concentrations mediates, others question this role of progesterone and suggest that progesterone only causes sperm hyperactivation with an accumulation by trapping.[109] Hyperactivation is activated by CatSper.[110,111] Furthermore, bourgeonal, for which human sperm express the receptor hOR17-4,[112] has been shown to mediate chemotactic human sperm motility in vitro.[113] Two other small studies have linked the olfactory sensitivity for bourgeonal to male infertility.[114,115] Hence it appears that thigmotaxis (physical contact with the walls of the microgrooves possibly mediated by surface charges), rheotaxis (swimming against a flow), the viscosity of the fluids of the female reproductive tract, and possibly thermotaxis facilitate sperm movement in the female reproductive tract, apart from passive transport mechanisms in the uterus.

Microfluidics as Advanced Sperm Selection Method

Since the principles of natural sperm selection have attracted more attention, the female reproductive tract has been recognized as microfluidic environment in recent years. As a result, microfluidics is currently a focal point of interest and research, and different types of microfluidic devices have been developed.[116-118] The sperm/semen compartment (inlet) can be separated from the sperm collection compartment (outlet) by confined micropores,[119,120] microchannels,[121,122] or microstructures[123] (Meissner, as per personal discussion in meeting in March

2022). Through the micropores, morphologically normal motile sperm will pass through and can thereby be separated from poorly motile and abnormal cells.[124,125] On the other hand, the microchannels and microstructures rather mimic the microgrooves found in the female reproductive tract, where sperm are swimming along the surfaces. Microfluidic sperm separation has further been shown to result in a significantly lower proportion of sperm with DNA fragmentation as compared to swim-up or density gradient centrifugation.[126,127]

While the general principle of sperm separation in a microfluidic system is the ability of sperm to swim against a laminar flow, i.e., rheotaxis,[94] the driving force for sperm separation can be passive, chemoattractant driven, flow driven, thermotaxis driven, or driven by multiple principles.[128] In passively driven devices, the sperm separation is based on the male germ cells' motility, thereby leaving less motile sperm behind the separating membrane, microchannels, or structures. This procedure is time dependent, with optimum results around 30 minutes of incubation being reported.[129] Xie et al.[130] developed a device that combined chemotaxis and sperm motility. The authors found that about 10% of the sperm were chemotactically responsive. In 2011, Ma and coworkers succeeded in IVF of murine oocytes and blastocyst development when sperm were separated and oocytes fertilized on one integrated dish.[131] Oocytes were positioned in the center and sperm in four inlet pools surrounding the oocyte chamber. Both the oocyte chamber and inlet pools were connected by microchannels. In order to create a constant slight flow in the separation chamber, various hydrostatic pressure-operated devices were developed,[116,132,133] with which sperm samples showing almost 100% motility could be obtained. On the other hand, using a device building up a temperature gradient, Li et al. found thermotactic responses in 5.7% to 10.6% of the sperm.[134]

Combination of Microfluidics with Other Techniques

In order to improve the selection of the most capable sperm, different microfluidic principles could be combined, though this will make the device more complicated and expensive for clinical use. First attempts to achieve this goal have been made by Ko et al.[135] by developing an advanced microfluidic chip that combines microfluidic technology with thermo- and chemotaxis. Results of this study show that murine sperm were attracted more, though not significantly, when thermo- and chemotactic stimuli were used in an integrated, combined manner. Using the same approach, Yan and coworkers[136] succeeded in separating sperm with increased motility by simultaneously responding to a temperature gradient and a progesterone gradient.

Artificial Intelligence

With the technological advancements of computer processors with increased computational speed and advanced software, AI systems based on deep-learning algorithms and artificial neuron networks have been developed and not only propelled science but also clinical applications, including reproductive medicine.[137,138] Although there were significant improvements since the inception of clinical assisted reproduction with the birth of Louise Brown in 1978, the selection of functional, good-quality gametes and embryos remains a challenge. Thus far the main focus of AI applications was on the evaluation and selection of oocytes and embryos,[139,140] semen parameters and analysis,[141-143] DNA damage,[144,145] and the identification of sperm with normal morphology.[146,147] More recent investigations used machine-learning AI systems to enhance sperm retrieval and selection for insemination.[148]

For sperm selection, several technologies have been described earlier. However, in order to select the sperm with the highest chance for successful pregnancy, these sperm have to be identified, a task for which the human eye by using a light microscope is not capable. Previous techniques such as selecting swim-up, density gradient centrifugation, or picking a normal spermatozoon for ICSI are suboptimal because not all features that make a good sperm are visible or the selection technique causes damage to the sperm. Therefore the aim of sperm selection for assisted reproduction should be to mimic the natural selection process in vitro and to identify the most fertilization-capable sperm in a non-consumptive manner. At this stage, microfluidics employing different sperm selection principles such as thermo- and/or chemotaxis integrating AI technology appears most suitable in order to increase the success rate of ART, which has remained at about 30% per treatment cycle over the years.[149]

Although challenging from the design, the most ideal solution could be a one-step chip, like an organ-on-a-chip device mimicking structure and function of organs[150-152] that not only integrates a microfluidic sperm selection system mimicking the natural sperm selection process in the female reproductive tract but also the fertilization step. Further, the technology must be time saving and cost effective enough that it can be adopted as a routine technique in an embryology laboratory. For the costs, the type of the device, the type of plastic used with the relevant toxicological aspects, and the relevant manufacturing procedures have to be considered.

Integrated Microfluidic System With Assisted Reproductive Technology

In a porcine model, Clark and coworkers[153] succeeded in significantly reducing the polyspermia rate using an integrated microfluidic IVF system. While polyspermia is a problem in porcine IVF, it is not in human IVF, where average polyspermia rates between 2% and 7% are reported.[154,155] In a mouse model, Han et al.[156] and Ma et al.[131] showed that all steps necessary for successful IVF can be performed simultaneously in one device that even allowed observation of individual embryo development. However, fertilization and embryo development (two-cell, four-cell, morula, and blastocyst) rates did not differ from the controls. This could be due to the small number of experiments conducted or due to using a standard mouse model, whereas in human IVF, many male patients present with compromised semen parameters. The latter is also a reason why many ART centers are performing ICSI rather than IVF and therefore the use of ICSI in nonmale factor cases is increasing.[157]

An integrated sperm separation/fertilization/embryo culture device would, apart from the more physiological selection of sperm, also offer benefits for the embryo as metabolic waste products would be removed and replaced with fresh medium. Fresh medium could then be continuously adapted to the physiological requirements, including changing nutritional and oxygen tension requirements that the embryo needs for normal development;[158-160] the advantage would be that such a system would need less handling with fewer disturbances outside the incubator. In addition, such device could also reduce human error and variability, embryo manipulation, and contamination, thereby increasing the success rate.[161,162]

Artificial Intelligence for Ovarian Stimulation, Oocyte Collection, and Embryo Culture

AI algorithms and predictive analytics can support effective clinical decision making for the management of ovarian stimulation during IVF and ICSI treatment. In the day-to-day management of IVF/ICSI treatment cycles, several variables are considered in making clinical decisions to ensure best clinical outcomes. These include the age, body mass index, hormone profiles, and antral follicle count to individualize gonadotropin stimulation protocols to optimize the response to ovarian stimulation and improve pregnancy outcomes.[163,164] During ovarian stimulation for IVF/ICSI, follicle diameters and hormone concentrations are carefully considered to aid decision making regarding dosage adjustment and decision to trigger. This often depends on the experience and expertise of the clinical team to make the most appropriate decisions to minimize errors and optimize treatment outcomes.

Recently, researchers have focused on the potential of AI to improve pregnancy outcomes in the IVF clinic. A study evaluated the accuracy of a clinical algorithm to predict important management decisions during ovarian stimulation for IVF. The researchers found that the algorithm performance for decisions to trigger/cancel, return, and days to follow-up was accurate and in agreement with clinical decisions by experienced clinical teams. However, they reported that the algorithm was not as accurate for dose adjustments. AI-based algorithms could therefore aid optimum decision making during IVF treatment.[165]

In another study, the authors compared 7866 patients undergoing IVF with ICSI to establish whether using a machine-learning algorithm model can optimize the timing of the trigger injection to maximize the yield of fertilized oocytes and usable blastocysts compared with the treating clinician's decision. They found that using the machine learning-assisted model for trigger decisions resulted in 1.430 more fertilized oocytes and 0.577 more usable blastocysts per stimulation as compared to clinical decision making only. The algorithm model's decision for trigger timing was based on the number of follicles measuring 16 to 20 mm in diameter, the number of follicles measuring 11 to 15 mm in diameter, and the estradiol level. The authors concluded that using the machine-learning algorithm to optimize the timing of the trigger injection may lead to a significant increase in the number of fertilized oocytes and usable blastocysts obtained from an IVF stimulation cycle compared with clinical decision making only.[166]

Oocyte Collection

AI-based methods are emerging as objective and efficient tools to select competent oocytes and embryos

with the goal of improving live birth rates. Machine learning can be applied to oocyte images to select competent oocytes before ICSI and help in identifying markers of cytoplasmic maturity.[167] Targosz et al. (2020) compared different types of convolutional neural networks for semantic oocyte segmentation. Semantic oocyte segmentation involves dividing an oocyte image into multiple segments such as cytoplasm, first polar body, zona pellucida, etc. They found that the top training accuracy reached about 85% for training patterns and 79% for validation.[168] Ongoing research has focused on evaluating oocytes with a view to predicting normal fertilization, development to the blastocyst stage, and assessment of implantation potential using static oocyte images.[167] In the future, AI-based techniques may also have applications in oocyte selection for in vitro maturation of oocytes and somatic cell nuclear transfer and reprogramming.

Embryo Culture

AI-based technology can assist trained embryologists to select the embryo with the highest implantation potential. Traditionally, embryo quality and selection of blastocysts for transfer have been based on visual assessment of morphology. AI algorithms can overcome the intra- and interoperator variability in traditional embryo grading and provide an objective way to standardize embryo culture systems and optimize assessment of embryo quality to aid embryo selection. This will in turn help to increase accuracy and decrease operator variability between different laboratories.[167] Automatic embryo developmental annotation systems have been introduced with the aim of providing fast, accurate, and reproducible methods of embryo assessment. Systems are being developed to assess accurately embryo morphology, nuclear abnormalities, and abnormal cellular development as predictors of embryo quality and implantation.[167]

AI algorithms and machine learning can facilitate analysis of large databases of morphokinetic data to predict embryo implantation potential. In a recent study, Feyeux et al.[169] reported the development and validation of automated software for the annotation of human embryo morphokinetic parameters based on gray level coefficient of variation and detection of zona pellucida thickness. Researchers have also examined whether a predictive model based on morphokinetic parameters and using advanced data mining and AI methods could accurately predict embryo implantation potential. Milewski et al.[170] used a combination of two data-mining methods, principal component analysis and artificial neural networks, to extract all available morphokinetic information from data. In another study, Bodri and colleagues used a combination of cleavage- and blastocyst-stage variables through hierarchical or data mining-based algorithms to successfully predict live birth. However, the authors suggested a lack of internal or external validation could affect the predictive capacities of their model in different datasets.[171]

Researchers have analyzed blastocyst images using AI techniques of segmentation, feature extraction, and principal component analysis to predict implantation potential. A recent retrospective cohort study examined whether novel embryo features could predict implantation potential as input data for an artificial neural network model. The authors included 637 patients from an oocyte donation program who underwent single-blastocyst transfer during 2 consecutive years. They found that novel parameters such as blastocyst expanded diameter and trophectoderm cell cycle length had statistically different values in implanted and nonimplanted embryos and their combination with conventional morphokinetic parameters is effective as input data for a predictive model based on AI.[172]

An AI approach based on deep neural networks to select high-quality embryos using many time-lapse images has been described. The authors developed a framework (STORK) to predict blastocyst quality and created a decision tree to incorporate patient age and embryo quality to predict the likelihood of pregnancy.[173] In another study, Bormann and colleagues evaluated the use of a deep CNN trained using single timepoint images of embryos and reported an accuracy of 90% in choosing the best embryo available.[174] Researchers have also suggested that AI training could be designed to be self-supervised. They showed that an adaptive adversarial neural network model was able to maintain adequate performance despite large variations in image quality compared with supervised learning models. They concluded that neural networks could be trained to focus on relevant features alone to improve the efficiency of AI models.[175]

In the future, AI-based methods can pave the way for the analysis of vast amounts of clinical, genetic, and embryological data to individualize patient treatments to optimize outcomes and ensure best practice. Multicenter randomized clinical trials are urgently required to evaluate the accuracy of AI models before routine use

in clinical practice is adopted. The efficiency and reproducibility of AI methods are limited by the size of the training datasets. Internal and external validation of different datasets are essential to improve the predictive capabilities of AI-based technology.

APPLICATIONS OF STEM CELL RESEARCH IN MALE FERTILITY PRESERVATION

Spermatogonial stem cells differentiate into spermatids and undergo maturation to spermatozoa. Young and adult males may suffer from loss of spermatogonial stem cells (SSCs) in the testes due to acquired or genetic causes, leading to testicular failure.[16] In addition, male cancer survivors may suffer long-term or permanent gonadal failure due to gonadotoxic cancer therapy.[176,177] Loss of SSCs is especially important in prepubertal boys undergoing gonadotoxic cancer treatments such as chemotherapy and radiotherapy as sperm cryopreservation is not a feasible option due to sexual immaturity in this age group.[164,176] Recently, researchers have explored the feasibility of restoring fertility through SSCs in males with testicular failure. Brinster and Zimmerman[178] were the first to demonstrate that stem cells isolated from testes of male mice could repopulate sterile testes when injected into seminiferous tubules. It has also been demonstrated that SSCs injected into the rete testes of prepubertal rhesus monkeys can undergo transformation into mature spermatozoa that have fertilization capacity.[179]

Ongoing studies have focused on the in vitro production of human SSCs for fertility preservation in prepubertal boys or in the treatment of adult males suffering from testicular failure. Although initial studies support the potential use of SSCs to restore fertility, currently researchers are focusing on techniques to improve the safety and efficacy of SSC transplantation.[180,181] It has been suggested that there could be epigenetic alterations in long-term cell culture of spermatogonia.[182] Research is therefore needed to assess the safety and efficacy of stem cell therapy and patterns of epigenetic alterations in long-term cell culture of in vitro-produced spermatogonia that could have a long-term effect on the health and well-being of the offspring.

SUMMARY

Since the birth of Louise Brown in 1978, reproductive medicine has made huge progress on the female as well as on the male side. On the andrological side, the invention of ICSI was a major breakthrough. Nevertheless, due to the fact that it is extremely difficult to identify the most suitable oocytes and spermatozoa rendering the highest success, the overall success rates remained relatively low. Therefore new technologies have been developed to isolate and identify the most functional spermatozoa, oocytes, and embryos. An important aspect here is also to make the semen analysis much more accurate and reliable as it is at the moment where scientists and clinicians not only have to deal with huge biological variations but also with individual variations between different technologists who do the analysis. For sperm, the separation techniques aim to mimic natural procedures that are taking place in the female reproductive tract. These include microfluidics and various forms of taxis, including rheo- and chemotaxis. First promising results have been obtained, but the techniques must still be optimized and made more usable in clinical practice. For ovarian stimulation and oocyte collection, encouraging results have been obtained using machine learning and AI. Similarly, these technologies have provided better results in embryo selection. Despite all this progress, these technologies have to be developed and optimized further and will include stem cell research, which might make it possible that in the future, fertility could be restored to infertile males by resetting spermatogenesis.

REFERENCES

1. Hindmarsh WL. Three cases of male infertility. *Aust Vet J.* 1941;17:21-23.
2. MacLeod J. The role of oxygen in the metabolism and motility of human spermatozoa. *Am J Physiol.* 1943;138:512-518.
3. Steptoe PC, Edwards RG. Birth after the reimplantation of a human embryo. *Lancet.* 1978;2:366.
4. Palermo G, Joris H, Devroey P, Van Steirteghem AC. Pregnancies after intracytoplasmic injection of single spermatozoon into an oocyte. *Lancet.* 1992;340:17-18.
5. Sato T, Katagiri K, Gohbara A, et al. In vitro production of functional sperm in cultured neonatal mouse testes. *Nature.* 2011;471:504-507.
6. Almeling R, Waggoner MR. More and less than equal: how men factor in the reproductive equation. *Gender Soc.* 2013;27:821-842.
7. Morin SJ, Scott RT. Knowledge gaps in male infertility: a reproductive endocrinology and infertility perspective. *Transl Androl Urol.* 2018;7(suppl 3):S283-S291.
8. Grace B, Shawe J, Johnson S, Stephenson J. You did not turn up... I did not realise I was invited...: understanding male attitudes towards engagement in fertility and reproductive health discussions. *Hum Reprod Open.* 2019; 2019(3):hoz014.
9. Dyer SJ, Abrahams N, Hoffman M, van der Spuy ZM. 'Men leave me as I cannot have children': women's experiences with involuntary childlessness. *Hum Reprod.* 2002;17:1663-1668.
10. Carlsen E, Giwercman A, Keiding N, Skakkebaek NE. Evidence for decreasing quality of semen during past 50 years. *BMJ.* 1992;305:609-613.
11. Virtanen HE, Jørgensen N, Toppari J. Semen quality in the 21st century. *Nat Rev Urol.* 2017;14:120-130.
12. Griffiths TA, Murdoch AP, Herbert M. Embryonic development in vitro is compromised by the ICSI procedure. *Hum Reprod.* 2000;15:1592-1596.
13. Alukal JP, Lamb DJ. Intracytoplasmic sperm injection (ICSI)—what are the risks? *Urol Clin North Am.* 2008; 35:277-288.
14. Basirat Z, Kashifard M, Golsorkhtabaramiri M, Mirabi P. Factors associated with spontaneous abortion following intracytoplasmic sperm injection (ICSI). *JBRA Assist Reprod.* 2019;23:230-234.
15. Wang L, Chen M, Yan G, Zhao S. DNA methylation differences between zona pellucida-bound and manually selected spermatozoa are associated with autism susceptibility. *Front Endocrinol (Lausanne).* 2021;12:774260.
16. Boulet SL, Mehta A, Kissin DM, Warner L, Kawwass JF, Jamieson DJ. Trends in use of and reproductive outcomes associated with intracytoplasmic sperm injection. *JAMA.* 2015;313:255-263.
17. Centers for Disease Control and Prevention. *Assisted Reproductive Technology National Summary Report.* 2016. Available at: https://www.cdc.gov/art/pdf/2016-report/ART-2016-National-Summary-Report.pdf.
18. Glenn TL, Kotlyar AM, Seifer DB. The impact of intracytoplasmic sperm injection in non-male factor infertility-A critical review. *J Clin Med.* 2021;10:2616.
19. Li Z, Wang AY, Bowman M, et al. ICSI does not increase the cumulative live birth rate in non-male factor infertility. *Hum Reprod.* 2018;33:1322-1330.
20. Miner MM, Heidelbaugh J, Paulos M, Seftel AD, Jameson J, Kaplan SA. The intersection of medicine and urology: an emerging paradigm of sexual function, cardiometabolic risk, bone health, and men's health centers. *Med Clin North Am.* 2018;102:399-415.
21. World Health Organization. *WHO Laboratory Manual for the Examination and Processing of Human Semen.* 6th ed. Geneva, Switzerland: World Health Organization; 2021. Licence: CC BY-NC-SA 3.0 IGO.
22. Practice Committee of the American Society for Reproductive Medicine. Diagnostic evaluation of the infertile

male: a committee opinion. *Fertil Steril.* 2015;103:e18-e25.

23. Baskaran S, Finelli R, Agarwal A, Henkel R. Diagnostic value of routine semen analysis in clinical andrology. *Andrologia.* 2021;53:e13614.

24. Wang C, Swerdloff RS. Limitations of semen analysis as a test of male fertility and anticipated needs from newer tests. *Fertil Steril.* 2014;102:1502-1507.

25. Douglas C, Parekh N, Kahn LG, Henkel R, Agarwal A. A novel approach to improving the reliability of manual semen analysis: a paradigm shift in the workup of infertile men. *World J Mens Health.* 2021;39:172-185.

26. Blickenstorfer K, Voelkle M, Xie M, Fröhlich A, Imthurn B, Leeners B. Are WHO recommendations to perform 2 consecutive semen analyses for reliable diagnosis of male infertility still valid? *J Urol.* 2019;201:783-791.

27. Mortimer ST, van der Horst G, Mortimer D. The future of computer-aided sperm analysis. *Asian J Androl.* 2015;17:545-553.

28. Amann RP, Waberski D. Computer-assisted sperm analysis (CASA): capabilities and potential developments. *Theriogenology.* 2014;81:5-17.

29. Agarwal A, Henkel R, Huang CC, Lee MS. Automation of human semen analysis using a novel artificial intelligence optical microscopic technology. *Andrologia.* 2019;51:e13440.

30. Agarwal A, Panner Selvam MK, Ambar RF. Validation of LensHooke® X1 PRO and computer-assisted semen analyzer compared with laboratory-based manual semen analysis. *World J Mens Health.* 2021;39:496-505.

31. Maroof S, Henkel R, Osmundson M, et al. Comparison of three methods of semen analysis: a novel at-home sperm test, a computer assisted assessment and an embryologist. *Hum Reprod.* 2022;37(suppl. 1):i55-i56.

32. Alameri M, Hasikin K, Kadri NA, et al. Multistage optimization using a modified Gaussian Mixture Model in sperm motility tracking. *Comput Math Methods Med.* 2021;2021:6953593. doi:10.1155/2021/6953593.

33. Riordon J, McCallum C, Sinton D. Deep learning for the classification of human sperm. *Comput Biol Med.* 2019;111:103342.

34. Yu S, Rubin M, Geevarughese S, Pino JS, Rodriguez HF, Asghar W. Emerging technologies for home-based semen analysis. *Andrology.* 2018;6:10-19.

35. Aitken RJ, Clarkson JS, Hargreave TB, Irvine DS, Wu FCW. Analysis of the relationship between defective sperm function and the generation of reactive oxygen species in cases of oligozoospermia. *J Androl.* 1989;10:214-220.

36. Agarwal A, Sharma RK, Nallella KP, Thomas Jr AJ, Alvarez JG, Sikka SC. Reactive oxygen species as an independent marker of male factor infertility. *Fertil Steril.* 2006;86:878-885.

37. Aitken RJ, Clarkson JS, Fishel S. Generation of reactive oxygen species, lipid peroxidation, and human sperm function. *Biol Reprod.* 1989;41:183-197.

38. Plante M, de Lamirande E, Gagnon C. Reactive oxygen species released by activated neutrophils, but not by deficient spermatozoa, are sufficient to affect normal sperm motility. *Fertil Steril.* 1994;62:387-393.

39. Parks JE, Lynch DV. Lipid composition and thermotropic phase behavior of boar, bull, stallion, and rooster sperm membranes. *Cryobiology.* 1992;29:255-266.

40. Henkel R. Leukocytes and oxidative stress: dilemma for sperm function and male fertility. *Asian J Androl.* 2011;13:43-52.

41. Lopes S, Jurisicova A, Sun JG, Casper RF. Reactive oxygen species: potential cause for DNA fragmentation in human spermatozoa. *Hum Reprod.* 1998;13:896-900.

42. O'Flaherty C, de Lamirande E, Gagnon C. Positive role of reactive oxygen species in mammalian sperm capacitation: triggering and modulation of phosphorylation events. *Free Radic Biol Med.* 2006;41:528-540.

43. Aitken RJ. Reactive oxygen species as mediators of sperm capacitation and pathological damage. *Mol Reprod Dev.* 2017;84:1039-1052.

44. Henkel R, Sandhu IS, Agarwal A. The excessive use of antioxidant therapy: a possible cause of male infertility? *Andrologia.* 2019;51:e13162.

45. Panner Selvam MK, Agarwal A, Henkel R, et al. The effect of oxidative and reductive stress on semen parameters and functions of physiologically normal human spermatozoa. *Free Radic Biol Med.* 2020;152:375-385.

46. Symeonidis EN, Evgeni E, Palapelas V, et al. Redox balance in male infertility: excellence through moderation-"Μέτρον ἄριστον". *Antioxidants.* 2021;10:1534.

47. Sies H. Oxidative stress: introductory remarks. In: Sies E, ed. *Oxidative Stress.* London: Academic Press; 1985:1-8.

48. Wendel A. Measurement of in vivo lipid peroxidation and toxicological significance. *Free Radic Biol Med.* 1987;3:355-358.

49. Castagne V, Lefevre K, Natero R, Clarke PG, Bedker DA. An optimal redox status for the survival of axotomized ganglion cells in the developing retina. *Neuroscience.* 1999;93:313-320.

50. Aitken RJ, Buckingham DW, West KM. Reactive oxygen species and human spermatozoa: analysis of the cellular mechanisms involved in luminol- and lucigenin-dependent chemiluminescence. *J Cell Physiol.* 1992;151:466-477.

51. Lewis SEM, Boyle PM, McKinney KA, Young IS, Thompson W. Total antioxidant capacity of seminal plasma is different in fertile and infertile men. *Fertil Steril.* 1995;64:868-870.

52. Esfandiari N, Sharma RK, Saleh RA, Thomas Jr AJ, Agarwal A. Utility of the nitroblue tetrazolium reduction test

for assessment of reactive oxygen species production by seminal leukocytes and spermatozoa. *J Androl.* 2003; 24:862-870.

53. Sharma RK, Pasqualotto FF, Nelson DR, Thomas Jr AJ, Agarwal A. The reactive oxygen species—total antioxidant capacity score is a new measure of oxidative stress to predict male infertility. *Hum Reprod.* 1999;14:2801-2807.

54. Drummen GP, van Liebergen LC, Op den Kamp JA, Post JA. C11-BODIPY(581/591), an oxidation-sensitive fluorescent lipid peroxidation probe: (micro)spectroscopic characterization and validation of methodology. *Free Radic Biol Med.* 2002;33:473-490.

55. Gomez E, Irvine DS, Aitken RJ. Evaluation of a spectrophotometric assay for the measurement of malondialdehyde and 4-hydroxyalkenals in human spermatozoa: relationships with semen quality and sperm function. *Int J Androl.* 1998;21:81-94.

56. Agarwal A, Sharma R, Roychoudhury S, Du Plessis S, Sabanegh E. MiOXSYS: a novel method of measuring oxidation reduction potential in semen and seminal plasma. *Fertil Steril.* 2016;106:566-573.

57. Agarwal A, Arafa M, Chandrakumar R, Majzoub A, Al-Said S, Elbardisi H. A multicenter study to evaluate oxidative stress by oxidation-reduction potential, a reliable and reproducible method. *Andrology.* 2017;5:939-945.

58. Agarwal A, Panner Selvam MK, Arafa M, et al. Multicenter evaluation of oxidation-reduction potential by the MiOXSYS in males with abnormal semen. *Asian J Androl.* 2019;21:1-5.

59. Henkel R, Morris A, Vogiatzi P, et al. Predictive value of seminal oxidation-reduction potential (ORP) analysis for reproductive outcomes of intracytoplasmic sperm injection (ICSI) cycles. *Reprod Biomed Online.* 2022;45(5):1007-1020. doi:10.1016/j.rbmo.2022.05.010.

60. Cohen J, Edwards R, Fehilly C, et al. In vitro fertilization: a treatment for male infertility. *Fertil Steril.* 1985;43:422-432.

61. Paulson JD, Polakoski KL. A glass wool column procedure for removing extraneous material from the human ejaculate. *Fertil Steril.* 1977;28:178-181.

62. van der Ven HH, Jeyendran RS, Al-Hasani S, et al. Glass wool column filtration of human semen: relation to swim-up procedure and outcome of IVF. *Hum Reprod.* 1988;3:85-88.

63. Ord T, Patrizio P, Marello E, Balmaceda JP, Asch RH. Mini-Percoll: a new method of semen preparation for IVF in severe male factor infertility. *Hum Reprod.* 1990; 5:987-989.

64. Palermo G, Joris H, Devroey P, Van Steirteghem AC. Pregnancies after intracytoplasmic injection of single spermatozoon into an oocyte. *Lancet.* 1992;340:17-18.

65. Henkel RR, Schill WB. Sperm preparation for ART. *Reprod Biol Endocrinol.* 2003;1:108.

66. Henkel R. Sperm preparation: state-of-the-art—physiological aspects and application of advanced sperm preparation methods. *Asian J Androl.* 2012;14:260-269.

67. Glander HJ, Schiller J, Süss R, Paasch U, Grunewald S, Arnhold J. Deterioration of spermatozoal plasma membrane is associated with an increase of sperm lyso-phosphatidylcholines. *Andrologia.* 2002;34:360-366.

68. Huszar G, Willetts M, Corrales M. Hyaluronic acid (Sperm Select) improves retention of sperm motility and velocity in normozoospermic and oligozoospermic specimens. *Fertil Steril.* 1990;54:1127-1134.

69. Parmegiani L, Cognigni GE, Bernardi S, Troilo E, Ciampaglia W, Filicori M. "Physiologic ICSI": Hyaluronic acid (HA) favors selection of spermatozoa without DNA fragmentation and with normal nucleus, resulting in improvement of embryo quality. *Fertil Steril.* 2010;93:598-604.

70. Chan PJ, Jacobson JD, Corselli JU, Patton WC. A simple zeta method for sperm selection based on membrane charge. *Fertil Steril.* 2006;85:481-486.

71. Bartoov B, Berkovitz A, Eltes F, et al. Pregnancy rates are higher with intracytoplasmic morphologically selected sperm injection than with conventional intracytoplasmic injection. *Fertil Steril.* 2003;80:1413-1419.

72. Berkovitz A, Eltes F, Lederman H, et al. How to improve IVF-ICSI outcome by sperm selection. *Reprod Biomed Online.* 2006;12:634-638.

73. Goswami G, Sharma M, Jugga D, Gouri DM. Can intracytoplasmic morphologically selected spermatozoa injection be used as first choice of treatment for severe male factor infertility patients? *J Hum Reprod Sci.* 2018;11:40-44.

74. Mangoli E, Khalili MA, Talebi AR, et al. IMSI procedure improves clinical outcomes and embryo morphokinetics in patients with different aetiologies of male infertility. *Andrologia.* 2019;51:e13340.

75. Troya J, Zorrilla I. Annexin V-MACS in infertile couples as method for separation of sperm without DNA fragmentation. *JBRA Assist Reprod.* 2015;19:66-69.

76. Hozyen M, Hasanen E, Elqusi K, et al. Reproductive outcomes of different sperm selection techniques for ICSI patients with abnormal sperm DNA fragmentation: a randomized controlled trial. *Reprod Sci.* 2022;29:220-228.

77. Prinosilova P, Kruger T, Sati L, et al. Selectivity of hyaluronic acid binding for spermatozoa with normal Tygerberg strict morphology. *Reprod Biomed Online.* 2009;18:177-183.

78. Yagci A, Murk W, Stronk J, Huszar G. Spermatozoa bound to solid state hyaluronic acid show chromatin structure with high DNA chain integrity: an acridine orange fluorescence study. *J Androl.* 2010;31:566-572.

79. Zini A, Meriano J, Kader K, Jarvi K, Laskin CA, Cadesky K. Potential adverse effect of sperm DNA damage on embryo quality after ICSI. *Hum Reprod.* 2005;20:3476-3480.

80. Salehi M, Afarinesh MR, Haghpanah T, Novin MG, Farifteh F. Impact of sperm DNA fragmentation on ICSI outcome and incidence of apoptosis of human pre-implantation embryos obtained from in vitro matured MII oocytes. *Biochem Biophys Res Commun.* 2019;510:110-115.

81. Leandri RD, Gachet A, Pfeffer J, et al. Is intracytoplasmic morphologically selected sperm injection (IMSI) beneficial in the first ART cycle? A multicentric randomized controlled trial. *Andrology.* 2013;1:692-697.

82. McDowell S, Kroon B, Ford E, Hook Y, Glujovsky D, Yazdani A. Advanced sperm selection techniques for assisted reproduction. *Cochrane Database Syst Rev.* 2014;28:CD010461.

83. Gatimel N, Parinaud J, Leandri RD. Intracytoplasmic morphologically selected sperm injection (IMSI) does not improve outcome in patients with two successive IVF-ICSI failures. *J Assist Reprod Genet.* 2016;33:349-355.

84. Lepine S, McDowell S, Searle LM, Kroon B, Glujovsky D, Yazdani A. Advanced sperm selection techniques for assisted reproduction. *Cochrane Database Syst Rev.* 2019;7:CD010461.

85. Miller D, Pavitt S, Sharma V, et al. Physiological, hyaluronan-selected intracytoplasmic sperm injection for infertility treatment (HABSelect): a parallel, two-group, randomised trial. *Lancet.* 2019;393:416-422.

86. Duran-Retamal M, Morris G, Achilli C, et al. Live birth and miscarriage rate following intracytoplasmic morphologically selected sperm injection vs intracytoplasmic sperm injection: an updated systematic review and meta-analysis. *Acta Obstet Gynecol Scand.* 2020;99(1):24-33. doi:10.1111/aogs.13703.

87. Williams M, Hill CJ, Scudamore I, Dunphy B, Cooke ID, Barratt CL. Sperm numbers and distribution within the human fallopian tube around ovulation. *Hum Reprod.* 1993;8:2019-2026.

88. Eisenbach M, Giojalas LC. Sperm guidance in mammals - an unpaved road to the egg. *Nat Rev Mol Cell Biol.* 2006;7:276-285.

89. Tournaye H, Verheyen G, Albano C, et al. Intracytoplasmic sperm injection versus in vitro fertilization: a randomized controlled trial and a meta-analysis of the literature. *Fertil Steril.* 2002;78:1030-1037.

90. Sakkas D, Ramalingam M, Garrido N, Barratt CLR. Sperm selection in natural conception: what can we learn from Mother Nature to improve assisted reproduction outcomes? *Hum Reprod Update.* 2015;21:711-726.

91. Mullins KJ, Saacke RG. Study of the functional anatomy of bovine cervical mucosa with special reference to mucus secretion and sperm transport. *Anat Rec.* 1989;225:106-117.

92. Suarez SS, Brockman K, Lefebvre R. Distribution of mucus and sperm in bovine oviducts after artificial insemination: the physical environment of the oviductal sperm reservoir. *Biol Reprod.* 1997;56:447-453.

93. Denissenko P, Kantsler V, Smith DJ, Kirkman-Brown J. Human spermatozoa migration in microchannels reveals boundary-following navigation. *Proc Natl Acad Sci USA.* 2012;109:8007-8010.

94. Miki K, Clapham DE. Rheotaxis guides mammalian sperm. *Curr Biol.* 2013;23:443-452.

95. Tung CK, Ardon F, Fiore AG, Suarez SS, Wu M. Cooperative roles of biological flow and surface topography in guiding sperm migration revealed by a microfluidic model. *Lab Chip.* 2014;14:1348-1356.

96. Kantsler V, Dunkel J, Blayney M, Goldstein RE. Rheotaxis facilitates upstream navigation of mammalian sperm cells. *Elife.* 2014;3:e02403.

97. Holt WV. Surface-bound sialic acid on ram and bull spermatozoa: deposition during epididymal transit and stability during washing. *Biol Reprod.* 1980;23:847-857.

98. Yanagimachi R, Noda YD, Fujimoto M, Nicolson GL. The distribution of negative surface charges on mammalian spermatozoa. *Am J Anat.* 1972;135:497-519.

99. Schröter S, Osterhoff C, McArdle W, Ivell R. The glycocalyx of the sperm surface. *Hum Reprod Update.* 1999;5:302-313.

100. Kirchhoff C, Hale G. Cell-to-cell transfer of glycosylphosphatidylinositol-anchored membrane proteins during sperm maturation. *Mol Hum Reprod.* 1996;2:177-184.

101. Razavi SH, Nasr-Esfahani MH, Deemeh MR, Shayesteh M, Tavalaee M. Evaluation of zeta and HA-binding methods for selection of spermatozoa with normal morphology, protamine content and DNA integrity. *Andrologia.* 2010;42:13-19.

102. Nasr-Esfahani MH, Deemeh MR, Tavalaee M, Sekhavati MH, Gourabi H. Zeta sperm selection improves pregnancy rate and alters sex ratio in male factor infertility patients: a double-blind, randomized clinical trial. *Int J Fertil Steril.* 2016;10:253-260.

103. Bahat A, Tur-Kaspa I, Gakamsky A, Giojalas LC, Breitbart H, Eisenbach M. Thermotaxis of mammalian sperm cells: a potential navigation mechanism in the female genital tract. *Nat Med.* 2003;9:149-150.

104. Eisenbach M. Sperm chemotaxis. *Rev Reprod.* 1999;4:56-66.

105. David A, Vilensky A, Nathan H. Temperature changes in the different parts of the rabbit's oviduct. *Int J Gynecol Obstet.* 1972;10:52-56.

106. Boryshpolets S, Pérez-Cerezales S, Eisenbach M. Behavioral mechanism of human sperm in thermotaxis: a role for hyperactivation. *Hum Reprod.* 2015;30:884-892.
107. Sun F, Bahat A, Gakamsky A, et al. Human sperm chemotaxis: both the oocyte and its surrounding cumulus cells secrete sperm chemoattractants. *Hum Reprod.* 2005;20:761-767.
108. Teves ME, Barbano F, Guidobaldi HA, Sanchez R, Miska W, Giojalas LC. Progesterone at the picomolar range is a chemoattractant for mammalian spermatozoa. *Fertil Steril.* 2006;86:745-749.
109. Jaiswal BS, Tur-Kaspa I, Dor J, Mashiach S, Eisenbach M. Human sperm chemotaxis: is progesterone a chemoattractant? *Biol Reprod.* 1999;60:1314-1319.
110. Lishko PV, Botchkina IL, Kirichok Y. Progesterone activates the principal Ca2+ channel of human sperm. *Nature.* 2011;471:387-391.
111. Strünker T, Goodwin N, Brenker C, et al. The CatSper channel mediates progesterone-induced Ca2+ influx in human sperm. *Nature.* 2011;471:382-386.
112. Parmentier M, Libert F, Schurmans S, et al. Expression of members of the putative olfactory receptor gene family in mammalian germ cells. *Nature.* 1992;355:453-455.
113. Spehr M, Gisselmann G, Poplawski A, et al. Identification of a testicular odorant receptor mediating human sperm chemotaxis. *Science.* 2003;299:2054-2058.
114. Ottaviano G, Zuccarello D, Menegazzo M, et al. Human olfactory sensitivity for bourgeonal and male infertility: a preliminary investigation. *Eur Arch Otorhinolaryngol.* 2013;270:3079-3086.
115. Sinding C, Kemper E, Spornraft-Ragaller P, Hummel T. Decreased perception of bourgeonal may be linked to male idiopathic infertility. *Chem Senses.* 2013;38:439-445.
116. Seo DB, Agca Y, Feng ZC, Critser JK. Development of sorting, aligning, and orienting motile sperm using microfluidic device operated by hydrostatic pressure. *Microfluid Nanofluid.* 2007;3:561-570.
117. Huang HY, Huang PW, Yao DJ. Enhanced efficiency of sorting sperm motility utilizing a microfluidic chip. *Microsyst Technol.* 2017;23:305-312.
118. Zaferani M, Cheong SH, Abbaspourrad A. Rheotaxis-based separation of sperm with progressive motility using a microfluidic corral system. *Proc Natl Acad Sci USA.* 2018;115:8272-8277.
119. Asghar W, Velasco V, Kingsley JL, et al. Selection of functional human sperm with higher DNA integrity and fewer reactive oxygen species. *Adv Healthc Mater.* 2014;3:1671-1679.
120. Quinn MM, Jalalian L, Ribeiro S, et al. Microfluidic sorting selects sperm for clinical use with reduced DNA damage compared to density gradient centrifugation with swim-up in split semen samples. *Hum Reprod.* 2018;33:1388-1393.
121. Nosrati R, Vollmer M, Eamer L, et al. Rapid selection of sperm with high DNA integrity. *Lab Chip.* 2014;14:1142-1150.
122. Xiao S, Riordon J, Simchi M, et al. FertDish: microfluidic sperm selection-in-a-dish for intracytoplasmic sperm injection. *Lab Chip.* 2021;21:775-783.
123. Kantsler V, Meissner M, Bukatin A, Denissenko P. Patent application for motile cell sorting device. Application number: 2020;WO 2020212695 A1.
124. Higuchi A, Yamamiya SI, Yoon BO, Sakurai M, Hara M. Peripheral blood cell separation through surface-modified polyurethane membranes. *J Biomed Mater Res A.* 2004;68:34-42.
125. Katigbak RD, Turchini GM, de Graaf SP, Kong L, Dumée LF. Review on sperm sorting technologies and sperm properties toward new separation methods via the interface of biochemistry and material science. *Adv Biosyst.* 2019;3:e1900079.
126. Shirota K, Yotsumoto F, Itoh H, et al. Separation efficiency of a microfluidic sperm sorter to minimize sperm DNA damage. *Fertil Steril.* 2016;105:315-321.
127. Pujol A, García-Peiró A, Ribas-Maynou J, et al. A microfluidic sperm-sorting device reduces the proportion of sperm with double-strand DNA fragmentation. *Fertil Steril.* 2019;112:e90.
128. Knowlton SM, Sadasivam M, Tasoglu S. Microfluidics for sperm research. *Trends Biotechnol.* 2015;33:221-229.
129. Tasoglu S, Safaee H, Zhang X, et al. Exhaustion of racing sperm in nature-mimicking microfluidic channels during sorting. *Small.* 2013;9:3374-3384.
130. Xie L, Ma R, Han C, et al. Integration of sperm motility and chemotaxis screening with a microchannel-based device. *Clin Chem.* 2010;56:1270-1278.
131. Ma R, Xie L, Han C, et al. In vitro fertilization on a single-oocyte positioning system integrated with motile sperm selection and early embryo development. *Anal Chem.* 2011;83:2964-2970.
132. Cho BS, Schuster TG, Zhu X, Chang D, Smith GD, Takayama S. Passively driven integrated microfluidic system for separation of motile sperm. *Anal Chem.* 2003;75:1671-1675.
133. Chen CY, Chiang TC, Lin CM, et al. Sperm quality assessment via separation and sedimentation in a microfluidic device. *Analyst.* 2013;138:4967-4974.
134. Li Z, Liu W, Qiu T, et al. The construction of an interfacial valve-based microfluidic chip for thermotaxis evaluation of human sperm. *Biomicrofluidics.* 2014;8:024102.

135. Ko YJ, Maeng JH, Hwang SY, Ahn Y. Design, fabrication, and testing of a microfluidic device for thermotaxis and chemotaxis assays of sperm. *SLAS Technol.* 2018;23:507-515.

136. Yan Y, Zhang B, Fu Q, Wu J, Liu R. A fully integrated biomimetic microfluidic device for evaluation of sperm response to thermotaxis and chemotaxis. *Lab Chip.* 2021;21:310-318.

137. Wang R, Pan W, Jin L, et al. Artificial intelligence in reproductive medicine. *Reproduction.* 2019;158:R139-R154.

138. Zaninovic N, Elemento O, Rosenwaks Z. Artificial intelligence: its applications in reproductive medicine and the assisted reproductive technologies. *Fertil Steril.* 2019;112:28-30.

139. Bormann CL, Curchoe CL, Thirumalaraju P, et al. Deep learning early warning system for embryo culture conditions and embryologist performance in the ART laboratory. *J Assist Reprod Genet.* 2021;38:1641-1646.

140. Dimitriadis I, Zaninovic N, Chavez Badiola A, Bormann CL. Artificial intelligence in the embryology laboratory: a review. *Reprod Biomed Online.* 2022;44(3):435-448. doi:10.1016/j.rbmo.2021.11.003.

141. Goodson SG, White S, Stevans AM, et al. CASAnova: a multiclass support vector machine model for the classification of human sperm motility patterns. *Biol Reprod.* 2017;97:698-708.

142. Agarwal A, Henkel R, Huang CC, Lee MS. Automation of human semen analysis using a novel artificial intelligence optical microscopic technology. *Andrologia.* 2019;51(11):e13440. doi:10.1111/and.13440.

143. Tsai FV, Zhuang B, Pong YH, Hsieh JT, Chang HC. Web- and artificial intelligence-based image recognition for sperm motility aalysis: verification study. *JMIR Med Inform.* 2020;8:e20031.

144. McCallum C, Riordon J, Wang Y, et al. Deep learning-based selection of human sperm with high DNA integrity. *Commun Biol.* 2019;2:250.

145. Dimitriadis I, Bormann CL, Kanakasabapathy MK, et al. Automated smartphone-based system for measuring sperm viability, DNA fragmentation, and hyaluronic binding assay score. *PLoS One.* 2019;14:e0212562.

146. Riordon J, McCallum C, Sinton D. Deep learning for the classification of human sperm. *Comput Biol Med.* 2019;111:103342.

147. Shaker F, Monadjemi SA, Naghsh-Nilchi AR. Automatic detection and segmentation of sperm head, acrosome and nucleus in microscopic images of human semen smears. *Comput Methods Programs Biomed.* 2016;132:11-20.

148. Kresch E, Efimenko I, Gonzalez D, Rizk PJ, Ramasamy R. Novel methods to enhance surgical sperm retrieval: a systematic review. *Arab J Urol.* 2021;19:227-237.

149. Wilkinson J, Bhattacharya S, Duffy JMN, et al. Reproductive medicine: still more ART than science? *BJOG.* 2019;126:138-141.

150. Zhang B, Radisic M. Organ-on-a-chip devices advance to market. *Lab Chip.* 2017;17(14):2395-2420.

151. Galan EA, Zhao H, Wang X, Dai Q, Huck WTS, Ma S. Intelligent mcrofluidics: the convergence of machine learning and microfluidics in materials science and biomedicine. *Matter.* 2020;3:1893-1922.

152. Wu Q, Liu J, Wang X, et al. Organ-on-a-chip: recent breakthroughs and future prospects. *Biomed Eng Online.* 2020;19:9.

153. Clark SG, Haubert K, Beebe DJ, Ferguson CE, Wheeler MB. Reduction of polyspermic penetration using biomimetic microfluidic technology during in vitro fertilization. *Lab Chip.* 2005;5:1229-1232.

154. Aoki VW, Peterson CM, Parker-Jones K, et al. Correlation of sperm penetration assay score with polyspermy rate in in-vitro fertilization. *J Exp Clin Assist Reprod.* 2005;2:3.

155. Xia P. Biology of polyspermy in IVF and its clinical indication. *Curr Obstet Gynecol Rep.* 2013;2:226-231.

156. Han C, Zhang Q, Ma R, et al. Integration of single oocyte trapping, in vitro fertilization and embryo culture in a microwell-structured microfluidic device. *Lab Chip.* 2010;10:2848-2854.

157. Dyer S, Chambers GM, de Mouzon J, et al. International Committee for Monitoring Assisted Reproductive Technologies world report: Assisted Reproductive Technology 2008, 2009 and 2010. *Hum Reprod.* 2016;31:1588-1609.

158. Filomeni G, Rotilio G, Ciriolo MR. Disulfide relays and phosphorylative cascades: partners in redox-mediated signaling pathways. *Cell Death Differ.* 2005;12:1555-1563.

159. Zander DL, Thompson JG, Lane M. Perturbations in mouse embryo development and viability caused by ammonium are more severe after exposure at the cleavage stages. *Biol Reprod.* 2006;74:288-294.

160. Ufer C, Wang CC, Borchert A, Heydeck D, Kuhn H. Redox control in mammalian embryo development. *Antioxid Redox Signal.* 2010;13:833-875.

161. Suh RS, Phadke N, Ohl DA, Takayama S, Smith GD. Rethinking gamete/embryo isolation and culture with microfluidics. *Hum Reprod Update.* 2003;9:451-461.

162. Meseguer M, Kruhne U, Laursen S. Full in vitro fertilization laboratory mechanization: toward robotic assisted reproduction? *Fertil Steril.* 2012;97:1277-1286.

163. Fanton M, Nutting V, Rothman A, et al. An interpretable machine learning model for individualized gonadotrophin starting dose selection during ovarian stimulation. *Reprod Biomed Online.* 2022;45(6):1152-1159. doi:10.1016/j.rbmo.2022.07.010.

164. Sadri-Ardekani H, Atala A. Testicular tissue cryopreservation and spermatogonial stem cell transplantation to restore fertility: from bench to bedside. *Stem Cell Res Ther.* 2014;5:68.

165. Letterie G, Mac Donald A. Artificial intelligence in in vitro fertilization: a computer decision support system for day-to-day management of ovarian stimulation during in vitro fertilization. *Fertil Steril.* 2020;114:1026-1031.

166. Hariton E, Chi EA, Chi G, et al. A machine learning algorithm can optimize the day of trigger to improve in vitro fertilization outcomes. *Fertil Steril.* 2021;116:1227-1235.

167. Zaninovic N, Rosenwaks Z. Artificial intelligence in human in vitro fertilization and embryology. *Fertil Steril.* 2020;114:914-920.

168. Targosz A, Przystałka P, Wiaderkiewicz R, Mrugacz G. Semantic segmentation of human oocyte images using deep neural networks. *Biomed Eng Online.* 2021;20:40.

169. Feyeux M, Reignier A, Mocaer M, et al. Development of automated annotation software for human embryo morphokinetics. *Hum Reprod.* 2020;35:557-564.

170. Milewski R, Kuczyńska A, Stankiewicz B, Kuczyński W. How much information about embryo implantation potential is included in morphokinetic data? A prediction model based on artificial neural networks and principal component analysis. *Adv Med Sci.* 2017;62:202-206.

171. Bodri D, Milewski R, Serna JY, et al. Predicting live birth by combining cleavage and blastocyst-stage time-lapse variables using a hierarchical and a data mining-based statistical model. *Reprod Biol.* 2018;18:355-360.

172. Bori L, Paya E, Alegre L, et al. Novel and conventional embryo parameters as input data for artificial neural networks: an artificial intelligence model applied for prediction of the implantation potential. *Fertil Steril.* 2020;114:1232-1241.

173. Khosravi P, Kazemi E, Zhan Q, et al. Deep learning enables robust assessment and selection of human blastocysts after in vitro fertilization. *NPJ Digit Med.* 2019;2:21.

174. Bormann CL, Kanakasabapathy MK, Thirumalaraju P, et al. Performance of a deep learning based neural network in the selection of human blastocysts for implantation. *Elife.* 2020;9:e55301.

175. Kanakasabapathy MK, Thirumalaraju P, Kandula H, et al. Adaptive adversarial neural networks for the analysis of lossy and domain-shifted datasets of medical images. *Nat Biomed Eng.* 2021;5:571-585.

176. Meistrich ML. Effects of chemotherapy and radiotherapy on spermatogenesis in humans. *Fertil Steril.* 2013;100:1180-186.

177. Saha S, Roy P, Corbitt C, Kakar SS. Application of stem cell therapy for infertility. *Cells.* 2021;10:1613.

178. Brinster RL, Zimmermann JW. Spermatogenesis following male germ-cell transplantation. *Proc Natl Acad Sci USA.* 1994;91:11298-11302.

179. Hermann BP, Sukhwani M, Winkler F, et al. Spermatogonial stem cell transplantation into rhesus testes regenerates spermatogenesis producing functional sperm. *Cell Stem Cell.* 2012;11:715-726.

180. Kilcoyne KR, Mitchell RT. Fertility preservation: testicular transplantation for fertility preservation: clinical potential and current challenges. *Reproduction.* 2019;158:F1-F14.

181. Faes K, Lahoutte T, Hoorens A, Tournaye H, Goossens E. In search of an improved injection technique for the clinical application of spermatogonial stem cell transplantation. *Reprod Biomed Online.* 2017;34:291-297.

182. Fend-Guella DL, von Kopylow K, Spiess AN, et al. The DNA methylation profile of human spermatogonia at single-cell- and single-allele-resolution refutes its role in spermatogonial stem cell function and germ cell differentiation. *Mol Hum Reprod.* 2019;25:283-294.

INDEX